THE COMPLETE FOOD COUNTER

With more than 3.5 million copies of their bestselling *Counter* books in print, Annette Natow and Jo-Ann Heslin share their professional knowledge with consumers to help guide them in making the best food choices when snacking, food shopping, preparing food, and eating out.

The nutrition experts have put together an indispensable encyclopedia of food values—in a one-volume, easy-to-use, and easy-to-carry reference that has every nutrition count you'll ever need:

- Calories
- Fat
- Protein
- Carbohydrate
- Fiber
- Cholesterol
- Sodium

Books by Annette B. Natow and Jo-Ann Heslin

Published by POCKET BOOKS

The Complete

FOOD COUNTER

Annette B. Natow, Ph.D., R.D.
and Jo-Ann Heslin, M.A., R.D.

POCKET BOOKS
New York   London   Toronto   Sydney   Singapore

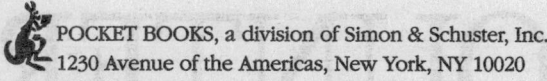 POCKET BOOKS, a division of Simon & Schuster, Inc.
1230 Avenue of the Americas, New York, NY 10020

Copyright © 1999, 2003 by Annette Natow and Jo-Ann Heslin

Originally published as a trade paperback in 1999 by Pocket Books. The 1999 edition of this work was titled *The Most Complete Food Counter*.

ISBN: 0-7434-5742-0

First Pocket Books printing of this revised edition January 2003

10 9 8 7 6 5 4 3 2 1

POCKET and colophon are registered trademarks of Simon & Schuster, Inc.

For information regarding special discounts for bulk purchases, please contact Simon & Schuster Special Sales at 1-800-456-6798 or business@simonandschuster.com

Cover design by Lisa B. Cohen

Printed in the U.S.A.

To our families, who support us through every project:
Harry, Allen, Irene, Sarah, Meryl, Laura, Marty, George,
Emily, Steven, Joe, Kristen, Brian, and Karen.

ACKNOWLEDGMENTS

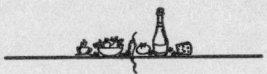

For graciously sharing their knowledge: Martin Lefkowitz, M.D., and Irene E. Rosenberg, M.D.

For all her support and help, our agent, Nancy Trichter.

Without the tireless cooperation of Steven Natow, M.D., and Stephen Llano, *The Complete Food Counter* would never have been completed.

A special thank you to our editor, Micki Nuding.

Our thanks also to all the food manufacturers who graciously shared their data.

". . . foods, though so numerous and so varied in form, can be reduced to rather simple terms."

Mary Swartz Rose, Ph.D.
Feeding the Family
The MacMillan Company, 1919

CONTENTS

PART ONE

Brand Name, Nonbranded (Generic) and Take-Out Foods

PART TWO

Restaurant Chains

INTRODUCTION

Calories, fat, cholesterol, protein, carbohydrate, fiber, sodium—the list is long. Because your body is working all the time (even when you're sleeping), you need a source of calories and other nutrients to keep you going. It's reassuring to know that it's easy to get all of these. Different foods have different assortments of nutrients: foods like meat and cheese are high in protein, fruits are high in carbohydrates, and whole wheat bread has lots of fiber. When you eat a variety of foods, it balances out so that you get all the nutrients you need. *The Complete Food Counter* is the most comprehensive nutrition resource, listing nutrition values for over 17,000 foods.

Calories (CALS)

You get calories from fat, protein, and carbohydrate in foods. Fat has the most calories of the three, more than twice as many as protein and carbohydrate. One teaspoon of olive oil (fat) has 40 calories, while a teaspoon of either sugar (carbohydrate) or unsweetened gelatin (protein) has only 16 calories.

Most men need about 2,400 calories a day, while most women need 1,800 or less. If a person is very active, calorie intake can go as high as 3,900 for men and 3,000 for women. Very few people need this many calories.

> ### Smart Stuff
>
> *Calories are a measure of the energy (heat) in food. When food is used or "burned" in the body, it gives off heat. The energy used by the body is measured as calories burned.*

Fat

Eating too much fat is not healthy. But some fat is needed by your body. How do you figure out how much to eat? A government recommendation, the Daily Value (DV), for a 2,000 calorie diet is 65 grams of fat or less each day. As a rule of thumb, if you are an average-weight, moderately active adult, and want a benchmark for your total fat grams each day, simply divide your weight in half.

It's now always easy to tell if a food is high in fat by looking at it. Some visible fat can be seen on slices of roast beef or bacon or in foods like butter, margarine, and oil. But in many foods, like milk, eggs, cheese, avocados, cookies, and nuts, the fat is not so obvious. That's when *The Complete Food Counter* comes in handy.

> ### Smart Stuff
>
> *Fat has an undeserved bad reputation. It's important in the body: providing energy; supplying essential fatty acids that the body cannot make; insulating the body and protecting vital organs; carrying fat soluble vitamins; forming part of cell membranes; and, just as important, making food taste good.*

Cholesterol (CHOL)

Although the body needs cholesterol to function normally, when the blood level gets too high, it's not healthy. Some of the cholesterol can be deposited in arteries, narrowing them and interfering with normal blood flow. Cholesterol is found in animal foods like meat, chicken, fish, milk, cheese, and eggs. It is also made in the body. Strict vegetarians, who eat no animal foods, make all the cholesterol they need. Most experts suggest that people limit their cholesterol intake to 200 milligrams or less a day.

Smart Stuff

Cholesterol is necessary and important for every cell in the body. It's part of cell membranes, and nerve and brain tissues, and is used to make vitamin D and important hormones.

Protein (PROT)

Protein is in every cell and substance in the body except urine and bile. It is used for growth, repair, and to replace cells worn out in daily living. Most experts recommend a protein intake of 51 to 64 grams a day for a woman weighing 140 pounds, and 62 to 77 grams for a man weighing 170 pounds. Since high protein foods are popular, many people eat much more than that amount. Proteins are found in both animal and vegetable foods. Meat, dairy, beans, and soy foods are excellent sources.

Smart Stuff

Protein is made up of smaller building blocks called amino acids. There are 20 amino acids that the body uses to build different proteins, the way the letters in an alphabet make up different words.

Carbohydrate (CARB)

Carbohydrates include sugars, starches, cellulose, and other fibers. The sugars and starches are digested and used in the body, while cellulose and fibers cannot be digested. A healthy carbohydrate intake is 50–60% of the calories eaten. In a 2,000 calorie diet, that would be equivalent to 250 to 300 grams of carbohydrate; 250 grams of carbohydrate equals 1000 calories, 300 grams equals 1200 calories.

Smart Stuff

SOURCES OF STARCH	SOURCES OF SUGAR
grains: wheat, rice, corn, oats, barley	fruits
	milk sugar (lactose)
legumes: peas, beans, lentils	syrup: corn, maple, molasses
yams	
vegetables	honey
bread	table sugar
pasta	jelly

Fiber

Fiber is the part of the plant that isn't digested. When you eat enough fiber it helps you avoid constipation and hemorrhoids, control weight, lower cholesterol, and protect against some cancers. Americans eat about 15 grams a day, half of the 25 to 30 grams recommended by experts.

Smart Stuff

Good sources of fiber are: whole wheat bread, pasta and cereal, fruits, vegetables, beans, and bran.

Sodium (SOD)

Sodium is an important mineral in the body, but you don't have to worry about getting too little. Almost all foods contain sodium, either naturally or as added salt. Table salt is a mixture of sodium and chloride, another mineral. Americans, on average, eat two to three teaspoons of salt a day. That's equal to 4,000 to 6,000 milligrams of sodium, which is about twice the recommended 2,400 milligrams. Even when the body loses a lot of salt through sweating, the salt is replaced quickly when food is eaten.

Smart Stuff

Most of your salt (sodium) intake doesn't come from the salt-shaker; 77% comes from convenience foods like frozen dinners, canned soups, mixes, sauces, and salad dressings you buy. Restaurant foods contain a lot of salt, too.

USING THE
COUNTER SECTION

The Complete Food Counter lists the calories, fat, cholesterol, protein, carbohydrate, fiber, and sodium content of over 17,000 foods. These are key nutrients for you to consider when you're choosing foods. Fat, cholesterol, and sodium are nutrients you may want to limit. You can be more liberal with the others, aiming for moderate amounts of calories, protein, and carbohydrate, and higher amounts of fiber. Recommended intakes for all nutrients counted are given in the introduction. There are still other nutrients needed for good health, but when you eat a variety of foods containing the nutrients listed in this counter, you will automatically get the other necessary nutrients.

Now, you will be able to compare your usual food selections with others that are available, so you can make the best choices. With this information at your fingertips, you'll find it easy to eat healthy. For example, when you want to select pizza, look up the pizza category on page 433. You will see over 150 listed so you can find the one that is best. A dash (—) appears in some entries. This means that no analysis was done for that nutrient. It is not the same as a "0," which means the nutrient is not in that food.

The Complete Food Counter has foods listed alphabetically. For each category, you will first find nonbranded (generic) foods listed in alphabetical order, followed by an alphabetical listing of brand name foods. The nonbranded listing will help you find values for foods when you do not see your favorite. Large categories are divided into subcategories such as canned, fresh, frozen and ready-to-eat, to make it easier to find what you're looking for. Many categories have a take-out subcategory. Look there for foods you take out or order in, because these foods are not nutrition labeled.

The Complete Food Counter is divided into two sections, Part One: Brand Name, Nonbranded (Generic) and Take-Out Foods, and Part Two: Restaurant Chains.

Most foods are listed alphabetically, but in some cases, foods are grouped by category. For example, a tuna salad sandwich is found in the sandwich category. Other group categories include:

Asian Food Page 20
   includes all types of Asian foods
   except egg rolls and sushi, which
   are found in separate categories

Deli Meats/Cold Cuts Page 240
   includes all sandwich meats
   except beef, chicken, ham, and
   turkey, which are found in
   separate categories

Dinner Page 244
   includes all by brand name,
   except pasta dinners, which are
   found in a separate category

In Part Two: Restaurant Chains, there are 80 national and regional restaurant, doughnut, ice cream, candy, and coffee chains listed.

DEFINITIONS

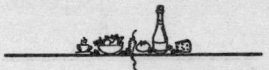

as prep (as prepared): refers to food that has been prepared according to package directions

lean and fat: describes meat with some fat on its edges that is not cut away before cooking, or poultry prepared with skin and fat as purchased

lean only: refers to lean meat that is trimmed of all visible fat or poultry without skin

shelf stable: refers to prepared products found on the supermarket shelf that are ready-to-eat or are to be heated and do not require refrigeration

take-out: describes prepared dishes that you purchase ready-to-eat; those included serve as a guide to the calorie, fat, cholesterol, protein, carbohydrate, fiber, and sodium values of similar products you may purchase

ABBREVIATIONS

avg	=	average
diam	=	diameter
fl	=	fluid
frzn	=	frozen
g	=	gram
in	=	inch
lb	=	pound
lg	=	large
med	=	medium
mg	=	milligram
oz	=	ounce
pkg	=	package
pt	=	pint
prep	=	prepared
qt	=	quart
reg	=	regular
sec	=	second
serv	=	serving
sm	=	small
sq	=	square
tbsp	=	tablespoon
tr	=	trace
tsp	=	teaspoon
w/	=	with
w/o	=	without
<	=	less than

NOTES

Cals = Calories

Prot = Protein
All protein values are given in grams (g).

Fat = Fat
All fat values of food are given in grams (g).

Carb = Carbohydrate
All carbohydrate values are given in grams (g).

Chol = Cholesterol
All cholesterol values are given in milligrams (mg).

Sod = Sodium
All sodium values are given in milligrams (mg).

Fiber = Fiber
All fiber values are given in grams (g).

tr (trace) = less than 1 gram of protein, fat, carbohydrate, or fiber, and less than 1 milligram of cholesterol or sodium.

— (dash) indicates data was not available.

0 (zero) indicates that there is none of the nutrient in that food.

Discrepancies in figures are due to rounding, product reformulation, and reevaluation. Labeling law allows rounding of values. Because much of the data is analysis data obtained directly from manufacturers, not from labels, in some cases our values may not be exactly the same as label information because they have not been rounded.

11

PART ONE

Brand Name, Nonbranded (Generic) and Take-Out Foods

FOOD	PORTION	CAL	PROT	FAT	CHOL	CARB	FIBER	SOD
ABALONE								
fresh fried	3 oz	161	17	6	80	9	–	502
raw	3 oz	89	15	1	72	5	–	255
ACEROLA								
fresh	1	2	tr	tr	0	tr	–	0
ACEROLA JUICE								
juice	1 cup	51	1	1	0	12	–	7
ADZUKI BEANS								
canned sweetened	1 cup	702	11	tr	0	163	–	646
dried cooked	1 cup	294	17	tr	0	57	–	18
yokan sliced	3¼ in slices	112	1	tr	0	26	–	36
AKEE								
fresh	3.5 oz	223	5	20	0	5	–	–
ALE (see BEER AND ALE, MALT)								
ALFALFA								
sprouts	1 cup	40	1	tr	0	1	–	2
sprouts	1 tbsp	1	tr	tr	0	tr	–	0
ALLIGATOR								
cooked	3 oz	126	28	2	57	0	0	66
ALLSPICE								
ground	1 tsp	5	tr	tr	0	1	–	1
ALMONDS								
almond butter honey & cinnamon	1 tbsp	96	3	8	0	4	–	2
almond butter w/ salt	1 tbsp	101	2	9	0	3	–	75
almond butter w/o salt	1 tbsp	101	2	10	0	3	–	2
almond meal	1 oz	116	11	5	0	8	–	2
almond paste	1 oz	127	3	8	0	12	–	3
dried unblanched	1 oz	167	6	15	0	6	–	3
dry roasted unblanched	1 oz	167	5	15	0	7	–	3

FOOD	PORTION	CAL	PROT	FAT	CHOL	CARB	FIBER	SOD
dry roasted unblanched salted	1 oz	167	5	15	0	7	—	260
dry roasted w/ salt	24 nuts (1 oz)	170	6	15	0	6	3	100
jordan almonds	10 (1.4 oz)	190	4	7	0	28	1	0
oil roasted blanched	1 oz	174	16	16	0	5	3	3
oil roasted blanched salted	1 oz	174	5	16	0	5	—	3
oil roasted unblanched	1 oz	176	6	16	0	5	—	3
praline	17 pieces (1.4 oz)	210	5	12	0	21	3	45
toasted unblanched	1 oz	167	6	14	0	7	3	3
Lance								
Smoked	1 pkg (0.8 oz)	130	6	10	0	4	3	125
Planters								
Almonds	1 oz	170	6	15	0	5	3	0
Gold Measure Slivered	1 pkg (2 oz)	340	12	31	0	11	4	0
Honey Roasted	1 oz	160	5	14	0	7	2	190

AMARANTH *(see also* CEREAL, COOKIES*)*

uncooked	1 cup (6.8 oz)	729	28	13	0	129	30	41

ANCHOVY

canned in oil	5	42	6	2	—	0	—	734
canned in oil	1 can (1.6 oz)	95	13	4	—	0	—	1651
fresh fillets	3 (0.4 oz)	21	2	1	—	tr	—	—
fresh raw	3 oz	62	17	4	—	0	—	88

ANGLERFISH

raw	3.5 oz	72	15	1	—	0	—	109

ANISE

seed	1 tsp	7	tr	tr	0	1	—	tr

ANTELOPE

roasted	3 oz	127	25	2	107	0	—	46

APPLE
CANNED

sliced sweetened	1 cup	136	tr	1	0	34	—	7

FOOD	PORTION	CAL	PROT	FAT	CHOL	CARB	FIBER	SOD
Del Monte								
Fruit Pleasures Pie Spiced Apples	½ cup (4.1 oz)	70	0	0	0	18	1	10
Luck's								
Fried Apples	½ cup (4.7 oz)	130	0	0	0	33	2	0
DRIED								
cooked w/ sugar	½ cup	116	tr	tr	0	29	–	27
cooked w/o sugar	½ cup	172	tr	tr	0	20	–	26
rings	10	155	1	tr	0	42	–	56
Sonoma								
Pieces	10–12 pieces (1.4 oz)	110	0	0	0	29	4	0
FRESH								
apple	1	81	tr	tr	0	21	3	1
w/o skin sliced	1 cup	62	tr	tr	0	16	2	0
w/o skin sliced & cooked	1 cup	91	tr	tr	0	23	–	1
w/o skin sliced & microwaved	1 cup	96	tr	tr	0	25	–	1
Chiquita								
Apple	1 med (5.4 oz)	80	0	0	0	22	5	0
Cool Cut								
Apples & Caramel Dip	1 pkg (4.25 oz)	180	1	5	5	32	3	80
Tastee								
Candy Apple	1 (3 oz)	160	3	5	0	26	4	20
Caramel Apple	1 (3 oz)	160	3	5	0	26	4	20
FROZEN								
sliced w/o sugar	½ cup	41	tr	tr	0	11	–	3
Stouffer's								
Escalloped	1 cup (6 oz)	180	0	3	0	37	3	70
TAKE-OUT								
baked	1 (5.3 oz)	126	tr	tr	0	33	3	1
baked no sugar	1 (5.9 oz)	82	tr	1	0	21	3	6
APPLE JUICE								
frzn as prep	1 cup	111	tr	tr	0	28	–	17
frzn not prep	6 oz	349	1	1	0	87	–	54
juice	1 cup	116	tr	tr	0	29	tr	7

FOOD	PORTION	CAL	PROT	FAT	CHOL	CARB	FIBER	SOD
After The Fall								
Organic	1 bottle (10 oz)	110	0	0	0	28	—	25
Vermont Apple	1 bottle (10 oz)	110	1	0	0	27	—	24
Vermont Apple	1 bottle (8 oz)	90	0	0	0	22	—	20
Apple & Eve								
100% Juice	8 fl oz	110	1	0	0	26	—	5
Cider	8 fl oz	110	1	0	0	27	—	10
Eden								
Organic Juice	8 oz	80	0	0	0	23	0	0
Everfresh								
Apple Juice	1 can (8 oz)	110	0	0	0	29	0	10
Hansen's								
Junior Juice 100%	1 box (4.23 oz)	60	0	0	0	15	1	0
Mott's								
100% Juice	8 fl oz	120	0	0	0	29	0	20
100% Juice	1 box (8 oz)	120	0	0	0	29	—	15
100% Natural	8 fl oz	120	0	0	0	29	0	20
Nantucket Nectars								
100% Pressed	8 oz	100	0	0	0	25	—	10
NutraBalance								
Plus Fibre	1 pkg (8 oz)	120	0	0	0	29	10	8
Ocean Spray								
100% Juice	8 oz	110	0	0	0	28	0	35
Swiss Miss								
Hot Apple Cider Mix	1 serv	84	tr	tr	0	20	1	58
Hot Apple Cider Mix Low Calorie	1 serv	14	0	0	0	3	0	78
Tropicana								
Season's Best	8 oz	110	tr	0	0	28	—	25
Turkey Hill								
Herbal Cider w/ Chamomile & Lemongrass	1 cup	100	—	0	0	24	—	—
Veryfine								
100% Juice	1 bottle (10 oz)	150	0	0	0	38	0	20
Juice-Ups	8 fl oz	120	0	0	0	30	0	35
White House								
Juice	8 oz	120	0	0	0	30	—	25

FOOD	PORTION	CAL	PROT	FAT	CHOL	CARB	FIBER	SOD
APPLESAUCE								
sweetened	½ cup	97	tr	tr	0	25	2	4
unsweetened	½ cup	53	tr	tr	0	14	2	2
Eden								
Organic	½ cup	50	0	0	0	15	2	15
Organic Sweet Cinnamon	½ cup	50	0	0	0	19	4	0
Mott's								
Single-Serve Cinnamon	1 pkg (4 oz)	100	0	0	0	26	–	0
Single-Serve Natural	1 pkg (4 oz)	50	0	0	0	12	–	0
Single-Serve Original	1 pkg (4 oz)	100	0	0	0	24	–	0
White House								
Applesauce	½ cup (4.4 oz)	90	0	0	0	23	2	15
Chunky	½ cup (4.4 oz)	90	0	0	0	23	2	15
Cinnamon	½ cup (4.5 oz)	100	0	0	0	25	2	15
Natural Plus	½ cup (4.4 oz)	70	0	0	0	15	2	15
APRICOT JUICE								
nectar	1 cup	141	1	tr	0	36	2	9
APRICOTS								
CANNED								
halves heavy syrup pack w/ skin	1 cup (9.1 oz)	214	1	tr	0	55	–	10
halves water pack w/ skin	1 cup (8.5 oz)	65	2	tr	0	16	–	7
halves water pack w/o skin	1 cup (8 oz)	51	2	tr	0	12	–	25
heavy syrup w/ skin	3 halves	70	tr	tr	0	18	–	3
juice pack w/ skin	3 halves	40	1	tr	0	10	–	3
light syrup w/ skin	3 halves	54	tr	tr	0	14	–	3
puree from heavy syrup pack w/ skin	¾ cup (9.1 oz)	214	1	tr	0	55	–	10
puree from light pack w/ skin	¾ cup (8.9 oz)	160	1	tr	0	42	–	10
puree from water pack w/ skin	¾ cup (8.5 oz)	65	2	tr	0	16	–	7
puree juice pack w/ skin	1 cup (8.7 oz)	119	2	tr	0	31	–	9

FOOD	PORTION	CAL	PROT	FAT	CHOL	CARB	FIBER	SOD
water pack w/ skin	3 halves	22	1	tr	0	5	–	2
water pack w/o skin	4 halves	20	1	tr	0	5	–	10
Del Monte								
Halves Unpeeled Lite	½ cup (4.3 oz)	60	0	0	0	16	1	10
Orchard Select Halves Unpeeled	½ cup (4.4 oz)	80	0	0	0	21	1	10
DRIED								
halves	10	83	1	tr	0	22	3	3
halves cooked w/o sugar	½ cup	106	2	tr	0	27	–	4
Sonoma								
Dried	10 pieces (1.4 oz)	120	2	0	0	31	1	0
FRESH								
apricots	3	51	1	tr	0	12	–	1
Chiquita								
Apricots	3 med (4 oz)	60	0	1	0	11	1	0
FROZEN								
sweetened	½ cup	119	1	tr	0	30	–	5
ARROWHEAD								
fresh boiled	1 med (⅓ oz)	9	1	tr	0	2	–	2
ARROWROOT								
flour	1 cup (4.5 oz)	457	tr	tr	0	113	4	3
ARTICHOKE								
CANNED								
Progresso								
Hearts	2 pieces (2.9 oz)	30	2	0	0	6	1	240
Hearts Marinated	2 pieces (1.1 oz)	170	0	5	0	2	0	110
S&W								
Marinated Hearts	2 pieces (1 oz)	20	0	2	0	2	1	80
FRESH								
boiled	1 med (4 oz)	60	4	tr	0	13	–	114
hearts cooked	½ cup	42	3	tr	0	9	–	80
FROZEN								
cooked	1 pkg (9 oz)	108	7	1	0	22	–	127
Birds Eye								
Hearts	½ cup	40	–	0	0	–	6	45

FOOD	PORTION	CAL	PROT	FAT	CHOL	CARB	FIBER	SOD
ARUGULA								
fresh	½ cup	2	tr	tr	0	tr	–	3
ASIAN FOOD *(see also* DINNER, EGG ROLLS, SUSHI*)*								
CANNED								
chow mein chicken	1 cup	95	7	tr	8	18	–	725
Chun King								
Beef Pepper Oriental BiPack	1 cup (8.8 oz)	98	10	2	14	13	3	865
Chow Mein Beef BiPack	1 cup (8.6 oz)	78	8	1	6	11	3	718
Chow Mein BiPack Chicken	1 cup (8.8 oz)	98	8	3	6	11	3	1123
Chow Mein Pork BiPack	1 cup (8.6 oz)	78	7	2	10	9	2	1183
Hot & Spicy Chicken BiPack	1 cup (8.6 oz)	98	8	3	19	11	1	857
Sweet & Sour Chicken BiPack	1 cup (8.9 oz)	161	7	2	25	29	3	687
La Choy								
Beef Pepper Oriental BiPack	1 cup (8.8 oz)	98	10	2	14	13	3	865
Chow Mein Beef BiPack	1 cup (8.6 oz)	78	8	1	6	11	3	718
Chow Mein Chicken PiBack	1 cup (8.9 oz)	98	8	3	6	11	3	1123
Chow Mein Shrimp BiPack	1 cup (8.6 oz)	52	4	1	4	9	3	965
Main Entree Chow Mein Chicken	1 cup (9.3 oz)	80	8	4	9	6	3	1325
Oriental Beef w/ Noodles BiPack	1 cup (8.8 oz)	156	18	3	17	18	4	896
Oriental Chicken w/ Noodles BiPack	1 cup (8.7 oz)	154	14	4	23	18	2	1100
Sweet & Sour Chicken BiPack	1 cup (8.9 oz)	161	7	2	25	29	3	687
Teriyaki Chicken BiPack	1 cup (8.6 oz)	109	8	3	20	15	3	1230

FOOD	PORTION	CAL	PROT	FAT	CHOL	CARB	FIBER	SOD
FRESH								
wonton wrappers	1	23	1	tr	1	5	–	46
Azumaya								
Round Wraps	10	160	6	1	10	31	1	370
Square Wraps	6	160	6	1	10	31	1	370
Wrappers Large Square	3	170	7	1	10	35	1	410
Nasoya								
Egg Roll Wrapper	3	170	7	1	10	35	1	410
Won Ton Wrappers	8	160	6	1	10	31	1	370
FROZEN								
Banquet								
Fried Rice w/ Chicken & Egg Rolls	1 meal (8.5 oz)	330	12	9	60	51	5	1270
Birds Eye								
Easy Recipe Creations Oriental Lo Mein as prep	2¼ cups (8.7 oz)	230	8	4	5	40	2	1200
Easy Recipe Creations Sesame Ginger Teriyaki as prep	2¼ cups (8.7 oz)	140	6	2	0	24	4	1230
Easy Recipe Creations Spicy Szechuan Cashews	2¼ cups (8.7 oz)	180	6	5	0	29	4	1410
Green Giant								
Create A Meal LoMein Stir Fry as prep	1¼ cups (10 oz)	320	30	70	60	35	4	980
Create A Meal Sweet & Sour Stir Fry as prep	1¼ cups (10 oz)	290	27	7	60	29	5	460
Create A Meal Szechuan Stir Fry as prep	1¼ cups (10 oz)	340	28	15	60	22	5	1280
Create A Meal Teriyaki Stir Fry as prep	1¼ cups (10 oz)	240	27	6	55	18	4	940

FOOD	PORTION	CAL	PROT	FAT	CHOL	CARB	FIBER	SOD
La Choy								
Beef Pepper Oriental	1 cup (7.1 oz)	151	8	1	10	30	2	714
Chow Mein Vegetable	1 cup (8.9 oz)	108	2	2	0	20	5	1135
Lean Cuisine								
Everyday Favorites Oriental Style Dumplings	1 pkg (9 oz)	300	10	6	20	51	2	520
Everyday Favorites Teriyaki Stir Fry	1 pkg (10 oz)	290	18	4	20	45	4	590
Rice Gourmet								
Chicken Teriyaki Rice Bowl	1 bowl (10.9 oz)	430	19	6	25	77	1	1210
Stouffer's								
Chicken Chow Mein w/ Rice	1 pkg (10.6 oz)	260	13	5	25	40	3	1090
Tyson								
Chicken Fried Rice Kit w/ Sauce	1 pkg (14 oz)	440	27	6	30	69	5	1810
Weight Watchers								
Smart Ones Chicken Chow Mein	1 pkg (9 oz)	200	12	2	25	34	3	570
Smart Ones Hunan Style Rice & Vegetables	1 pkg (10.34 oz)	280	7	0	0	45	5	630
Smart Ones King Pao Noodles & Vegetables	1 pkg (10 oz)	250	8	8	5	37	5	650
Smart Ones Spicy Szechaun Style Vegetables & Chicken	1 pkg (9 oz)	220	11	2	10	39	3	730
TAKE-OUT								
buddha's delight w/ cellophane noodles fat choi jai	1 serv (7.6 oz)	211	7	4	tr	44	2	772
cha siu bao steamed buns w/ chicken filling	1 (2.3 oz)	160	5	3	15	26	tr	300

FOOD	PORTION	CAL	PROT	FAT	CHOL	CARB	FIBER	SOD
chicken teriyaki	¾ cup	399	30	27	92	7	–	2190
chicken teriyaki w/ rice	1 serv (11 oz)	430	19	6	25	77	1	1210
chop suey w/ beef & pork	1 cup	300	26	17	68	13	–	1053
chop suey w/ pork	1 cup	375	19	29	62	29	2	1378
chow mein chicken	1 cup	255	31	10	75	10	–	718
chow mein pork	1 cup	425	32	24	89	21	3	1673
chow mein shrimp	1 cup	221	13	10	55	21	3	1658
chow mein vegetable	1 serv (8 oz)	90	3	3	0	15	4	1010
filipino chicken adobo	1 serv (15 oz)	555	33	26	116	45	1	468
fried rice	6.6 oz	249	4	6	–	48	2	–
fried rice w/ egg	6.7 oz	395	8	20	–	49	2	–
phad thai	1 serv (9.2 oz)	232	11	9	0	30	1	426
sesame seed paste bun	1 (2.5 oz)	220	5	6	0	39	2	53
shrimp chips	1¼ cups (1 oz)	140	2	6	0	19	0	240
shu mai chicken & vegetable dumplings	6 (3.6 oz)	160	10	5	35	18	1	910
spring roll	1 (3.5 oz)	112	12	2	–	37	5	670
sweet & sour pork	1 serv (8 oz)	250	6	8	30	37	2	1500
sweet red bean bun	1 (2.5 oz)	130	4	1	0	38	2	95
szechuan chicken w/ lo mein	1 cup (5.3 oz)	190	10	1	5	35	0	560
wonton fried	½ cup (1 oz)	111	2	8	31	8	1	147
wonton soup	1 cup	205	16	3	89	26	1	322

ASPARAGUS
CANNED
spears	½ cup	24	3	1	0	3	–	–

Del Monte
Cuts & Tips	½ cup (4.4 oz)	20	2	0	0	3	1	420
Spears Extra Long	½ cup (4.4 oz)	20	2	0	0	3	1	420
Spears Tender Young	½ cup (4.4 oz)	20	2	0	0	3	1	420
Tips Hand Selected	½ cup (4.4 oz)	20	2	0	0	3	1	420

Green Giant
Cut Spears	½ cup (4.2 oz)	20	2	0	0	3	1	420
Cut Spears 50% Less Sodium	½ cup (4.2 oz)	20	2	0	0	3	1	210

FOOD	PORTION	CAL	PROT	FAT	CHOL	CARB	FIBER	SOD
Extra Long Spears	4.5 oz	20	2	0	0	3	1	400
Spears	4.5 oz	20	2	0	0	3	1	450
LeSueur								
Spears Extra Large	4.5 oz	20	2	0	0	3	1	440
Owatonna								
Spears Cut	½ cup	20	–	0	0	–	–	–
S&W								
Green	6 pieces (4.5 oz)	15	2	0	0	4	1	260
FRESH								
cooked	4 spears	14	2	tr	0	3	–	7
cooked	½ cup	22	2	tr	0	4	–	10
raw	½ cup	16	2	tr	0	3	–	2
raw	4 spears	14	1	tr	0	3	–	1
FROZEN								
cooked	4 spears	17	2	tr	0	3	–	2
cooked	1 pkg (10 oz)	82	9	1	0	14	–	12
Birds Eye								
Cuts	½ cup	25	–	0	0	–	2	5
Spears	3 oz	20	–	0	0	–	1	5
Green Giant								
Harvest Fresh Cuts	⅔ cup (3 oz)	25	2	0	0	4	1	85
ATEMOYA								
fresh	½ cup	94	1	1	–	24	–	2
AVOCADO								
fresh	1	324	4	31	0	15	–	21
fresh mashed	1 cup	370	5	35	0	17	–	24
Chiquita								
Fresh	⅓ med (1 oz)	55	1	5	0	3	3	0
TAKE-OUT								
guacamole	1 serv (2.2 oz)	105	1	10	0	5	2	187
BACON								
breakfast strips cooked	3 strips	156	10	12	36	tr	0	714
gammon lean & fat grilled	4.2 oz	274	35	15	–	0	0	–
pan fried	3 strips	109	6	9	16	tr	0	303
Armour								
Star cooked	1 strip	38	–	3	6	–	–	185

FOOD	PORTION	CAL	PROT	FAT	CHOL	CARB	FIBER	SOD
Black Label								
Center Cut cooked	3 slices (0.5 oz)	70	5	6	15	0	0	260
Cooked	2 slices (0.5 oz)	80	5	7	15	0	0	330
Low Salt cooked	2 slices (0.5 oz)	80	5	7	15	0	0	230
Health Is Wealth								
Uncured Sliced	2 slices (0.5 oz)	70	3	7	10	0	—	380
Hormel								
Bacon Bits	1 tbsp (7 g)	30	3	2	5	0	0	250
Bacon Pieces	1 tbsp (7 g)	25	3	2	10	0	0	180
Microwave cooked	2 slices (0.5 oz)	70	5	5	15	0	0	230
Old Smokehouse								
Cooked	2 slices (0.5 oz)	80	5	7	15	0	0	280
Oscar Mayer								
Bacon Bits	1 tbsp (0.2 oz)	25	3	2	5	0	0	220
Bacon Pieces	1 tbsp (0.2 oz)	25	2	2	5	0	0	170
Center Cut cooked	2 slices (0.4 oz)	70	4	5	15	0	0	270
Cooked	2 slices (0.5 oz)	70	4	6	15	0	0	290
Lower Sodium cooked	2 slices (0.5 oz)	70	5	5	15	1	0	200
Thick Cut cooked	1 slice (0.4 oz)	60	4	5	10	0	0	250
Range Brand								
Cooked	2 slices (0.7 oz)	100	7	9	20	0	0	460
Ready Crisp								
Fully Cooked	3 slices (0.5 oz)	70	4	6	15	0	—	270
Red Label								
Cooked	2 slices (0.5 oz)	80	5	7	15	0	0	330
BACON SUBSTITUTES								
bacon substitute	1 strip	25	1	2	0	1	—	117
Bac-Os								
Chips or Bits	1½ tbsp (7 g)	30	3	2	0	2	0	120
Lightlife								
Fakin' Bacon Bits	1 tsp	45	1	1	0	1	0	25
Smart Bacon	2 strips (0.8 oz)	45	6	2	0	2	0	360
Louis Rich								
Turkey Bacon	1 slice (0.5 oz)	35	2	3	15	0	0	180
Morningstar Farms								
Breakfast Strips	2 (0.5 oz)	60	2	5	0	2	tr	220
Worthington								
Stripples	2 strips (0.5 oz)	60	2	5	0	2	tr	220

FOOD	PORTION	CAL	PROT	FAT	CHOL	CARB	FIBER	SOD
BAGEL								
cinnamon raisin	1 (3½ in)	194	7	1	0	39	—	229
cinnamon raisin toasted	1 (3½ in)	194	7	1	0	39	—	229
egg	1 (3½ in)	197	8	2	17	38	—	359
egg toasted	1 (3½ in)	197	8	2	17	38	—	358
oat bran	1 (3½ in)	181	8	1	0	38	—	360
oat bran toasted	1 (3½ in)	181	8	1	0	38	—	360
onion	1 (3½ in)	195	8	1	0	38	2	379
plain	1 (3½ in)	195	8	1	0	38	2	379
plain toasted	1 (3½ in)	195	8	1	0	38	2	379
poppy seed	1 (3½ in)	195	8	1	0	38	2	379
Amy's Organic								
Cinnamon Raisin	1 (3.5 oz)	240	8	2	0	52	3	480
Plain	1 (3.5 oz)	230	8	2	0	48	2	490
Poppy Seed	1 (3.5 oz)	230	8	2	0	48	2	480
Sesame	1 (3.5 oz)	240	8	2	0	48	2	480
Otis Spunkmeyer								
Barnstormin' Blueberry	1 (3.6 oz)	250	10	3	0	50	3	390
Barnstormin' Cinnamon Raisin	1 (3.6 oz)	230	9	2	0	47	3	370
Barnstormin' Onion	1 (3.6 oz)	230	9	2	0	47	3	370
Barnstormin' Plain	1 (3.6 oz)	240	10	3	0	49	3	390
Pepperidge Farm								
Mini	1 (1.4 oz)	120	5	0	0	24	tr	190
Plain	1 (3.5 oz)	290	11	1	0	60	2	480
Sara Lee								
Blueberry	1 (2.8 oz)	210	8	1	0	41	2	570
Cinnamon Raisin	1 (2.8 oz)	220	8	1	0	45	3	320
Egg	1 (2.8 oz)	210	7	1	0	44	2	460
Oat Bran	1 (2.8 oz)	210	8	1	0	42	3	570
Onion	1 (2.8 oz)	210	7	0	0	44	2	540
Plain	1 (2.8 oz)	210	8	1	0	43	2	500
Poppy Seed	1 (2.8 oz)	210	8	1	0	41	2	570
Sesame Seed	1 (2.8 oz)	210	8	2	0	42	2	530
Thomas'								
Everything	1 (3.6 oz)	300	10	4	0	56	3	510
Multi-Grain	1 (3.6 oz)	280	11	2	0	55	4	460
Plain	1 (3.6 oz)	280	10	2	0	56	2	530

FOOD	PORTION	CAL	PROT	FAT	CHOL	CARB	FIBER	SOD
Uncle B's								
Plain	1 (2.8 oz)	210	8	1	0	41	2	310
Wonder								
Blueberry	1 (3 oz)	210	7	1	0	43	1	450
Cinnamon Raisin	1 (3 oz)	210	8	1	0	42	2	360
Onion	1 (3 oz)	210	8	1	0	43	1	340
Plain	1 (3 oz)	210	8	1	0	43	2	350
Rye	1 (3 oz)	220	9	1	0	42	2	520
Wheat	1 (3 oz)	210	8	1	0	43	2	350

BAKING POWDER

FOOD	PORTION	CAL	PROT	FAT	CHOL	CARB	FIBER	SOD
baking powder	1 tsp	2	0	0	0	1	–	488
low sodium	1 tsp	5	0	0	0	2	–	4
Calumet								
Baking Powder	¼ tsp (1 g)	0	0	0	0	0	0	100

BAKING SODA

FOOD	PORTION	CAL	PROT	FAT	CHOL	CARB	FIBER	SOD
baking soda	1 tsp	0	0	0	0	0	–	1259

BALSAM PEAR

FOOD	PORTION	CAL	PROT	FAT	CHOL	CARB	FIBER	SOD
leafy tips cooked	½ cup	10	1	tr	0	2	–	4
leafy tips raw	½ cup	7	1	tr	0	1	–	3
pods cooked	½ cup	12	1	tr	0	3	–	4

BAMBOO SHOOTS

FOOD	PORTION	CAL	PROT	FAT	CHOL	CARB	FIBER	SOD
canned sliced	1 cup	25	2	1	0	4	–	9
fresh	½ cup	21	2	tr	0	1	–	3
fresh cooked	½ cup	15	2	tr	0	2	–	5
Chun King								
Bamboo Shoots	2 tbsp (0.8 oz)	3	tr	tr	0	1	tr	0
La Choy								
Bamboo Shoots	2 tbsp (0.8 oz)	3	tr	tr	0	1	tr	0

BANANA

FOOD	PORTION	CAL	PROT	FAT	CHOL	CARB	FIBER	SOD
banana chips	1 oz	147	1	10	0	17	2	2
fresh	1	105	1	tr	0	27	2	1
fresh mashed	1 cup	207	2	1	0	53	4	2
powder	1 tbsp	21	tr	tr	0	5	–	0
Chiquita								
Fresh	1 med (4.4 oz)	110	1	0	0	29	4	0
Rainforest Farms								
Slices Dried	5 slices (1.3 oz)	60	1	0	0	12	–	10

FOOD	PORTION	CAL	PROT	FAT	CHOL	CARB	FIBER	SOD
BARBECUE SAUCE								
barbecue	1 cup	188	5	5	0	32	–	2038
Bull's Eye								
Original	2 tbsp	50	–	0	0	–	–	–
Healthy Choice								
Hickory	2 tbsp (1.1 oz)	26	tr	0	0	6	tr	229
Hot & Spicy	2 tbsp (1.1 oz)	25	tr	0	0	6	tr	229
Original	2 tbsp (1.1 oz)	25	tr	0	0	6	tr	229
House Of Tsang								
Hong Kong	1 tbsp (0.6 oz)	10	0	0	0	2	0	150
Hunt's								
Bold Hickory	2 tbsp (1.2 oz)	47	tr	tr	0	11	1	283
Bold Original	2 tbsp (1.2 oz)	46	tr	tr	0	11	1	315
Hickory & Brown Sugar	2 tbsp (1.3 oz)	75	tr	tr	0	18	1	382
Honey Hickory	2 tbsp (1.2 oz)	54	1	tr	0	12	1	411
Honey Mustard	2 tbsp (1.2 oz)	48	tr	tr	0	12	1	450
Hot & Spicy	2 tbsp (1.2 oz)	48	tr	tr	0	12	1	450
Light Original	2 tbsp (1.2 oz)	23	tr	tr	0	6	1	169
Mesquite	2 tbsp (1.2 oz)	40	1	tr	0	9	1	361
Mild	2 tbsp (1.2 oz)	41	tr	tr	0	10	1	381
Mild Dijon	2 tbsp (1.2 oz)	39	tr	tr	0	9	tr	400
Open Range Original	2 tbsp (1.2 oz)	39	1	tr	0	9	1	333
Open Range Premier	2 tbsp (1.3 oz)	56	1	tr	0	13	1	415
Open Range Smokey	2 tbsp (1.2 oz)	37	tr	tr	0	9	1	423
Original	2 tbsp (1.2 oz)	40	tr	tr	0	9	1	410
Teriyaki	2 tbsp (1.2 oz)	46	1	tr	0	11	1	351
Kraft								
Char-Grill	2 tbsp (1.3 oz)	60	0	0	0	13	0	460
Extra Rich Original	2 tbsp (1.2 oz)	50	0	0	0	12	0	440
Hickory Smoke	2 tbsp (1.2 oz)	40	0	0	0	9	0	420
Hickory Smoke Onion Bits	2 tbsp (1.2 oz)	45	0	0	0	11	0	360
Honey	2 tbsp (1.3 oz)	50	0	0	0	13	0	360
Honey Hickory	2 tbsp (1.3 oz)	60	0	0	0	14	0	370
Honey Mustard	2 tbsp (1.3 oz)	60	0	0	0	13	0	300
Hot	2 tbsp (1.2 oz)	40	0	0	0	9	0	520
Hot Hickory Smoke	2 tbsp (1.2 oz)	40	0	0	0	9	0	380
Kansas City Style	2 tbsp (1.2 oz)	50	0	0	0	11	0	310
Mesquite Smoke	2 tbsp (1.2 oz)	40	0	0	0	9	0	420

FOOD	PORTION	CAL	PROT	FAT	CHOL	CARB	FIBER	SOD
Molasses	2 tbsp (1.3 oz)	70	0	0	0	16	0	390
Onion Bits	2 tbsp (1.2 oz)	45	0	0	0	11	0	360
Original	2 tbsp (1.2 oz)	40	0	0	0	9	0	420
Roasted Garlic	2 tbsp (1.2 oz)	50	0	0	0	12	0	360
Spicy Honey	2 tbsp (1.3 oz)	60	0	0	0	14	0	360
Teriyaki	2 tbsp (1.3 oz)	60	tr	1	0	12	0	440
Thick'N Spicy Brown Sugar	2 tbsp (1.2 oz)	60	0	0	0	15	0	350
Thick'N Spicy Hickory Bacon	2 tbsp (1.2 oz)	60	0	1	0	13	0	570
Thick'N Spicy Hickory Smoke	2 tbsp (1.2 oz)	50	0	0	0	12	0	450
Thick'N Spicy Honey	2 tbsp (1.3 oz)	60	0	0	0	13	0	360
Thick'N Spicy Honey Mustard	2 tbsp (1.3 oz)	60	0	0	0	14	0	310
Thick'N Spicy Kansas City Style	2 tbsp (1.3 oz)	60	0	0	0	14	0	310
Thick'N Spicy Mesquite Smoke	2 tbsp (1.2 oz)	50	0	0	0	12	0	440
McIlhenny								
Sauce	2 tbsp (1.1 oz)	70	tr	5	0	6	tr	290
Muir Glen								
Garlic Mesquite	2 tbsp (1.3 oz)	40	0	0	0	6	tr	265
Hot & Smoky	2 tbsp (1.2 oz)	40	0	0	0	6	tr	265
Original	2 tbsp (1.2 oz)	40	0	0	0	6	tr	265
BARLEY								
flour	1 cup (5.2 oz)	511	15	2	0	110	15	6
malt flour	1 cup (5.7 oz)	585	17	3	0	127	12	18
pearled cooked	1 cup (5.5 oz)	193	4	1	0	44	6	5
pearled uncooked	1 cup (7 oz)	704	20	2	0	155	31	18
BARRACUDA								
fresh	3 oz	122	14	8	66	0	0	57
BASIL								
fresh chopped	2 tbsp	1	tr	tr	0	tr	—	0
ground	1 tsp	4	tr	tr	0	1	—	tr
leaves fresh	5	1	tr	tr	0	tr	—	0
BASS								
freshwater raw	3 oz	97	16	3	58	0	—	59

FOOD	PORTION	CAL	PROT	FAT	CHOL	CARB	FIBER	SOD
sea cooked	3 oz	105	20	2	45	0	–	74
sea raw	3 oz	82	16	2	35	0	–	58
striped baked	3 oz	105	19	3	87	0	–	75

BAY LEAF

crumbled	1 tsp	2	tr	tr	0	tr	–	tr

BEANS (see also individual names)
CANNED

FOOD	PORTION	CAL	PROT	FAT	CHOL	CARB	FIBER	SOD
baked beans plain	½ cup	118	6	1	0	26	10	504
baked beans vegetarian	½ cup	118	6	1	0	26	10	504
baked beans w/ beef	½ cup	161	8	5	29	22	–	632
baked beans w/ franks	½ cup	182	9	8	8	20	9	551
baked beans w/ pork	½ cup	133	7	2	9	25	7	522
baked beans w/ pork & sweet sauce	½ cup	140	7	2	9	26	7	423
baked beans w/ pork & tomato sauce	½ cup	123	7	1	9	24	7	554
refried beans	½ cup	134	8	1	–	23	–	534
B&M								
99% Fat Free Baked Beans	½ cup (4.6 oz)	160	8	1	0	31	7	220
Baked w/ Honey	½ cup (4.7 oz)	170	8	2	0	30	8	450
Barbeque Baked Beans	½ cup (4.6 oz)	210	8	1	0	42	9	570
Brick Oven Baked	½ cup (4.6 oz)	180	8	2	5	32	7	390
Extra Hearty Baked	½ cup (4.6 oz)	190	8	2	<5	36	8	450
Bush's								
Barbecue	½ cup (4.6 oz)	160	6	1	0	32	6	510
Maple Cured Bacon	½ cup (4.6 oz)	150	7	1	0	28	7	620
Vegetarian	½ cup (4.6 oz)	130	6	0	0	24	6	550
Chi-Chi's								
Refried	½ cup (4.2 oz)	100	5	1	0	18	4	580
Refried Beans Fat Free	½ cup (4.2 oz)	120	5	0	0	17	4	570
Refried Beans Vegetarian	½ cup (4.2 oz)	100	5	1	0	18	4	580

FOOD	PORTION	CAL	PROT	FAT	CHOL	CARB	FIBER	SOD
Eden								
Organic Baked w/ Sorghum & Mustard	½ cup (4.6 oz)	150	8	0	0	27	7	130
Friend's								
Original Baked	½ cup (4.6 oz)	170	8	1	<5	32	7	390
Gebhardt								
Chili	½ cup (4.6 oz)	134	7	1	0	31	7	630
Refried Jalapeno	½ cup (4.5 oz)	105	7	3	1	19	6	380
Refried No Fat	½ cup (4.5 oz)	92	7	tr	0	20	6	480
Refried Traditional	½ cup (4.5 oz)	109	6	3	1	20	6	497
Refried Vegetarian	½ cup (4.5 oz)	118	8	2	tr	21	7	550
Green Giant								
Pork And Beans w/ Tomato Sauce	½ cup (4.5 oz)	120	5	1	0	23	4	490
Spicy Chili	½ cup (4.5 oz)	110	6	1	0	20	5	490
Three Bean Salad	½ cup (4.2 oz)	90	3	0	0	20	4	490
Health Valley								
Honey Baked	½ cup	110	7	0	0	25	7	135
Honey Baked No Salt	½ cup	110	7	0	0	25	7	25
Heartland								
Iron Kettle Baked	½ cup (4.6 oz)	150	5	1	<5	29	5	400
Hormel								
Beans & Wieners	1 can (7.5 oz)	290	11	12	50	34	6	1310
Hunt's								
Big John's Beans & Fixin's	½ cup (4.7 oz)	127	7	4	3	23	6	590
Homestyle Country Kettle	½ cup (4.6 oz)	152	7	2	1	31	7	425
Homestyle Special Recipe	½ cup (4.7 oz)	185	7	3	1	36	8	687
Mix & Serve	½ cup (4.7 oz)	125	2	3	1	30	8	575
Pork & Beans	½ cup (4.6 oz)	157	6	5	2	27	7	621
Pork & Beans	½ cup (4.5 oz)	130	6	1	tr	28	4	516
Kid's Kitchen								
Microwave Meals Beans & Weiners	1 cup (7.5 oz)	310	13	13	45	37	8	760

FOOD	PORTION	CAL	PROT	FAT	CHOL	CARB	FIBER	SOD
Old El Paso								
Mexe-Beans	½ cup (4.6 oz)	110	7	1	0	19	7	630
Refried	½ cup (4.2 oz)	110	6	2	<5	17	5	500
Refried Fat Free	½ cup (4.4 oz)	110	6	0	0	20	6	480
Refried Spicy	½ cup (4.3 oz)	140	6	3	<5	22	6	560
Refried Vegetarian	½ cup (4.1 oz)	100	6	1	0	16	6	490
Refried w/ Cheese	½ cup (4.2 oz)	130	7	4	5	18	6	500
Refried w/ Green Chilies	½ cup (4.3 oz)	110	6	1	<5	19	6	720
Refried w/ Sausage	½ cup (4.1 oz)	200	7	13	10	14	8	360
Open Range								
Ranch	½ cup (4.4 oz)	124	6	3	1	23	8	628
Pringles								
Vegetarian	1 cup (7.9 oz)	250	11	1	0	48	9	840
Rosarita								
3 Bean Recipe Bacon & Jalapeno	½ cup (4.6 oz)	117	8	2	1	22	5	543
3 Bean Recipe Chiles & Chicken	½ cup (4.6 oz)	115	7	1	1	22	4	517
3 Bean Recipe Chilies & Chorizo	½ cup (4.6 oz)	111	8	2	1	19	4	591
3 Bean Recipe Onions & Peppers	½ cup (4.6 oz)	104	7	1	1	20	5	539
Fiesta Beans Bacon & Jalapenos	½ cup (4.6 oz)	117	8	2	1	22	5	543
Fiesta Beans Chicken & Chilies	½ cup (4.6 oz)	115	7	1	1	22	4	517
Fiesta Beans Chilies & Chorizo	½ cup (4.6 oz)	110	8	2	1	19	4	591
Fiesta Beans Onions & Peppers	½ cup (4.6 oz)	104	8	1	1	20	5	539
Refried Bacon	½ cup (4.5 oz)	116	6	3	1	19	8	489
Refried Green Chile	½ cup (4.5 oz)	110	6	3	1	20	7	495
Refried Low Fat Black	½ cup (4.5 oz)	107	8	1	0	23	7	569
Refried Nacho Cheese	½ cup (4.5 oz)	108	8	2	2	19	6	574
Refried No Fat	½ cup (4.5 oz)	120	7	0	0	28	6	570
Refried No Fat Green Chiles & Lime	½ cup (4.5 oz)	101	8	tr	0	22	8	565

FOOD	PORTION	CAL	PROT	FAT	CHOL	CARB	FIBER	SOD
Refried No Fat w/ Zesty Salsa	½ cup (4.5 oz)	105	6	tr	0	24	6	599
Refried Onion	½ cup (4.5 oz)	114	6	3	1	21	6	508
Refried Spicy	½ cup (4.5 oz)	118	7	3	0	22	6	574
Refried Traditional	½ cup (4.5 oz)	108	5	1	0	19	5	510
Refried Vegetarian	½ cup (4.5 oz)	237	15	5	tr	42	13	1101
S&W								
Barbecue Beans Ranch Recipe	½ cup (4.5 oz)	100	6	2	0	25	8	640
Taco Bell								
Home Originals Fat Free Refried Beans	½ cup (4.6 oz)	110	7	0	0	21	6	460
Home Originals Fat Free Refried Beans w/ Mild Chilies	½ cup (4.5 oz)	110	7	0	0	20	5	480
Home Originals Refried Beans	½ cup (4.7 oz)	140	5	3	0	23	7	530
Van Camp								
Baked Fat Free	½ cup (4.6 oz)	132	6	tr	0	29	5	505
Baked Original	½ cup (4.7 oz)	143	7	1	1	29	6	535
Baked Southern Style Sauteed Onion	½ cup (4.8 oz)	145	6	1	1	35	8	555
Baked Sweet Hickory & Bacon	1 can (4.8 oz)	143	6	1	tr	32	6	471
Beanee Weenee BBQ	1 cup (7.7 oz)	290	14	12	35	36	7	970
Beanee Weenee Baked	1 cup (9.1 oz)	410	18	14	40	58	10	1210
Beanee Weenee Microwave	1 cup (7.5 oz)	260	14	11	35	29	6	1020
Beanee Weenee Original	1 cup (9.1 oz)	320	16	14	40	35	8	1240
Beanee Weenee Zestful	1 cup (7.7 oz)	300	14	12	35	40	7	1030
Brown Sugar	½ cup (4.6 oz)	170	7	3	5	31	6	410
Pork And Beans	½ cup (4.6 oz)	110	6	2	0	23	6	490
Vegetarian	½ cup (4.6 oz)	110	6	1	0	23	5	400

FOOD	PORTION	CAL	PROT	FAT	CHOL	CARB	FIBER	SOD
FROZEN								
Natural Touch								
Nine Bean Loaf	1 in slice (3 oz)	160	8	8	<5	13	5	350
MIX								
Melting Pot								
Terrazza Napoli Mixed Beans	1 cup	200	9	2	<5	41	2	460
TAKE-OUT								
baked beans	½ cup	190	7	6	6	27	—	532
barbecue beans	3.5 oz	120	4	tr	0	26	—	460
four bean salad	3.5 oz	100	4	tr	0	20	—	280
refried beans	½ cup	43	2	2	2	5	—	104
three bean salad	¾ cup	230	5	11	0	31	1	500

BEAN SPROUTS (see ALFALFA, SPROUTS)

BEAR

simmered	3 oz	220	28	11	—	0	—	—

BEAVER

roasted	3 oz	140	30	6	—	0	—	50
simmered	3 oz	141	23	5	—	0	—	39

BEECHNUTS

dried	1 oz	164	2	14	0	10	—	—

BEEF (see also BEEF DISHES, VEAL)

CANNED								
corned beef	1 oz	71	—	4	24	—	—	—
corned beef	3 oz	85	10	5	—	0	—	—
Armour								
Chopped Beef	2 oz	170	7	15	40	2	0	810
Corned Beef	2 oz	120	15	7	50	1	0	490
Potted Meat	1 can (3 oz)	120	12	7	75	0	0	750
Tripe	3 oz	90	18	2	125	0	0	100
Hormel								
Corned Beef	2 oz	120	15	7	50	0	0	490
Cubed Beef	½ cup (4.9 oz)	130	25	3	60	0	0	600
Potted Meat	4 tbsp (2 oz)	100	7	8	50	0	0	610
Treet								
Luncheon Loaf	2 oz	130	6	11	50	3	0	740

FOOD	PORTION	CAL	PROT	FAT	CHOL	CARB	FIBER	SOD
Luncheon Loaf 50% Less Fat	2 oz	110	6	8	45	4	0	750
DRIED								
Armour								
Sliced	7 slices (1 oz)	60	8	2	25	2	0	1370
Hormel								
Pillow Pack	10 slices (1 oz)	45	8	1	20	0	0	1010
FRESH								
bottom round lean & fat trim 0 in braised	3 oz	193	26	26	82	0	–	43
brisket whole lean & fat trim 0 in braised	3 oz	247	23	17	79	0	–	55
brisket whole lean & fat trim ¼ in braised	3 oz	327	27	27	80	0	–	52
corned beef brisket cooked	3 oz	213	15	16	83	tr	–	964
eye of round lean & fat trim ¼ in Select roasted	3 oz	184	23	10	61	0	–	51
flank lean & fat trim 0 in braised	3 oz	224	23	14	62	0	–	60
flank lean & fat trim 0 in broiled	3 oz	192	22	11	58	0	–	69
ground extra lean broiled medium	3 oz	217	22	14	71	0	–	59
ground extra lean broiled well done	3 oz	225	24	14	84	0	–	70
ground extra lean fried medium	3 oz	216	21	14	69	0	–	59
ground extra lean fried well done	3 oz	224	24	14	79	0	–	69
ground extra lean raw	4 oz	265	21	19	78	0	–	75
ground lean broiled medium	3 oz	231	21	16	74	0	–	65

FOOD	PORTION	CAL	PROT	FAT	CHOL	CARB	FIBER	SOD
ground lean broiled well done	3 oz	238	24	15	86	0	—	76
ground regular broiled medium	3 oz	246	20	18	76	0	—	70
ground regular broiled well done	3 oz	248	23	17	86	0	—	79
ground low-fat w/ carrageenan raw	4 oz	160	20	7	53	tr	—	70
porterhouse steak lean only trim ¼ in Prime broiled	3 oz	185	24	9	68	0	—	56
rib large end lean & fat trim 0 in roasted	3 oz	300	20	24	72	0	—	55
rib large end lean & fat trim ¼ in broiled	3 oz	295	18	24	69	0	—	54
rib large end lean & fat trim ¼ in roasted	3 oz	310	19	25	72	0	—	54
rib small end lean & fat trim 0 in broiled	3 oz	252	21	18	70	0	—	54
rib small end lean & fat trim ¼ in broiled	3 oz	285	20	22	71	0	—	53
rib small end lean & fat trim ¼ in roasted	3 oz	295	19	24	71	0	—	53
short loin top loin lean & fat trim ¼ in Select broiled	1 steak (6.3 oz)	473	46	31	140	0	—	114
shortribs lean & fat Choice braised	3 oz	400	18	36	80	0	—	43
t-bone steak lean & fat trim ¼ in Choice broiled	3 oz	253	21	18	70	0	—	52

FOOD	PORTION	CAL	PROT	FAT	CHOL	CARB	FIBER	SOD
tenderloin lean & fat trim ¼ in Choice broiled	3 oz	208	23	12	72	0	–	52
tip round lean & fat trim ¼ in Choice roasted	3 oz	210	23	13	70	0	–	53
top round lean & fat trim 0 in Select braised	3 oz	170	30	5	77	0	–	38
top sirloin lean & fat trim ¼ in Choice broiled	3 oz	228	23	14	76	0	–	53
tripe raw	4 oz	111	16	4	107	0	–	52
Healthy Choice								
Ground Extra Lean	4 oz	130	22	4	55	2	0	230
Laura's Lean								
Eye Of Round	4 oz	140	–	4	60	–	–	40
Flank Steak	4 oz	140	–	5	50	–	–	45
Ground 92% Lean	4 oz	160	–	9	60	–	–	70
Ground Round 94% Lean	4 oz	140	–	5	60	–	–	50
Ribeye Steak	4 oz	140	–	5	60	–	–	40
Sirloin Tip Round	4 oz	120	–	3	65	–	–	50
Sirloin Top Butt	4 oz	140	–	5	60	–	–	45
Strip Steak	4 oz	140	–	4	55	–	–	45
Tenderloins	4 oz	140	–	6	65	–	–	45
Top Round	4 oz	130	–	3	55	–	–	45
Maverick Ranch								
Ground Round Extra Lean	4 oz	130	24	4	60	0	–	65
Organic Valley								
Extra Lean Ground	3 oz	130	18	6	55	0	0	55
Extra Lean Patties	1 (3.2 oz)	130	19	6	60	0	0	55
FROZEN								
patties broiled medium	3 oz	240	21	17	80	0	–	66
READY-TO-EAT								
smoked beef cooked	1 sausage (1.4 oz)	134	–	12	29	–	–	–

FOOD	PORTION	CAL	PROT	FAT	CHOL	CARB	FIBER	SOD
Alpine Lace								
Roast Beef 97% Fat Free	2 oz	70	13	2	40	1	0	200
Boar's Head								
Corned Beef Brisket	2 oz	80	12	4	40	0	0	460
Eye Round Pepper Seasoned	2 oz	90	14	3	40	0	0	130
Italian Style Oven Roasted Top Round	2 oz	80	12	2	40	2	0	350
Roast Beef Cajun	2 oz	80	14	3	35	0	0	200
Top Round Deluxe	2 oz	90	14	3	30	0	0	80
Top Round Oven Roasted No Salt Added	2 oz	90	14	3	30	0	0	40
Healthy Choice								
Deli-Thin Roast Beef	6 slices (2 oz)	60	11	2	25	1	0	520
Fresh-Trak Roast Beef	1 slice (1 oz)	30	5	1	10	0	0	260
Jordan's								
Healthy Trim 97% Fat Free Roast Beef Medium	1 slice (1 oz)	30	6	1	20	0	0	130
Healthy Trim 97% Fat Free Roast Beef Rare	1 slice (1 oz)	30	6	1	20	0	0	130
Tyson								
Beef Strips Seasoned	1 serv (3 oz)	140	20	6	55	1	0	420
TAKE-OUT								
roast beef medium	2 oz	70	12	2	30	0	–	210
roast beef rare	2 oz	70	12	2	30	0	–	210

BEEF DISHES
CANNED

FOOD	PORTION	CAL	PROT	FAT	CHOL	CARB	FIBER	SOD
corned beef hash	3 oz	155	10	10	–	9	–	–
Armour								
Corned Beef Hash	1 cup (8.3 oz)	440	19	30	100	23	2	840
Corned Beef Hash w/ Peppers & Onions	1 cup (8.3 oz)	270	19	30	100	23	3	1220

FOOD	PORTION	CAL	PROT	FAT	CHOL	CARB	FIBER	SOD
Roast Beef Hash	1 cup (8.4 oz)	400	20	25	95	23	3	1460
Roast Beef In Gravy	½ cup (4.6 oz)	150	25	4	75	3	0	640
Stew	1 cup (8.6 oz)	220	8	12	30	21	2	1250
Dinty Moore								
Meatball Stew	1 cup (8.4 oz)	250	13	15	40	17	2	1120
Sliced Potatoes & Beef	1 can (7.5 oz)	230	10	9	35	28	4	1080
Stew	1 cup (8.2 oz)	230	11	14	40	16	2	950
Hormel								
Beef Goulash	1 can (7.5 oz)	230	13	11	50	19	3	1040
Roast Beef w/ Gravy	2 oz	60	11	2	30	1	0	280
Mary Kitchen								
Corned Beef Hash	1 cup (8.3 oz)	410	21	27	80	22	2	1020
Corned Beef Hash 50% Reduced Fat	1 cup (8.3 oz)	280	19	12	65	25	3	1070
Roast Beef Hash	1 cup (8.3 oz)	390	21	24	70	22	2	790
Sausage Hash	1 cup (8.3 oz)	410	20	27	85	23	2	1020
FROZEN								
Banquet								
Sandwich Toppers Creamed Chipped Beef	1 pkg (4 oz)	120	7	6	25	8	0	700
Sandwich Toppers Gravy & Salisbury Steak	1 pkg (5 oz)	210	9	16	25	8	2	790
Sandwich Toppers Gravy & Sliced Beef	1 pkg (4 oz)	70	8	2	25	5	0	440
MIX								
Hamburger Helper								
BBQ Beef as prep	1 cup	320	21	10	55	37	1	760
Beef Pasta as prep	1 cup	270	20	10	50	26	1	910
Beef Romanoff as prep	1 cup	280	20	10	50	27	0	890
Beef Stew as prep	1 cup	260	18	10	50	26	2	760
Beef Taco as prep	1 cup	280	19	10	50	31	2	960
Beef Teriyaki as prep	1 cup	290	18	10	50	34	2	990
Cheddar & Broccoli as prep	1 cup	350	22	15	60	33	0	830
Cheddar Melt as prep	1 cup	310	20	12	55	31	1	890

FOOD	PORTION	CAL	PROT	FAT	CHOL	CARB	FIBER	SOD
Cheddar'n Bacon as prep	1 cup	330	23	15	65	27	2	980
Cheeseburger Macaroni as prep	1 cup	360	23	16	65	33	1	940
Cheesy Hashbrowns as prep	1 cup	400	21	19	60	39	2	530
Cheesy Italian as prep	1 cup	320	22	14	60	28	1	920
Cheesy Shells as prep	1 cup	330	21	15	60	30	tr	840
Chili Macaroni as prep	1 cup	290	20	10	55	30	2	870
Fettuccine Alfredo as prep	1 cup	300	20	13	55	26	0	860
Four Cheese Lasagne as prep	1 cup	330	21	14	55	31	0	860
Italian Parmesan w/ Rigatoni as prep	1 cup	300	20	11	50	31	tr	870
Lasagne as prep	1 cup	270	19	10	50	29	2	1000
Meat Loaf as prep	⅙ loaf	270	24	14	110	11	0	580
Meaty Spaghetti & Cheese as prep	1 cup	290	20	10	50	30	1	970
Mushroom & Wild Rice as prep	1 cup	310	20	12	55	30	2	880
Nacho Cheese as prep	1 cup	320	22	13	55	30	tr	930
Pizza Pasta w/ Cheese Topping as prep	1 cup	280	19	10	50	31	2	750
Pizzabake as prep	⅙ pie	270	17	10	45	28	tr	720
Potatoes Au Gratin as prep	1 cup	280	18	13	55	25	2	730
Potatoes Stroganoff as prep	1 cup	250	17	11	50	23	2	870
Reduced Sodium Cheddar Spirals as prep	1 cup	300	20	13	55	27	0	590
Reduced Sodium Italian Herby as prep	1 cup	270	19	10	50	29	2	630
Reduced Sodium Southwestern Beef as prep	1 cup	300	20	10	50	32	2	620
Rice Oriental as prep	1 cup	280	18	10	50	32	0	990

FOOD	PORTION	CAL	PROT	FAT	CHOL	CARB	FIBER	SOD
Salisbury as prep	1 cup	270	19	10	50	26	1	790
Spaghetti as prep	1 cup	270	19	10	50	27	1	940
Stroganoff as prep	1 cup	320	21	13	55	30	0	830
Swedish Meatballs as prep	1 cup	290	19	14	55	25	2	780
Three Cheeses as prep	1 cup	340	21	15	55	32	tr	830
Zesty Italian as prep	1 cup	300	20	10	50	32	2	580
Zesty Mexican as prep	1 cup	280	19	10	50	31	2	690
READY-TO-EAT								
Thomas E. Wilson								
Roast Beef In Brown Gravy	1 serv + gravy (3.5 oz)	160	22	6	55	3	0	1210
SHELF-STABLE								
Dinty Moore								
Microwave Cup Corned Beef Hash	1 pkg (7.5 oz)	350	19	22	60	19	2	850
Microwave Cup Hearty Burger Stew	1 pkg (7.5 oz)	240	12	13	40	19	3	930
Microwave Cup Stew	1 pkg (7.5 oz)	190	11	10	40	15	2	900
Hormel								
Microcup Meals Stew	1 cup (7.5 oz)	190	11	10	35	15	2	900
Lunch Bucket								
Beef Stew	1 pkg (7.5 oz)	170	6	9	25	17	2	810
TAKE-OUT								
beef bourguignon	1 serv (7 oz)	254	23	16	128	3	1	212
bubble & squeak	5 oz	186	2	13	–	16	3	–
bulgoghi korean grilled beef	1 serv (5.2 oz)	256	23	15	67	5	tr	834
cornish pasty	1 (8 oz)	847	20	52	–	79	3	–
greek moussaka	1 serv (8.5 oz)	450	24	33	179	12	1	763
irish stew	1 cup (7 oz)	280	23	16	–	10	–	–
kebab indian	1 (5.4 oz)	553	47	40	–	2	–	–
kheena	6.7 oz	781	34	71	–	1	tr	–
koftas	5	280	18	22	–	3	tr	–
samosa	2 (4 oz)	652	6	62	–	20	2	–
shepherds pie	1 serv (7 oz)	282	16	16	70	20	2	840
steak & kidney pie w/ top crust	1 slice (5 oz)	400	21	26	–	23	1	–

FOOD	PORTION	CAL	PROT	FAT	CHOL	CARB	FIBER	SOD
stew	6 oz	208	17	13	–	6	1	–
stew w/ vegetables	1 cup	220	16	11	71	15	–	292
stroganoff	¾ cup	260	14	19	69	43	–	503
swiss steak	4.6 oz	214	23	9	61	10	2	139
toad in the hole	1 (4.7 oz)	383	10	29	–	23	1	–

BEEFALO

roasted	3 oz	160	26	5	49	0	–	70

BEER AND ALE

alcohol free beer	7 fl oz	50	1	tr	–	11	–	3
ale brown	10 oz	77	1	0	–	8	0	–
ale pale	10 oz	88	1	0	–	12	0	–
beer light	12 oz can	100	tr	0	0	5	–	10
beer regular	12 oz can	146	1	0	0	13	–	19
lager	10 oz	80	1	0	–	4	0	–
pilsener lager beer	7 fl oz	85	1	tr	–	13	–	4
stout	10 oz	102	1	0	–	6	0	–
Amstel								
Light	12 oz	95	–	0	0	–	–	–
Anheuser Busch								
Natural Light	12 oz	110	–	0	0	–	–	–
Bud								
Light	12 oz	108	–	0	0	–	–	–
Guiness								
Kaliber nonalcholic	12 oz	43	–	0	0	–	–	–
Michelob								
Light	12 oz	134	–	0	0	–	–	–
Miller								
Lite	12 oz	96	–	0	0	–	–	–
Molson								
Light	12 oz	109	–	0	0	–	–	–
Piels								
Light	12 oz	136	–	0	0	–	–	–
Schmidts								
Light	12 oz	96	–	0	0	–	–	–

BEET JUICE

juice	7 oz	72	2	0	0	16	–	400

FOOD	PORTION	CAL	PROT	FAT	CHOL	CARB	FIBER	SOD
BEETS								
CANNED								
harvard	½ cup	89	1	tr	0	22	—	199
pickled	½ cup	75	1	tr	0	19	—	301
sliced	½ cup	27	1	tr	0	6	—	—
Del Monte								
Pickled Crinkle Style Sliced	½ cup (4.5 oz)	80	1	0	0	19	2	380
Sliced	½ cup (4.3 oz)	35	1	0	0	8	2	290
Whole	½ cup (4.3 oz)	35	1	0	0	8	2	290
Green Giant								
Harvard	⅓ cup (3.1 oz)	60	tr	0	0	15	2	270
Sliced	½ cup (4.2 oz)	35	1	0	0	8	2	260
Sliced No Salt Added	½ cup (4.2 oz)	35	1	0	0	8	2	60
Whole	½ cup (4.2 oz)	35	1	0	0	8	2	260
LeSueur								
Baby Whole	½ cup (4.3 oz)	35	1	0	0	8	2	260
S&W								
Julienne	½ cup (4.3 oz)	30	1	0	0	7	1	230
Pickled Sliced	1 oz	15	0	0	0	4	1	50
Pickled Whole	1 oz	15	0	0	0	4	1	50
Sliced	½ cup (4.3 oz)	30	1	0	0	7	1	230
Whole Small	½ cup (4.3 oz)	30	1	0	0	7	1	230
FRESH								
greens cooked	½ cup	20	2	tr	0	4	—	173
greens raw	½ cup	4	tr	tr	0	1	—	38
greens raw chopped	½ cup	4	tr	tr	0	1	—	38
raw sliced	½ cup (2.4 oz)	29	1	tr	0	7	—	53
sliced cooked	½ cup (3 oz)	38	1	tr	0	9	—	65
whole cooked	2 (3.5 oz)	44	2	tr	0	10	—	77
whole raw	2 (5.7 oz)	70	3	tr	0	16	—	126

BEVERAGES *(see BEER AND ALE, CHAMPAGNE, COFFEE, DRINK MIXERS, ENERGY DRINKS, FRUIT DRINKS, ICED TEA, LIQUOR/LIQUEUR, MALT, MILKSHAKE, SODA, TEA/HERBAL TEA, WATER, WINE)*

BISCUIT

FOOD	PORTION	CAL	PROT	FAT	CHOL	CARB	FIBER	SOD
MIX								
buttermilk	1 (2 oz)	191	4	7	—	28	1	544
plain	1 (2 oz)	191	4	7	—	28	1	544

FOOD	PORTION	CAL	PROT	FAT	CHOL	CARB	FIBER	SOD
Bisquick								
Buttermilk	½ cup	150	2	6	0	21	–	320
Cheese Garlic	½ cup	160	2	7	0	22	–	360
Cinnamon Swirl	½ cup	150	2	4	0	30	–	330
Mix	⅓ cup (1.4 oz)	160	3	6	0	25	–	400
Reduced Fat	⅓ cup	140	3	3	0	27	tr	500
Kentucky Kernel								
Biscuit	¼ cup (1 oz)	171	3	5	0	28	1	659
READY-TO-EAT								
oatcakes	2 (4 oz)	115	3	5	–	16	1	–
REFRIGERATED								
buttermilk	1 (1 oz)	98	2	4	0	14	–	341
plain	1 (1 oz)	98	2	4	–	14	tr	341
1869 Brand								
Buttermilk	1 (1.1 oz)	100	2	5	0	12	0	320
Hungry Jack								
Butter Tastin' Flaky	1 (1.2 oz)	100	2	5	0	14	0	350
Cinnamon & Sugar	1 (1.2 oz)	110	2	4	0	17	tr	280
Flaky	1 (1.2 oz)	100	2	5	0	14	0	360
Flaky Buttermilk	1 (1.2 oz)	100	2	5	0	14	0	360
Pillsbury								
Big Country Butter Tastin'	1 (1.2 oz)	100	2	4	0	13	0	360
Big Country Buttermilk	1 (1.2 oz)	100	2	4	0	14	0	360
Big Country Southern Style	1 (1.2 oz)	100	2	4	0	14	0	360
Buttermilk	1 (2.2 oz)	150	4	2	0	29	tr	540
Country	1 (2.2 oz)	150	4	2	0	29	tr	540
Grands Blueberry	1 (2.1 oz)	210	4	9	0	29	tr	510
Grands Butter Tastin'	1 (2.1 oz)	200	4	10	0	24	tr	620
Grands Buttermilk	1 (2.1 oz)	200	4	10	0	24	tr	620
Grands Buttermilk Reduced Fat	1 (2.1 oz)	190	4	7	0	27	tr	620
Grands Extra Rich	1 (2.1 oz)	220	4	12	0	25	tr	580
Grands Flaky	1 (2.1 oz)	200	4	9	0	25	tr	580
Grands Golden Corn	1 (1.2 oz)	210	4	10	0	26	tr	600
Grands HomeStyle	1 (2.1 oz)	210	4	10	0	25	tr	620
Grands Southern Style	1 (2.1 oz)	200	4	10	0	24	tr	620

FOOD	PORTION	CAL	PROT	FAT	CHOL	CARB	FIBER	SOD
Southern Style Flakey	1 (1.2 oz)	100	2	5	0	14	0	360
Tender Layer Buttermilk	1 (2.2 oz)	160	4	5	0	27	tr	520
TAKE-OUT								
buttermilk	1 (2 oz)	212	4	10	2	27	—	348
plain	1 (35 g)	276	4	34	5	13	—	584
tea biscuit	1 (3 oz)	210	5	3	0	30	1	370
w/ egg	1 (4.8 oz)	316	11	20	233	24	—	654
w/ egg & bacon	1 (5.2 oz)	458	17	31	353	29	1	999
w/ egg & ham	1 (6.7 oz)	442	20	27	300	30	4	1382
w/ egg & sausage	1 (6.3 oz)	581	19	39	302	41	1	1141
w/ egg & steak	1 (5.2 oz)	410	18	28	272	21	—	888
w/ egg cheese & bacon	1 (5.1 oz)	477	16	31	261	33	—	1260
w/ ham	1 (4 oz)	386	13	18	25	44	1	1433
w/ sausage	1 (4.4 oz)	485	12	32	35	40	1	1071
w/ steak	1 (4.9 oz)	455	13	26	25	44	—	795

BISON
roasted	3 oz	122	24	2	70	0	—	48

BLACK BEANS
dried cooked	1 cup	227	15	1	0	41	—	1
Bean Cuisine								
Pasta & Beans Mediterranean Black Beans & Fusilli	1 serv	210	7	1	0	30	4	10
Eden								
Organic	½ cup (4.6 oz)	100	7	0	0	18	6	15
Green Giant								
Black Beans	½ cup (4.5 oz)	50	6	0	0	18	5	400
Old El Paso								
Black Beans	½ cup (4.6 oz)	100	7	1	0	17	7	400
Refried	½ cup (4.2 oz)	120	6	2	0	18	6	340
Progresso								
Black Beans	½ cup (4.6 oz)	110	7	1	0	17	7	400

BLACKBERRIES
canned in heavy syrup	½ cup	118	2	tr	0	30	—	3

FOOD	PORTION	CAL	PROT	FAT	CHOL	CARB	FIBER	SOD
fresh	½ cup	37	1	tr	0	9	3	0
unsweetened frzn	1 cup	97	2	1	0	24	–	2

BLACKBERRY JUICE
Clear Fruit

Blackberry Rush	8 oz	90	0	0	0	23	–	0

Everfresh

Clear Fruit Blackberry Rush	8 oz	90	0	0	0	23	–	0

Kool-Aid

Scary Blackberry Ghoul-Aid Drink as prep w/ sugar	1 serv (8 oz)	100	0	0	0	25	0	0

BLACKEYE PEAS
CANNED

w/pork	½ cup	199	7	4	17	40	–	840

Eden

Organic	½ cup (4.6 oz)	90	6	1	0	16	4	25

Green Giant

Blackeye Peas	½ cup (4.4 oz)	90	6	0	0	16	3	250

DRIED

cooked	1 cup	198	13	1	0	36	16	6

Hurst

HamBeens California w/ Ham	1 serv	120	8	1	0	22	7	73

FROZEN
Birds Eye

Blackeye Peas	½ cup (2.8 oz)	110	7	1	0	21	4	10

BLINTZE
Golden

Cheese	1 (2.1 oz)	80	6	2	15	13	2	135

TAKE-OUT

cheese	1 (2.7 oz)	160	5	9	65	15	tr	240

BLUEBERRIES

canned in heavy syrup	1 cup	225	2	1	0	56	–	9
fresh	1 cup	82	1	1	0	20	–	9
unsweetened frzn	1 cup	78	1	1	0	19	–	1

FOOD	PORTION	CAL	PROT	FAT	CHOL	CARB	FIBER	SOD
Sonoma								
Dried	¼ cup (1.3 oz)	140	1	0	0	33	5	0
Tree Of Life								
Organic	1 cup (5 oz)	80	1	0	0	20	2	0

BLUEBERRY JUICE

After The Fall

| Maine Coast | 1 cup (8 oz) | 90 | 0 | 0 | 0 | 25 | 0 | 20 |

BLUEFIN

| fillet baked | 4.1 oz | 186 | 30 | 6 | 88 | 0 | – | 90 |

BLUEFISH

| fresh baked | 3 oz | 135 | 22 | 5 | 64 | 0 | – | 65 |

BOAR

| wild roasted | 3 oz | 136 | 24 | 4 | – | 0 | – | – |

BOK CHOY *(see CABBAGE)*

BONITO

| fresh | 3 oz | 117 | 20 | 4 | – | 0 | 0 | – |

BORAGE

| fresh chopped cooked | 3½ oz | 25 | 2 | 1 | 0 | 4 | – | 88 |
| raw chopped | ½ cup | 9 | 1 | tr | 0 | 1 | – | 35 |

BOTTLED WATER *(see WATER)*

BOYSENBERRIES

| in heavy syrup | 1 cup | 226 | 3 | tr | 0 | 57 | – | 9 |
| unsweetened frzn | 1 cup | 66 | 1 | tr | 0 | 16 | – | 2 |

BRAINS

beef pan-fried	3 oz	167	11	13	1696	0	–	134
beef simmered	3 oz	136	9	11	1746	0	–	102
lamb braised	3 oz	124	11	9	1737	0	–	114
lamb fried	3 oz	232	14	19	2128	0	–	133
pork braised	3 oz	117	10	8	2169	0	0	77
veal braised	3 oz	115	10	8	2635	0	–	133
veal fried	3 oz	181	12	14	1802	0	–	150
Armour								
Pork Brains In Milk Gravy	⅔ cup (5.5 oz)	150	16	5	3500	10	0	550

FOOD	PORTION	CAL	PROT	FAT	CHOL	CARB	FIBER	SOD
BRAN								
corn	1 cup (2.7 oz)	170	6	1	0	65	65	5
oat	½ cup (1.6 oz)	116	8	3	0	31	7	2
oat cooked	½ cup (3.8 oz)	44	4	1	0	13	3	1
rice	½ cup (2.1 oz)	187	8	12	0	29	12	3
wheat	½ cup (2 oz)	63	5	1	0	19	12	1
Hodgson Mill								
Oat	¼ cup (1.4 oz)	120	6	3	0	23	6	3
Quaker								
Oat Bran	½ cup (1.4 oz)	150	7	3	0	25	6	0
BRAZIL NUTS								
dried unblanched	1 oz	186	4	19	0	4	–	0
BREAD								
CANNED								
boston brown	1 slice (1.6 oz)	88	2	1	–	20	2	284
B&M								
Brown Bread	½ in slice (2 oz)	130	3	1	0	29	2	390
Brown Bread Raisins	½ in slice (2 oz)	130	3	1	0	29	2	360
FROZEN								
Marie Callender's								
Cornbread & Honey Butter	1 piece + butter	210	2	11	15	28	1	370
Original Garlic	1 piece	190	4	8	<5	23	2	330
Parmesan & Romano Garlic	1 piece	200	5	10	5	23	2	430
New York								
Garlic	1 slice (2 oz)	190	3	8	0	27	1	390
Garlic Reduced Fat	1 slice (2 oz)	160	4	4	0	29	1	340
Texas Garlic Toast	1 in slice (1.4 oz)	160	3	9	0	17	1	260
Pepperidge Farm								
Garlic	1 slice (1.8 oz)	170	5	10	30	15	1	270
Garlic Sourdough 30% Reduced Fat	1 slice (1.8 oz)	170	6	7	5	22	2	310
Monterey Jack Jalapeno Cheese	1 slice (2 oz)	145	5	11	41	22	4	279
Mozzeralla Garlic Cheese	1 slice (2 oz)	201	6	10	40	21	1	280

FOOD	PORTION	CAL	PROT	FAT	CHOL	CARB	FIBER	SOD
MIX								
cornbread	1 piece (2 oz)	189	4	6	37	29	1	467
Hodgson Mill								
European Cheese & Herb	¼ cup (1.2 oz)	130	5	1	0	21	tr	250
Honey Whole Wheat	¼ cup (1.2 oz)	120	5	1	0	22	2	160
Zia Foods								
Cornbread Blue Cornmeal	1 piece (1.2 oz)	110	–	6	41	–	–	–
READY-TO-EAT								
baguette whole wheat	2 oz	140	6	0	0	29	1	360
challah	1 slice (2 oz)	160	3	3	0	29	1	250
cracked wheat	1 slice	65	2	1	–	12	1	135
egg	1 slice (1.4 oz)	115	4	2	20	19	–	197
french	1 slice (1 oz)	78	3	1	0	15	1	172
french	1 loaf (1 lb)	1270	43	18	0	230	–	2633
gluten	1 slice	47	2	tr	0	8	–	104
italian	1 loaf (1 lb)	1255	41	4	0	256	–	2656
italian	1 slice (1 oz)	81	3	1	0	15	1	175
navajo fry	1 (10.5 in diam)	527	11	15	0	85	–	1112
navajo fry	1 (5 in diam)	296	6	9	0	48	–	625
oat bran	1 slice	71	3	1	0	12	1	122
oat bran reduced calorie	1 slice	46	2	1	0	10	–	81
oatmeal	1 slice	73	2	1	–	13	1	162
oatmeal reduced calorie	1 slice	48	2	1	0	10	–	89
pita	1 reg (2 oz)	165	5	1	0	33	1	322
pita	1 sm (1 oz)	78	3	tr	0	16	1	152
pita whole wheat	1 reg (2 oz)	170	6	2	0	35	5	340
pita whole wheat	1 sm (1 oz)	76	3	1	0	16	2	151
protein	1 slice	47	2	tr	0	8	–	104
pumpernickel	1 slice	80	3	1	0	15	2	215
raisin	1 slice	71	2	1	0	14	–	101
rice bran	1 slice	66	1	1	0	12	–	119
rye	1 slice	83	3	1	0	16	2	211
rye reduced calorie	1 slice	47	2	1	0	9	–	93
seven grain	1 slice	65	3	1	0	12	2	127

FOOD	PORTION	CAL	PROT	FAT	CHOL	CARB	FIBER	SOD
sourdough	1 slice (1 oz)	78	3	1	0	15	1	172
vienna	1 slice (1 oz)	78	3	1	0	15	1	172
wheat reduced calorie	1 slice	46	2	1	—	10	3	117
wheat berry	1 slice	65	2	1	0	12	1	132
wheat bran	1 slice	89	3	1	0	17	3	175
wheat germ	1 slice	74	3	1	—	14	—	157
white	1 slice	67	2	1	0	12	1	135
white reduced calorie	1 slice	48	2	1	0	10	2	104
white toasted	1 slice	67	2	1	0	13	—	136
white cubed	1 cup	80	2	1	0	15	—	154
whole wheat	1 slice	70	3	1	—	13	2	149
Arnold								
Country Buttermilk	1 slice (1.3 oz)	110	4	2	0	20	1	180
Country Wheat	1 slice (1.3 oz)	100	4	2	0	19	1	190
Natural 100% Whole Wheat	1 slice (1.3 oz)	90	4	1	0	16	3	170
Raisin Cinnamon	1 slice (1 oz)	80	2	2	0	15	1	95
Bread Du Jour								
French	3 in slice (2 oz)	140	5	1	0	26	1	310
Damascus								
Mountain Shepard Lahvash	⅓ loaf (2 oz)	135	5	0	0	28	2	90
Pita	1 (2 oz)	130	6	0	0	29	2	150
Pita Whole Wheat	1 (2 oz)	160	6	0	0	32	3	230
Wraps Honey Wheat	½ wrap (2 oz)	130	5	0	0	28	1	150
Wraps Plain	½ wrap (2 oz)	130	5	0	0	29	1	150
Wraps Spinach	1 (2 oz)	280	10	0	0	56	2	460
Wraps Tomato	1 12-inch (4 oz)	240	10	0	0	58	2	440
Home Pride								
Wheat	1 slice (1 oz)	80	2	1	0	14	1	190
La Mexicana								
Wraps Chocolate	1 (1.3 oz)	120	4	3	0	18	1	360
Wraps Southwestern Mild Chili	1 (1.3 oz)	120	4	4	0	18	1	360
Wraps Spinach	1 (1.3 oz)	120	4	4	0	18	1	360
Wraps Tomato Basil	1 (1.3 oz)	120	4	4	0	18	1	360
Meditarranean Magic								
Focaccia	⅕ loaf (1.8 oz)	140	4	2	0	27	tr	550

FOOD	PORTION	CAL	PROT	FAT	CHOL	CARB	FIBER	SOD
Milton's								
Healthy Multi-Grain	1 slice (1.4 oz)	110	3	1	0	24	3	150
Pepperidge Farm								
Apple Cinammon	1 slice (1 oz)	80	4	2	0	15	1	120
Deli Swirl Rye & Pump	1 slice (1.1 oz)	80	3	1	0	15	1	220
Farmhouse Hearty White	1 slice (1.5 oz)	110	5	2	<5	20	tr	260
Farmhouse Sourdough	1 slice (1.5 oz)	110	4	2	0	20	1	220
Natural Whole Grain Whole Wheat	1 slice (1.2 oz)	90	4	1	0	16	2	135
Natural Whole Grain Honey Oat	1 slice (1.2 oz)	90	4	2	0	15	2	135
Sandwich Pocket Wheat	1 (2 oz)	160	6	1	0	30	3	260
Sandwich Pocket White	1 (2 oz)	150	6	1	0	30	2	290
Swirl Cinnamon	1 slice (1 oz)	90	2	3	0	15	1	110
Swirl Raisin Cinnamon	1 slice (1 oz)	80	3	2	0	14	1	105
Stroehmann								
100% Whole Wheat	1 slice (1.3 oz)	90	5	1	0	17	2	180
D'Italiano Italian No Seeds	1 slice (1 oz)	80	2	1	0	15	tr	170
D'Italiano Italian Seeded	1 slice (1 oz)	80	2	1	0	15	tr	170
Family White	1 slice (0.8 oz)	65	2	1	0	13	0	135
Homestyle Split Top Wheat	1 slice (0.8 oz)	60	2	0	0	13	tr	110
Homestyle Split Top White	1 slice (0.8 oz)	65	2	1	0	12	1	110
Honey Cracked Wheat	1 slice (1.2 oz)	80	3	1	0	16	1	170
King White	1 slice (0.8 oz)	65	2	1	0	13	0	135
Potato	1 slice (1.2 oz)	100	3	2	0	19	tr	170
Ranch White	1 slice (0.8 oz)	65	2	1	0	13	0	135
Rye	1 slice (1.1 oz)	80	3	1	0	15	tr	180
Rye w/ Caraway	1 slice (1.1 oz)	80	3	1	0	15	tr	170
Twelve Grain	1 slice (1.2 oz)	90	3	1	0	17	1	140

FOOD	PORTION	CAL	PROT	FAT	CHOL	CARB	FIBER	SOD
Valley Lahvosh								
Valley Wraps	1 (1 oz)	100	4	1	0	19	1	125
ZA								
Pit-Za Hearty Multi-Grain	1/9 bread (2 oz)	130	5	2	0	25	2	210
Pit-Za Salt-Free Garlic Whole Wheat	1/9 bread (2 oz)	150	7	1	0	28	3	10
REFRIGERATED								
Pillsbury								
Crusty French Loaf	1/5 loaf (2.2 oz)	150	5	2	0	27	tr	390
Grands Wheat	1 (2.1 oz)	200	4	8	0	27	2	600
TAKE-OUT								
chapatis as prep w/ fat	1 bread (1.6 oz)	95	3	2	3	18	3	180
chapatis as prep w/o fat	1 (2 ½ oz)	141	5	1	–	31	5	–
cornbread	2 in x 2 in (1.4 oz)	107	4	2	28	18	–	276
cornstick	1 (1.3 oz)	101	2	4	30	13	tr	195
focaccia onion	1 piece (4.6 oz)	282	6	10	0	43	2	536
focaccia rosemary	1 piece (3.5 oz)	251	6	7	0	40	2	535
focaccia tomato olive	1 piece (4.7 oz)	270	6	8	0	42	2	683
garlic bread	2 slices (2 oz)	190	3	8	0	27	1	290
irish soda bread	1 slice (2 oz)	174	4	3	11	34	–	239
naan	1 bread (3.5 oz)	286	7	9	46	43	2	546
papadums fried	2 (1.5 oz)	81	4	4	–	9	2	–
paratha	1 bread (2.1 oz)	201	4	10	27	23	2	268

BREAD COATING

FOOD	PORTION	CAL	PROT	FAT	CHOL	CARB	FIBER	SOD
Don's Chuck Wagon								
Chicken Baking Mix	¼ cup (1 oz)	95	3	0	0	21	1	850
Fish & Chips Mix	¼ cup (1 oz)	100	3	0	0	21	1	740
Fish Mix	¼ cup (1 oz)	95	4	0	0	21	1	940
Mushroom Batter Mix	¼ cup (1 oz)	95	3	0	0	21	1	990
Onion Ring Mix	¼ cup (1 oz)	100	3	0	0	21	1	690
Seafood Bake & Fry Mix	¼ cup (1 oz)	95	2	0	0	21	1	990

FOOD	PORTION	CAL	PROT	FAT	CHOL	CARB	FIBER	SOD
Luzianne								
Cajun Chicken Coating Mix	2 tbsp (1 oz)	100	3	1	0	20	1	1260
Mrs. Dash								
Crispy Coating	2 tbsp (0.6 oz)	65	5	1	0	10	–	3
Oven Fry								
Extra Crispy For Chicken	⅛ pkg (0.5 oz)	60	2	1	0	10	0	420
Extra Crispy For Pork	⅛ pkg (0.5 oz)	60	2	2	0	11	0	340
Shake 'N Bake								
Buffalo Wings	¹⁄₁₀ pkg (0.4 oz)	40	0	1	0	8	0	300
Classic Italian Chicken or Pork	⅛ pkg (0.4 oz)	40	1	1	0	7	0	270
Country Mild Recipe	⅛ pkg (0.3 oz)	35	0	2	0	5	0	240
Glazes Barbecue Chicken Or Pork	⅛ pkg (0.4 oz)	45	0	1	0	9	0	410
Glazes Honey Mustard Chicken Or Pork	⅛ pkg (0.4 oz)	45	0	1	0	9	0	300
Glazes Tangy Honey Chicken Or Pork	⅛ pkg (0.4 oz)	45	0	1	0	9	0	300
Home Style Flour Recipe For Chicken	⅛ pkg (0.4 oz)	40	tr	1	0	7	0	470
Hot & Spicy Chicken Or Pork	⅛ pkg (0.4 oz)	40	1	1	0	7	0	170
Original For Chicken	⅛ pkg (0.4 oz)	40	1	1	0	7	0	220
Original For Fish	¼ pkg (0.7 oz)	80	2	2	0	14	tr	350
Original For Pork	⅛ pkg (0.4 oz)	45	1	1	0	8	0	230
BREAD MACHINE MIX								
Fleischmann's								
Apple Cinnamon	⅛ loaf	160	5	1	0	32	2	160
Cinnamon Raisin	⅛ loaf	160	5	1	0	33	2	170
Country White	⅛ loaf (1.6 oz)	170	6	3	0	31	2	170
Cranberry Orange	⅛ loaf	150	2	2	0	33	2	150
Honey Oatmeal	⅛ loaf	160	5	1	0	33	3	270
Italian Herb	⅛ loaf	160	5	2	0	29	2	310
Sourdough	⅛ loaf	150	5	2	0	29	2	160
Stoneground Wheat	⅛ loaf	160	5	1	0	32	3	180

FOOD	PORTION	CAL	PROT	FAT	CHOL	CARB	FIBER	SOD
Sassafras								
Apricot Oatmeal	1 slice (1.4 oz)	140	5	1	0	29	2	190
BREADCRUMBS								
dry	1 cup	426	14	6	–	78	5	930
dry seasonsed	1 cup (4 oz)	441	17	3	–	85	5	3180
fresh	⅔ cup	76	4	1	0	14	1	153
Progresso								
Garlic & Herb	¼ cup (1 oz)	100	4	2	0	18	1	530
Italian Style	¼ cup (1 oz)	110	4	2	0	20	1	430
Parmesan	¼ cup (1 oz)	100	4	2	0	17	1	870
Plain	¼ cup (1 oz)	110	4	2	0	19	1	210
BREADFRUIT								
fresh	¼ small	99	1	tr	0	26	–	2
seeds cooked	1 oz	48	2	1	0	9	–	–
seeds raw	1 oz	54	2	2	0	8	–	–
seeds roasted	1 oz	59	2	tr	0	11	–	–
BREADNUTTREE SEEDS								
dried	1 oz	104	2	tr	0	23	–	–
BREADSTICKS								
onion poppyseed	1	64	2	1	10	11	–	69
plain	1 sm	25	1	1	0	4	–	66
plain	1	41	1	1	0	7	–	66
Bread Du Jour								
Original	1 (1.9 oz)	130	5	1	0	25	1	290
Sourdough	1 (1.9 oz)	130	5	1	0	25	1	280
New York								
Garlic Soft	1 (1.5 oz)	140	3	4	0	23	1	220
Pillsbury								
Soft	1 (1.4 oz)	110	3	2	0	19	tr	290
Soft Garlic & Herb	1 (2.1 oz)	180	4	7	0	25	tr	580
Stella D'Oro								
Garlic	1 (0.4 oz)	40	1	1	0	7	0	60
Grissini Style Fat Free	3 (0.5 oz)	60	2	0	0	12	0	130
Original	1 (0.4 oz)	45	1	1	0	7	0	40
Potato 'N Onion	1 (0.4 oz)	45	1	1	0	8	0	210
Roasted Garlic	1 (0.4 oz)	45	1	1	0	8	tr	210
Sesame	1 (0.4 oz)	50	1	3	0	7	tr	45

FOOD	PORTION	CAL	PROT	FAT	CHOL	CARB	FIBER	SOD
Snack Stix Cracked Pepper	4 (0.5 oz)	70	2	2	0	11	0	290
Snack Stix Salted	4 (0.5 oz)	70	2	2	0	11	0	290
Sodium Free	1 (0.4 oz)	45	1	1	0	7	0	0
Wheat	1 (0.3 oz)	40	1	1	0	6	0	20

BREAKFAST BAR *(see* CEREAL BARS, ENERGY BARS*)*

BREAKFAST DRINKS *(see also* ENERGY DRINKS, NUTRITION SUPPLEMENTS*)*

FOOD	PORTION	CAL	PROT	FAT	CHOL	CARB	FIBER	SOD
orange drink powder	3 rounded tsp	93	0	0	0	24	–	4
orange drink powder as prep w/water	6 oz	86	0	0	0	22	–	9
Carnation								
Instant Breakfast Vanilla as prep w/ skim milk	1 serv	220	13	1	5	39	–	220
Instant Breakfast Vanilla as prep w/ whole milk	1 serv	280	13	8	35	39	–	220

BROAD BEANS

FOOD	PORTION	CAL	PROT	FAT	CHOL	CARB	FIBER	SOD
canned	1 cup	183	14	1	0	32	–	1161
dried cooked	1 cup	186	13	1	0	33	–	8
fresh cooked	3½ oz	56	5	tr	0	10	–	41

BROCCOFLOWER

FOOD	PORTION	CAL	PROT	FAT	CHOL	CARB	FIBER	SOD
fresh raw	½ cup (1.8 oz)	16	1	tr	0	3	–	12

BROCCOLI
FRESH

FOOD	PORTION	CAL	PROT	FAT	CHOL	CARB	FIBER	SOD
chinese broccoli (gai lan) cooked	1 cup (3.1 oz)	19	1	1	0	3	2	6
chopped cooked	½ cup	22	2	tr	0	4	2	20
raw chopped	½ cup	12	1	tr	0	2	1	12
FROZEN								
chopped cooked	½ cup	25	3	tr	0	5	–	22
spears cooked	½ cup	25	3	tr	0	5	3	22
spears cooked	10 oz pkg	69	8	tr	0	13	4	60
Amy's Organic								
Pocket Sandwich Broccoli & Cheese	1 (4.5 oz)	270	8	10	15	37	3	560

FOOD	PORTION	CAL	PROT	FAT	CHOL	CARB	FIBER	SOD
Birds Eye								
Chopped	⅓ cup	25	–	0	0	–	2	15
Cuts	½ cup	25	–	0	0	–	3	30
Florets	1 cup (3 oz)	25	2	0	0	4	2	35
In Cheese Sauce	½ cup (4 oz)	70	3	4	5	7	2	500
Green Giant								
Butter Sauce	4 oz	50	2	2	<5	7	2	330
Cheese Sauce	⅔ cup (3.9 oz)	70	3	3	<5	9	2	520
Chopped	¾ cup (2.8 oz)	25	2	0	0	4	2	25
Cuts	1 cup (2.9 oz)	25	2	0	0	4	2	25
Harvest Fresh Cut	⅔ cup (3.2 oz)	25	2	0	0	4	2	150
Harvest Fresh Spears	3.5 oz	25	2	0	0	4	2	125
Select Florets	1⅓ cups (2.9 oz)	25	2	0	0	4	2	25
Select Spears	3 oz	25	2	0	0	4	2	25
Health Is Wealth								
Broccoli Munchees	2 (1 oz)	60	2	2	0	10	1	170
Stouffer's								
Au Gratin	1 serv (4 oz)	100	5	4	10	10	2	450
Tree Of Life								
Cuts	1 cup (3.1 oz)	25	2	0	0	4	2	20

BROWNIE

FROZEN

FOOD	PORTION	CAL	PROT	FAT	CHOL	CARB	FIBER	SOD
Greenfield								
Fat Free Homestyle	1 (1.3 oz)	110	2	0	0	27	0	60
Otis Spunkmeyer								
Blue Yonder w/ Walnuts	1 (2 oz)	230	3	10	20	34	2	170
Weight Watchers								
Brownie A La Mode	1 (3.14 oz)	190	5	4	30	33	2	190
Double Fudge Brownie Parfait	1 (5.3 oz)	190	6	3	5	39	2	170
MIX								
plain	1 (1.2 oz)	139	1	7	9	20	1	83
plain low calorie	1 (0.8 oz)	84	1	2	0	16	1	21
Betty Crocker								
Chocolate Chunk as prep	1	180	1	9	21	25	–	90
Dark Chocolate Fudge as prep	1	170	1	7	21	24	–	120

FOOD	PORTION	CAL	PROT	FAT	CHOL	CARB	FIBER	SOD
Dark Chocolate w/ Syrup as prep	1	170	2	7	21	25	—	105
Fudge as prep	1	170	1	7	21	23	—	100
German Chocolate Coconut Pecan Filling as prep	1	200	1	8	21	29	1	115
Hot Fudge as prep	1	170	2	8	21	23	—	105
Original as prep	1	180	1	6	21	27	—	135
Peanut Butter as prep	1	180	3	8	21	23	—	105
Stir'n Bake w/ Mini Kisses as prep	1 serv	220	2	7	0	38	1	160
Turtle w/ Caramel & Pecans as prep	1	170	1	8	21	25	—	95
Walnut as prep	1	180	2	9	21	23	—	90
Estee								
Brownie Mix as prep	2	100	tr	4	0	23	1	0
No Pudge!								
Cappuccino Fudge	1	100	2	0	0	21	tr	90
Mint Fudge	½ cup	100	2	0	0	21	tr	90
Original Fudge	1	100	2	0	0	21	tr	90
Raspberry Fudge	1	100	2	0	0	21	tr	90
Sweet Rewards								
Low Fat Fudge as prep	1	130	2	3	0	27	1	115
Reduced Fat Supreme as prep	1	140	2	3	21	27	—	110
READY-TO-EAT								
plain	1 sm (1 oz)	115	1	5	5	18	1	88
plain	1 lg (2 oz)	227	3	9	10	36	1	175
w/ nuts	1 (1 oz)	100	1	4	14	16	—	59
Dolly Madison								
Fudge	1 (3 oz)	330	3	11	45	54	1	190
Entenmann's								
Little Bites	3 (2.2 oz)	290	3	16	45	37	1	200
Ultimate Fudge	1 (1.6 oz)	220	3	13	50	27	2	60
Greenfield								
Blondie Fat Free Apple Spice	1 (1.3 oz)	110	2	0	0	26	0	60
Health Valley								
Bar w/ Fudge Filling	1 bar	110	3	0	0	26	4	30

FOOD	PORTION	CAL	PROT	FAT	CHOL	CARB	FIBER	SOD
Hostess								
Brownie Bites	3 (1.3 oz)	170	2	9	30	21	1	80
Fudge	1 (3 oz)	330	3	11	45	54	1	190
Light	1 (1.4 oz)	140	1	3	1	28	1	80
Lance								
Fudge Nut	1 (2.25 oz)	340	3	13	20	56	2	180
Little Debbie								
Brownie Lights	1 (2 oz)	190	3	3	0	39	1	200
Brownie Loaves	1 (2.1 oz)	260	3	15	40	31	1	160
Fudge	1 pkg (2.1 oz)	270	2	13	15	39	tr	170
Tastykake								
Fudge Walnut	1 (3 oz)	370	5	17	80	52	1	150
Tom's								
Fudge Nut	1 pkg (2.5 oz)	300	3	13	5	45	0	95
REFRIGERATED								
Toll House								
Brownie Dough	½ pkg (1.5 oz)	180	2	7	15	26	2	160
TAKE-OUT								
plain	1, 2 in sq (2.1 oz)	243	3	10	10	39	—	153

BRUSSELS SPROUTS

FOOD	PORTION	CAL	PROT	FAT	CHOL	CARB	FIBER	SOD
FRESH								
cooked	½ cup	30	2	tr	0	7	3	17
cooked	1 sprout	8	1	tr	0	2	—	4
raw	½ cup	19	1	tr	0	4	—	11
raw	1 sprout	8	1	tr	0	2	1	5
FROZEN								
cooked	½ cup	33	3	tr	0	6	—	18
Birds Eye								
Brussels Sprouts	11 sprouts	35	3	0	0	7	3	15
Green Giant								
Butter Sauce	⅔ cup (3.6 oz)	60	3	2	<5	9	4	270

BUCKWHEAT

FOOD	PORTION	CAL	PROT	FAT	CHOL	CARB	FIBER	SOD
groats roasted cooked	1 cup (5.9 oz)	647	6	1	0	34	5	7
groats roasted uncooked	1 cup (5.7 oz)	567	19	4	0	123	17	18

BUFFALO

FOOD	PORTION	CAL	PROT	FAT	CHOL	CARB	FIBER	SOD
water buffalo roasted	3 oz	111	23	2	52	0	—	48

FOOD	PORTION	CAL	PROT	FAT	CHOL	CARB	FIBER	SOD
BULGUR								
cooked	1 cup (6.3 oz)	151	7	tr	0	34	8	9
uncooked	1 cup (4.9 oz)	479	17	2	0	106	26	24
Hodgson Mill								
Bulgur w/ Soygrits	¼ cup (1.4 oz)	120	6	1	0	24	1	0
BURBOT (FISH)								
fresh baked	3 oz	98	65	1	65	0	–	106
BURDOCK ROOT								
cooked	1 cup	110	3	tr	0	26	–	5
raw	1 cup	85	2	tr	0	20	–	6
BUTTER *(see also BUTTER BLENDS, BUTTER SUBSTITUTES)*								
clarified butter	3½ oz	876	tr	99	256	0	–	–
ghee cow's milk	1 tbsp	126	–	14	39	–	0	0
ghee vegetable oil	1 tbsp	126	–	14	0	–	0	0
stick	1 stick (4 oz)	813	1	92	248	tr	–	937
stick	1 pat (5 g)	36	tr	4	11	tr	–	41
whipped	4 oz	542	1	61	165	tr	–	625
whipped	1 pat (4 g)	27	tr	3	8	tr	–	31
Breakstone's								
Salted	1 tbsp (0.5 oz)	100	0	11	30	0	–	85
Hotel Bar								
Stick	1 tbsp (0.5 oz)	100	0	11	30	0	–	90
Keller's								
European	1 tbsp (0.5 oz)	100	0	11	30	0	0	0
Land O Lakes								
Salted	1 tbsp (0.5 oz)	100	0	11	30	0	–	85
Ultra Creamy Salted	1 tbsp (0.5 oz)	110	0	12	30	0	–	85
Organic Valley								
Butter	1 tbsp (0.5 oz)	100	0	11	30	0	0	75
Unsalted	1 tbsp (0.5 oz)	110	0	12	30	0	0	0
BUTTER BEANS								
CANNED								
Green Giant								
Butter Beans	½ cup (4.5 oz)	90	6	0	0	16	4	450
Van Camp								
Butter Beans	½ cup (4.6 oz)	110	8	1	0	22	7	430

FOOD	PORTION	CAL	PROT	FAT	CHOL	CARB	FIBER	SOD
FROZEN								
Birds Eye								
Speckled	½ cup (2.7 oz)	100	6	0	0	20	4	130
BUTTER BLENDS								
stick	1 stick	811	1	91	99	1	–	1013
Brummel & Brown								
Spread Made w/ Yogurt	1 tbsp (0.5 oz)	50	0	5	0	0	–	90
BUTTER SUBSTITUTES								
Molly McButter								
Cheese	1 tsp	5	0	0	0	1	–	125
Light Sodium	1 tsp	5	0	0	0	1	–	90
Natural Butter	1 tsp	5	0	0	0	1	–	180
Roasted Garlic	1 tsp	5	0	0	0	1	–	125
Mrs. Bateman's								
Butterlike Baking Butter	1 tbsp (0.5 oz)	36	0	1	<5	8	0	20
Butterlike Saute Butter	1 tbsp (0.5 oz)	40	0	2	5	8	0	60
BUTTERBUR								
canned fuki chopped	1 cup	3	tr	tr	0	tr	–	5
fresh fuki	1 cup	13	tr	tr	0	3	–	7
BUTTERFISH								
baked	3 oz	159	19	9	71	0	–	97
fillet baked	1 oz	47	6	3	21	0	–	29
BUTTERNUTS								
dried	1 oz	174	7	16	0	3	–	0
BUTTERSCOTCH *(see also CANDY)*								
Hershey								
Chips	1 tbsp (0.5 oz)	80	tr	4	0	10	–	10
Nestle								
Morsels	1 tbsp	80	0	4	0	9	0	15
CABBAGE *(see also COLESLAW)*								
chinese bok choy shredded cooked	½ cup	10	1	tr	0	2	–	29
chinese pak-choi raw shredded	½ cup	5	1	tr	0	1	–	23

FOOD	PORTION	CAL	PROT	FAT	CHOL	CARB	FIBER	SOD
chinese pe-tsai raw shredded	1 cup	12	1	tr	0	2	–	7
chinese pe-tsai shredded cooked	1 cup	16	2	tr	0	3	–	11
danish raw	1 head (2 lbs)	228	13	2	0	49	18	164
danish raw shredded	½ cup (1.2 oz)	9	1	tr	0	2	tr	6
danish shredded cooked	½ cup (2.6 oz)	17	1	tr	0	3	1	6
green raw	1 head (2 lbs)	228	2	12	0	49	18	164
green raw shredded	½ cup (1.2 oz)	9	1	tr	0	2	tr	6
green shredded cooked	½ cup (2.6 oz)	17	1	tr	0	3	1	6
napa cooked	1 cup (3.8 oz)	13	1	tr	0	2	0	12
red raw shredded	½ cup	10	tr	tr	0	2	1	4
red shredded cooked	½ cup	16	1	tr	0	3	–	6
savoy raw shredded	½ cup	10	1	tr	0	2	–	10
savoy shredded cooked	½ cup	18	1	tr	0	4	–	17
TAKE-OUT								
korean kimchee	½ cup	22	2	tr	0	4	4	–
stuffed cabbage	1 (6 oz)	373	25	22	95	18	–	1007
sweet & sour red cabbage	4 oz	61	1	3	–	8	3	–
CACTUS								
napoles fresh sliced	½ cup (1.5 oz)	7	1	tr	0	1	–	9
pricklypear fresh	1 cup (5.3 oz)	56	2	1	0	13	4	–
CAKE (see also CAKE MIX)								
angelfood	1 cake (11.9 oz)	876	20	3	0	197	5	2548
apple crisp	1 recipe 6 serv (29.6 oz)	1377	15	31	1	273	–	1537
battenburg cake	1 slice (2 oz)	204	3	10	–	28	1	–
boston cream pie	⅙ cake (3.2 oz)	232	2	8	34	40	1	132
carrot w/ cream cheese icing	1 cake 10 in diam	6175	63	328	1183	775	–	4470
cheesecake	⅙ cake (2.8 oz)	256	4	18	44	20	2	165
cheesecake	1 cake 9 in diam	3350	60	213	2053	317	–	2464
coffeecake fruit	⅛ cake (1.8 oz)	156	3	5	–	26	–	192

FOOD	PORTION	CAL	PROT	FAT	CHOL	CARB	FIBER	SOD
crumpet	1 (2.3 oz)	131	4	1	0	31	2	535
eccles cake	1 slice (2 oz)	285	2	16	–	36	1	–
eclair	1 (1.4 oz)	149	2	10	–	15	tr	–
fruitcake	1 piece (1.5 oz)	139	1	4	2	27	–	116
jelly roll lemon filled	1 slice (3 oz)	210	3	2	35	48	tr	300
madeira cake	1 slice (1 oz)	98	1	4	–	15	1	–
pound	1/10 cake (1 oz)	117	2	6	66	15	–	119
pound fat free	1 cake (12 oz)	961	18	4	0	208	–	1158
sponge	1/12 cake (1.3 oz)	110	2	1	39	23	–	93
sponge cake dessert shell	1 (0.8 oz)	75	2	1	33	16	0	165
tiramisu	1 cake (4.4 lbs)	5732	101	421	2395	439	3	1107
treacle tart	1 slice (2.5 oz)	258	3	10	–	42	1	–
Baby Watson								
Cheesecake	1 slice (3 oz)	260	4	18	65	19	tr	150
Carousel								
New York Cheese Cake	1 cake (3 oz)	250	4	19	95	16	1	180
Dolly Madison								
Angel Food	1 slice (2.1 oz)	160	3	2	0	34	1	190
Apple Crumb	1 (1.6 oz)	160	2	5	15	28	0	160
Banana Dream Flip	1 (3.5 oz)	390	3	16	30	59	1	240
Bear Claw	1 (2.75 oz)	270	5	10	25	40	1	330
Carrot	1 (4 oz)	360	4	8	0	67	1	500
Chocolate Snack Squares	1 (1.6 oz)	210	2	10	10	28	0	150
Cinnamon Buttercrumb	1 (1.6 oz)	170	2	6	15	28	0	170
Cinnamon Buttercrumb Low Fat	1 (1.5 oz)	140	1	2	0	29	0	150
Cinnamon Stix	1 (1.3 oz)	170	1	9	15	21	0	140
Creme Cakes	2 (1.9 oz)	210	1	8	25	32	0	230
Cupcakes Chocolate	1 (2 oz)	210	2	7	5	35	1	330
Cupcakes Spice	1 (2 oz)	230	2	10	20	33	0	160
Dunkin' Stix	1 (1.3 oz)	170	1	9	15	20	0	130
Frosty Angel	1 (3.5 oz)	330	4	6	0	65	1	270
Holiday Cupcakes	1 (1.9 oz)	180	1	3	5	35	0	190
Honey Bun	1 (3.7 oz)	440	6	25	15	49	1	260
Koo Koos	1 (1.8 oz)	200	1	9	5	29	0	90

FOOD	PORTION	CAL	PROT	FAT	CHOL	CARB	FIBER	SOD
Mini Coconut Loaf	1 (3.5 oz)	350	3	10	5	62	1	350
Mini Pound Cake	1 (3.2 oz)	310	5	11	15	48	1	390
Raspberry Square	1 (1.8 oz)	190	1	8	5	28	0	110
Sweet Roll Apple	1 (2.2 oz)	200	3	6	5	33	0	240
Sweet Roll Cherry	1 (2.2 oz)	210	3	6	10	34	1	180
Sweet Roll Cinnamon	1 (2.2 oz)	230	3	7	10	36	1	200
Texas Cinnamon Bun	1 (4.2 oz)	440	7	15	25	69	1	410
Zingers Devil's Food	2 (2.6 oz)	270	2	8	5	46	1	230
Zingers Lemon	1 (1.4 oz)	150	1	6	5	22	0	90
Zingers Raspberry	1 (1.4 oz)	150	1	6	5	22	0	90
Zingers Yellow	2 (2.5 oz)	280	2	8	5	50	1	160
Drake's								
Coffee Cake Low Fat	1 (1.1 oz)	110	1	2	10	21	0	110
Mini Coffee Cakes	4 (1.83 oz)	220	3	9	18	33	1	140
Yodel's	1 (1 oz)	150	2	9	5	16	—	65
Dutch Mill								
Dessert Shells Chocolate Covered	1 (0.5 oz)	80	1	5	0	8	0	—
Entenmann's								
Apple Puffs	1 (3 oz)	270	2	13	0	37	1	230
Cupcakes Light Chocolate Creme Filled	1 (2 oz)	160	1	0	0	39	1	150
Hot Cross Buns	1 (2.3 oz)	230	4	7	20	37	2	160
Stollen Fruit	⅛ cake (2 oz)	210	3	7	15	34	1	125
Greenfield								
Blondie Fat Free Chocolate Chip	1 (1.3 oz)	110	2	0	0	27	0	60
Hostess								
Angel Food	⅛ cake (2 oz)	160	3	2	0	33	1	180
Chocodiles	1 (1.6 oz)	240	2	11	20	33	1	180
Chocolicious	1 (1.6 oz)	190	1	7	10	30	1	210
Coffee Crumb	1 (1.1 oz)	130	1	5	10	19	0	110
Crumb Cake Light	1 (1 oz)	100	1	2	0	18	0	130
Cupcakes Chocolate	1 (1.8 oz)	180	2	6	5	30	1	290
Cupcakes Orange	1 (1.5 oz)	160	1	5	10	27	0	160
Cupcakes Light Chocolate	1 (1.6 oz)	140	2	2	0	29	1	190

FOOD	PORTION	CAL	PROT	FAT	CHOL	CARB	FIBER	SOD
Ding Dongs	2 (2.7 oz)	360	3	19	15	44	2	240
Ho Ho's	2 (2 oz)	250	2	12	20	34	1	150
Honey Bun Glazed	1 (2.7 oz)	320	4	19	15	34	1	210
Honey Bun Iced	1 (3.4 oz)	410	5	24	10	42	1	270
Shortcake Dessert Cups	1 (1 oz)	100	1	2	15	17	0	120
Sno Balls	1 (1.8 oz)	180	1	5	5	31	1	190
Suzy Q's	1 (2 oz)	230	2	9	10	35	1	270
Sweet Roll Cherry	1 (2.2 oz)	210	3	6	10	34	1	180
Sweet Roll Cinnamon	1 (2.2 oz)	230	3	7	10	36	1	200
Twinkies	1 (1.5 oz)	150	1	5	20	25	0	200
Twinkies Light	1 (1.5 oz)	130	1	2	10	27	0	190
Jell-O								
Dessert Delights Cheesecake	1 bar (1.4 oz)	160	2	7	5	20	tr	100
Dessert Delights Chocolate Fudge Pudding	1 bar (1.4 oz)	150	2	6	0	23	1	80
Kellogg's								
Pop-Tarts Apple Cinnamon	1 (1.8 oz)	210	2	6	0	37	1	180
Pop-Tarts Blueberry	1 (1.8 oz)	210	2	5	0	36	1	190
Pop-Tarts Brown Sugar Cinnamon	1 (1.8 oz)	210	3	6	0	35	1	190
Pop-Tarts Cherry	1 (1.8 oz)	200	2	5	0	37	1	180
Pop-Tarts Chocolate Graham	1 (1.8 oz)	210	3	6	0	35	1	230
Pop-Tarts Frosted Apple Cinnamon	1 (1.8 oz)	190	2	3	0	39	1	230
Pop-Tarts Frosted Blueberry	1 (1.8 oz)	200	2	5	0	37	1	170
Pop-Tarts Frosted Brown Sugar Cinnamon	1 (1.8 oz)	210	3	7	0	34	1	180
Pop-Tarts Frosted Cherry	1 (1.8 oz)	200	2	5	0	38	1	170
Pop-Tarts Frosted Chocolate Vanilla Creme	1 (1.8 oz)	200	3	5	0	37	1	220

FOOD	PORTION	CAL	PROT	FAT	CHOL	CARB	FIBER	SOD
Pop-Tarts Frosted Chocolate Fudge	1 (1.8 oz)	200	3	5	0	37	1	220
Pop-Tarts Frosted Grape	1 (1.8 oz)	200	2	5	0	38	1	170
Pop-Tarts Frosted Raspberry	1 (1.8 oz)	210	2	5	0	37	1	170
Pop-Tarts Frosted S'mores	1 (1.8 oz)	200	3	6	0	36	1	200
Pop-Tarts Frosted Strawberry	1 (1.8 oz)	200	2	5	0	38	1	170
Pop-Tarts Frosted Wild Berry	1 (2 oz)	210	2	5	0	39	1	170
Pop-Tarts Frosted Wild Watermelon	1 (2 oz)	210	2	5	0	39	1	170
Pop-Tarts Low Fat Blueberry	1 (1.8 oz)	190	2	3	0	39	1	230
Pop-Tarts Low Fat Cherry	1 (1.8 oz)	190	2	3	0	39	1	230
Pop-Tarts Low Fat Frosted Chocolate Fudge	1 (1.8 oz)	190	3	3	0	39	2	270
Pop-Tarts Low Fat Frosted Strawberry	1 (1.8 oz)	190	2	3	0	39	1	210
Pop-Tarts Low Fat Strawberry	1 (1.8 oz)	190	2	3	0	39	1	230
Pop-Tarts Strawberry	1 (1.8 oz)	200	2	5	0	37	1	190
Lance								
Dunking Sticks	1 (2.75 oz)	180	2	10	<5	22	tr	130
Fig Cake	½ piece (2.1 oz)	110	1	2	0	21	1	70
Fig Cake Fat Free	½ piece (2.1 oz)	100	1	0	0	22	1	85
Honey Bun	1 (3 oz)	330	4	13	0	47	4	200
Pecan Twirls	1 pkg (2 oz)	220	3	9	5	32	1	140
Swiss Rolls	1 (2.5 oz)	170	1	9	10	23	tr	130
Little Debbie								
Angel Cakes Lemon	1 (1.6 oz)	130	2	1	0	29	0	135
Angel Cakes Raspberry	1 (1.6 oz)	130	2	1	0	29	0	125

FOOD	PORTION	CAL	PROT	FAT	CHOL	CARB	FIBER	SOD
Banana Nut Loaves	1 (1.9 oz)	220	2	10	10	31	tr	220
Banana Twins	1 (2.2 oz)	250	2	10	10	39	0	170
Be My Valentine Chocolate	1 (2.2 oz)	280	2	13	0	38	1	140
Be My Valentine Vanilla	1 (2.2 oz)	290	2	14	0	38	0	125
Blueberry Loaves	1 (2 oz)	220	3	10	0	29	tr	200
Chocolate Chip	1 (2.4 oz)	310	2	15	0	41	tr	210
Christmas Tree Cake	1 pkg (1.5 oz)	190	1	10	0	26	0	100
Coconut Creme	1 (1.7 oz)	210	1	10	0	30	0	140
Coffee Cake Apple	1 (2.1 oz)	230	2	7	10	39	0	190
Cupcake Creme Filled Chocolate	1 (1.6 oz)	180	2	9	5	26	tr	135
Cupcake Creme Filled Orange	1 (1.7 oz)	210	1	10	0	29	0	110
Cupcake Creme Filled Strawberry	1 (1.7 oz)	210	1	10	0	29	tr	100
Devil Cremes	1 (1.6 oz)	190	1	8	0	29	0	170
Devil Squares	1 (2.2 oz)	270	2	13	0	39	1	180
Easter Basket Cake Chocolate	1 (2.4 oz)	300	3	14	0	40	tr	160
Easter Basket Cake Vanilla	1 (2.5 oz)	320	2	10	0	43	0	150
Fall Party Cake Chocolate	1 (2.4 oz)	290	2	14	0	42	tr	170
Fall Party Cake Vanilla	1 (2.5 oz)	310	2	15	0	44	0	170
Fancy Cakes	1 (2.4 oz)	300	1	15	0	42	0	190
Frosted Fudge	1 (1.5 oz)	200	2	10	<5	25	tr	105
Golden Cremes	1 (1.5 oz)	150	1	5	10	26	0	120
Holiday Cake Roll Cherry Creme	1 (2.1 oz)	260	2	12	13	37	tr	170
Holiday Snack Cake Chocolate	1 (2.4 oz)	300	3	14	0	41	1	150
Holiday Snack Cake Vanilla	1 (2.5 oz)	320	2	15	0	41	0	180
Honey Bun	1 (1.8 oz)	220	3	13	<5	24	tr	170
Pecan Spinwheels	1 (1 oz)	110	1	4	0	16	0	80
Snack Cake Chocolate	1 (2.5 oz)	310	2	15	0	44	1	180

FOOD	PORTION	CAL	PROT	FAT	CHOL	CARB	FIBER	SOD
Strawberry Shortcake Roll	1 (2.1 oz)	230	1	8	15	41	0	230
Swiss Rolls	1 (2.1 oz)	270	2	12	15	38	1	140
Zebra Cakes	1 (2.6 oz)	330	2	16	0	45	0	160
Marie Callender's								
Cobbler Apple	1 serv (4.25 oz)	370	2	20	0	45	2	170
Cobbler Berry	1 serv (4.25 oz)	370	3	21	<5	41	1	220
Cobbler Cherry	1 serv (4.25 oz)	380	3	19	5	50	0	240
Cobbler Peach	1 serv (4.25 oz)	380	3	18	0	47	0	240
Natural Touch								
Toaster Square Blueberry	1 (2.8 oz)	180	6	2	0	33	6	65
Toaster Squares Date Walnut	1 (2.8 oz)	200	6	3	0	36	8	50
Nature's Choice								
Toaster Pastries Fat Free Apple Cinnamon	1 (1.9 oz)	180	3	0	0	41	4	180
Toaster Pastries Fat Free Blueberry	1 (1.9 oz)	180	3	0	0	41	4	180
Toaster Pastries Fat Free Raspberry	1 (1.9 oz)	180	3	0	0	41	3	190
Toaster Pastries Fat Free Strawberry	1 (1.9 oz)	180	3	0	0	41	3	190
Toaster Pastries Low Fat Cherry	1 (1.9 oz)	180	3	3	0	36	3	30
Toaster Pastries Low Fat Frosted Blueberry	1 (1.9 oz)	190	3	2	0	42	3	40
Toaster Pastries Low Fat Frosted Chocolate	1 (1.9 oz)	200	3	3	0	42	3	45
Toaster Pastries Low Fat Frosted Cinnamon	1 (1.9 oz)	190	3	2	0	42	3	40
Toaster Pastries Low Fat Frosted Strawberry	1 (1.9 oz)	190	3	2	0	42	3	40

FOOD	PORTION	CAL	PROT	FAT	CHOL	CARB	FIBER	SOD
Toaster Pastries Low Fat Peach Apricot	1 (1.9 oz)	180	3	3	0	36	3	30
Pepperidge Farm								
Apple Turnover	1 (3.1 oz)	330	4	14	0	48	6	180
Blueberry Turnover	1 (3.1 oz)	340	4	16	0	45	6	200
Cherry Turnover	1 (3.1 oz)	320	4	13	0	46	6	190
Large Layer Chocolate Fudge	⅛ cake (2.4 oz)	260	3	11	30	31	1	160
Large Layer Coconut	⅛ cake (2.4 oz)	260	2	11	35	35	0	115
Large Layer Vanilla	⅛ cake (2.4 oz)	250	2	11	25	35	0	120
Mini Turnover Apple	1 (1.4 oz)	140	2	8	0	15	1	80
Mini Turnover Cherry	1 (1.4 oz)	140	2	8	0	16	1	70
Mini Turnover Strawberry	1 (1.4 oz)	140	2	7	0	18	0	100
Peach Turnover	1 (3.1 oz)	340	4	15	0	47	6	180
Raspberry Turnover	1 (3.1 oz)	330	4	14	0	47	6	190
Philadelphia								
Snack Bars Classic Cheesecake	1 (1.5 oz)	200	2	13	35	17	0	85
Pillsbury								
Apple Turnovers	1 (2 oz)	170	2	8	0	23	tr	310
Cherry Turnovers	1 (2 oz)	180	2	8	0	24	0	310
Sara Lee								
Cheesecake 25% Reduced Fat	¼ cake (4.2 oz)	310	9	13	70	40	2	310
Cheesecake Cherry Cream	¼ cake (4.7 oz)	350	6	12	35	55	2	310
Cheesecake Chocolate Chip	¼ cake (4.2 oz)	410	8	21	65	47	2	300
Cheesecake French	⅙ cake (3.9 oz)	350	5	21	20	24	1	280
Cheesecake French Strawberry	⅙ cake (4.3 oz)	320	4	14	20	43	1	230
Cheesecake Strawberry Cream	¼ cake (4.7 oz)	330	6	12	40	49	2	330
Coffee Cake Butter Streusel	⅙ cake (1.9 oz)	220	4	12	35	25	1	240
Coffee Cake Crumb	⅛ cake (2 oz)	220	3	9	15	32	1	210
Coffee Cake Pecan	⅙ cake (1.9 oz)	230	4	12	25	24	1	170

FOOD	PORTION	CAL	PROT	FAT	CHOL	CARB	FIBER	SOD
Coffee Cake Raspberry	1/6 cake (1.9 oz)	220	3	8	15	27	1	220
Coffee Cake Reduced Fat Cheese	1/6 cake (1.9 oz)	180	3	6	20	28	0	230
Layer Cake Coconut	1/8 cake (2.8 oz)	260	2	14	15	33	1	210
Layer Cake Double Chocolate	1/8 cake (2.8 oz)	260	3	13	10	33	2	230
Layer Cake Fudge Golden	1/8 cake (2.8 oz)	260	2	13	15	34	1	200
Layer Cake German Chocolate	1/8 cake (2.9 oz)	280	3	14	15	35	1	250
Layer Cake Vanilla	1/8 cake (2.8 oz)	260	2	14	15	32	0	210
Original Cheesecake	1/4 cake (4.2 oz)	350	7	18	50	39	1	320
Pound Cake All Butter	1/4 cake (2.7 oz)	320	4	16	85	38	1	280
Pound Cake Chocolate Swirl	1/4 cake (2.9 oz)	330	5	16	75	42	tr	350
Pound Cake Family Size	1/6 cake (2.7 oz)	310	4	17	75	36	1	360
Pound Cake Reduced Fat	1/4 cake (2.7 oz)	280	4	11	65	42	tr	350
Pound Cake Strawberry Swirl	1/4 cake (2.9 oz)	290	4	11	60	44	tr	140
Strawberry Shortcake	1/8 cake (2.5 oz)	180	2	7	15	27	1	140
SnackWell's								
Streusal Squares Apple Cinnamon	1 (1.5 oz)	150	1	3	0	31	tr	90
Streusal Squares Cherry	1 (1.5 oz)	150	1	3	0	31	tr	110
Tastykake								
Banana Creamie	1 (1.5 oz)	170	1	7	5	25	0	105
Bear Claw Appled	1 (3 oz)	280	4	7	0	50	0	320
Bear Claw Cinnamon	1 (3 oz)	300	5	8	0	53	tr	310
Big Texas	1 (3 oz)	300	5	9	0	51	tr	360
Breakfast Bun Chocolate Raisin	1 (3.2 oz)	330	5	8	0	59	1	320
Bunny Trail Treats	1 (1.3 oz)	150	1	6	30	25	0	105
Chocolate Creamie	1 (1.5 oz)	180	1	8	15	25	0	120
Chocolate Krimpies	2 (2.2 oz)	240	3	10	45	38	1	250
Coffee Roll Glazed	1 (3 oz)	300	5	9	0	51	tr	360

FOOD	PORTION	CAL	PROT	FAT	CHOL	CARB	FIBER	SOD
Coffee Roll Vanilla	1 (3.2 oz)	320	5	9	0	56	tr	360
Cupcakes	2 (2.1 oz)	200	2	5	10	37	1	240
Cupcakes Butter Cream Cream Filled Iced	2 (2.2 oz)	240	2	8	10	40	1	250
Cupcakes Chocolate Cream Filled Iced	2 (2.2 oz)	230	2	8	10	39	1	240
Cupcakes Low Fat Chocolate Cream Filled	2 (2.2 oz)	200	3	3	0	42	1	250
Cupcakes Low Fat Vanilla Cream Filled	2 (2.2 oz)	190	2	2	0	42	0	210
Cupid Kake	1 (1.3 oz)	150	1	6	30	25	0	105
Honey Bun Glazed	1 (3.2 oz)	350	5	17	10	47	0	210
Honey Bun Iced	1 (3.2 oz)	350	5	17	10	47	0	210
Junior Chocolate	1 (3.3 oz)	330	4	12	80	54	1	180
Junior Coconut	1 (3.3 oz)	310	3	8	75	54	0	180
Junior Koffee Kake	1 (2.5 oz)	270	3	9	45	42	1	200
Junior Pound Kake	1 (3 oz)	320	5	13	100	45	1	320
Kandy Kakes Chocolate	3 (2 oz)	250	2	13	0	35	2	90
Kandy Kakes Coconut	2 (2.7 oz)	330	3	18	5	43	2	105
Kandy Kakes Peanut Butter	2 (1.3 oz)	190	3	9	10	21	1	85
Koffee Kake Cream Filled	2 (2 oz)	240	2	10	30	35	0	130
Koffee Kake Low Fat Apple	2 (2 oz)	170	2	2	0	34	1	170
Koffee Kake Low Fat Lemon	2 (2 oz)	180	2	3	10	36	0	180
Koffee Kake Low Fat Raspberry	2 (2 oz)	170	2	2	0	36	1	180
Kreepy Kakes	2 (2.2 oz)	240	2	8	20	38	0	230
Kreme Krimpies	2 (2 oz)	230	2	9	55	34	0	200
Krimpets Butterscotch Iced	2 (2 oz)	210	2	5	60	38	0	220
Krimpets Jelly Fillled	2 (2 oz)	190	2	3	45	38	1	170

FOOD	PORTION	CAL	PROT	FAT	CHOL	CARB	FIBER	SOD
Krimpets Strawberry	2 (2 oz)	210	2	5	65	37	0	220
Kringle Kake	1 (1.3 oz)	150	1	6	30	25	0	105
Santa Snacks	2 (2.2 oz)	240	2	8	20	38	0	230
Sparkle Kake	1 (1.3 oz)	150	1	6	30	25	0	105
Tasty Tweets	2 (2.2 oz)	240	2	8	20	38	0	230
Tropical Delight Coconut	2 (2 oz)	190	3	9	30	26	0	230
Tropical Delight Guava	2 (2 oz)	190	2	7	15	30	0	200
Tropical Delight Papaya	2 (2 oz)	200	2	7	20	32	0	220
Tropical Delight Pineapple	2 (2 oz)	200	2	7	20	32	0	220
Vanilla Creamie	1 (1.5 oz)	190	1	9	35	25	0	115
Witchy Treat	1 (1.3 oz)	150	1	6	30	24	0	90
Tom's								
Honey Bun	1 pkg (3 oz)	360	4	20	10	41	2	200
Honey Bun Jelly Filled	1 pkg (4 oz)	490	6	29	0	52	2	490
Marble Pound	1 pkg (2.5 oz)	300	4	16	50	35	1	380
Texas Cinnamon Roll	1 pkg (4 oz)	360	7	6	0	71	0	470
Tortuga								
Cayman Island Rum Cake	1 piece (2 oz)	194	2	9	0	27	0	198
Weight Watchers								
Chocolate Raspberry Royale	1 (3.5 oz)	190	4	3	20	38	2	220
Chocolate Eclair	1 (2.1 oz)	150	2	4	30	25	1	170
Danish Coffee Cake Apple Cinnamon	1 piece (1.9 oz)	160	3	3	0	30	1	170
Danish Coffee Cake Cheese	1 piece (1.9 oz)	160	4	3	5	29	1	200
Danish Coffee Cake Raspberry	1 piece (1.9 oz)	160	4	3	0	30	1	170
Double Fudge	1 piece (2.75 oz)	190	4	4	25	36	2	200
French Style Cheesecake	1 piece (3.9 oz)	170	7	4	15	28	2	230
New York Style Cheesecake	1 piece (2.5 oz)	150	6	5	15	21	1	140
Strawberry Parfait Royale	1 (5.24 oz)	180	5	2	10	35	0	100

FOOD	PORTION	CAL	PROT	FAT	CHOL	CARB	FIBER	SOD
Triple Chocolate Eclair	1 (2.14 oz)	160	3	5	30	25	1	190
TAKE-OUT								
angelfood	1/12 cake (1 oz)	73	2	tr	0	16	1	212
apple crisp	½ cup (5 oz)	230	37	5	0	46	–	257
baklava	1 oz	126	2	9	23	10	1	78
basbousa namoura	1 piece (1 oz)	60	2	3	0	–	2	144
boston cream pie	1/6 cake (3.3 oz)	293	4	12	43	43	1	309
carrot w/ cream cheese icing	1/12 cake (3.9 oz)	484	5	29	60	52	–	273
cheesecake w/ cherry topping	1/12 cake (5 oz)	359	6	23	106	33	–	254
chocolate w/ chocolate frosting	1/8 cake (2.2 oz)	235	3	11	–	35	2	213
coffeecake cheese	1/6 cake (2.7 oz)	258	5	12	–	38	1	257
coffeecake crumb topped cheese	1/6 cake (2.7 oz)	258	5	12	–	38	1	257
coffeecake crumb topped cinnamon	1/9 cake (2.2 oz)	263	4	15	20	29	2	221
cream puff w/ custard filling	1 (4.6 oz)	336	9	20	174	30	–	444
eclair w/ chocolate icing & custard filling	1	205	–	10	35	–	–	–
french apple tart	1 (3.5 oz)	302	4	15	60	37	2	326
fruitcake	1/36 cake (2.9 oz)	302	3	10	24	54	3	121
gingerbread	1/9 cake (2.6 oz)	264	3	12	24	36	2	242
panettone	1/12 cake (2.9 oz)	300	6	12	90	43	2	120
petit fours	2 (0.9 oz)	120	1	7	0	15	0	15
pineapple upside down	1/9 cake (4 oz)	367	4	14	25	58	–	367
pound fat free	1 oz	80	2	tr	0	17	–	96
pound cake	1 slice (1 oz)	120	2	5	32	15	–	96
sacher torte	1 slice (2.2 oz)	240	4	11	50	30	4	120
sheet cake w/ white frosting	1/9 cake	445	4	14	70	77	–	275
strudel apple	1 piece (2½ oz)	195	2	8	–	29	2	191
tiramisu	1 piece (5.1 oz)	409	7	30	171	31	tr	79

FOOD	PORTION	CAL	PROT	FAT	CHOL	CARB	FIBER	SOD
trifle w/ cream	6 oz	291	4	16	–	34	1	–
yellow w/ vanilla frosting	⅛ cake (2.2 oz)	239	2	9	–	38	–	220

CAKE ICING
Betty Crocker

FOOD	PORTION	CAL	PROT	FAT	CHOL	CARB	FIBER	SOD
HomeStyle Mix Coconut Pecan as prep	2 tbsp	160	tr	2	0	21	tr	5
HomeStyle Mix White Fluffy as prep	6 tbsp	100	tr	0	0	24	–	60
Party Frosting Chocolate w/ Stars	2 tbsp (1.2 oz)	140	0	5	0	22	–	90
Rich & Creamy Butter Cream	2 tbsp (1.3 oz)	140	0	5	0	23	–	75
Rich & Creamy Cherry	2 tbsp (1.2 oz)	140	0	5	0	23	–	75
Rich & Creamy Chocolate	2 tbsp (1.2 oz)	130	0	5	0	21	–	90
Rich & Creamy Cream Cheese	2 tbsp (1.2 oz)	140	0	5	0	23	–	80
Rich & Creamy Dark Chocolate	2 tbsp (1.3 oz)	130	1	6	0	23	1	90
Rich & Creamy French Vanilla	2 tbsp (1.2 oz)	140	0	5	0	23	–	70
Rich & Creamy Milk Chocolate	2 tbsp (1.3 oz)	130	0	5	0	21	–	90
Rich & Creamy Rainbow Chip	2 tbsp (1.2 oz)	140	0	5	0	23	–	65
Rich & Creamy Vanilla	2 tbsp (1.2 oz)	140	0	5	0	23	–	70
Toppers Milk Chocolate	2 tbsp (1.2 oz)	130	0	5	0	22	–	85
Toppers Vanilla	2 tbsp (1.2 oz)	140	0	5	0	24	–	70

Duncan Hines

FOOD	PORTION	CAL	PROT	FAT	CHOL	CARB	FIBER	SOD
Chocolate Creamy Homestyle	2 tbsp	130	0	5	0	20	2	95
Milk Chocolate Creamy Homestyle	2 tbsp	130	0	5	0	20	1	95

FOOD	PORTION	CAL	PROT	FAT	CHOL	CARB	FIBER	SOD
Vanilla Creamy Homestyle	2 tbsp	140	0	5	0	22	1	60
Estee								
Frosting as prep	⅓ pkg	100	0	0	0	20	0	0
Sweet Rewards								
Ready-To-Spread Reduced Fat Chocolate	2 tbsp (1.2 oz)	120	tr	2	0	24	—	55
Ready-To-Spread Reduced Fat Vanilla	2 tbsp (1.2 oz)	130	0	2	0	27	—	60

CAKE MIX

FOOD	PORTION	CAL	PROT	FAT	CHOL	CARB	FIBER	SOD
angelfood	10 in cake (20.9 oz)	1535	36	2	0	350	9	3036
angelfood	½₂ cake (1.8 oz)	129	3	tr	0	29	1	255
carrot w/o frosting	2 layers (29.6 oz)	2886	43	133	—	395	—	3001
carrot w/o frosting	½₂ cake (2.5 oz)	239	4	11	—	33	—	249
cheesecake no-bake	⅛ cake (3.5 oz)	271	6	13	—	35	2	377
chocolate pudding type w/o frosting	½₂ cake (2.7 oz)	270	4	14	—	34	—	402
chocolate pudding type w/o frosting	2 layers (32.4 oz)	3234	43	172	—	409	—	4815
chocolate w/o frosting	2 layers (26.8 oz)	2393	44	92	425	384	—	4464
chocolate w/o frosting	½₂ cake (2.3 oz)	198	4	8	35	32	—	370
chocolate w/o frosting low sodium	½₀ cake (1.3 oz)	116	1	3	0	23	—	130
coffeecake crumb topped cinnamon	⅛ cake (2 oz)	178	3	5	28	30	2	236
devil's food w/o frosting	½₂ cake (2.3 oz)	198	4	8	35	32	—	370
devil's food w/ chocolate frosting	½₆ cake	235	3	8	37	40	—	181
devil's food w/ chocolate frosting	1 cake 9 in diam	3755	49	136	598	645	—	2900

FOOD	PORTION	CAL	PROT	FAT	CHOL	CARB	FIBER	SOD
fudge w/o frosting	1/12 cake (2.3 oz)	198	4	8	35	32	–	370
german chocolate pudding type w/ coconut nut frosting	1/12 cake (3.9 oz)	404	4	21	53	55	–	369
gingerbread	1/9 cake (2.4 oz)	207	3	7	24	34	2	307
gingerbread	1 cake 8 in sq	1575	18	39	6	291	–	1733
lemon w/o frosting no sugar low sodium	1/10 cake (1.3 oz)	118	1	3	0	23	–	83
marble pudding type w/o frosting	1/12 cake (2.6 oz)	253	3	12	53	35	–	242
marble pudding type w/o frosting	2 layers (30.6 oz)	3021	36	148	638	412	–	2884
white pudding type w/o frosting	2 layers (29 oz)	2915	30	123	–	427	–	3654
white pudding type w/o frosting	1/12 cake (2.4 oz)	244	3	10	–	36	–	305
white w/o frosting	1/12 cake (2.2 oz)	190	3	5	–	34	–	301
white w/o frosting	2 layer cake (26 oz)	2265	30	57	–	410	–	3593
white w/o frosting no sugar low sodium	1/10 cake (1.3 oz)	118	1	3	0	23	–	83
yellow pudding-type w/o frosting	1/12 cake (2.6 oz)	257	3	12	–	35	–	317
yellow pudding-type w/o frosting	2 layers (31 oz)	3084	40	139	–	421	–	3800
yellow w/ chocolate frosting	1/16 cake	235	3	8	36	40	–	157
yellow w/o frosting	1/12 cake (2.2 oz)	202	3	6	37	34	–	299
yellow w/o frosting	2 layers (26.5 oz)	2415	35	71	437	411	–	3580
yellow w/ chocolate frosting	1 cake 9 in diam	3895	40	175	609	620	–	3080
Betty Crocker								
Angel Food Fat Free	1/12 cake	140	3	0	0	32	–	320
Angel Food Fat Free Confetti as prep	1/12 cake	150	3	0	0	34	–	320

FOOD	PORTION	CAL	PROT	FAT	CHOL	CARB	FIBER	SOD
Cheesecake Chocolate Chip as prep	⅛ cake	410	3	28	99	32	1	230
Cheesecake Original as prep	⅛ cake	400	2	27	102	30	–	240
Cheesecake Strawberry Swirl as prep	⅛ cake	380	2	25	96	32	–	220
Pineapple Upside Down as prep	⅙ cake	420	2	14	36	64	–	280
Quick Bread Banana	1/12 cake	170	2	7	36	25	–	190
Quick Bread Cinnamon Streusel as prep	1/14 cake	180	3	7	30	26	–	150
Quick Bread Cranberry Orange as prep	1/12 cake	170	2	6	36	29	–	170
Quick Bread Lemon Poppy Seed as prep	1/12 cake	170	2	7	36	25	–	150
Stir'n Bake Carrot Cake w/ Cream Cheese Frosting as prep	⅙ cake	260	2	7	–	46	–	290
Stir'n Bake Coffee Cake w/ Cinnamon Streusel as prep	⅙ cake	230	2	2	12	36	–	120
Stir'n Bake Yellow w/ Chocolate Frosting as prep	⅙ cake	240	2	7	9	43	1	240
SuperMoist Butter Pecan as prep	1/12 cake	240	1	10	54	35	–	260
SuperMoist Butter Yellow as prep	1/12 cake	260	2	11	75	36	–	270
SuperMoist Carrot as prep	1/10 cake	320	2	15	63	42	–	340

FOOD	PORTION	CAL	PROT	FAT	CHOL	CARB	FIBER	SOD
SuperMoist Cherry Chip	⅒ cake	300	2	13	63	41	–	330
SuperMoist Chocolate Fudge as prep	⅟₁₂ cake	270	2	12	54	35	1	320
SuperMoist Golden Vanilla as prep	⅟₁₂ cake	240	1	10	54	35	–	270
SuperMoist Lemon as prep	⅟₁₂ cake	240	1	10	54	35	–	270
SuperMoist Milk Chocolate as prep	⅟₁₂ cake	240	2	10	54	34	1	290
SuperMoist Pineapple as prep	⅟₁₂ cake	250	1	7	54	25	–	270
SuperMoist Spice as prep	⅟₁₂ cake	240	1	10	54	36	–	270
SuperMoist Strawberry as prep	⅟₁₂ cake	250	1	10	39	35	–	260
SuperMoist White as prep	⅟₁₂ cake	230	2	14	0	34	–	290
SuperMoist White Light as prep	⅒ cake	210	2	3	0	43	–	380
Bisquick								
Mix	⅓ cup (1.4 oz)	160	3	6	0	25	–	400
Reduced Fat	⅓ cup (1.4 oz)	140	3	3	0	27	tr	500
Dromedary								
Date Bread	⅟₁₁ cake (2 oz)	190	2	7	0	29	1	288
Date Nut Roll	½ in slice	80	1	2	–	13	–	160
Gingerbread	1 piece (2 in x 2 in)	100	1	2	–	19	–	190
Pound	½ in slice	150	2	6	–	21	–	160
Duncan Hines								
Angel Food as prep	⅟₁₂ pkg (1.3 oz)	140	4	0	0	31	1	310
Butter Recipe Golden as prep	⅟₁₂ cake	320	3	16	80	42	–	190
Cupcake Yellow as prep	1	180	1	0	6	29	–	140

FOOD	PORTION	CAL	PROT	FAT	CHOL	CARB	FIBER	SOD
Dark Chocolate Fudge as prep	1/12 cake	290	4	15	55	34	–	360
Devil's Food Moist Deluxe as prep	1/12 cake (1.5 oz)	290	4	15	55	34	1	360
French Vanilla	1/12 cake (1.5 oz)	250	3	11	55	–	–	290
Fudge Marble Moist Deluxe as prep	1/12 cake (1.5 oz)	250	3	17	45	36	0	290
Lemon Supreme Moist Deluxe	1/12 cake (1.5 oz)	250	3	17	55	36	0	290
White Moist Deluxe as prep	1/12 cake	190	3	6	0	34	–	300
Yellow Moist Deluxe as prep	1/12 cake (1.5 oz)	250	3	17	55	36	–	270
Yellow Moist Deluxe as prep	1/12 cake	250	3	11	55	36	–	290
Estee								
Chocolate as prep	1/5 cake	190	2	4	0	36	1	240
White as prep	1/5 cake	200	2	4	0	38	tr	170
Hodgson Mill								
Gingerbread Whole Wheat	1/4 cup (1 oz)	110	2	0	0	24	2	260
Jell-O								
No Bake Cherry Cheesecake as prep	1/8 cake (4.8 oz)	340	5	12	5	52	tr	400
No Bake Double Layer Chocolate as prep	1/8 cake (4.4 oz)	260	4	12	<5	34	1	410
No Bake Double Layer Cookies And Creme as prep	1/8 cake (4.5 oz)	390	5	19	<5	51	1	480
No Bake Double Layer Lemon as prep	1/8 cake (4.4 oz)	260	4	12	<5	36	tr	370
No Bake Homestyle Cheesecake as prep	1/6 cake (4.6 oz)	360	7	15	10	50	tr	550
No Bake Peanut Butter Cup as prep	1/8 cake (3.8 oz)	380	5	23	<5	41	1	380

FOOD	PORTION	CAL	PROT	FAT	CHOL	CARB	FIBER	SOD
No Bake Strawberry Cheesecake as prep	⅛ cake (4.8 oz)	340	5	12	5	52	tr	400
Real Cheesecake as prep	⅛ cake (4.6 oz)	360	7	16	5	47	1	510
Sweet Rewards								
Reduced Fat White as prep	½ cake	180	2	3	0	36	—	300
Reduced Fat Yellow as prep	½ cake	200	2	5	30	37	—	280

CALABAZA
fresh	½ cup	32	1	tr	—	8	—	3

CALZONE
TAKE-OUT
cheese	1 (12 oz)	1020	48	54	100	86	8	1760

CANADIAN BACON
grilled	1 pkg (6 oz)	257	34	12	81	2	0	2149
Boar's Head								
Canadian Bacon	2 oz	70	12	3	30	1	0	560
Hormel								
Sandwich Style	3 slices (2 oz)	70	10	3	30	0	0	640
Oscar Mayer								
Canandian Bacon	2 slices (1.6 oz)	50	8	2	25	0	0	620
Yorkshire Farms								
Uncured	3 oz	100	17	4	44	9	—	350

CANADIAN BACON SUBSTITUTES
Yves
Canadian Veggie Bacon	1 serv (2 oz)	80	17	1	0	1	1	480

CANDY (see also CHEWING GUM, MARSHMALLOW)
candied cherries	1 (4 g)	12	0	tr	0	3	—	—
candied citron	1 oz	89	tr	tr	0	23	—	82
candied lemon peel	1 oz	90	tr	tr	0	23	—	14
candied orange peel	1 oz	90	tr	tr	0	23	—	14
candied pineapple slice	1 slice (2 oz)	179	tr	tr	0	45	—	—
dark chocolate	1 oz	150	1	10	0	16	—	5
gumdrops	10 sm (0.4 oz)	135	0	0	0	35	—	15

FOOD	PORTION	CAL	PROT	FAT	CHOL	CARB	FIBER	SOD
gumdrops	10 lg (3.8 oz)	420	0	0	0	108	–	48
jelly beans	10 sm (0.4 oz)	40	0	tr	0	10	–	3
marzipan	1 oz	128	3	7	0	15	2	5
peanuts chocolate covered	1 cup (5.2 oz)	773	19	50	13	74	–	61
peanuts chocolate covered	10 (1.4 oz)	208	5	13	4	20	–	16
pretzels chocolate covered	1 oz	130	2	5	–	20	–	–
pretzels chocolate covered	1 (0.4 oz)	50	1	2	–	8	–	10
sesame crunch	20 pieces (1.2 oz)	181	4	12	0	18	–	–
100 Grand								
Bar	1 bar (1.5 oz)	200	2	8	10	30	tr	75
3 Musketeers								
Bar	2 fun size (1.2 oz)	140	1	4	5	25	0	60
Bar	1 (2.1 oz)	260	2	8	5	46	1	110
5th Avenue								
Snack Size	1 bar (0.58)	80	1	4	0	10	–	25
Almond Joy								
Snack Size	1 (0.68 oz)	90	tr	5	0	11	–	30
Andes								
Chocolate Covered Mint Patties	1 (0.5 oz)	60	0	1	0	13	0	2
Baby Ruth								
Bar	1 bar (2.1 oz)	270	4	13	0	36	2	130
Fun Size	1 bar (1 oz)	130	3	6	0	17	tr	60
Barricini								
Dark Chocolate Raspberry Creme Shells	1 piece (0.3 oz)	47	0	3	0	5	0	4
Bittyfinger								
Bars	2	170	2	7	0	27	tr	85
Body Smarts								
Chocolate Peanut Crunch	2 bars (1.8 oz)	210	5	6	<5	34	2	70
Breath Savers								
Sugar Free Mint Cinnamon	1 piece (2 g)	10	0	0	0	2	–	0

FOOD	PORTION	CAL	PROT	FAT	CHOL	CARB	FIBER	SOD
Sugar Free Peppermint	1 piece (2 g)	10	0	0	0	2	–	0
Sugar Free Spearmint	1 piece (2 g)	10	0	0	–	2	–	0
Sugar Free Wintergreen	1 piece (2 g)	10	0	0	–	2	–	0
Butterfinger								
BB's	1 pkg (1.7 oz)	230	2	9	0	33	1	95
Bar	1 (2.1 oz)	270	3	11	0	42	1	130
Fun Size	1 bar	100	1	4	0	15	0	45
Cape Cod Provisions								
Cranberry Bog Frogs	3 pieces (1.9 oz)	250	3	12	7	34	tr	65
Carmello								
Snack Size	1 (0.66 oz)	90	1	4	<5	12	–	20
Charleston Chew								
Chocolate	½ bar	120	–	3	–	–	–	–
Strawberry	½ bar	120	–	3	–	–	–	–
Vanilla	½ bar	120	–	3	–	–	–	–
Charms								
Blow Pop	1 (0.6 oz)	70	0	0	0	17	–	0
Lollipop Sour	1 (0.6 oz)	70	0	0	0	18	–	0
Lollipop Sweet	1 (0.6 oz)	70	0	0	0	18	–	0
Chunky								
Bar	1 (1.4 oz)	210	3	11	5	24	1	20
Crunch								
Fun Size	4 bars	210	2	11	10	26	tr	60
Del Monte								
Radical Raizins Cinnamon	1 pkg (0.7 oz)	70	0	0	0	18	0	0
Radical Raizins Rainbow	1 pkg (0.7 oz)	70	0	0	0	18	0	0
Dove								
Dark Chocolate	¼ bar (1.5 oz)	230	2	14	5	26	3	0
Dark Chocolate	1 bar (1.3 oz)	200	2	12	5	22	2	0
Dark Chocolate Miniatures	7 (1.5 oz)	220	2	14	5	26	2	0
Milk Chocolate	1 bar (1.3 oz)	200	2	12	5	22	1	25
Milk Chocolate	¼ bar (1.5 oz)	230	3	13	10	25	1	30
Milk Chocolate Miniatures	7 (1.5 oz)	230	3	13	10	25	1	30

FOOD	PORTION	CAL	PROT	FAT	CHOL	CARB	FIBER	SOD
Dream								
Caramel & Nougat In Milk Chocolate	1 bar (1 oz)	90	1	3	<5	21	1	70
Estee								
Caramels Vanilla & Chocolate	5	115	1	5	0	26	0	65
Dark Chocolate	½ bar (1.4 oz)	200	2	14	10	23	0	10
Milk Chocolate	½ bar (1.4 oz)	230	4	17	20	17	0	65
Milk Chocolate w/ Almonds	½ bar (1.4 oz)	230	4	17	20	16	0	65
Milk Chocolate w/ Crisp Rice	½ bar (1.2 oz)	370	7	26	30	29	0	110
Milk Chocolate w/ Fruit & Nuts	½ bar (1.4 oz)	220	4	16	20	18	0	65
Mint Chocolate	½ bar (1.4 oz)	200	2	14	10	23	0	10
Peanut Brittle	⅓ box (1.3 oz)	160	3	9	10	28	1	115
Peanut Butter Cups	5	200	5	12	<5	19	1	70
Sugar Free Assorted Fruit	5	30	0	0	0	16	0	0
Sugar Free Assorted Mint	5	30	0	0	0	16	0	0
Sugar Free Butterscotch	2	25	0	0	0	12	0	50
Sugar Free Fruit Gum Drops	23	80	0	0	0	36	0	0
Sugar Free Gourmet Jelly Beans	26	70	0	0	0	24	0	30
Sugar Free Gummy Apple Rings	5	70	0	0	0	28	0	5
Sugar Free Gummy Bears Assorted Fruit	17	100	3	0	0	30	0	5
Sugar Free Licorice Gum Drops	11	90	1	0	0	36	0	65
Sugar Free Peppermint Swirl	3	30	0	0	0	14	0	0
Sugar Free Sour Citrus Slices	9	60	0	0	0	30	0	50
Sugar Free Toffee	5	30	0	0	0	16	0	0

FOOD	PORTION	CAL	PROT	FAT	CHOL	CARB	FIBER	SOD
Sugar Free Tropical Fruit	5	30	0	0	0	16	0	0
Favorite Brands								
Candy Corn	24 pieces (1.4 oz)	150	0	0	—	37	—	110
Cinnamon Imperials	52 (0.5 oz)	80	0	0	—	14	—	5
Circus Peanuts	5 pieces (1.6 oz)	160	1	0	—	39	—	10
Gummallo Apple Ring	5 pieces (1.4 oz)	120	2	0	—	27	—	0
Gummallo Peach Ring	5 pieces (1.4 oz)	120	2	0	—	27	—	5
Gummi Bears	18 pieces (1.4 oz)	130	2	0	—	30	—	15
Gummi Dinos	7 pieces (1.3 oz)	120	2	0	—	28	—	15
Gummi Worms	4 pieces (1.4 oz)	130	2	0	—	29	—	15
Jelly Beans	13 (1.4 oz)	150	0	0	—	37	—	20
Marshmallow Eggs	3 (1.3 oz)	140	0	0	—	34	—	10
Neon Worms	4 pieces (1.4 oz)	120	2	0	—	28	—	0
Sour Gummi Bears	16 pieces (1.4 oz)	110	2	0	—	26	—	0
Sour Gummi Worms	4 pieces (1.6 oz)	130	2	0	—	29	—	0
Ferrero Rocher								
Candy	2 pieces (0.9 oz)	150	2	10	0	11	0	24
Godiva								
Chocolatier Dark Chocolate w/ Raspberry	1 bar (1.5 oz)	220	2	11	3	28	0	10
Chocolatier Milk Chocolate	1 bar (1.5 ox)	230	3	13	10	26	0	30
Mochaccino Mousse	2 pieces (1.25 oz)	210	2	15	4	17	0	10
Truffles Assorted	2 pieces (1.5 oz)	220	2	13	10	24	0	15
Goetze's								
Cow Tales	1 pkg (1 oz)	110	1	3	tr	20	tr	40
Goldenberg's								
Peanut Chews	3 pieces (1.3 oz)	180	4	9	0	22	1	40
Goo Goo Supreme								
With Pecans	1 pkg (1.5 oz)	188	2	5	0	34	4	51
Goobers								
Peanuts	1 pkg (1.38 oz)	210	4	13	5	20	1	15
Haviland								
Chocolate Covered Thin Mints	6 (1.5 oz)	170	1	5	0	33	1	5

FOOD	PORTION	CAL	PROT	FAT	CHOL	CARB	FIBER	SOD
Hershey								
Amazin'Fruit Gummy Candy	1 snack pkg (0.7 oz)	60	1	0	0	15	—	25
Bar	1 (0.6 oz)	100	2	6	0	9	—	5
Candy-Coated Milk Chocolate Eggs	4 pieces	90	1	5	<5	12	—	10
Cookies 'n' Mint	1 bar (0.6 oz)	90	1	5	<5	11	—	30
Hugs	1 piece	25	0	2	0	3	—	0
Hugs w/ Almonds	1 piece	25	0	2	0	3	—	0
Kisses	1	25	0	2	0	3	—	0
Kisses w/ Almond	1	25	tr	2	0	3	—	0
Milk Chocolate	1 bar (0.6 oz)	90	1	5	<5	10	—	15
Milk Chocolate w/ Almonds	1 bar (0.6 oz)	100	2	6	<5	9	—	15
Miniature Milk Chocolate	1 (0.3 oz)	45	tr	3	0	5	—	5
Nuggets Cookies 'n' Creme	1 (0.35 oz)	50	tr	3	0	5	—	20
Nuggets Cookies 'n' Mint	1 (0.35 oz)	50	tr	3	0	6	—	15
Nuggets Milk Chocolate	1 (0.35 oz)	50	tr	3	0	6	—	10
Nuggets Milk Chocolate w/ Almonds	1 (0.35 oz)	50	tr	3	0	5	—	10
PayDay Snack Size	1 (0.66 oz)	90	2	5	—	11	—	75
Pot Of Gold Solitaires	5 pieces	90	2	6	<5	8	—	10
ReeseSticks Snack Size	2 pieces (1.2 oz)	190	3	11	0	19	1	85
Special Dark Miniature	1 (0.3 oz)	45	0	2	0	5	—	0
Sweet Escapes Chocolate Toffee Crisp	1 bar (0.66 oz)	80	1	4	<5	12	—	40
Sweet Escapes Peanut Butter Crispy	1 bar (0.7 oz)	70	1	3	0	12	—	75

FOOD	PORTION	CAL	PROT	FAT	CHOL	CARB	FIBER	SOD
Sweet Escapes Triple Chocolate Wafer	1 bar (0.7 oz)	80	tr	3	0	14	–	30
Tastetations Butterscotch	3 pieces (0.6 oz)	60	0	2	<5	12	–	85
Tastetations Caramel	3 pieces (0.6 oz)	60	0	2	<5	12	–	85
Tastetations Chocolate	3 pieces (0.6 oz)	60	0	1	<5	12	–	30
Tastetations Chocolate Mint	3 pieces (0.6 oz)	60	0	2	<5	12	–	30
Tastetations Peppermint	3 pieces (0.6 oz)	60	0	0	0	15	–	15
Jolly Rancher								
Lollipops All Flavors	1 (0.6 oz)	60	0	0	0	16	–	10
Joyva								
Halvah	1.5 oz	240	4	16	0	16	2	80
Halvah Chocolate Covered	1 bar (2 oz)	380	5	23	0	20	3	95
Jells Raspberry	3 pieces (1.6 oz)	200	0	3	0	25	tr	15
Junior Mints								
Snack Size	1 pkg (0.7 oz)	75	tr	1	0	16	0	5
Just Born								
Hot Tamales	1 pkg (2.1 oz)	220	0	0	0	55	–	25
Mike and Ike Berry Fruits	1 pkg (2.1 oz)	220	0	0	0	55	–	85
Mike and Ike Cherry & Bubble Gum	1 pkg (2.1 oz)	220	0	0	0	55	–	25
Mike and Ike Chewy Grape	1 pkg (2.1 oz)	220	0	0	0	55	–	25
Mike and Ike Lemon Watermelon	1 pkg (2.1 oz)	220	0	0	0	55	–	25
Mike and Ike Original	1 pkg (1.2 oz)	220	0	0	0	55	–	25
Mike and Ike Strawberry & Banana	1 pkg (2.1 oz)	220	0	0	0	55	–	25
Mike and Ike Tropical Fruits	1 pkg (2.1 oz)	220	0	0	0	55	–	25
Super Hot Tamales	1 pkg (2.1 oz)	220	0	0	0	55	–	25
Teenee Beanee Assorted Fruits	36 pieces (1.4 oz)	150	0	0	0	36	–	15

FOOD	PORTION	CAL	PROT	FAT	CHOL	CARB	FIBER	SOD
Teenee Beanee Berry Berry	36 pieces (1.4 oz)	150	0	0	0	36	—	15
Teenee Beanee Tropical Mix	36 pieces (1.4 oz)	150	0	0	0	36	—	15
Kit Kat								
Bar	1 (0.56 oz)	80	1	4	0	10	—	10
Krackel								
Bar	1 (0.6 oz)	90	1	5	<5	11	—	25
Miniature	1 (0.3 oz)	45	tr	3	0	5	—	10
Lance								
Chocolaty Peanut Bar	1 (2 oz)	290	9	15	0	32	2	90
Cinnamon Chews	1 pkg (1.06 oz)	120	0	1	0	28	0	0
Fruit Chews	1 pkg (1.06 oz)	120	0	1	0	28	0	0
Gum Ball Pops	1 (0.45 oz)	45	0	0	0	12	tr	0
K-Nuts	4 pieces (1.5 oz)	240	4	15	5	23	0	130
Mint Chews	1 pkg (1.06 oz)	120	0	1	0	28	0	0
Peanut Bar	1 (1.75 oz)	270	10	15	0	23	2	80
Pop-A-Lance	1 piece (0.42 oz)	45	0	0	0	11	0	0
Popcorn'n'Carmel	1 bar (0.75 oz)	90	0	0	0	20	0	120
Starlight Mints	3 pieces (1 oz)	60	0	0	0	15	0	0
Strawberry Chews	1 pkg (1.06 oz)	120	0	1	0	28	0	0
Suckers	3 pieces (0.5 oz)	50	0	0	0	13	0	6
Whistle Pop	1 (0.67 oz)	70	0	0	0	19	tr	0
Lifesavers								
Big Tablet Candy Cane	4 pieces (0.5 oz)	60	0	0	0	16	—	0
Cards 'N Candy	4 pieces (0.4 oz)	40	0	0	0	10	—	0
Christmas Tin	4 pieces (0.5 oz)	60	0	0	0	16	—	20
Egg-Sortment	1 roll (0.4 oz)	40	0	0	0	10	—	0
Gummi Bunnies	3 pkg (1.6 oz)	140	3	0	0	34	—	0
Gummi Savers Five Flavor	1 roll (1.5 oz)	130	2	0	0	32	—	0
Gummi Savers Five Flavor	1 pkg (1.8 oz)	160	3	0	0	38	—	0
Gummi Savers Mixed Berry	1 roll (1.5 oz)	130	2	0	0	32	—	0
Gummi Savers Mixed Berry	1 pkg (1.8 oz)	160	3	0	0	38	—	0

FOOD	PORTION	CAL	PROT	FAT	CHOL	CARB	FIBER	SOD
Gummi Savers Tangy Fruits	1 roll (1.5 oz)	130	2	0	0	32	—	0
Gummi Savers Tangy Fruits	1 pkg (1.8 oz)	160	3	0	0	38	—	0
Gummi Savers Variety	2 pkg (1.3 oz)	120	2	0	0	27	—	0
Gummi Savers Wacky Frootz	1 roll (1.5 oz)	130	2	0	0	32	—	0
Gummi Savers Wacky Frootz	1 pkg (1.8 oz)	160	3	0	0	38	—	0
Gummi Shapes Barnum's Animals	1 pkg (0.8 oz)	70	1	0	0	18	—	0
Holes Five Flavor	20 pieces (5 g)	20	0	0	0	5	—	0
Holes Island Fruit	20 pieces (5 g)	20	0	0	0	5	—	0
Holes Sour 'N Sweet	16 pieces (5 g)	20	0	0	0	5	—	0
Holes Sunshine Fruits	20 pieces (0.2 oz)	20	0	0	0	5	—	0
Holes Super Tart	20 pieces (5 g)	20	0	0	0	5	—	0
Holes Wild Fruits	20 pieces (5 g)	20	0	0	<5	5	—	0
Lollipops Candy Cane	1 (0.4 oz)	40	0	0	0	10	—	0
Lollipops Christmas	1 (0.4 oz)	40	0	0	0	10	—	0
Lollipops Easter	1 (0.4 oz)	40	0	0	0	10	—	0
Lollipops Fruit Flavors	1 (0.4 oz)	45	0	0	0	11	0	0
Lollipops Swirled Flavors	1 (0.4 oz)	40	0	0	0	10	—	0
Lollipops Valentine	1 (0.4 oz)	40	0	0	0	10	—	0
Roll Butter Rum	2 pieces (5 g)	20	0	0	0	5	—	20
Roll Candy Cane	4 pieces (0.4 oz)	40	0	0	0	10	—	0
Roll Cryst-O-Mint	2 pieces (5 g)	20	0	0	0	5	—	0
Roll Five Flavor	2 pieces (5 g)	20	0	0	0	5	—	0
Roll Fruits On Fire	2 pieces (5 g)	20	0	0	0	5	—	0
Roll Pep-O-Mint	3 pieces (5 g)	20	0	0	0	5	—	0
Roll Spear-O-Mint	3 pieces (5 g)	20	0	0	0	5	—	0
Roll Sunshine Fruits	2 pieces (5 g)	20	0	0	0	5	—	0
Roll Tangy Fruit Swirl	2 pieces (5 g)	20	0	0	0	5	—	0

FOOD	PORTION	CAL	PROT	FAT	CHOL	CARB	FIBER	SOD
Roll Tangy Fruit Watermelon	1 piece (5 g)	20	0	0	0	5	—	0
Roll Tangy Fruits	2 pieces (5 g)	20	0	0	0	5	—	0
Roll Tropical Fruits	2 pieces (5 g)	20	0	0	0	5	—	0
Roll Wild Cherry	1 piece (5 g)	20	0	0	0	5	—	0
Roll Wild Flavors	2 pieces (5 g)	20	0	0	0	5	—	0
Roll Wild Sour Berries	2 pieces (5 g)	20	0	0	0	5	—	0
Roll Wint-O-Green	3 pieces (5 g)	20	0	0	0	5	—	0
Sack'it Butter Rum	4 pieces (0.5 oz)	60	0	0	0	15	—	65
Sack'it Five Flavor	4 pieces (0.5 oz)	60	0	0	0	16	—	0
Sack'it Holiday Tin	4 pieces (0.5 oz)	60	0	0	0	16	—	65
Sack'it Pep-O-Mint	4 pieces (0.5 oz)	60	0	0	0	16	—	0
Sack'it Tangy Fruits	4 pieces (0.5 oz)	60	0	0	0	16	—	0
Sack'it Wild Cherry	4 pieces (0.5 oz)	60	0	0	0	16	—	0
Sack'it Wint-O-Green	4 pieces (0.5 oz)	60	0	0	0	16	—	0
Sugar Free Iced Mint	1 piece (2 g)	10	0	0	0	2	—	0
Sugar Free Vanilla Mint	1 piece (2 g)	10	0	0	0	2	—	0
Valentine Book	2 pieces (5 g)	20	0	0	0	5	—	20
Lindt								
Truffles Milk Chocolate	3 pieces (1.3 oz)	210	2	17	5	15	tr	20
M&M's								
Almond	1.5 oz	220	4	12	5	24	2	20
Almond	1 pkg (1.3 oz)	200	3	11	5	21	2	20
Mint	1 pkg (1.7 oz)	230	2	10	10	34	1	35
Mint	1.5 oz	200	2	9	5	30	1	30
Peanut	½ bag king size (1.6 oz)	240	4	12	5	28	2	25
Peanut	1 fun size (0.7 oz)	110	2	5	5	13	1	10
Peanut	1 pkg (1.7 oz)	250	5	13	5	30	2	25
Peanut	1.5 oz	220	4	11	5	25	2	20
Peanut Butter	1 fun size (0.7 oz)	110	2	6	0	12	1	45
Peanut Butter	1.5 oz	220	4	12	5	25	2	90
Peanut Butter	1 pkg (1.6 oz)	240	5	13	5	27	2	100
Plain	1 pkg fun size	100	1	4	5	15	0	15
Plain	½ pkg king size (1.6 oz)	220	2	9	5	32	1	30

FOOD	PORTION	CAL	PROT	FAT	CHOL	CARB	FIBER	SOD
Plain	1.5 oz	200	2	9	5	30	1	30
Plain	1 pkg (1.7 oz)	230	2	10	6	34	1	35
Mars								
Almond Bar	2 fun size (1.3 oz)	190	3	10	5	23	1	55
Almond Bar	1 bar (1.8 oz)	240	3	13	5	31	1	70
Milk Duds								
Snack Size	4 boxes (1.3 oz)	160	1	6	0	26	0	70
Milky Way								
Bar	2 fun size (1.4 oz)	180	2	7	5	28	0	60
Bar	⅓ king size	160	1	6	5	24	0	50
Bar	1 (2.1 oz)	280	2	11	5	43	1	90
Dark	1 fun size (0.7 oz)	90	1	3	0	14	0	35
Dark	1 bar (1.8 oz)	220	1	8	5	36	1	85
Miniature	5 (1.5 oz)	190	2	7	5	30	0	65
Mounds								
Bar	1 (0.68 oz)	90	tr	5	0	11	–	30
Mr. Goodbar								
Miniature	1 (0.3 oz)	45	tr	3	0	4	–	0
Necco								
Bridge Mix	¼ cup (1.5 oz)	180	2	9	5	27	tr	35
Chocolate Covered Raisins	30 pieces (1.5 oz)	170	1	7	0	30	1	35
Malted Milk Balls	11 pieces (1.5 oz)	180	1	6	0	28	tr	35
Mint	1 piece	12	–	tr	0	–	–	–
SkyBar	1 bar (1.5 oz)	190	2	9	5	28	0	45
Nestle								
Buncha Crunch	1 pkg (1.4 oz)	90	2	10	10	26	tr	60
Crunch	1 bar (1.55 oz)	230	2	12	10	29	tr	65
Crunch Disk	1 (1.2 oz)	180	2	9	5	22	tr	50
Crunchkins	5 pieces	190	2	10	5	24	tr	45
Jingles Milk Chocolate Butterfinger	5 pieces	180	2	8	<5	26	tr	55
Jingles Milk Chocolate Crunch	7 pieces	220	2	11	10	28	tr	65
Jingles White Crunch	7 pieces	230	3	14	10	24	0	80
Milk Chocolate	1 bar (1.45 oz)	220	2	13	10	26	tr	25
Nesteggs Milk Chocolate Butterfinger	5 pieces	210	3	10	5	28	tr	55

FOOD	PORTION	CAL	PROT	FAT	CHOL	CARB	FIBER	SOD
Nesteggs Milk Chocolate Crunch	5 pieces	190	2	10	5	24	tr	45
Nesteggs White Crunch	7 pieces	230	3	14	10	24	0	75
Pearson's Egg Nog	2 pieces	60	0	2	0	11	0	40
Treasures Butterfinger	3 pieces	180	2	9	5	24	tr	40
Treasures Crunch	4 pieces (1.4 oz)	210	2	11	10	26	tr	60
Treasures Peanut Butter	4 pieces	250	4	17	5	23	1	90
Turtles	2 pieces (1.2 oz)	160	2	9	<5	20	tr	40
Turtles Bite Size	1 piece (0.4 oz)	50	1	2	1	6	tr	11
White Crunch	1 bar (1.4 oz)	220	3	13	10	23	0	70
Newman's Own								
Organic Peanut Butter Cups Dark Chocolate	3 pieces (1.2 oz)	180	3	12	0	18	tr	55
Organic Peanut Butter Cups Milk Chocolate	3 pieces (1.2 oz)	180	4	12	0	18	tr	70
Organic Peppermint Cups	3 pieces (1.2 oz)	180	2	12	0	20	tr	15
Organics Espresso Sweet Dark Chocolate	1 bar (1.2 oz)	190	2	12	0	19	0	10
Nibs								
Cherry	1 pkg (0.49 oz)	45	0	0	0	11	—	30
Licorice	1 pkg (0.49 oz)	40	0	0	0	10	—	75
Nips								
Butter Rum	2 pieces	60	0	2	0	11	0	40
Caramel	2 pieces	60	0	2	0	11	0	40
Chocolate	2 pieces	60	0	2	0	11	0	40
Chocolate Parfait	2 pieces	60	0	2	0	10	0	30
Coffee	2 pieces	50	0	2	0	10	0	40
Vanilla Almond Cafe	2 pieces	50	0	1	0	10	0	40
Oh Henry!								
Bar	1 (1.8 oz)	120	2	5	<5	16	0	60
Palmer								
Milk Chocolate Lollipop	1 (0.9 oz)	130	1	7	4	16	2	35

FOOD	PORTION	CAL	PROT	FAT	CHOL	CARB	FIBER	SOD
Pearson's								
Irish Cream Parfait	2 pieces	60	0	2	0	10	0	30
Mint Patties	5 (1.3 oz)	150	tr	3	0	31	tr	70
Pez								
Candy	1 roll (0.3 oz)	35	0	0	0	9	–	0
Candy Sugar Free	1 roll (0.3 oz)	30	0	0	0	8	–	0
Planters								
Original Peanut Bar	1 pkg (1.6 oz)	230	6	14	0	22	2	70
Raisinets								
Candy	1 pkg (1.58 oz)	200	2	8	<5	31	1	15
Fun Size	3 pkg (1.7 oz)	200	2	8	5	43	2	15
Reese's								
Eggs	1 (0.6 oz)	90	2	5	0	9	–	65
FastBreak	1 bar (2 oz)	270	5	13	<5	34	2	180
Nutrageous	1 (0.6 oz)	90	2	5	0	9	–	25
Peanut Butter Cups	1 (0.28 oz)	40	tr	3	0	4	–	25
Pieces	25 (0.7 oz)	100	3	4	0	12	–	30
ReeseSticks	2 pieces (1.2 oz)	190	3	11	0	19	1	85
Peanut Butter								
Rokeach								
Cotton Candy	2 cups (1 oz)	110	0	0	0	28	0	0
Rolo								
Caramels In Milk Chocolate	3 pieces (0.64 oz)	90	tr	4	<5	12	–	40
Russell Stover								
Assorted Creams	3 pieces (1.4 oz)	180	1	7	<5	29	0	50
Peanut Butter & Grape Jelly	1 piece (0.8 oz)	100	2	6	<5	10	tr	30
Peanut Butter & Red Raspberry Cups	2 (1.2 oz)	140	3	9	<5	14	tr	40
Pecan Delights	1 pkg (1.8 oz)	250	3	17	10	22	2	60
Pecan Roll	1 (1.75 oz)	260	3	18	<5	23	2	80
S'mores	3 (1.4 oz)	210	2	12	<5	22	tr	80
Sugar Free Peanut Butter Cups	4 pieces (1.3 oz)	200	5	13	0	17	2	140
Sugar Free Pecans & Caramel	2 pieces (1.2 oz)	170	2	12	0	17	0	30
Simply Lite								
Sugar Free Li'l Bits Chocolately	36 pieces (1.4 oz)	130	3	5	0	28	1	55

FOOD	PORTION	CAL	PROT	FAT	CHOL	CARB	FIBER	SOD
Sugar Free Li'l Bits Peanut Buttery	36 pieces (1.4 oz)	140	4	5	0	26	1	50
Sugar Free Patteez	5 pieces (1.3 oz)	110	1	3	0	29	1	10
Skittles								
Original	2 pkg fun size (1.6 oz)	180	0	2	0	41	0	5
Original	1 pkg (2.8 oz)	250	0	3	0	55	0	10
Original	½ king size (1.3 oz)	150	0	2	0	34	0	5
Original	1.5 oz	170	0	2	0	38	0	5
Tropical	1 bag (2.2 oz)	250	0	3	0	56	0	10
Tropical	1.5 oz	170	0	2	0	38	0	5
Tropical	2 bags fun size (1.4 oz)	160	0	2	0	36	0	5
Wild Berry	2 bags fun size (1.4 oz)	160	0	2	0	36	0	5
Wild Berry	1.5 oz	170	0	2	0	38	0	5
Wild Berry	1 bag (2.2 oz)	250	0	3	0	56	0	10
Smucker's								
Fruit Fillers Strawberry	1 pkg (0.9 oz)	80	1	0	0	19	–	25
Jelly Beans	1 pkg (0.7 oz)	70	0	0	0	18	0	10
Snickers								
Bar	2 bars fun size (1.4 oz)	190	3	9	5	24	1	100
Bar	1 bar (2.1 oz)	280	4	14	10	36	1	150
Bar	⅓ king size (1.2 oz)	170	3	8	5	21	1	85
Cruncher	3 fun size (1.4 oz)	230	4	13	5	25	1	140
Miniatures	4 (1.3 oz)	170	3	8	5	22	1	90
Munch Bar	1 (1.4 oz)	230	6	15	10	17	2	150
Peanut Butter	1 bar (2 oz)	310	6	20	5	28	1	150
Sno Caps								
Candies	1 pkg (2.3 oz)	300	2	13	0	48	3	0
Starburst								
California Fruits	8 pieces (1.4 oz)	160	0	3	0	33	0	20
California Fruits	1 stick (2.1 oz)	240	0	5	2	48	0	35
Original Fruits	⅓ king size (1.2 oz)	140	0	3	0	28	0	20
Original Fruits	1 stick (2.1 oz)	240	0	5	0	48	0	35
Original Fruits	8 pieces (1.4 oz)	160	0	3	0	33	0	20
Strawberry Fruits	8 pieces (1.4 oz)	160	0	3	0	33	0	20
Strawberry Fruits	1 stick (2.1 oz)	240	0	5	0	48	0	35

FOOD	PORTION	CAL	PROT	FAT	CHOL	CARB	FIBER	SOD
Tropical Fruits	1 stick (2.1 oz)	240	0	5	0	48	0	35
Tropical Fruits	8 pieces (1.4 oz)	160	0	3	0	33	0	20
Steel's								
Salt Water Taffy Assorted	3 pieces (1 oz)	90	0	1	0	22	0	50
Sugar Babies								
Tidbits	1 pkg	180	–	2	–	–	–	–
Swedish Fish								
Original	19 pieces (1.4 oz)	160	0	0	0	39	0	25
Sweet'N Low								
Sugar Free Butter Toffee	4 pieces (0.5 oz)	30	0	1	<5	15	–	80
Sugar Free Butterscotch	1 piece	7	0	0	0	4	–	0
Sugar Free Cinnamon	1 piece	7	0	0	0	4	–	0
Sugar Free Fancy Fruit	1 piece	7	0	0	0	4	–	0
Sugar Free Fruit Flavors	1 piece	7	0	0	0	4	–	0
Sugar Free Hard Candy Coffee	4 pieces (0.5 oz)	30	0	0	0	14	–	20
Sugar Free Peppermint	1 piece	7	0	0	0	4	–	0
Sugar Free Soft Candy Fruitie Flavors	1 piece	11	tr	tr	–	4	–	0
Sugar Free Soft Candy Tropical Flavors	1 piece	11	tr	tr	–	4	–	0
Sugar Free Watermelon	1 piece	7	0	0	0	4	–	0
Sugar Free Wild Cherry	1 piece	7	0	0	0	4	–	0
Symphony								
Bar	1 (0.6 oz)	100	1	6	<5	10	–	15
W/ Almonds & Chocolate Chips	1 bar (0.6 oz)	90	1	6	<5	9	–	25
Tobler								
Orange Dark Chocolate	5 pieces (1.5 oz)	240	2	13	<5	28	3	10

FOOD	PORTION	CAL	PROT	FAT	CHOL	CARB	FIBER	SOD
Tom's								
Cherry Sours	1 pkg (2.25 oz)	210	0	0	0	53	0	30
Jelly Beans	1 pkg (2.25 oz)	230	0	0	0	58	0	30
Twix								
Caramel	1 pkg (2 oz)	280	3	14	5	37	0	115
Caramel	1 fun size (0.5 oz)	80	1	4	0	10	0	30
Caramel	1 (1 oz)	140	1	7	0	19	0	60
Caramel	1 king size (0.8 oz)	120	1	6	0	15	1	45
Peanut Butter	1 (0.9 oz)	130	3	8	0	13	1	70
Twizzlers								
Cherry	1 piece	35	0	0	0	9	—	35
Chocolate	1 piece	30	0	0	0	7	—	35
Licorice	1 piece	35	0	0	0	9	—	60
Pull'n'Peel Cherry	1 piece (1 oz)	90	1	0	0	19	—	70
Strawberry	1 piece	35	0	0	0	9	—	30
Very Special								
Chocolate Bottles Liquor Filled	3 pieces (1 oz)	150	1	6	0	24	2	10
Whatchamacallit								
Bar	1 (0.58 oz)	80	1	4	0	10	—	35
York								
Chocolate Covered Peppermint Bites	15 pieces (1 oz)	150	1	3	0	31	tr	20
Peppermint Patty	1 (0.49 oz)	50	0	1	0	11	—	0
CANTALOUPE								
dried	3.5 pieces (1.4 oz)	140	0	0	0	34	1	110
fresh cubed	1 cup	57	1	tr	0	13	1	14
fresh half	½	94	2	1	0	22	2	23
Chiquita								
Wedge	¼ med (4.7 oz)	50	0	0	0	12	1	25
CARAWAY								
seed	1 tsp	7	tr	tr	0	1	—	tr
CARDAMOM								
ground	1 tsp	6	tr	tr	0	1	—	tr
CARDOON								
fresh cooked	3½ oz	22	1	tr	0	5	—	176
raw shredded	½ cup	36	1	tr	0	4	—	151

FOOD	PORTION	CAL	PROT	FAT	CHOL	CARB	FIBER	SOD
CARIBOU								
roasted	3 oz	142	25	4	93	0	—	51
CARISSA								
fresh	1	12	tr	tr	0	3	—	1
CAROB								
carob mix	3 tsp	45	tr	0	0	11	—	12
carob mix as prep w/ whole milk	9 oz	195	8	8	33	23	—	132
flour	1 tbsp	14	tr	tr	0	7	—	3
flour	1 cup	185	5	1	0	92	—	36
CARP								
fresh	3 oz	108	15	5	56	0	—	42
fresh cooked	3 oz	138	19	6	72	0	—	54
fresh cooked	1 fillet (6 oz)	276	39	12	143	0	—	107
roe raw	1 oz	37	7	tr	103	tr	—	—
roe salted in olive oil	2 tbsp (1 oz)	40	—	—	100	6	0	1400
CARROT JUICE								
canned	6 oz	73	2	tr	0	17	—	54
CARROTS								
CANNED								
slices	½ cup	17	tr	tr	0	4	1	176
slices low sodium	½ cup	17	tr	tr	0	4	1	31
Del Monte								
Sliced	½ cup (4.3 oz)	35	0	0	0	8	3	300
Green Giant								
Sliced	½ cup (4.2 oz)	25	tr	0	0	6	2	380
LeSueur								
Baby Whole	½ cup (4.2 oz)	35	tr	0	0	8	3	410
S&W								
Julienne	½ cup (4.3 oz)	30	1	0	0	5	2	390
Sliced	½ cup (4.3 oz)	30	1	0	0	5	2	390
Whole Small	½ cup (4.3 oz)	30	1	0	0	5	2	390
FRESH								
baby raw	1 (½ oz)	6	tr	tr	0	1	—	5
raw	1 (2.5 oz)	31	1	tr	0	7	2	25
raw shredded	½ cup	24	1	tr	0	6	2	19
slices cooked	½ cup	35	1	tr	0	8	—	52

FOOD	PORTION	CAL	PROT	FAT	CHOL	CARB	FIBER	SOD
Dole								
Shredded	1 cup (3 oz)	40	1	0	0	9	2	45
FROZEN								
slices cooked	½ cup	26	1	tr	0	6	—	43
Birds Eye								
Baby Whole	½ cup	40	—	0	0	—	2	45
Sliced	½ cup	35	—	0	0	—	3	45
Green Giant								
Harvest Fresh Baby	⅔ cup (3 oz)	20	0	0	0	5	2	70
Select Baby Cut	¾ cup (2.8 oz)	30	tr	0	0	7	3	40
CASABA								
cubed	1 cup	45	2	tr	0	11	—	20
fresh	¹⁄₁₀	43	1	tr	0	10	—	20
CASHEWS								
cashew butter w/o salt	1 tbsp	94	3	8	0	4	—	2
dry roasted salted	1 oz	163	4	13	0	9	—	213
dry roasted w/ salt	18 nuts (1 oz)	160	4	13	0	9	1	180
oil roasted	1 oz	163	5	14	0	8	—	5
oil roasted salted	1 oz	163	5	14	0	8	—	209
Frito Lay								
Salted	1 oz	180	5	15	0	7	1	190
Lance								
Cashews	1 pkg (1⅛ oz)	200	6	16	0	8	3	90
Planters								
Fancy Oil Roasted	1 oz	170	5	14	0	8	1	120
Fancy Oil Roasted	1 pkg (2 oz)	340	9	29	0	16	3	240
Halves Lightly Salted Oil Roasted	1 oz	160	4	13	0	9	2	55
Honey Roasted	1 oz	150	4	12	0	11	1	120
Honey Roasted	1 pkg (2 oz)	310	9	24	0	23	3	240
Munch'N Go Honey Roasted	1 pkg (2 oz)	310	9	24	0	23	3	240
Munch'N Go Singles Oil Roasted	1 pkg (2 oz)	330	10	28	0	16	3	240
Oil Roasted	1 pkg (1 oz)	160	5	14	0	8	1	120
Oil Roasted	1 pkg (1.5 oz)	250	7	21	0	12	2	240
CASSAVA								
raw	3½ oz	120	3	tr	0	27	—	8

FOOD	PORTION	CAL	PROT	FAT	CHOL	CARB	FIBER	SOD
CATFISH								
channel breaded & fried	3 oz	194	15	11	69	7	–	238
channel raw	3 oz	99	15	4	49	0	–	54
CATSUP *(see KETCHUP)*								
CAULIFLOWER								
FRESH								
cooked	½ cup (2.2 oz)	14	1	tr	0	3	1	9
flowerets cooked	3 (2 oz)	12	1	tr	0	2	1	8
flowerets raw	3 (2 oz)	14	1	tr	0	3	1	17
green cooked	1½ cup (3.2 oz)	29	3	tr	0	6	3	21
green raw	1 head 7 in diam	158	15	2	0	31	16	118
green raw	1 cup (2.2 oz)	20	2	tr	0	4	2	15
green raw floweret	1 (0.9 oz)	8	1	tr	0	2	1	6
raw	½ cup (1.8 oz)	13	1	tr	0	3	1	15
FROZEN								
cooked	½ cup	17	1	tr	0	3	–	16
Birds Eye								
Frzn	½ cup	20	–	0	0	–	2	15
Green Giant								
Cheese Sauce	½ cup (3.5 oz)	60	2	3	<5	8	2	510
Florets	1 cup (2.8 oz)	25	2	0	0	4	2	25
CAVIAR								
black	1 oz	71	7	5	165	1	–	420
black	1 tbsp	40	4	3	94	1	–	240
red	1 tbsp	40	4	3	94	1	–	240
red	1 oz	71	7	5	165	1	–	420
CELERIAC								
fresh cooked	3½ oz	25	1	tr	0	6	–	61
raw	½ cup	31	1	tr	0	7	–	78
CELERY								
diced cooked	½ cup	13	1	tr	0	3	–	68
fresh	1 stalk (1.3 oz)	6	tr	tr	0	1	1	35
raw diced	½ cup	10	tr	tr	0	2	1	52
seed	1 tsp	8	tr	tr	0	1	–	3
CELTUCE								
raw	3½ oz	22	1	tr	0	4	–	11

FOOD	PORTION	CAL	PROT	FAT	CHOL	CARB	FIBER	SOD
CEREAL								
bran flakes	¾ cup (1 oz)	90	4	1	0	22	–	264
corn flakes	1¼ cup (1 oz)	110	2	tr	0	24	–	351
corn flakes low sodium	1 cup (0.9 oz)	100	2	tr	0	22	tr	3
corn grits white regular or quick as prep	¾ cup (6.4 oz)	109	3	tr	0	24	tr	0
corn grits yellow regular & quick not prep	1 cup (5.5 oz)	579	14	2	0	124	3	2
crispy rice	1 cup (1 oz)	111	2	tr	0	25	tr	206
crispy rice low sodium	1 cup (0.9 oz)	105	1	tr	0	23	tr	3
farina as prep w/ water	¾ cup (6.1 oz)	88	2	tr	0	19	2	0
farina not prep	1 tbsp (0.4 oz)	40	1	tr	0	9	tr	0
granola	½ cup (2.1 oz)	285	9	15	0	32	6	15
oatmeal instant w/ cinnamon & spice as prep w/ water	1 pkg (5.6 oz)	177	5	2	0	35	3	280
oatmeal instant w/ raisins & spice as prep w/ water	1 cup (5.5 oz)	161	4	2	0	32	2	226
oatmeal instant w/ bran & raisins as prep w/ water	1 pkg (6.8 oz)	158	5	2	0	30	6	248
oatmeal istant as prep w/ water	1 cup (8.2 oz)	138	6	2	0	24	4	377
oatmeal regular & quick as prep w/ water	¾ cup (6.1 oz)	149	5	2	0	19	3	2
oatmeal regular & quick not prep	⅓ cup (0.9 oz)	104	4	2	0	18	3	1
oatmeal instant cooked w/o salt	1 cup	145	6	2	0	25	–	2
oatmeal quick cooked w/o salt	1 cup	145	6	2	0	25	–	2

FOOD	PORTION	CAL	PROT	FAT	CHOL	CARB	FIBER	SOD
oatmeal regular cooked w/o salt	1 cup	145	6	2	0	25	–	2
puffed rice	1 cup (0.5 oz)	56	1	tr	0	13	tr	0
puffed wheat	1 cup (0.4 oz)	44	2	tr	0	10	1	0
shredded mini wheats	1 cup (1.1 oz)	107	3	1	0	24	3	3
shredded wheat rectangular	1 biscuit (0.8 oz)	85	3	tr	0	19	2	0
shredded wheat round	2 biscuits (1.3 oz)	136	4	1	0	31	4	1
sugar-coated corn flakes	¾ cup (1 oz)	110	1	1	0	26	–	230
whole wheat hot natural as prep w/ water	¾ cup (6.4 oz)	113	4	1	0	25	3	0
Albers								
Hominy Quick Grits uncooked	¼ cup	140	3	1	0	31	1	0
Alpen								
Corn Flakes	1 serv (1 oz)	110	2	tr	–	25	tr	2
No Salt No Sugar	1 serv (2 oz)	200	7	3	–	34	6	35
Regular	1 serv (2 oz)	200	7	3	–	37	4	100
Barbara's Bakery								
Apple Cinnamon O's	¾ cup	110	3	1	0	24	2	90
Bite Size Shredded Oats	1¼ cups (2 oz)	220	6	3	0	46	6	260
Cinnamon Puffins	1¼ cup (2 oz)	100	2	1	0	26	6	150
Cocoa Crunch Stars	1 cup (1 oz)	110	2	1	0	26	1	140
Frosted Corn Flakes	1 cup (1 oz)	110	2	1	0	27	4	100
Fruit Juice Sweetened Breakfast O's	1 cup (1 oz)	120	5	2	0	22	3	115
Fruit Juice Sweetened Brown Rice Crisps	1 cup (1 oz)	120	2	1	0	25	1	125
Fruit Juice Sweetened Corn Flakes	1 cup (1 oz)	110	2	0	0	26	2	130

FOOD	PORTION	CAL	PROT	FAT	CHOL	CARB	FIBER	SOD
GrainShop	⅔ cup (1 oz)	90	3	1	0	24	8	110
Honey Crunch Stars	1 cup (1 oz)	110	2	0	0	26	2	50
Honey Nut Toasted O's	¾ cup	120	3	2	0	23	2	90
Organic Fruity Punch	1 cup (1 oz)	110	2	1	0	26	0	120
Organic Soy Essence	¾ cup (1 oz)	100	3	1	0	25	5	110
Puffins	¾ cup (0.9 oz)	90	2	1	0	23	5	190
Shredded Spoonfuls	¾ cup (1.1 oz)	110	5	2	0	23	4	200
Shredded Wheat	2 biscuits (1.4 oz)	140	4	1	0	31	5	0
General Mills								
Basic 4	1 cup (1.9 oz)	200	4	2	0	42	3	320
Boo Berry	1 cup (1 oz)	120	1	1	0	27	—	210
Cheerios	1 cup (1 oz)	110	3	2	0	22	3	280
Cheerios Apple Cinnamon	¾ cup (1 oz)	120	2	2	0	25	1	120
Cheerios Frosted	1 cup (1 oz)	120	2	1	0	25	1	210
Cheerios Honey Nut	1 cup (1 oz)	120	3	2	0	24	2	270
Cheerios Multi Grain	1 cup (1 oz)	110	3	1	0	24	3	200
Cheerios Team	1 cup (1 oz)	120	2	1	0	25	1	210
Chex Corn	1 cup (1 oz)	110	2	0	0	26	0	280
Chex Honey Nut	¾ cup	120	1	1	0	26	—	220
Chex Morning Mix Cinnamon	1 pkg (1.1 oz)	130	2	4	0	24	1	180
Chex Morning Mix Fruit & Nut	1 pkg (1.1 oz)	180	2	4	0	24	1	190
Chex Morning Mix Honey Nut	1 pkg (1.1 oz)	130	2	4	0	24	1	190
Chex Multi-Bran	1 cup (2 oz)	200	4	2	0	49	8	380
Chex Rice	1¼ cup (1.1 oz)	120	2	0	0	27	0	290
Cinnamon Grahams	¾ cup (1 oz)	120	1	1	0	26	1	240
Cinnamon Toast Crunch	¾ cup (1 oz)	130	1	4	1	24	1	210
Cocoa Puffs	1 cup (1 oz)	120	1	1	0	26	—	170
Cookie Crisp	1 cup (1 oz)	120	1	1	0	26	0	180
Count Chocula	1 cup (1 oz)	120	1	1	0	26	0	180
Country Corn Flakes	1 cup (1 oz)	120	2	0	0	26	—	270
Fiber One	½ cup (1 oz)	60	2	1	0	24	14	130
Franken Berry	1 cup (1 oz)	120	1	1	0	27	—	210
French Toast Crunch	¾ cup (1 oz)	120	1	1	0	26	0	180

FOOD	PORTION	CAL	PROT	FAT	CHOL	CARB	FIBER	SOD
Gold Medal Raisin Bran	1⅓ cups (1.9 oz)	170	5	2	0	41	6	330
Golden Grahams	¾ cup (1 oz)	120	1	1	0	25	1	270
Harmony	1¼ cups (1.9 oz)	200	5	4	0	44	2	350
Honey Nut Clusters	1 cup (1.9 oz)	210	4	3	0	46	3	270
Kaboom	1¼ cup (1 oz)	120	2	1	0	24	1	290
Kix	1⅓ cup (1 oz)	120	2	1	0	26	1	270
Kix Berry Berry	¾ cup (1 oz)	120	1	2	0	26	0	180
Lucky Charms	1 cup (1 oz)	120	2	1	0	25	1	210
Nature Valley Low Fat Fruit Granola	⅔ cup (1.9 oz)	210	4	3	0	44	3	210
Newquick	¾ cup (1 oz)	120	1	2	0	25	–	190
Oatmeal Crisp Almond	1 cup (1.9 oz)	220	5	5	0	42	4	240
Oatmeal Crisp Apple Cinnamon	1 cup (1.9 oz)	210	5	2	0	45	4	250
Oatmeal Crisp Raisin	1 cup (1.9 oz)	210	5	2	0	44	4	220
Para Su Familia Cinnamon Stars	1 cup (1 oz)	120	1	1	0	28	–	240
Para Su Familia Fruitis	1 cup (1 oz)	120	1	1	0	25	–	210
Para Su Familia Raisin Bran	1¼ cups (2 oz)	170	5	2	0	41	6	320
Raisin Nut Bran	¾ cup (1.9 oz)	200	4	4	0	41	4	250
Reese's Puffs	¾ cup	130	2	3	0	23	0	170
Snack'N Dash Cinnamon Toast Crunch	1 pkg (1.2 oz)	140	2	4	0	27	1	230
Snack'N Dash Honey Nut Cheerios	1 pkg (1 oz)	110	3	1	0	23	2	250
Snack'N Dash Lucky Charms	1 pkg (1 oz)	110	2	1	0	24	1	100
Sunrise Organic	¾ cup (1 oz)	110	1	1	0	26	1	190
Total Brown Sugar & Oat	¾ cup (1 oz)	110	2	1	0	23	1	200
Total Corn Flakes	1⅓ cup (1 oz)	110	2	0	0	24	–	210
Total Raisin Bran	1 cup (1.9 oz)	170	4	1	0	41	5	240

FOOD	PORTION	CAL	PROT	FAT	CHOL	CARB	FIBER	SOD
Total Whole Grain	¾ cup (1 oz)	110	2	1	0	23	3	190
Trix	1 cup (1 oz)	120	1	1	0	27	1	190
Wheat Hearts	¼ cup (1.3 oz)	130	5	1	0	26	2	0
Wheaties	1 cup (1 oz)	110	3	1	0	24	3	220
Wheaties Energy Crunch	1 cup (1.9 oz)	210	6	3	0	42	4	310
Wheaties Frosted	¾ cup (1 oz)	110	1	1	0	27	—	200
Wheaties Raisin Bran	1 cup (1.9 oz)	180	4	1	0	45	5	250
Grainfield's								
Brown Rice	1 serv (1 oz)	110	3	1	—	24	tr	4
Crisp Rice	1 serv (1 oz)	112	3	tr	—	25	tr	3
Raisin Bran	1 serv (1 oz)	90	2	2	—	20	2	4
Wheat Flakes	1 serv (1 oz)	100	3	1	—	20	2	2
Health Valley								
10 Bran O's Apple Cinnamon	¾ cup	100	3	0	0	23	3	90
Bran w/ Apples & Cinnamon	¾ cup	160	5	0	0	41	7	10
Golden Flax	½ cup	190	6	3	0	38	6	30
Granola 98% Fat Free Date Almond	⅔ cup	180	5	1	0	43	6	90
Healthy Crunches & Flakes Almond	¾ cup	130	3	0	0	31	4	35
Healthy Crunches & Flakes Apple Cinnamon	¾ cup	130	3	0	0	31	4	35
Healthy Crunches & Flakes Honey Crunch	¾ cup	130	3	0	0	31	4	35
Hot Cereal Cups Amazing Apple!	1 pkg	220	9	2	0	43	4	230
Hot Cereal Cups Banana Gone Nuts	1 pkg	240	10	3	0	45	4	240
Hot Cereal Cups Maple Madness!	1 pkg	240	9	2	0	47	4	290
Hot Cereal Cups Terrific 10 Grain!	1 pkg	220	12	3	0	41	5	210
Oat Bran O'S	¾ cup	100	3	0	0	23	3	90

FOOD	PORTION	CAL	PROT	FAT	CHOL	CARB	FIBER	SOD
Organic Amaranth Flakes	¾ cup	100	3	0	0	24	4	35
Organic Blue Corn Bran Flakes	¾ cup	100	3	0	0	24	4	10
Organic Bran w/ Raisin	¾ cup	160	5	0	0	40	6	10
Organic Fiber 7 Flakes	¾ cup	100	3	0	0	24	4	15
Organic Healthy Fiber Flakes	¾ cup	100	3	0	0	23	4	10
Organic Oat Bran Flakes	¾ cup	100	3	0	0	24	4	15
Organic Oat Bran Flakes w/ Raisins	¾ cup	110	3	0	0	26	4	15
Puffed Honey Sweetened Corn	1 cup	110	2	0	0	28	2	0
Puffed Honey Sweetened Crisp Brown Rice	1 cup	110	1	0	0	28	2	0
Raisin Bran Flakes	1¼ cup	190	5	0	0	47	5	90
Real Oat Bran	½ cup	200	6	3	0	34	5	90
Healthy Choice								
Almond Crunch w/ Raisins	1 cup (2 oz)	210	5	3	0	46	5	230
Golden Multi-Grain Flakes	¾ cup (1.1 oz)	110	3	0	0	26	3	180
Toasted Brown Sugar Squares	1 cup (2 oz)	190	5	1	0	44	5	5
Hodgson Mill								
Cracked Wheat	¼ cup (1.4 oz)	110	4	1	0	26	8	0
Multi Grain w/ Flaxseed & Soy	⅓ cup (1.4 oz)	160	7	3	0	25	6	0
Kashi								
Breakfast Pilaf as prep	½ cup (4.9 oz)	170	6	3	0	30	6	15
Go Apple Spice	½ cup (4.9 oz)	270	7	3	0	56	6	0
Go Banana Almond	½ cup (4.9 oz)	280	7	4	0	57	6	5
Go Berry Tart	½ cup (4.9 oz)	260	7	3	0	55	6	5
Go Blueberry Bliss	½ cup (4.9 oz)	260	7	3	0	55	6	5

FOOD	PORTION	CAL	PROT	FAT	CHOL	CARB	FIBER	SOD
Go Cherry Vanilla	½ cup (4.9 oz)	260	7	3	0	54	6	15
Go Just Peachy	½ cup (4.9 oz)	260	7	3	0	54	6	0
GoLean	¾ cup (1.4 oz)	120	8	1	0	28	10	35
Good Friends	¾ cup (1 oz)	90	3	1	0	24	8	70
Honey Puffed	1 cup (1 oz)	120	3	1	0	25	2	6
Medley	½ cup (1 oz)	100	4	1	0	20	2	50
Pillows Apple	¾ cup (1.9 oz)	200	3	1	0	45	2	30
Pillows Chocolate	¾ cup (1.9 oz)	200	3	1	0	45	2	50
Pillows Strawberry Crisp	¾ cup (1.9 oz)	200	3	1	0	46	2	25
Puffed	1 cup (0.9 oz)	70	3	tr	0	13	2	0
Kellogg's								
All-Bran	½ cup (1.1 oz)	80	4	1	0	24	10	65
All-Bran Bran Buds	⅓ cup (1 oz)	80	3	1	0	24	13	210
All-Bran Extra Fiber	½ cup (0.9 oz)	50	3	1	0	20	13	120
Apple Jacks	1 cup (1.2 oz)	120	2	0	0	30	1	150
Cocoa Frosted Flakes	¾ cup (1.1 oz)	120	1	0	0	28	0	210
Cocoa Krispies	¾ cup (1.1 oz)	120	1	1	0	27	0	220
Complete Oat Bran Flakes	¾ cup (1 oz)	110	4	1	0	23	4	270
Complete Wheat Bran Flakes	¾ cup (1 oz)	90	3	1	0	23	5	220
Corn Flakes	1 cup (1 oz)	100	2	0	0	24	1	300
Corn Pops K-Sentials	1 oz	100	1	0	0	25	0	110
Cracklin' Oat Bran	¾ cup (1.7 oz)	190	4	7	0	35	6	170
Crispix	1 cup (1 oz)	110	2	0	0	25	1	210
Froot Loops K-Sentials	1 oz	100	2	1	0	24	0	130
Frosted Flakes	¾ cup (1.1 oz)	120	1	0	0	28	1	200
Granola Low Fat	½ cup (1.7 oz)	190	4	3	0	39	3	120
Honey Crunch Corn Flakes	¾ cup (1.1 oz)	120	2	1	0	26	1	210
Just Right Crunchy Nuggets	1 cup (2 oz)	210	4	2	0	46	3	320
Just Right Fruit & Nut	1 cup (2.1 oz)	220	4	2	0	49	3	280
Low Fat w/ Raisins	⅔ cup (2.1 oz)	220	5	3	0	47	3	150
Mini-Wheat Frosted	1 cup (1.8 oz)	180	5	1	0	41	5	5
Mini-Wheat Strawberry Squares	¾ cup (1.8 oz)	170	4	1	0	40	5	15

FOOD	PORTION	CAL	PROT	FAT	CHOL	CARB	FIBER	SOD
Mini-Wheats Apple Cinnamon Squares	¾ cup (1.9 oz)	180	4	1	0	44	5	20
Mini-Wheats Blueberry Squares	¾ cup (1.9 oz)	180	4	1	0	43	5	20
Mini-Wheats Frosted Bite Size	24 pieces (2.1 oz)	200	6	1	0	48	6	5
Mini-Wheats Raisin Squares	¾ cup (1.9 oz)	180	5	1	0	42	5	5
Mueslix Apple & Almond Crunch	¾ cups (1.9 oz)	200	5	5	0	39	5	260
Mueslix Raisin & Almond	⅔ cup (1.9 oz)	200	5	3	0	41	4	160
Nutri-Grain Almond Raisin	1¼ cup (1.7 oz)	180	4	3	0	38	4	170
Nutri-Grain Golden Wheat	¾ cup (1 oz)	100	3	1	0	23	4	210
Product 19	1 cup (1 oz)	100	2	0	0	25	1	210
Raisin Bran	1 cup (2.1 oz)	200	6	2	0	47	8	370
Rice Krispies	1¼ cup (1.2 oz)	120	2	0	0	29	0	350
Rice Krispies Razzle Dazzle	¾ cup (1 oz)	110	1	0	0	25	0	170
Rice Krispies Treats	¾ cup (1 oz)	120	1	2	0	26	0	190
Smacks	¾ cup (1 oz)	100	2	1	0	24	1	50
Smart Start	1 cup (1.8 oz)	180	3	1	0	43	2	310
Special K	1 cup (1.1 oz)	110	6	0	0	21	1	220
Kolln								
Crispy Oats	1 cup (1.8 oz)	190	5	3	0	40	2	210
Oat Bran Crunch	⅔ cup (2.1 oz)	220	10	5	0	41	9	0
Oat Muesli Fruit	¾ cup (2 oz)	200	6	5	0	39	4	15
Lundberg								
Purely Organic Hot'n Creamy Rice	⅓ cup	190	4	2	0	43	3	0
McCann's								
Irish Oatmeal	1 oz	110	5	2	0	20	3	0
Morning Traditions								
Banana Nut Crunch	1 cup (2 oz)	250	5	6	0	43	4	240
Blueberry Morning	1¼ cup (1.9 oz)	220	4	3	0	43	2	250

FOOD	PORTION	CAL	PROT	FAT	CHOL	CARB	FIBER	SOD
Cranberry Almond Crunch	1 cup (1.9 oz)	220	4	3	0	44	3	200
Great Grains Crunchy Pecan	⅔ cup (1.9 oz)	220	5	6	0	38	4	190
Great Grains Raisins Dates & Pecans	⅔ cup (1.9 oz)	210	4	5	0	39	4	160
Nabisco								
100% Bran	⅓ cup (1 oz)	80	4	1	0	23	8	120
Cream Of Wheat Instant as prep	1 cup	120	3	0	–	25	1	0
Cream Of Wheat Quick as prep	1 cup	120	3	0	–	25	1	–
Cream Of Wheat Regular as prep	1 cup	120	3	0	–	25	1	0
Frosted Shredded Wheat Bite Size	1 cup (1.8 oz)	190	4	1	0	44	5	10
Honey Nut Shredded Wheat Bite Size	1 cup (1.8 oz)	200	5	2	0	43	4	40
Original Shredded Wheat	2 biscuits (1.6 oz)	160	5	1	0	38	5	0
Original Shredded Wheat 'N Bran	1¼ cup (2.1 oz)	200	7	1	0	47	8	0
Original Shredded Wheat Spoon Size	1 cup (1.7 oz)	170	5	1	0	41	5	0
Nutri-Grain								
Almond Raisin	1¼ cup (2 oz)	200	4	3	0	43	4	200
Golden Wheat	¾ cup (1.1 oz)	100	3	1	0	24	4	220
Post								
Alpha-Bits	1 cup (1 oz)	130	3	2	0	27	1	210
Alpha-Bits Marshmallow	1 cup (1 oz)	120	2	1	0	25	0	160
Bran Flakes	¾ cup (1 oz)	100	3	1	0	24	5	220
Cocoa Pebbles	¾ cup (1 oz)	120	1	1	0	26	0	160
Fruit & Fibre Dates Raisins & Walnuts	1 cup (1.9 oz)	210	4	3	0	42	5	250
Fruit & Fibre Peaches Raisins & Almonds	1 cup (1.9 oz)	210	4	3	0	42	5	260
Fruity Pebbles	¾ cup (1 oz)	110	tr	1	0	24	0	160
Golden Crisp	¾ cup (1 oz)	110	1	0	0	25	0	40
Grape-Nuts	¾ cup (1 oz)	100	3	1	0	24	3	140

FOOD	PORTION	CAL	PROT	FAT	CHOL	CARB	FIBER	SOD
Grape-Nuts Flakes	¾ cup (1 oz)	100	3	1	0	24	3	140
Honey Bunches Of Oats	¾ cup (1 oz)	120	2	2	0	25	1	190
Honey Bunches Of Oats w/ Almonds	¾ cup (1.1 oz)	130	3	3	0	24	1	180
Honeycomb	1⅓ cups (1 oz)	110	2	1	0	26	tr	220
Post Toasties	1 cup (1 oz)	100	2	0	0	24	1	270
Raisin Bran	1 cup (2 oz)	190	4	1	0	47	8	300
Selects Blueberry Morning	¾ cup (1.3 oz)	140	2	2	0	30	2	150
Waffle Crisp	1 cup (1 oz)	130	2	3	0	24	0	120
Quaker								
Instant Grits Original	1 pkg (1 oz)	100	2	0	0	22	1	300
Multigrain	½ cup (1.4 oz)	130	5	2	0	29	5	10
Oatmeal Instant	1 pkg (1 oz)	100	4	2	0	19	3	80
Oatmeal Instant Apples & Cinnamon	1 pkg (1.2 oz)	130	3	2	0	27	3	170
Oatmeal Instant Bananas & Cream	1 pkg (1.2 oz)	130	3	3	0	26	2	170
Oatmeal Instant Blueberries & Cream	1 pkg (1.2 oz)	130	3	3	0	26	2	160
Oatmeal Instant Cinnamon & Spice	1 pkg (1.6 oz)	170	4	2	0	35	3	250
Oatmeal Instant Kid's Choice Cookie'n Cream	1 pkg (1.5 oz)	160	4	3	0	31	2	200
Oatmeal Instant Kid's Choice S'mores	1 pkg (1.5 oz)	160	4	3	0	32	2	220
Oatmeal Instant Maple & Brown Sugar	1 pkg (1.5 oz)	160	4	2	0	32	3	260
Oatmeal Instant Peaches & Cream	1 pkg (1.2 oz)	140	3	3	0	27	2	170
Oatmeal Instant Raisin & Spice	1 pkg (1.5 oz)	150	3	2	0	33	3	250

FOOD	PORTION	CAL	PROT	FAT	CHOL	CARB	FIBER	SOD
Oatmeal Instant Raisin Date & Walnut	1 pkg (1.3 oz)	140	3	3	0	27	3	240
Oatmeal Instant Strawberries & Cream	1 pkg (1.2 oz)	140	3	3	0	27	2	170
Oatmeal Nutrition for Women Golden Brown Sugar	1 pkg (1.6 oz)	170	5	2	0	33	3	310
Oatmeal Quick'n Hearty Microwave	1 pkg (1 oz)	110	4	2	0	19	2	150
Oatmeal Quick'n Hearty Microwave Apple Spice	1 pkg (1.6 oz)	170	4	2	0	35	3	280
Oatmeal Quick'n Hearty Microwave Honey Bran	1 pkg (1.4 oz)	150	4	2	0	30	3	250
Oats Old Fashion	½ cup (1.4 oz)	150	5	3	0	27	4	0
Oats Quick	½ cup (1.4 oz)	150	5	3	0	27	4	0
Oats Steel Cut	½ cup (1.4 oz)	150	5	3	0	27	4	0
Whole Wheat Hot Natural	½ cup (1.4 oz)	130	5	1	0	30	4	0
Sunbelt								
Berry Basic	½ cup (1.9 oz)	220	6	6	0	40	5	200
Granola Banana Nut	½ cup (1.9 oz)	250	5	9	0	37	4	60
Granola Cinnamon Raisins	½ cup (1.9 oz)	200	5	3	0	42	4	80
Granola Fruit & Nut	½ cup (1.9 oz)	240	4	7	0	40	3	70
Muesli 5 Whole Grains	½ cup (1.9 oz)	210	4	2	0	44	3	70
Uncle Sam								
Cereal	1 cup (1.9 oz)	190	7	1	0	38	10	135
Weetabix								
Cereal	2 biscuits (1.2 oz)	100	3	1	–	21	3	106
Wheatena								
Cereal	⅓ cup (1.4 oz)	150	5	1	0	33	5	0

CEREAL BARS (see also ENERGY BARS, NUTRITION SUPPLEMENTS)

Barbara's Bakery

FOOD	PORTION	CAL	PROT	FAT	CHOL	CARB	FIBER	SOD
Nature's Choice Apple Cinnamon	1 bar (1.3 oz)	120	2	2	0	27	2	75

FOOD	PORTION	CAL	PROT	FAT	CHOL	CARB	FIBER	SOD
Nature's Choice Blueberry	1 bar (⅓ oz)	120	2	2	0	27	2	75
Nature's Choice Cherry	1 bar (1.3 oz)	120	2	2	0	27	2	75
Nature's Choice Granola Carob Chip	1 bar (0.7 oz)	80	2	2	0	16	2	5
Nature's Choice Granola Cinnamon & Raisin	1 bar (0.7 oz)	80	2	2	0	16	3	5
Nature's Choice Granola Oats 'N Honey	1 bar (0.7 oz)	80	2	2	0	15	2	5
Nature's Choice Granola Peanut Butter	1 bar (0.7 oz)	80	2	3	0	14	2	5
Nature's Choice Raspberry	1 bar (1.3 oz)	120	2	2	0	27	2	75
Nature's Choice Strawberry	1 bar (1.3 oz)	120	2	2	0	27	2	75
Nature's Choice Triple Berry	1 bar (1.3 oz)	120	2	2	0	27	2	75
Cap'n Crunch								
Bar	1 (0.8 oz)	90	1	2	0	17	–	105
Berries Bar	1 (0.8 oz)	90	–	2	0	17	–	110
Dolly Madison								
Apple	1 (1.3 oz)	120	1	2	0	25	1	90
Blueberry	1 (1.3 oz)	120	1	2	0	25	1	90
Raspberry	1 (1.3 oz)	120	1	2	0	24	1	100
Strawberry	1 (1.3 oz)	120	1	2	0	24	1	100
Entenmann's								
Apple Cinnamon	1 (1.3 oz)	140	1	3	0	25	tr	85
Blueberry	1 (1.3 oz)	140	1	3	0	25	tr	90
Oatmeal Apple Cinnamon	1 (1.3 oz)	140	1	3	0	27	1	110
Oatmeal Apple Raisin	1 (1.3 oz)	140	1	3	0	27	1	110
Raspberry	1 (1.3 oz)	140	1	3	0	27	1	110
Strawberry	1 (1.3 oz)	140	1	3	0	25	tr	90

FOOD	PORTION	CAL	PROT	FAT	CHOL	CARB	FIBER	SOD
Estee								
Rice Crunchie Chocolate	1 (0.7 oz)	50	1	0	0	15	tr	40
Rice Crunchie Chocolate Chip	1 (0.7 oz)	50	1	0	0	15	0	40
Rice Crunchie Peanut Butter	1 (0.7 oz)	60	1	1	0	15	0	35
Rice Crunchie Vanilla	1 (0.7 oz)	60	1	0	0	14	0	35
General Mills								
Milk 'N Cereal Bars Chex	1 bar (1.6 oz)	160	6	4	0	26	–	150
Milk 'N Cereal Bars Cinnamon Toast Crunch	1 bar (1.6 oz)	180	6	4	0	30	1	160
Glenny's								
Chocolate Crunch Creamy Low Fat	1 bar (1.75 oz)	190	3	3	0	36	4	113
Chocolate Crunch Roasted Peanut	1 bar (1.75 oz)	200	4	4	0	36	6	100
Chocolate Crunch Toasted Almond	1 bar (1.75 oz)	200	4	4	0	36	6	100
Health Valley								
98% Fat Free Raisin Cinnamon	⅔ cup	180	5	1	0	43	6	90
98% Fat Free Tropical	⅔ cup	180	5	1	0	43	6	90
Blueberry	1	140	2	0	0	35	3	5
Breakfast Bakes Apple Cinnamon	1 bar	110	2	0	0	26	3	25
Breakfast Bakes California Strawberry	1 bar	110	2	0	0	26	3	25
Breakfast Bakes Mountain Blueberry	1 bar	110	2	0	0	26	3	25
Breakfast Bakes Red Raspberry	1 bar	110	2	0	0	26	3	25
Chocolate Chip	1	140	2	0	0	35	3	5
Crisp Rice Bars Apple Cinnamon	1	110	1	0	0	26	1	5

FOOD	PORTION	CAL	PROT	FAT	CHOL	CARB	FIBER	SOD
Crisp Rice Bars Orange Date	1	110	1	0	0	26	1	5
Crisp Rice Bars Tropical Fruit	1	110	1	0	0	26	1	5
Date Almond	1	140	2	0	0	35	3	5
Fiber 7 Flakes w/ Strawberry	1 bar	110	2	0	0	26	3	25
O's Almond	¾ cup	120	3	0	0	26	3	90
O's Apple Cinnamon	¾ cup	120	3	0	0	26	3	90
O's Honey Crunch	¾ cup	120	3	0	0	26	3	90
Oat Bran Flakes w/ Blueberry	1 bar	110	2	0	0	26	3	25
Raisin	1	140	2	0	0	35	3	5
Raisin Bran Flakes w/ Apple Raisin	1 bar	110	2	0	0	26	3	25
Raspberry	1	140	2	0	0	35	3	5
Strawberry	1	140	2	0	0	35	3	5
Hershey's								
Crisy Rice Snacks Peanut Butter	1 bar (0.5 oz)	60	1	2	0	9	tr	57
Hostess								
Apple	1 (1.3 oz)	120	1	2	0	25	1	90
Banana Nut	1 (1.3 oz)	120	2	2	0	25	2	80
Blueberry	1 (1.3 oz)	120	1	2	0	25	1	90
Raspberry	1 (1.3 oz)	120	1	2	0	24	1	100
Strawberry	1 (1.3 oz)	120	1	2	0	24	1	100
Kellogg's								
Nutri-Grain Apple Cinnamon	1 (1.3 oz)	140	2	3	0	27	1	110
Nutri-Grain Blueberry	1 (1.3 oz)	140	2	3	0	27	1	110
Nutri-Grain Cherry	1 (1.3 oz)	140	2	3	0	27	1	110
Nutri-Grain Mixed Berry	1 (1.3 oz)	140	2	3	0	27	1	110
Nutri-Grain Peach	1 (1.3 oz)	140	2	3	0	27	1	110
Nutri-Grain Raspberry	1 (1.3 oz)	140	2	3	0	27	1	110
Nutri-Grain Strawberry	1 (1.3 oz)	140	2	3	0	27	1	110

FOOD	PORTION	CAL	PROT	FAT	CHOL	CARB	FIBER	SOD
Nutri-Grain Twists Low Fat Apple Cinnamon	1 (1.3 oz)	140	1	3	0	27	1	105
Nutri-Grain Twists Low Fat Banana Strawberry	1 (1.3 oz)	140	1	3	0	26	1	100
Nutri-Grain Twists Low Fat Strawberry Blueberry	1 (1.3 oz)	140	1	3	0	27	1	110
Rice Krispies Treats	1 (0.8 oz)	90	1	2	0	18	0	100
Rice Krispies Treats Cocoa	1 (0.8 oz)	100	1	4	0	16	0	105
Rice Krispies Treats Peanut Butter Chocolate	1 (0.8 oz)	110	2	4	0	16	0	100
Kudos								
Chocolate Coated Chocolate Chip	1	120	1	5	0	20	1	75
Chocolate Coated Peanut Butter	1	90	1	3	0	17	1	105
Low Fat Blueberry	1 (0.7 oz)	90	1	2	0	15	1	90
Snickers	1	100	1	4	0	16	0	105
With M&M's	1	90	1	3	0	17	1	105
Little Debbie								
Raspberry	1 (1.3 oz)	130	1	3	0	28	tr	75
S'mores Granola Treats	1 (1 oz)	130	2	5	0	21	1	45
Strawberry	1 (1.3 oz)	130	1	3	0	28	tr	75
Nabisco								
Nutter Butter Granola Bar	1 (1 oz)	120	2	8	0	21	tr	45
Oreo Granola Bar	1 (1 oz)	120	2	4	0	21	1	65
Nature Valley								
Low Fat Chewy Orchard Blend	1 bar (1 oz)	110	2	2	0	22	1	65
Nature's Choice								
Carob Chip	1 bar (0.7 oz)	80	2	3	0	16	2	5
Cinnamon & Raisin	1 bar (0.7 oz)	80	2	2	0	16	3	5

FOOD	PORTION	CAL	PROT	FAT	CHOL	CARB	FIBER	SOD
Fat Free Apple	1 bar (1.3 oz)	110	2	0	0	27	2	90
Fat Free Blueberry	1 bar (1.3 oz)	110	2	0	0	27	2	90
Fat Free Cranberry	1 bar (1.3 oz)	110	2	0	0	27	2	110
Fat Free Peach	1 bar (1.3 oz)	110	2	0	0	27	2	90
Fat Free Raspberry	1 bar (1.3 oz)	110	2	0	0	27	2	110
Fat Free Strawberry	1 bar (1.3 oz)	110	2	0	0	27	2	110
Low Fat Triple Berry	1 bar (1.3 oz)	130	2	2	0	28	2	190
Low Fat Very Cherry	1 bar (1.3 oz)	130	2	2	0	28	2	190
Oats 'n Honey	1 bar (0.7 oz)	80	2	2	0	15	2	5
Peanut Butter	1 bar (0.7 oz)	80	2	3	0	14	2	5
Nutri-Grain								
Fruit-full Squares Apple	1 (1.7 oz)	180	3	4	0	35	1	95
Fruit-full Squares Banana	1 (1.7 oz)	190	3	5	0	35	1	95
Fruit-full Squares Cinnamon Raisin	1 (1.7 oz)	180	3	4	0	35	1	95
Quaker								
Chewy Chocolate Chip	1 (1 oz)	120	2	4	0	21	1	70
Chewy Cookies 'n Cream	1 (1 oz)	110	2	3	0	22	1	80
Chewy Peanut Butter Chocolate Chunk	1 (1 oz)	120	2	3	0	20	1	105
Chewy Graham Slam Chocolate Chip	1 (1 oz)	110	2	2	0	22	1	75
Chewy Graham Slam Peanut Butter	1 (1 oz)	110	2	2	0	22	1	80
Chewy Low Fat Chocolate Chunk	1 (1 oz)	110	2	2	0	22	1	80
Chewy Low Fat Oatmeal Raisin	1 (1 oz)	110	1	2	0	22	1	70
Chewy Low Fat S'mores	1 (1 oz)	110	1	2	0	22	1	80
Fruit & Oatmeal Apple Cinnamon	1 (1.3 oz)	130	1	3	0	26	1	95
Fruit & Oatmeal Low Fat Cherry Cobbler	1 (1.3 oz)	140	2	3	0	26	1	95

FOOD	PORTION	CAL	PROT	FAT	CHOL	CARB	FIBER	SOD
Fruit & Oatmeal Low Fat Strawberry	1 (1.3 oz)	140	2	3	0	26	1	125
Fruit & Oatmeal Low Fat Strawberry Banana	1 (1.3 oz)	130	1	3	0	26	tr	100
Fruit & Oatmeal Low Fat Strawberry Cheesecake	1 (1.3 oz)	130	2	3	0	26	tr	125
SnackWell's								
Country Fruit Medley	1 (1.3 oz)	130	1	3	0	27	tr	75
Fat Free Apple Cinnamon	1 (1.3 oz)	120	1	0	0	28	1	115
Fat Free Blueberry	1 (1.3 oz)	120	1	0	0	28	1	85
Fat Free Strawberry	1 (1.3 oz)	120	1	0	0	28	1	115
Hearty Fruit'n Grain Crisp Autumn Apple	1 (1.3 oz)	130	1	3	0	25	1	95
Hearty Fruit'n Grain Mixed Berry	1 (1.3 oz)	120	1	3	0	25	1	95
Hearty Fruit'n Grain Orchard Cherry	1 (1.3 oz)	130	1	5	0	26	1	90
Sunbelt								
Apple	1 (1.3 oz)	130	1	3	0	28	tr	75
Blueberry	1 (1.3 oz)	130	1	3	0	28	tr	75
Chewy Granola Almond	1 (1 oz)	130	2	7	0	17	1	65
Chewy Granola Apple Cinnamon	1 (1.2 oz)	140	2	3	0	28	2	105
Chewy Granola Chocolate Chip	1 (1.2 oz)	160	2	7	0	23	2	70
Chewy Granola Oatmeal Raisin	1 (1.2 oz)	130	2	3	0	27	1	100
Chewy Granola Oats & Honey	1 (1 oz)	120	2	5	0	19	1	65
Granola Fudge Dipped Chocolate Chip	1 (1.5 oz)	200	2	10	0	27	2	70

FOOD	PORTION	CAL	PROT	FAT	CHOL	CARB	FIBER	SOD
Granola Fudge Dipped Macaroon	1 (1.4 oz)	190	2	10	0	24	1	65
Weight Watchers								
Apple Cinnamon	1 (1 oz)	100	1	2	0	21	2	95
Blueberry	1 (1 oz)	100	1	2	0	21	1	90
Raspberry	1 (1 oz)	100	1	2	0	21	2	90

CHAMPAGNE

FOOD	PORTION	CAL	PROT	FAT	CHOL	CARB	FIBER	SOD
sekt german champagne	3.5 fl oz	84	tr	0	0	5	–	–

CHAYOTE

FOOD	PORTION	CAL	PROT	FAT	CHOL	CARB	FIBER	SOD
fresh cooked	1 cup	38	1	1	0	8	–	1
raw	1 (7 oz)	49	2	1	0	11	–	8
raw cut up	1 cup	32	1	tr	0	7	–	198

CHEESE *(see also* CHEESE DISHES, CHEESE SUBSTITUTES, COTTAGE CHEESE, CREAM CHEESE, NEUFCHATEL*)*

FOOD	PORTION	CAL	PROT	FAT	CHOL	CARB	FIBER	SOD
american	1 oz	93	6	7	18	2	–	337
american cheese food	1 pkg (8 oz)	745	45	56	145	17	–	2700
american cheese spread	1 jar (5 oz)	412	23	30	78	12	–	1910
american cold pack	1 pkg (8 oz)	752	45	56	144	19	–	2193
american cheese spread	1 oz	82	5	6	16	2	–	381
beaufort	1 oz	115	8	9	34	tr	0	128
bel paese	1 oz	112	7	9	–	0	–	–
blue	1 oz	100	6	8	21	1	–	396
blue crumbled	1 cup (4.7 oz)	477	29	39	102	3	–	1884
brick	1 oz	105	7	8	27	1	–	159
brie	1 oz	95	8	8	28	tr	–	178
cacio di roma sheep's milk cheese	1 oz	130	8	10	30	0	–	170
caerphilly	1.4 oz	150	9	13	–	0	0	–
camembert	1 oz	85	6	7	20	tr	–	239
camembert	1 wedge (1⅓ oz)	114	8	9	27	tr	–	320
cantal	1 oz	105	7	9	26	tr	0	269
caraway	1 oz	107	7	8	–	1	–	196
chabichou	1 oz	95	6	8	23	tr	0	189
chaource	1 oz	83	5	7	20	tr	0	230

FOOD	PORTION	CAL	PROT	FAT	CHOL	CARB	FIBER	SOD
cheddar	1 oz	114	7	9	30	tr	–	176
cheddar low fat	1 oz	49	9	2	6	1	–	174
cheddar low sodium	1 oz	113	7	9	28	1	–	6
cheddar reduced fat	1.4 oz	104	13	6	–	0	0	–
cheddar shredded	1 cup	455	28	37	119	1	–	701
cheshire	1 oz	110	7	9	29	1	–	198
cheshire reduced fat	1.4 oz	108	13	6	–	tr	0	–
colby	1 oz	112	7	9	27	1	–	171
colby low fat	1 oz	49	9	2	6	1	–	174
colby low sodium	1 oz	113	7	9	28	1	–	6
comte	1 oz	114	8	9	34	tr	0	105
coulommiers	1 oz	88	6	7	23	tr	0	195
crottin	1 oz	105	6	9	23	tr	0	133
derby	1.4 oz	161	10	14	–	0	0	–
edam	1 oz	101	7	8	25	tr	–	274
edam reduced fat	1.4 oz	92	13	4	–	tr	0	–
emmentaler	1 oz	115	8	9	26	tr	–	129
feta	1 oz	75	4	6	25	1	–	316
fontina	1 oz	110	7	9	33	tr	–	–
frais	1.6 oz	51	3	3	–	3	0	–
gjetost	1 oz	132	3	8	–	12	–	170
gloucester double	1.4 oz	162	10	14	–	0	0	–
goat fresh	1 oz	23	1	2	5	tr	0	18
goat hard	1 oz	128	9	10	30	1	–	98
goat semisoft	1 oz	103	6	8	22	1	–	146
goat soft	1 oz	76	5	6	13	tr	–	104
gorgonzola	1 oz	107	5	9	–	tr	–	–
gouda	1 oz	101	7	8	32	1	–	232
gruyere	1 oz	117	8	9	31	tr	–	95
lancashire	1.4 oz	149	9	12	–	0	0	–
leicester	1.4 oz	160	10	14	–	0	0	–
limburger	1 oz	93	8	8	26	tr	–	227
lymeswold	1.4 oz	170	6	16	–	tr	0	–
maroilles	1 oz	97	6	8	26	tr	0	300
monterey	1 oz	106	7	9	–	tr	–	152
morbier	1 oz	99	7	8	23	tr	0	283
mozzarella	1 lb	1276	88	98	356	10	–	1692
mozzarella	1 oz	80	6	6	22	1	–	106

FOOD	PORTION	CAL	PROT	FAT	CHOL	CARB	FIBER	SOD
mozzarella low moisture	1 oz	90	6	7	25	1	—	118
mozzarella low moisture part skim	1 oz	79	8	5	15	1	—	150
mozzarella part skim	1 oz	72	7	5	16	1	—	132
muenster	1 oz	104	7	9	27	tr	—	178
parmesan grated	1 oz	129	12	9	22	1	—	528
parmesan grated	1 tbsp (5 g)	23	2	2	4	tr	—	93
parmesan hard	1 oz	111	10	7	19	1	—	454
picodon	1 oz	99	6	8	23	tr	0	—
pimento	1 oz	106	6	9	27	tr	—	405
pont l'eveque	1 oz	86	6	7	20	tr	0	191
port du salut	1 oz	100	7	8	35	tr	—	151
provolone	1 oz	100	7	8	20	1	—	248
pyrenees	1 oz	101	6	8	26	tr	0	235
quark 20% fat	1 oz	33	4	1	5	1	—	10
quark 40% fat	1 oz	48	3	3	11	1	—	10
quark made w/ skim milk	1 oz	22	4	tr	tr	1	—	11
queso anego	1 oz	106	6	9	30	1	—	321
queso asadero	1 oz	101	6	8	30	1	—	186
queso chichuahua	1 oz	106	6	8	30	2	—	175
queso fresco	1 oz	41	4	2	—	1	0	—
queso manchego	1 oz	107	8	8	27	tr	0	341
queso panela	1 oz	74	6	5	—	1	0	—
raclette	1 oz	102	7	8	26	tr	0	217
reblochon	1 oz	88	6	7	23	tr	0	240
ricotta part skim	½ cup (4.4 oz)	171	14	10	38	6	—	155
ricotta part skim	1 cup (8.6 oz)	340	28	19	76	13	—	307
ricotta whole milk	1 cup (8.6 oz)	428	28	32	124	7	—	207
ricotta whole milk	½ cup (4.4 oz)	216	14	16	63	4	—	104
romadur 40% fat	1 oz	83	7	6	—	tr	—	—
romano	1 oz	110	9	8	29	1	—	340
roquefort	1 oz	105	6	9	26	1	—	513
rouy	1 oz	95	7	8	23	tr	0	138
saint marcellin	1 oz	94	5	8	23	tr	0	171
saint nectaire	1 oz	97	6	8	23	tr	0	169
saint paulin	1 oz	85	7	6	20	tr	0	174

FOOD	PORTION	CAL	PROT	FAT	CHOL	CARB	FIBER	SOD
sainte maure	1 oz	99	6	8	23	tr	0	411
selles sur cher	1 oz	93	5	8	20	tr	0	181
stilton blue	1.4 oz	164	9	14	–	0	0	–
stilton white	1.4 oz	145	8	13	–	0	0	–
swiss	1 oz	107	8	8	26	1	–	74
swiss cheese food	1 pkg (8 oz)	734	50	55	186	10	–	3523
swiss processed	1 oz	95	7	7	24	1	–	388
tilsit	1 oz	96	7	7	29	1	–	213
tome	1 oz	92	6	7	23	tr	0	231
triple creme	1 oz	113	3	11	34	tr	0	86
vacherin	1 oz	92	5	8	23	tr	0	129
wensleydale	1.4 oz	151	9	13	–	0	0	–
whey cheese	1 oz	126	4	8	–	9	0	146
yogurt cheese	1 oz	20	–	0	7	–	–	–
yogurt cheese	1 oz	80	6	7	15	0	0	60
Alouette								
Garlic & Herbs	2 tbsp (0.8 oz)	70	1	7	30	1	0	135
Alpine Lace								
American Jalapeno Peppers	1 slice (1 oz)	80	6	6	20	2	0	260
American Less Fat Less Sodium White	1 slice (1 oz)	50	6	6	20	2	0	200
American Less Fat Less Sodium Yellow	1 slice (1 oz)	80	6	6	20	2	0	200
Cheddar Reduced Fat	1 slice (1 oz)	70	8	5	15	1	0	170
Colby Reduced Fat	1 slice (1 oz)	80	9	5	15	1	0	115
Fat Free Parmesan	2 tsp (5 g)	10	1	0	0	0	0	65
Feta Reduced Fat	1 oz	50	5	3	10	1	0	370
Feta Reduced Fat Sun Dried Tomato & Basil	1 oz	50	5	3	10	1	0	370
Goat Reduced Fat	1 oz	40	2	3	5	tr	0	130
Mozzarella Reduced Fat	1 oz	70	8	3	10	1	0	200
Muenster Reduced Sodium	1 slice (1 oz)	100	7	9	25	1	0	85

FOOD	PORTION	CAL	PROT	FAT	CHOL	CARB	FIBER	SOD
Provolone Smoked Reduced Fat	1 slice (1 oz)	70	9	5	15	1	0	120
Swiss Reduced Fat	1 slice (1 oz)	90	8	6	20	1	0	35
Boar's Head								
American	1 oz	100	6	9	25	1	0	380
Baby Swiss	1 oz	110	7	9	25	tr	0	135
Canadian Cheddar	1 oz	110	7	10	35	0	0	170
Double Glouster Yellow	1 oz	110	7	10	35	0	0	200
Havarti	1 oz	110	6	10	35	0	0	210
Havarti w/ Dill	1 oz	110	6	10	35	0	0	210
Havarti w/ Jalapeno	1 oz	110	6	10	35	0	0	210
Lacey Swiss	1 oz	90	9	6	15	0	0	35
Longhorn Colby	1 oz	110	7	9	30	tr	0	170
Monerey Jack	1 oz	100	6	9	25	0	0	170
Monerey Jack w/ Jalapeno	1 oz	100	6	9	25	0	0	170
Mozzarella	1 oz	90	6	7	25	tr	0	140
Muenster	1 oz	100	6	8	25	0	0	180
Muenster Low Sodium	1 oz	100	6	8	20	0	0	75
Provolone Picante Sharp	1 oz	100	7	8	25	1	0	250
Swiss	1 oz	110	8	8	20	tr	0	65
Swiss No Salt Added	1 oz	110	8	8	25	tr	0	10
Borden								
Lite Line Mozzarella	1 oz	50	—	2	—	—	—	—
Lite Line Sharp Cheddar	1 oz	50	—	2	—	—	—	—
Lite Line Swiss	1 oz	50	—	2	—	—	—	—
Breakstone's								
Ricotta	¼ cup (2.2 oz)	110	7	8	25	3	0	90
Cabot								
Cheddar	1 oz	110	7	9	30	tr	0	180
Cheddar Five Peppercorn	1 oz	110	7	9	30	tr	0	180
Cheddar Mediterranean	1 oz	110	7	9	30	tr	0	180

FOOD	PORTION	CAL	PROT	FAT	CHOL	CARB	FIBER	SOD
Cheddar Sundried Tomato Basil	1 oz	110	7	9	30	tr	0	180
Cheddar Toasted Onion & Chive	1 oz	110	7	9	30	tr	0	180
Cheddar Light 50% Reduced Fat	1 oz	70	8	5	15	1	0	170
Cheddar Light 50% Reduced Fat Jalapeno	1 oz	70	8	5	15	1	0	170
Cheddar Light 50% Reduced Fat Tomato Basil	1 oz	70	8	5	15	1	0	170
Cheddar Light 75% Reduced Fat	1 oz	60	9	3	10	1	0	200
Dehydrated Cheddar Powder	2 tsp (5 g)	25	1	2	5	1	0	210
Monterey Jack	1 oz	110	7	9	30	tr	0	170
Cedar Grove								
Marble Colby	1 oz	110	7	9	30	0	0	185
Organic Tomato Basil Cheddar	1 oz	110	7	9	30	0	0	185
Cheez Whiz								
Light	2 tbsp (1.2 oz)	80	6	3	15	6	0	540
Churney								
Diet Snack Cheddar Flavored	1 oz	70	–	3	10	–	–	–
Diet Snack Port Wine Flavored	1 oz	70	–	3	10	–	–	–
Cracker Barrel								
Baby Swiss	1 oz	110	7	9	25	0	0	110
Cheddar Extra Sharp	1 oz	120	6	10	30	0	0	180
Cheddar Marbled Sharp	1 oz	110	7	9	30	tr	0	180
Cheddar New York Aged	1 oz	120	6	10	30	0	0	180
Cheddar Sharp	1 oz	120	6	10	30	0	0	180
Cheddar Vermont Sharp	1 oz	110	7	9	30	tr	0	180
Reduced Fat Cheddar Extra Sharp	1 oz	90	7	6	20	tr	0	240

FOOD	PORTION	CAL	PROT	FAT	CHOL	CARB	FIBER	SOD
Reduced Fat Cheddar Sharp	1 oz	90	7	6	20	tr	0	240
Reduced Fat Cheddar Vermont Sharp	1 oz	90	7	6	20	tr	0	240
Whipped Spreadable Cream Cheese & Sharp Cheddar	2 tbsp (0.9 oz)	80	3	8	20	tr	0	180
Di Giorno								
Parmesan Grated	2 tsp (5 g)	25	2	2	5	0	0	85
Parmesan Shredded	2 tsp (5 g)	20	2	2	5	0	0	75
Romano Grated	2 tsp (5 g)	25	2	2	5	0	0	90
Romano Shredded	2 tsp (5 g)	20	2	2	5	0	0	70
Fleurs De France								
Brie	3.5 oz	311	21	25	—	tr	tr	200
Friendship								
Farmer	2 tbsp (1 oz)	50	5	3	10	0	0	120
Handi-Snacks								
Cheez'n Breadsticks	1 pkg (1.1 oz)	120	4	6	15	12	0	320
Cheez'n Crackers	1 pkg (1.1 oz)	110	3	7	15	9	0	300
Cheez'n Pretzels	1 pkg (1 oz)	100	4	5	15	11	tr	410
Mozzarella String Cheese	1 piece (1 oz)	80	7	6	20	0	0	240
Nacho Stix'n Cheez	1 pkg (1.1 oz)	110	4	6	15	11	0	320
Healthy Choice								
American Singles White	1 slice (0.7 oz)	30		0	<5	2	—	290
American Singles Yellow	1 slice (0.7 oz)	30		0	<5	2	—	290
Cheddar Fancy Shreds	¼ cup (1 oz)	45	9	0	<5	2	—	200
Cheddar Shreds	¼ cup (1 oz)	45	9	0	<5	2	—	200
Loaf	1 in cube (1 oz)	35	8	0	<5	3	—	390
Mexican Shreds	¼ cup (1 oz)	45	9	0	<5	2	—	200
Mozzarella	1 oz	45	10	0	<5	1	—	200
Mozzarella Fancy Shreds	¼ cup (1 oz)	45	9	0	<5	2	—	200
Mozzarella Shreds	¼ cup (1 oz)	45	9	0	<5	2	—	200
Mozzarella String Cheese	1 stick (1 oz)	45	9	0	<5	1	—	200

FOOD	PORTION	CAL	PROT	FAT	CHOL	CARB	FIBER	SOD
Pizza Fancy Shreds	¼ cup (1 oz)	45	9	0	<5	2	–	200
Pizza String	1 stick (1 oz)	45	10	0	<5	1	–	200
Hollow Road Farms								
Sheep's Milk	1 oz	45	3	3	15	1	–	65
Kraft								
Cheddar Extra Sharp	1 oz	120	6	10	30	0	0	180
Cheddar Medium	1 oz	110	7	9	30	tr	0	180
Cheddar Mild	1 oz	110	7	9	30	tr	0	180
Cheddar Sharp	1 oz	120	6	10	30	0	0	180
Cheddary Melts Medium Cheddar	1 oz	110	5	9	30	2	0	390
Cheddary Melts Mild Cheddar	1 oz	110	5	9	30	2	0	390
Cheddary Melts Shreds Medium Cheddar	¼ cup (1.1 oz)	120	6	9	30	2	0	420
Cheddary Melts Shreds Mild Cheddar	¼ cup (1.1 oz)	120	6	9	30	2	0	420
Cheese Food w/ Garlic	1 oz	90	5	7	20	2	0	370
Cheese Food w/ Jalapeno Peppers	1 oz	90	5	7	20	2	0	370
Colby	1 oz	110	7	9	30	tr	0	180
Colby Monterey Jack	1 oz	110	7	9	30	0	0	180
Deluxe American	1 oz	100	6	9	25	tr	0	430
Deluxe American White	1 oz	100	6	9	25	tr	0	430
Deluxe Singles American	1 (1 oz)	110	6	9	30	tr	0	460
Deluxe Singles American	1 (0.7 oz)	70	4	6	15	tr	0	310
Deluxe Singles Pimento	1 (1 oz)	100	6	8	25	tr	0	430
Deluxe Singles Swiss	1 (1 oz)	90	6	7	25	0	0	410
Deluxe Singles Swiss	1 slice (0.7 oz)	70	5	5	20	0	0	310
Free Grated	2 tsp (5 g)	15	tr	0	0	3	0	75

FOOD	PORTION	CAL	PROT	FAT	CHOL	CARB	FIBER	SOD
Free Shredded Cheddar	¼ cup (0.9 oz)	40	9	0	<5	1	0	270
Free Shredded Mozzarella	¼ cup (1 oz)	45	9	0	<5	2	tr	340
Grated Parm Plus! Garlic Herb	2 tsp (5 g)	15	tr	0	0	2	0	110
Grated Parm Plus! Zesty Red Pepper	2 tsp (5 g)	15	tr	0	0	2	0	110
Grated Parmesan	2 tsp (5 g)	20	2	2	5	0	0	85
Grated Romano	2 tsp (5 g)	20	2	2	<5	0	0	70
Marbled Cheddar Mild	1 oz	110	7	9	30	tr	0	180
Marbled Cheddar & Monterey Jack	1 oz	110	7	9	30	tr	0	190
Marbled Cheddar & Whole Milk Mozzarella	1 oz	100	6	8	25	tr	0	190
Marbled Colby Monterey Jack	1 oz	110	7	9	30	0	0	180
Monterey Jack	1 oz	110	6	9	30	0	0	190
Monterey Jack w/ Jalapeno Peppers	1 oz	110	7	9	30	tr	0	190
Mozzarella Part Skim Low Moisture	1 oz	80	8	5	15	tr	0	200
Mozzarella String Cheese Low Moisture Part Skim	1 piece (1 oz)	80	7	6	20	0	0	240
Pizza Shredded Four Cheese	¼ cup (0.9 oz)	90	6	7	20	tr	0	220
Pizza Shredded Mozzarella & Cheddar	⅓ cup (1.1 oz)	120	7	9	30	1	0	220
Pizza Shredded Mozzarella & Provolone w/ Smoke Flavor	¼ cup (0.9 oz)	90	6	7	20	tr	0	200

FOOD	PORTION	CAL	PROT	FAT	CHOL	CARB	FIBER	SOD
Reduced Fat Cheddar Mild	1 oz	90	7	6	20	tr	0	240
Reduced Fat Cheddar Sharp	1 oz	90	7	6	20	tr	0	240
Reduced Fat Colby	1 oz	80	7	6	20	0	0	220
Reduced Fat Monterey Jack	1 oz	80	7	6	20	tr	0	240
Shredded Cheddar Medium	¼ cup (0.9 oz)	100	6	8	30	tr	0	170
Shredded Cheddar Mild	¼ cup (0.9 oz)	100	6	8	30	tr	0	170
Shredded Cheddar Sharp	1 oz (0.9 oz)	110	6	9	25	tr	0	170
Shredded Cheddar & Monterey Jack	¼ cup (0.9 oz)	100	6	8	25	tr	0	170
Shredded Colby & Monterey Jack	¼ cup (0.9 oz)	100	6	8	25	tr	0	170
Shredded Hearty Italian	⅓ cup (1.1 oz)	100	7	8	25	2	0	230
Shredded Italian Style Classic Garlic	⅓ cup (1.1 oz)	100	7	8	25	2	tr	240
Shredded Italian Style Mozzarelle & Parmesan	⅓ cup (1.1 oz)	100	7	8	25	1	0	240
Shredded Lower Fat Cheddar Mild	¼ cup (0.9 oz)	80	7	6	20	tr	0	220
Shredded Lower Fat Cheddar Sharp	¼ cup (0.9 oz)	80	7	6	20	tr	0	220
Shredded Lower Fat Colby & Monterey Jack	¼ cup (0.9 oz)	80	7	5	15	tr	0	210
Shredded Lower Fat Mozzarella	⅓ cup (1.1 oz)	80	9	5	15	tr	0	210
Shredded Lower Fat Pizza Cheese	⅓ cup (1.1 oz)	90	9	6	20	1	0	240

FOOD	PORTION	CAL	PROT	FAT	CHOL	CARB	FIBER	SOD
Shredded Mexican Style Cheddar & Monterey Jack	⅓ cup (1.1 oz)	120	7	10	30	tr	0	200
Shredded Mexican Style Four Cheese	⅓ cup (1.1 oz)	120	7	10	30	tr	0	210
Shredded Mexican Style Taco Cheese	⅓ cup (1.1 oz)	120	7	10	30	1	0	240
Shredded Monterey Jack	¼ cup (0.9 oz)	100	6	8	25	tr	0	170
Shredded Parmesan	2 tsp (5 g)	20	2	2	2	0	0	75
Shredded Part Skim Mozzarella	¼ cup (1.1 oz)	90	8	6	20	tr	0	220
Shredded Swiss	¼ cup (0.9 oz)	100	7	8	25	tr	0	25
Shredded Whole Milk Mozzarella	¼ cup (1.1 oz)	100	7	8	25	1	0	220
Shredded Finely Cheddar Mild	¼ cup (1.1 oz)	120	7	10	30	tr	0	190
Shredded Finely Cheddar Sharp	¼ cup (1.1 oz)	120	7	10	30	tr	0	190
Shredded Finely Colby & Monterey Jack	¼ cup (1 oz)	110	7	9	30	tr	0	190
Shredded Finely Lower Fat Cheddar Mild	⅓ cup (1.1 oz)	100	8	7	20	1	0	260
Shredded Finely Lower Fat Cheddar Sharp	⅓ cup (1.1 oz)	100	8	7	20	1	0	260
Shredded Finely Part Skim Mozzarella	¼ cup (1.1 oz)	90	8	6	20	tr	0	220
Shredded Finely Swiss	¼ cup (0.9 oz)	110	7	8	25	tr	0	45
Singles American	1 (1.2 oz)	110	6	8	25	3	0	460
Singles American	1 (0.7 oz)	60	3	5	15	2	0	260

FOOD	PORTION	CAL	PROT	FAT	CHOL	CARB	FIBER	SOD
Singles American	1 (0.6 oz)	60	3	5	15	2	0	260
Singles Mild Mexican	1 (0.7 oz)	70	4	5	15	2	0	280
Singles Monterey	1 slice (0.7 oz)	70	4	5	15	2	0	290
Singles Pimento	1 (0.7 oz)	60	4	5	15	1	0	260
Singles Reduced Fat American	1 (0.7 oz)	50	5	3	10	2	0	320
Singles Reduced Fat American White	1 (0.7 oz)	50	4	3	10	2	0	320
Singles Sharp	1 slice (0.7 oz)	70	4	6	20	tr	0	300
Singles Swiss	1 slice (0.7 oz)	70	4	5	15	1	0	320
Singles Nonfat American	1 (0.7 oz)	30	4	0	<5	3	0	270
Singles Nonfat American White	1 (0.7 oz)	30	4	0	<5	3	0	270
Singles Nonfat Sharp Cheddar	1 (0.7 oz)	35	5	0	<5	3	0	300
Singles Nonfat Swiss	1 slice (0.7 oz)	30	5	0	<5	3	0	270
Slices Cheddar Mild	1 (1 oz)	110	7	9	30	tr	0	180
Slices Colby	1 (1.6 oz)	180	11	14	45	tr	0	290
Slices Part Skim Mozzarella	1 (1.6 oz)	130	12	8	25	tr	0	320
Slices Part Skim Mozzarella	1 (1.5 oz)	120	12	8	25	tr	0	310
Slices Provolone Smoke Flavor	1 (1.5 oz)	150	11	11	35	tr	0	370
Slices Swiss	1 (1.5 oz)	170	12	13	45	tr	0	45
Slices Swiss	1 (1.3 oz)	150	10	12	40	tr	0	65
Slices Swiss	1 (0.8 oz)	90	6	7	25	0	0	40
Slices Swiss	1 (1.6 oz)	180	12	14	45	tr	0	45
Slices Swiss Aged	1 (1.5 oz)	170	12	13	45	tr	0	75
Slices Deli-Thin Part Skim Mozzarella	1 (1 oz)	80	8	5	15	tr	0	200
Slices Deli-Thin Swiss	1 (0.8 oz)	90	6	7	25	0	0	40
Slices Deli-Thin Swiss Aged	1 (0.8 oz)	90	6	7	25	0	0	40
Slices Reduced Fat Swiss	1 (1.3 oz)	130	11	9	25	tr	0	90
Spread Bacon	2 tbsp (1.1 oz)	90	5	8	25	tr	0	570

FOOD	PORTION	CAL	PROT	FAT	CHOL	CARB	FIBER	SOD
Spread Olive & Pimento	2 tbsp (1.1 oz)	70	2	6	20	3	0	220
Spread Pimento	2 tbsp (1.1 oz)	80	2	6	20	3	0	170
Spread Pineapple	2 tbsp (1.1 oz)	70	2	5	15	4	0	115
Spread Roka Brand Blue	2 tbsp (1.1 oz)	90	5	8	25	tr	0	520
Swiss	1 oz	110	8	9	30	0	0	50
Land O Lakes								
American	1 slice (0.7 oz)	80	4	6	20	1	0	320
American Jalapeno	1 slice (0.6 oz)	70	3	6	15	1	0	320
American Light	1 oz	70	7	5	20	2	0	400
American Reduced Salt	1 oz	110	6	9	30	tr	0	270
American Sharp	2 slices (1 oz)	100	5	9	30	1	0	420
American & Swiss	1 slice (0.6 oz)	70	4	5	15	1	0	310
Baby Swiss	1 oz	110	6	9	25	0	0	125
Chedarella	1 oz	100	7	8	25	0	0	200
Cheddar	1 oz	100	6	9	30	tr	0	180
Cheddar Extra Sharp	1 oz	110	6	8	30	tr	0	360
Cheddar Sharp	1 oz	110	7	9	30	tr	0	180
Cheese Spread Golden Velvet	1 oz	80	5	6	20	2	0	370
Colby	1 oz	110	7	9	30	tr	0	180
Jalapeno Light	1 oz	70	7	4	15	1	0	400
Monterey Jack	1 oz	110	6	8	30	tr	0	170
Monterey Jack Hot Pepper	1 oz	110	6	8	30	tr	0	140
Mozzarella	1 oz	80	7	6	15	tr	0	190
Muenster	1 oz	100	6	8	25	0	0	220
Parmesan Grated	1 tbsp	35	3	4	10	0	0	95
Provolone	1 oz	100	7	8	20	tr	0	240
Swiss	1 oz	110	8	8	25	tr	0	75
Swiss Light	1 oz	80	9	4	15	tr	0	60
Lifetime								
Cheddar Fat Free	1 oz	40	8	0	<5	1	0	220
Cheddar Fat Free Lactose Free	1 oz	40	8	0	<5	1	0	220
Garden Vegetable Fat Free	1 oz	40	8	0	<5	1	0	220

FOOD	PORTION	CAL	PROT	FAT	CHOL	CARB	FIBER	SOD
Jalapeno Jack Fat Free	1 oz	40	8	0	<5	1	0	220
Jalapeno Jack Fat Free Lactose Free	1 oz	40	8	0	<5	1	0	220
Mild Mexican Fat Free	1 oz	40	8	0	<5	1	0	220
Monterey Jack Fat Free	1 oz	40	8	0	<5	1	0	220
Mozzarella Fat Free	1 oz	40	8	0	<5	1	0	220
Mozzarella Fat Free Lactose Free	1 oz	40	8	0	<5	1	0	220
Onions & Chives Fat Free	1 oz	40	8	0	<5	1	0	220
Sharp Cheddar Fat Free	1 oz	40	8	0	<5	1	0	220
Smoked Cheddar Fat Free	1 oz	40	8	0	<5	1	0	220
Swiss Fat Free	1 oz	40	8	0	<5	1	0	220
Light N'Lively								
Singles American	1 (0.7 oz)	45	5	3	10	2	0	280
Northfield								
Naturally Slender	1 oz	90	–	7	10	–	–	–
Old English								
American Sharp	1 slice (1 oz)	100	6	9	30	tr	0	460
Organic Valley								
Aged Swiss Unpasteurized	1 oz	100	8	8	25	tr	0	60
Cheddar Reduced Fat Low Sodium	1 oz	90	8	6	15	1	0	135
Cheddar Sharp & Mild	1 oz	110	7	9	25	1	0	190
Cheddar Sharp & Mild Unpasteurized	1 oz	110	7	9	25	1	0	190
Colby	1 oz	110	7	9	28	1	0	175
Colby Unpasteurized	1 oz	110	7	9	28	1	0	175
Farmer Reduced Fat	1 oz	90	7	6	15	1	0	110
Feta	1 oz	90	6	7	20	0	0	180

FOOD	PORTION	CAL	PROT	FAT	CHOL	CARB	FIBER	SOD
Monterey Jack	1 oz	100	6	8	20	1	0	170
Monterey Jack Reduced Fat	1 oz	80	8	5	15	1	0	170
Mozzarella Part Skim	1 oz	80	8	5	16	1	0	170
Muenster	1 oz	100	6	8	25	1	0	165
Pepper Jack	1 oz	110	6	9	20	1	0	160
Provolone	1 oz	100	7	8	20	1	0	245
String Part Skim	1 oz	80	8	5	16	1	0	170
Wisconsin Raw Milk Cheese	1 oz	100	6	8	20	1	0	170
Polly-O								
String Lite	1 piece (1 oz)	60	7	3	10	tr	0	230
President								
Feta Fat Free	1 oz	30	6	0	0	2	0	450
Rouge Et Noir								
Breakfast	1 oz	86	5	7	–	1	–	–
Brie	1 oz	86	5	7	–	1	–	–
Camembert	1 oz	86	5	7	–	1	–	–
Schloss	1 oz	86	5	7	–	1	–	–
Sargento								
Blue Crumbled	¼ cup (1 oz)	100	6	8	20	1	0	380
Cheddar	1 slice (1 oz)	110	6	9	30	1	0	160
Cheddar Shredded	¼ cup (1 oz)	110	6	9	30	1	0	160
Cheese For Nachos & Tacos Shredded	¼ cup (1 oz)	110	6	9	25	1	0	240
Cheese For Pizza Shredded	¼ cup (1 oz)	90	7	6	20	0	0	210
Cheese For Tacos Shredded	¼ cup (1 oz)	110	6	9	25	1	0	220
Colby	1 slice (1 oz)	110	6	9	30	0	0	190
Colby-Jack Shredded	¼ cup (1 oz)	110	6	9	25	tr	0	190
Jarlsberg	1 slice (1.2 oz)	120	9	9	20	1	0	160
Monterey Jack	1 slice (1 oz)	100	6	9	30	0	0	190
Monterey Jack Shredded	¼ cup (1 oz)	100	6	9	30	0	0	190
MooTown Snackers Cheddar	1 piece (0.8 oz)	100	5	8	25	1	0	130
MooTown Snackers Cheddar Mild Light	1 piece (0.8 oz)	60	7	4	10	tr	0	170

FOOD	PORTION	CAL	PROT	FAT	CHOL	CARB	FIBER	SOD
MooTown Snackers Cheese & Pretzels	1 pkg (0.9 oz)	90	3	3	10	12	0	320
MooTown Snackers Colby-Jack	1 piece (0.8 oz)	90	5	8	20	tr	0	160
MooTown Snackers Pizza Cheese & Sticks	1 pkg (1 oz)	100	3	4	10	13	0	260
MooTown Snackers String	1 piece (0.8 oz)	70	6	5	15	tr	0	170
MooTown Snackers String Light	1 piece (0.8 oz)	60	7	3	10	tr	0	200
Mozzarella	1 slice (1.5 oz)	130	11	9	25	2	0	230
Mozzarella Shredded	¼ cup (1 oz)	80	7	6	15	1	0	150
Muenster	1 slice (1 oz)	100	6	9	25	tr	0	200
Parmesan Grated	1 tbsp (5 g)	25	2	2	<5	0	0	75
Parmesan Shredded	¼ cup (1 oz)	110	9	7	25	1	0	300
Parmesan & Romano Shredded	¼ cup (1 oz)	110	9	7	25	1	0	340
Parmesan & Romano Grated	1 tbsp (5 g)	25	2	2	<5	0	0	70
Pizza Double Cheese Shredded	¼ cup (1 oz)	90	7	6	20	1	0	150
Preferred Light Cheddar Mild Shredded	¼ cup (1 oz)	70	8	5	10	tr	0	200
Preferred Light Cheese For Tacos Shredded	¼ cup (1 oz)	70	8	5	15	tr	0	240
Preferred Light Mozzarella	1 slice (1.5 oz)	90	11	5	15	0	0	230
Preferred Light Mozzarella Shredded	¼ cup (1 oz)	70	8	3	10	tr	0	140
Preferred Light Swiss	1 slice (1 oz)	80	9	4	15	tr	0	50
Provolone	1 slice (1 oz)	100	7	8	25	0	0	190
Recipe Blend 4 Cheese Mexican Shredded	¼ cup (1 oz)	110	6	9	25	tr	0	200

FOOD	PORTION	CAL	PROT	FAT	CHOL	CARB	FIBER	SOD
Recipe Blend 6 Cheese Italian Shredded	¼ cup (1 oz)	90	7	7	20	0	0	180
Ricotta Light	¼ cup (2.2 oz)	60	5	3	15	3	0	55
Ricotta Old Fashioned	¼ cup (2.2 oz)	90	7	6	25	3	0	75
Ricotta Part-Skim	¼ cup (2.2 oz)	80	7	5	20	2	0	75
Swiss	1 slice (0.7 oz)	80	6	6	20	0	0	30
Swiss Shredded	¼ cup (1 oz)	110	8	8	30	0	0	40
Swiss Wafer Thin	2 slices (1 oz)	110	5	9	25	0	0	40
Smart Beat								
American Fat Free	1 slice (0.6 oz)	25	4	0	0	3	—	180
Lactose Free Fat Free	1 slice (0.6 oz)	25	4	0	0	3	—	180
Mellow Cheddar Fat Free	1 slice (0.6 oz)	25	4	0	0	3	—	180
Sharp Cheddar Fat Free	1 slice (0.6 oz)	25	4	0	0	3	—	220
Sorrento								
Mozzarella Part Skim Jalapeno	1 oz	80	8	5	15	1	0	180
Tree Of Life								
Cheddar 33% Reduced Fat Organic Milk	1 oz	90	8	6	15	1	—	135
Colby	1 oz	110	7	9	30	1	—	170
Colby Organic Milk	1 oz	120	7	10	30	1	—	190
Farmer Part-Skim Organic Milk	1 oz	90	7	6	15	1	—	110
Jalapeno Organic Milk	1 oz	110	6	9	20	1	—	190
Monterey Jack 35% Reduced Fat Organic Milk	1 oz	80	8	5	15	1	—	190
Monterey Jack Organic Milk	1 oz	100	6	8	20	1	—	185
Mozzarella Organic Milk	1 oz	80	8	5	16	1	—	170

FOOD	PORTION	CAL	PROT	FAT	CHOL	CARB	FIBER	SOD
Muenster Organic Milk	1 oz	100	6	8	25	1	–	185
Provolone	1 oz	100	7	8	20	1	–	250
Velveeta								
Light	1 oz	60	5	3	10	3	0	440
Shredded	¼ cup (1.3 oz)	130	8	9	30	3	0	500
Shredded Mild Mexican w/ Jalapeno Pepper	¼ cup (1.3 oz)	120	8	9	30	3	0	520
Spread	1 oz	90	5	6	25	3	0	420
Spread Hot Mexican	1 oz	90	5	6	20	3	0	420
Spread Mild Mexican	1 oz	90	5	6	25	3	0	420
Weight Watchers								
Cheddar Mild Yellow	1 oz	80	8	5	15	1	0	180
Cheddar Sharp Yellow	1 oz	80	8	5	15	1	0	180
Fat Free Grated Italian Topping	1 tbsp	20	2	0	0	2	0	60
Fat Free Reduced Sodium Yellow	2 slices (0.75 oz)	30	5	0	0	3	0	160
Fat Free Sharp Cheddar	2 slices (0.75 oz)	30	5	0	0	3	0	320
Fat Free Swiss	2 slices (0.75 oz)	30	5	0	0	2	0	320
Fat Free White	2 slices (0.75 oz)	30	5	0	0	3	0	320
Fat Free Yellow	2 slices (0.75 oz)	30	5	0	0	3	0	320
Wholesome Valley								
Organic American Reduced Fat	1 slice (0.7 oz)	50	4	3	10	2	0	290

CHEESE DISHES

FROZEN
Banquet

FOOD	PORTION	CAL	PROT	FAT	CHOL	CARB	FIBER	SOD
Mozzeralla Nuggets	6	260	9	18	40	19	1	1060
Health Is Wealth								
Mozzarella Sticke	2 (1.3 oz)	120	5	5	15	14	0	250
Stouffer's								
Welsh Rarebit	½ cup (2.5 oz)	120	5	9	20	5	0	280
TAKE-OUT								
cheese omelette as prep w/ 2 eggs	1 (6.8 oz)	519	31	44	–	tr	0	–

FOOD	PORTION	CAL	PROT	FAT	CHOL	CARB	FIBER	SOD
fondue	½ cup (3.8 oz)	247	15	15	49	4	–	142
fried mozzarella sticks	9	840	–	–	–	–	–	–
souffle	1 serv (7 oz)	504	23	38	370	18	1	848

CHEESE SUBSTITUTES

mozzarella	1 oz	70	3	3	0	7	–	194
Sargento								
Cheddar Shredded	¼ cup (1 oz)	90	5	7	0	2	0	420
Mozzarella Shredded	¼ cup (1 oz)	80	6	6	0	tr	0	320
Yves								
Good Slice American	1 slice (0.7 oz)	35	4	2	0	0	0	290
Good Slice Cheddar	1 slice (0.7 oz)	35	4	2	0	1	1	280
Good Slice Jalapeno Jack	1 slice (0.7 oz)	35	4	2	0	0	0	250
Good Slice Mozzarella	1 slice (0.7 oz)	30	4	2	0	0	0	270
Good Slice Swiss	1 slice (0.7 oz)	35	4	2	0	1	0	260

CHERIMOYA

fresh	1	515	7	2	0	131	–	–

CHERRIES
CANNED

sour in heavy syrup	½ cup	232	2	tr	0	60	–	18
sour in light syrup	½ cup	189	2	tr	0	49	–	18
sour water packed	1 cup	87	2	tr	0	22	–	17
sweet in heavy syrup	½ cup	107	1	tr	0	27	–	3
sweet in light syrup	½ cup	85	1	tr	0	22	–	3
sweet juice pack	½ cup	68	1	tr	0	17	–	3
sweet water pack	½ cup	57	1	tr	0	15	–	2
Del Monte								
Dark Pitted In Heavy Syrup	½ cup (4.2 oz)	100	1	0	0	24	1	10

DRIED

Sonoma								
Pitted	¼ cup (1.4 oz)	140	1	0	0	34	2	0

FRESH

sour	1 cup	51	1	tr	0	13	–	3
sweet	10	49	1	1	0	11	–	0

FOOD	PORTION	CAL	PROT	FAT	CHOL	CARB	FIBER	SOD
Chiquita								
Cherries	21	90	2	1	0	22	9	0
FROZEN								
sour unsweetened	1 cup	72	1	1	0	17	—	1
sweet sweetened	1 cup	232	3	tr	0	58	—	3

CHERRY JUICE

FOOD	PORTION	CAL	PROT	FAT	CHOL	CARB	FIBER	SOD
After The Fall								
Black Cherry	1 can (12 oz)	170	0	0	0	42	0	20
Capri Sun								
Wild Cherry Drink	1 pkg (7 oz)	100	0	0	0	30	0	20
Eden								
Montmorency Juice	8 oz	140	1	1	0	33	0	30
Juicy Juice								
Drink	1 box (4.23 oz)	70	0	0	0	17	0	10
Drink	1 box (8.5 oz)	140	0	0	0	34	0	15
Kool-Aid								
Black Cherry Drink as prep w/ sugar	1 serv (8 oz)	100	0	0	0	25	0	15
Bursts Cherry Drink	1 (7 oz)	100	0	0	0	25	0	30
Splash Drink	1 serv (8 oz)	110	0	0	0	29	0	35
Sugar Free Drink Mix as prep	1 serv (8 oz)	5	0	0	0	0	0	5
Mott's								
Cherry	1 box (8 oz)	120	0	0	0	31	—	15
Ocean Spray								
Black Cherry Blast	8 oz	140	0	0	0	33	0	35
Veryfine								
Juice-Ups	8 fl oz	130	0	0	0	33	0	15

CHERVIL

FOOD	PORTION	CAL	PROT	FAT	CHOL	CARB	FIBER	SOD
seed	1 tsp	1	tr	tr	0	tr	—	tr

CHESTNUTS

FOOD	PORTION	CAL	PROT	FAT	CHOL	CARB	FIBER	SOD
chinese cooked	1 oz	44	1	tr	0	10	—	1
chinese dried	1 oz	103	2	tr	0	23	—	2
chinese raw	1 oz	64	1	tr	0	14	—	1
chinese roasted	1 oz	68	1	tr	0	15	—	1
cooked	1 oz	37	1	tr	0	8	—	8
creme de marrons	1 oz	73	1	tr	0	18	1	1
dried peeled	1 oz	105	1	1	0	22	—	11

FOOD	PORTION	CAL	PROT	FAT	CHOL	CARB	FIBER	SOD
japanese cooked	1 oz	16	tr	tr	0	4	–	1
japanese dried	1 oz	102	1	tr	0	23	–	10
japanese raw	1 oz	44	1	tr	0	10	–	4
japanese roasted	1 oz	57	1	tr	0	13	–	–
raw peeled	1 oz	56	tr	tr	0	13	–	1
roasted	2 to 3 (1 oz)	70	1	1	0	15	–	1
roasted	1 cup	350	5	3	0	76	–	3

CHEWING GUM

FOOD	PORTION	CAL	PROT	FAT	CHOL	CARB	FIBER	SOD
bubble gum	1 block (8 g)	27	0	0	0	8	–	0
stick	1 (3 g)	10	0	0	0	3	–	0
Aquafresh								
Peppermint	2 pieces	5	0	0	0	2	–	0
Arm & Hammer								
Dental Care Spearmint or Peppermint	2 pieces (2.5 g)	5	0	0	0	2	–	30
Beech-Nut								
Peppermint	1 stick (3 g)	10	0	0	0	2	0	0
Spearmint	1 stick (3 g)	10	0	0	0	2	0	0
Big Red								
Stick	1	10	tr	tr	0	2	–	0
Bubble Yum								
Bananaberry Split	1 piece (0.3 oz)	25	0	0	0	6	–	0
Cotton Candy	1 piece (0.3 oz)	25	0	0	0	6	–	0
Grape	1 piece (0.3 oz)	25	0	0	0	6	–	0
Luscious Lime	1 piece (0.3 oz)	25	0	0	0	6	–	0
Regular	1 piece (0.3 oz)	25	0	0	0	6	0	0
Sour Apple	1 piece (0.3 oz)	25	0	0	0	6	1	0
Sour Cherry	1 piece (0.3 oz)	25	0	0	0	6	0	0
Sugarless	1 piece (0.2 oz)	15	0	0	–	3	–	0
Sugarless Grape	1 piece (0.2 oz)	15	0	0	–	3	–	0
Sugarless Peppermint	1 piece (0.2 oz)	15	0	0	–	3	–	0
Sugarless Strawberry	1 piece (0.2 oz)	15	0	0	–	3	–	0
Sugarless Variety	1 piece (0.2 oz)	15	0	0	–	3	–	0
Variety Pack	1 piece (0.3 oz)	25	0	0	0	6	0	0
Watermelon	1 piece (0.3 oz)	25	0	0	0	6	0	0
Wild Strawberry	1 piece (0.3 oz)	25	0	0	0	6	0	0
*Care*Free*								
Sugarless Bubble Gum	1 stick (3 g)	10	0	0	–	2	–	0

FOOD	PORTION	CAL	PROT	FAT	CHOL	CARB	FIBER	SOD
Sugarless Cinnamon	1 piece (3 g)	5	0	0	–	2	–	0
Sugarless Peppermint	1 piece (3 g)	5	0	0	–	2	–	0
Sugarless Spearmint	1 piece (3 g)	5	0	0	–	2	–	0
Sugarless Wild Cherry	1 stick (3 g)	10	0	0	0	2	–	0
Dentyne								
Ice Peppermint	2 pieces (3 g)	5	0	0	0	2	–	0
Doublemint								
Chewing Gum	1 piece	10	tr	tr	0	2	–	0
Extra Sugar Free								
Cinnamon	1 piece	8	tr	tr	0	tr	–	0
Spearmint & Peppermint	1 stick	8	tr	tr	0	tr	–	0
Winter Fresh	1 piece	8	tr	tr	0	tr	–	0
Freedent								
Spearmint Peppermint & Cinnamon	1 stick	10	tr	tr	0	3	–	0
Fruit Stripe								
Bubble Gum Jumbo Pack	1 stick (3 g)	10	0	0	0	2	0	0
Variety Pack Chewing & Bubble Gum	1 stick (3 g)	10	0	0	0	2	0	0
Hubba Bubba								
Bubble Gum Cola	1 piece	23	tr	tr	0	6	–	0
Bubble Gum Sugarfree Grape	1 piece	13	tr	tr	0	tr	–	0
Bubble Gum Sugarfree Original	1 piece	14	tr	tr	0	tr	–	0
Original	1 piece	23	tr	tr	0	6	–	0
Strawberry Grape Raspberry	1 piece	23	tr	tr	0	6	–	0
Juicy Fruit								
Stick	1	10	tr	tr	0	2	–	0
Lance								
Big Red Cinnamon	1 piece (3 g)	10	0	0	0	2	0	0
Double Bubble	1 piece (7 g)	25	0	0	0	6	0	0
Double Mint	1 piece (3 g)	10	0	0	0	2	0	0

FOOD	PORTION	CAL	PROT	FAT	CHOL	CARB	FIBER	SOD
Stick*Free								
Sugarless Peppermint	1 stick (3 g)	10	0	0	–	2	–	0
Sugarless Spearmint	1 stick (3 g)	10	0	0	–	2	–	0
Winterfresh								
Stick	1 stick (3 g)	10	0	0	0	2	–	0
Wrigley's								
Spearmint	1 stick	10	tr	tr	0	2	–	0

CHIA SEEDS

dried	1 oz	134	5	7	0	14	–	–

CHICKEN *(see also* CHICKEN DISHES, CHICKEN SUBSTITUTES, DINNER, HOT DOGS*)*

FOOD	PORTION	CAL	PROT	FAT	CHOL	CARB	FIBER	SOD
CANNED								
chicken spread	1 tbsp	25	2	2	–	1	–	–
chicken spread	1 oz	55	4	3	–	2	–	–
chicken spread barbeque flavored	1 oz	55	4	3	–	2	–	–
w/ broth	½ can (2.5 oz)	117	15	6	–	0	–	357
w/ broth	1 can (5 oz)	234	31	11	–	0	–	714
FRESH								
broiler/fryer back w/ skin batter dipped & fried	½ back (2.5 oz)	238	16	16	63	7	–	228
broiler/fryer back w/ skin floured & fried	1.5 oz	146	12	9	39	3	–	40
broiler/fryer back w/ skin roasted	1 oz	96	8	7	28	0	–	28
broiler/fryer back w/ skin stewed	½ back (2.1 oz)	158	14	11	48	0	–	39
broiler/fryer back w/o skin fried	½ back (2 oz)	167	17	9	54	3	–	58
broiler/fryer breast w/ skin batter dipped & fried	½ breast (4.9 oz)	364	35	18	119	13	–	385
broiler/fryer breast w/ skin batter dipped & fried	2.9 oz	218	21	11	72	8	–	231

FOOD	PORTION	CAL	PROT	FAT	CHOL	CARB	FIBER	SOD
broiler/fryer breast w/ skin roasted	½ breast (3.4 oz)	193	29	8	83	0	–	69
broiler/fryer breast w/ skin roasted	2 oz	115	17	5	49	0	–	41
broiler/fryer breast w/ skin stewed	½ breast (3.9 oz)	202	30	8	83	0	–	68
broiler/fryer breast w/o skin fried	½ breast (3 oz)	161	29	4	78	tr	–	68
broiler/fryer breast w/o skin roasted	½ breast (3 oz)	142	27	3	73	0	–	63
broiler/fryer breast w/o skin stewed	2 oz	86	17	2	44	0	–	36
broiler/fryer dark meat w/ skin floured & fried	3.9 oz	313	30	19	101	4	–	98
broiler/fryer dark meat w/ skin roasted	3.5 oz	256	26	16	92	0	–	88
broiler/fryer dark meat w/ skin stewed	3.9 oz	256	26	16	90	0	–	77
broiler/fryer dark meat w/o skin fried	1 cup (5 oz)	334	41	16	135	4	–	136
broiler/fryer dark meat w/o skin roasted	1 cup (5 oz)	286	38	14	130	0	–	130
broiler/fryer dark meat w/o skin stewed	1 cup (5 oz)	269	36	13	123	0	–	104
broiler/fryer dark meat w/o skin stewed	3 oz	165	22	8	76	0	–	64
broiler/fryer drumstick w/ skin floured & fried	1 (1.7 oz)	120	13	7	44	1	–	44
broiler/fryer drumstick w/ skin roasted	1 (1.8 oz)	112	14	6	48	0	–	47

FOOD	PORTION	CAL	PROT	FAT	CHOL	CARB	FIBER	SOD
broiler/fryer drumstick w/ skin stewed	1 (2 oz)	116	14	6	48	0	–	43
broiler/fryer drumstick w/o skin fried	1 (1.5 oz)	82	12	3	40	0	–	40
broiler/fryer drumstick w/o skin roasted	1 (1.5 oz)	76	12	2	41	0	–	42
broiler/fryer drumstick w/o skin stewed	1 (1.6 oz)	78	13	3	40	0	–	37
broiler/fryer leg w/ skin batter dipped & fried	1 (5.5 oz)	431	34	26	142	14	–	442
broiler/fryer leg w/ skin floured & fried	1 (3.9 oz)	285	30	16	105	3	–	99
broiler/fryer leg w/ skin roasted	1 (4 oz)	265	30	15	105	0	–	99
broiler/fryer leg w/ skin stewed	1 (4.4 oz)	275	30	16	105	0	–	92
broiler/fryer leg w/o skin fried	1 (3.3 oz)	195	27	9	93	1	–	90
broiler/fryer leg w/o skin roasted	1 (3.3 oz)	182	26	8	89	0	–	87
broiler/fryer leg w/o skin stewed	1 (3.5 oz)	187	26	8	90	0	–	78
broiler/fryer light meat w/ skin floured & fried	2.7 oz	192	24	9	68	1	–	60
broiler/fryer light meat w/ skin roasted	2.8 oz	175	23	9	67	0	–	59
broiler/fryer light meat w/ skin stewed	3.2 oz	181	9	9	66	0	–	57

FOOD	PORTION	CAL	PROT	FAT	CHOL	CARB	FIBER	SOD
broiler/fryer light meat w/o skin fried	1 cup (5 oz)	268	46	8	125	1	–	114
broiler/fryer light meat w/o skin roasted	1 cup (5 oz)	242	43	6	118	0	–	108
broiler/fryer light meat w/o skin stewed	1 cup (5 oz)	223	40	6	107	0	–	91
broiler/fryer neck w/ skin stewed	1 (1.3 oz)	94	7	7	27	0	–	20
broiler/fryer neck w/o skin stewed	1 (.6 oz)	32	4	1	14	0	–	12
broiler/fryer skin batter dipped & fried	from ½ chicken (6.7 oz)	748	20	55	140	44	–	1105
broiler/fryer skin batter dipped & fried	4 oz	449	12	33	84	26	–	663
broiler/fryer skin floured & fried	from ½ chicken (2 oz)	281	24	24	41	5	–	30
broiler/fryer skin floured & fried	1 oz	166	6	14	24	3	–	18
broiler/fryer skin roasted	from ½ chicken (2 oz)	254	11	23	46	0	–	36
broiler/fryer skin stewed	from ½ chicken (2.5 oz)	261	11	24	45	0	–	40
broiler/fryer thigh w/ skin batter dipped & fried	1 (3 oz)	238	19	14	80	8	–	248
broiler/fryer thigh w/ skin floured & fried	1 (2.2 oz)	162	17	9	60	2	–	55
broiler/fryer thigh w/ skin roasted	1 (2.2 oz)	153	16	10	58	0	–	52
broiler/fryer thigh w/ skin stewed	1 (2.4 oz)	158	16	10	57	0	–	49
broiler/fryer thigh w/o skin fried	1 (1.8 oz)	113	15	5	53	1	–	49

FOOD	PORTION	CAL	PROT	FAT	CHOL	CARB	FIBER	SOD
broiler/fryer thigh w/o skin roasted	1 (1.8 oz)	109	13	6	49	0	—	46
broiler/fryer thigh w/o skin stewed	1 (1.9 oz)	107	14	5	49	0	—	41
broiler/fryer w/ skin floured & fried	½ chicken (11 oz)	844	90	47	283	10	—	264
broiler/fryer w/ skin fried	½ chicken (16.4 oz)	1347	81	81	404	44	—	1360
broiler/fryer w/ skin roasted	½ chicken (10.5 oz)	715	82	41	263	0	—	244
broiler/fryer w/ skin stewed	½ chicken (11.7 oz)	730	82	42	262	0	—	224
broiler/fryer w/ skin neck & giblets roasted	1 chicken (1.5 lbs)	1598	183	90	730	tr	—	536
broiler/fryer w/ skin neck & giblets stewed	1 chicken (1.6 lbs)	1625	184	93	726	tr	—	494
broiler/fryer w/o skin fried	1 cup	307	43	13	131	2	—	127
broiler/fryer w/o skin roasted	1 cup (5 oz)	266	41	10	125	0	—	120
broiler/fryer w/o skin stewed	1 oz	54	7	3	22	0	—	18
broiler/fryer w/o skin stewed	1 cup (5 oz)	248	38	9	116	0	—	98
broiler/fryer wing w/ skin batter dipped & fried	1 (1.7 oz)	159	10	11	39	5	—	157
broiler/fryer wing w/ skin floured & fried	1 (1.1 oz)	103	8	7	26	1	—	25
broiler/fryer wing w/ skin roasted	1 (1.2 oz)	99	9	7	29	0	—	28
broiler/fryer wing w/ skin stewed	1 (1.4 oz)	100	9	7	28	0	—	27
capon w/ skin neck & giblets roasted	1 chicken (3.1 lbs)	3211	402	165	1458	1	—	704

FOOD	PORTION	CAL	PROT	FAT	CHOL	CARB	FIBER	SOD
cornish hen w/ skin roasted	1 hen (8 oz)	595	51	42	299	0	–	146
cornish hen w/o skin & bone roasted	1 hen (3.8 oz)	144	25	4	113	0	–	67
cornish hen w/o skin & bone roasted	½ hen (2 oz)	72	13	2	57	0	–	34
cornish hen w/skin roasted	½ hen (4 oz)	296	25	21	149	0	–	73
roaster dark meat w/o skin roasted	1 cup (5 oz)	250	33	12	104	0	–	133
roaster light meat w/o skin roasted	1 cup (5 oz)	214	38	6	105	0	–	71
roaster w/ skin neck & giblets roasted	1 chicken (2.4 lbs)	2363	257	140	1003	1	–	760
roaster w/ skin roasted	½ chicken (1.1 lbs)	1071	115	64	365	0	–	349
roaster w/o skin roasted	1 cup (5 oz)	469	9	28	160	0	–	105
stewing dark meat w/o skin stewed	1 cup (5 oz)	361	39	21	132	0	–	133
stewing w/ skin neck & giblets stewed	1 chicken (1.3 lbs)	1636	157	107	603	tr	–	419
stewing w/ skin stewed	6.2 oz	507	34	34	140	0	–	130
stewing w/ skin stewed	½ chicken (9.2 oz)	744	70	49	205	0	–	190
Perdue								
Boneless Skinless Breasts Cooked	3 oz	110	25	2	70	0	–	30
Boneless Breast Roasted Garlic Herb	1 piece (3 oz)	90	18	1	50	3	–	620
Breaded Breast Strips Barbecue	3 oz	120	12	1	30	16	–	720
Breaded Breast Strips Hot & Spicy	3 oz	110	12	1	30	13	–	930
Breaded Breast Strips Original	3 oz	120	14	1	35	14	–	750
Burger Cooked	1 (3 oz)	160	17	10	110	0	–	55

FOOD	PORTION	CAL	PROT	FAT	CHOL	CARB	FIBER	SOD
Chicken Breast Seasoned Italian Cooked	1 piece (3 oz)	90	18	1	50	3	—	610
Chicken Breast Seasoned Lemon Pepper Cooked	1 piece (3 oz)	90	18	1	50	3	—	610
Chicken Breast Seasoned Teriyaki Cooked	1 piece (3 oz)	90	18	1	50	3	—	560
Ground Cooked	3 oz	170	18	11	125	0	—	50
Ground Breast Cooked	3 oz	80	19	1	55	0	—	60
Honey Rotisserie Dark Meat	3 oz	200	12	16	80	1	—	300
Honey Rotisserie White Meat	3 oz	140	19	8	70	1	—	290
Oven Stuffer Dark Meat Roasted	3 oz	210	18	15	100	0	—	60
Oven Stuffer Drumstick Roasted	1 (3.6 oz)	190	22	11	120	0	—	100
Oven Stuffer White Meat Roasted	3 oz	170	21	9	80	0	—	50
Oven Stuffer Wingette Roasted	3 (3.4 oz)	220	21	15	120	0	—	80
Seasoned Roasting Chicken Toasted Garlic Dark Meat	3 oz	190	16	14	100	1	—	330
Seasoned Roasting Chicken Toasted Garlic White Meat	3 oz	160	19	9	75	1	—	320
Seasoned Strips Parmesan Garlic cooked	3 oz	100	20	2	55	2	—	710

FOOD	PORTION	CAL	PROT	FAT	CHOL	CARB	FIBER	SOD
Seasoned Strips Savory Classic cooked	3 oz	90	19	1	55	1	—	500
Seasoned Strips Spicy Fiesta cooked	3 oz	140	16	7	75	3	—	630
Split Breast Cooked	1 piece (6.8 oz)	370	48	20	180	0	—	100
Thin Sliced Breast Rosemary Garlic Thyme	1 piece (3 oz)	90	20	2	60	1	—	820
Thin Sliced Breast Tomato Herb	1 piece (3 oz)	90	20	2	60	1	—	740
Whole Dark Meat cooked	3 oz	150	17	16	110	0	—	55
Whole White Meat Cooked	3 oz	170	21	10	85	0	0	45
Wings Roasted	2 (3.2 oz)	210	19	15	115	0	—	75
Tyson								
Broth Marinated Breast Filet	1 (4.7 oz)	140	26	4	70	0	0	330
Broth Marinated Drums	2 (4 oz)	140	17	7	90	0	0	290
Broth Marinated Thighs	1 (4.9 oz)	380	17	34	110	1	0	350
Broth Marinated Wings	4 pieces (4.2 oz)	240	20	18	95	0	0	340
Chicken Broccoli & Cheese	1 piece (5.9 oz)	320	20	16	50	23	3	670
Chicken Stuffed w/ Wild Rice & Mushroom	1 piece (5.9 oz)	300	23	12	50	25	1	860
Cordon Bleu	1 piece (5.9 oz)	350	25	17	55	24	3	640
Cornish Hen	1 serv (4 oz)	180	18	12	130	0	0	65
Kiev	1 piece (5.9 oz)	460	20	32	115	24	2	570
Wampler								
Breast Tenders	4 oz	130	27	2	70	0	—	55
FROZEN								
Banquet								
Breast Nuggets	7	280	13	20	40	11	1	500

FOOD	PORTION	CAL	PROT	FAT	CHOL	CARB	FIBER	SOD
Breast Patties Grilled Honey BBQ	1	110	13	5	40	3	0	440
Breast Patties Grilled Honey Mustard	1	120	13	5	25	5	0	500
Breast Tenders Our Original	3	250	12	15	40	15	tr	480
Breast Tenders Southern	3 pieces	260	12	16	40	16	1	460
Country Fried	1 serv (3 oz)	270	14	18	65	13	1	620
Fat Free Baked Breast Patties	1	100	9	0	20	15	1	400
Fried Our Original	1 serv (3 oz)	280	14	18	65	15	1	830
Honey BBQ Skinless Fried	1 serv (3 oz)	230	18	13	55	9	1	480
Hot 'n Spicy Fried	1 serv (3 oz)	260	14	18	65	13	1	730
Nuggets Our Original	6	270	14	19	35	12	1	540
Nuggets Southern Fried	5	270	12	18	35	16	2	570
Patties Our Orignal	1	190	7	14	30	10	1	440
Patties Southern Fried	1	190	8	12	25	10	tr	430
Skinless Fried	1 serv (3 oz)	220	18	13	65	7	2	480
Smokehouse Big Wings	2 (.6 oz)	200	14	17	70	4	0	300
Southern Fried	1 serv (3 oz)	280	14	18	65	15	1	700
Wings Firehouse Big	2	190	14	14	70	1	0	650
Wings Honey BBQ	4	380	31	24	70	15	1	570
Wings Hot & Spicy	4 pieces	280	18	20	90	9	tr	450
Country Skillet								
Bites	5	270	12	16	20	18	1	720
Breast Tenders	3	240	11	14	25	16	1	450
Chunks	5	270	12	18	20	18	1	720
Fried	3 oz	270	14	18	65	13	1	620
Nuggets	10	280	14	17	25	16	1	610
Patties	1	190	9	12	20	12	1	490
Southern Fried Chunks	5	270	11	18	20	17	1	550
Southern Fried Patties	1	190	9	12	20	12	1	440

FOOD	PORTION	CAL	PROT	FAT	CHOL	CARB	FIBER	SOD
Health Is Wealth								
Nuggets	4 (3 oz)	150	14	6	40	9	0	180
Patties	1 (3 oz)	150	13	6	40	9	0	180
Tenders	3 (3 oz)	130	14	3	35	11	0	230
Kid Cuisine								
Dino Mite Nuggets	4 pieces	300	11	23	40	10	1	540
Radical Racin' Nuggets w/ Cheese	4 pieces	300	11	23	35	12	tr	620
Sensible Chef								
Fried Breast	1 (3 oz)	200	21	10	55	8	2	310
Weaver								
Breast Strips	3 pieces (3.3 oz)	210	14	11	35	13	2	430
Breast Tenders	5 pieces (3 oz)	220	14	15	35	8	1	290
Croquettes	1 serv (3.5 oz)	290	11	18	45	22	2	540
Dutch Frye Nuggets	5 pieces (3.3 oz)	280	14	20	45	12	2	410
Honey Battered Tenders	5 pieces (2.9 oz)	230	12	15	35	12	1	380
Hot Wings Buffalo Style	3 pieces (2.7 oz)	190	18	13	95	0	0	370
Mini Drums Crispy	5 pieces (3.3 oz)	250	14	16	40	14	1	410
Nuggets	4 pieces (2.7 oz)	210	11	15	35	9	1	360
Patties	1 (2.6 oz)	180	10	11	30	10	1	430
Rondelet	1 (2.6 oz)	170	10	10	20	10	1	410
Rondelet Dutch Frye	1 (2.6 oz)	230	11	16	35	10	1	360
Rondelet Italian	1 (2.6 oz)	210	10	14	20	12	1	470
READY-TO-EAT								
chicken roll light meat	1 pkg (6 oz)	271	33	13	85	4	—	992
chicken roll light meat	2 oz	90	11	4	28	1	—	331
poultry salad sandwich spread	1 tbsp (13 g)	109	2	2	4	1	—	49
poultry salad sandwich spread	1 oz	238	3	4	9	2	—	107
Banquet								
Fat Free Baked Breast Tenders	3	120	13	0	30	16	2	480

FOOD	PORTION	CAL	PROT	FAT	CHOL	CARB	FIBER	SOD
Boar's Head								
Breast Hickory Smoked	2 oz	60	11	1	30	tr	0	440
Breast Oven Roasted	2 oz	50	11	1	30	tr	0	420
Breast Bar B Q Sauce Basted	2 oz	60	11	1	30	3	0	490
Butterball								
Crispy Baked Breasts Italian Style Herb	1 piece (0.5 oz)	190	17	6	55	16	1	710
Crispy Baked Breasts Lemon Pepper	1 piece (0.5 oz)	200	16	7	50	16	tr	420
Crispy Baked Breasts Original	1 piece (0.5 oz)	180	16	6	45	16	1	500
Crispy Baked Breasts Parmesan	1 piece (0.5 oz)	200	17	7	55	16	tr	650
Crispy Baked Breasts Southwestern	1 piece (0.5 oz)	170	17	6	35	13	2	590
Tenders Baked Breast	3 pieces	170	14	6	35	15	1	410
Tenders Hickory Smoked Grilled	4 pieces + sauce	160	17	5	50	12	1	570
Tenders Oriental Grilled	4 pieces + sauce	160	17	5	45	12	1	560
Carl Buddig								
Chicken Sliced	1 pkg (2.5 oz)	110	12	7	40	1	—	680
Lean Slices Honey Smoked Breast	1 pkg (2.5 oz)	70	12	1	30	3	—	630
Lean Slices Roasted Breast	1 pkg (2.5 oz)	60	13	1	30	1	—	630
Chicken By George								
Cajun	1 breast (4 oz)	130	21	4	60	3	0	700
Caribbean Grill	1 breast (4 oz)	150	22	4	60	8	0	550
Garlic & Herb	1 breast (4 oz)	120	21	3	60	3	0	600
Italian Bleu Cheese	1 breast (4 oz)	130	20	5	60	2	0	790
Lemon Herb	1 breast (4 oz)	120	20	3	60	3	0	800
Lemon Oregano	1 breast (4 oz)	130	20	4	50	3	0	600
Mesquite Barbecue	1 breast (4 oz)	130	21	3	60	5	0	700
Mustard Dill	1 breast (4 oz)	140	20	5	60	2	0	650
Roasted	1 breast (4 oz)	110	20	3	55	1	0	500

FOOD	PORTION	CAL	PROT	FAT	CHOL	CARB	FIBER	SOD
Teriyaki	1 breast (4 oz)	130	21	3	55	6	0	530
Tomato Herb w/ Basil	1 breast (4 oz)	140	20	5	60	5	0	630
Healthy Choice								
Deli-Thin Oven Roasted Breast	6 slices (2 oz)	45	11	0	25	0	0	410
Deli-Thin Smoked Breast	6 slices (2 oz)	60	11	2	30	1	0	420
Fresh-Trak Oven Roasted Breast	1 slice (1 oz)	30	6	1	15	0	0	290
Oven Roasted Breast	1 slice (1 oz)	25	6	0	15	0	0	220
Smoked Breast	1 slice (1 oz)	35	6	1	15	0	0	220
Louis Rich								
Carving Board Classic Baked	2 slices (1.6 oz)	45	9	1	25	2	0	510
Carving Board Grilled	2 slices (1.6 oz)	45	9	1	25	2	0	510
Deli-Thin Oven Roasted Breast	4 slices (1.8 oz)	50	10	1	25	1	0	620
Oven Roasted Deluxe Breast	1 slice (1 oz)	30	5	1	15	1	0	330
Oscar Mayer								
Free Oven Roasted Breast	4 slices (1.8 oz)	45	10	0	25	1	0	650
Perdue								
Breast Cutlets Homestyle	1 (2.9 oz)	110	14	1	35	12	–	730
Breast Cutlets Italian Style	1 (2.9 oz)	120	15	2	40	11	–	690
Breast Filets In Barbecue Sauce	1 piece + 3 tbsp sauce (5.9 oz)	200	24	1	70	24	–	1100
Breast Strips In Garlic & Herb Sauce	1 serv (5 oz)	100	18	1	50	4	2	1010
Breast Strips In Marinara Sauce	1 serv (5 oz)	120	18	3	50	5	–	1130
Breast Strips In Teriyaki Sauce	1 serv (5 oz)	190	20	1	50	26	–	1660
Carved Breast Honey Roasted	½ cup (2.5 oz)	100	18	2	45	2	–	450

FOOD	PORTION	CAL	PROT	FAT	CHOL	CARB	FIBER	SOD
Carved Breast Original Roasted	½ cup (2.5 oz)	90	19	2	50	1	—	500
Cutlets Cooked	1 (3.5 oz)	220	15	11	55	15	—	600
Nuggets	5 (3.4 oz)	210	15	11	50	15	—	580
Nuggets Chicken & Cheese	5 (3.4 oz)	230	15	13	55	15	—	670
Short Cuts Italian	½ cup (2.5 oz)	100	19	3	60	0	—	380
Short Cuts Lemon Pepper	½ cup (2.5 oz)	100	19	3	60	1	—	490
Short Cuts Southwestern	½ cup (2.5 oz)	100	18	3	60	1	—	410
Shady Brook								
Slow Roasted Breast	2 oz	60	12	1	30	—	—	400
Tyson								
Breaded Breast Chunks	6 pieces (2.9 oz)	230	9	16	20	13	1	440
Breaded Breast Fillet	2 pieces (2.8 oz)	180	12	8	25	15	1	440
Breaded Breast Pattie	1 (2.6 oz)	190	11	12	25	9	1	320
Breaded Breast Tenders	5 pieces (3 oz)	220	14	15	35	8	1	290
Breaded Chicken Chunks	6 pieces (3 oz)	220	13	14	40	11	0	480
Chick'n Quick Chick'n Cheddar	1 patty (2.6 oz)	220	11	14	40	12	0	270
Chicken Bits Southern Fried	6 pieces (2.9 oz)	260	11	19	40	11	1	540
Chicken Strips	1 serv (3 oz)	90	20	1	45	0	0	240
Chicken Strips Southwestern	1 serv (3 oz)	110	18	3	40	2	0	400
Country Fried Chicken Fritter	5 pieces (2.9 oz)	260	11	18	40	13	1	470
Drumsticks Hot BBQ Style	2 (3.5 oz)	160	22	7	100	3	1	620
Glazed Grilled Breast Pattie	1 (2.7 oz)	120	12	7	40	1	0	440
Grilled Chicken Pattie	1 (2.9 oz)	170	13	12	55	1	0	340
Nuggets Breaded White Meat	6 pieces (2.9 oz)	250	11	18	35	12	1	450
Patties Southern Fried	1 (2.9 oz)	260	11	19	40	11	1	540
Roasted Drumsticks	3 (5.6 oz)	320	44	15	230	2	0	1200

FOOD	PORTION	CAL	PROT	FAT	CHOL	CARB	FIBER	SOD
Roasted Drumsticks w/o Skin	2 (3.3 oz)	140	22	5	120	1	0	730
Roasted Half Chicken	1 serv (3 oz)	160	16	11	75	1	0	490
Roasted Whole Chicken	1 serv (3 oz)	160	16	11	75	1	0	490
Roasted Breast Boneless w/o Skin	1 (3.7 oz)	130	26	3	70	1	0	580
Roasted Breast Half w/o Skin	1 (4.3 oz)	150	30	3	80	1	0	660
Roasted Half Breast w/ Skin	1 (5.1 oz)	260	34	13	110	1	0	670
Roasted Half Chicken w/o Skin	1 serv (3 oz)	120	17	6	75	1	0	510
Roasted Tabasco Wings	3 (3 oz)	190	16	13	100	1	1	520
Roasted Thigh w/ Skin	1 (3.6 oz)	270	19	21	120	1	0	650
Roasted Thigh w/o Skin	1 (2.9 oz)	150	19	8	95	1	0	560
Roll White Meat	2 oz	90	10	6	25	0	0	440
Southern Fried Breaded Breast Pattie	1 (2.6 oz)	180	11	12	30	8	0	360
Southern Fried Breast Fillets	2 pieces (3.4 oz)	210	15	11	30	14	1	480
Southern Fried Chunks	6 pieces (2.9 oz)	260	11	19	40	11	1	540
Tenders Breaded Honey Battered	5 pieces (2.9 oz)	230	12	15	35	12	1	380
Tenders Breaded Pattie	3 pieces (3.2 oz)	100	13	0	0	11	1	540
Thick'n Crispy Pattie	1 (2.6 oz)	200	10	14	40	10	1	320
Wings BBQ	3 pieces (3.2 oz)	200	19	13	110	2	0	330
Wings Hot N'Spicy	4 (3.2 oz)	210	18	14	100	1	0	1020
Wings Teriyaki	4 pieces (3.4 oz)	190	21	12	120	2	2	210
Wings Of Fire	4 pieces (3.4 oz)	220	20	15	110	1	0	560
TAKE-OUT								
oven roasted breast of chicken	2 oz	60	11	1	25	0	–	470

FOOD	PORTION	CAL	PROT	FAT	CHOL	CARB	FIBER	SOD
CHICKEN DISHES								
CANNED								
Bumble Bee								
Chicken Salad	1 pkg (3.5 oz)	230	10	10	25	25	0	540
Dinty Moore								
Noodles & Chicken	1 can (7.5 oz)	180	7	8	30	19	1	1010
Stew	1 cup (8.5 oz)	220	12	11	40	16	2	980
FROZEN								
White Castle								
Grilled Chicken Sandwich	2 (4 oz)	250	17	9	20	24	5	490
Grilled Chicken Sandwich w/ Sauce	2 (4.8 oz)	290	17	9	20	33	5	600
MIX								
Chicken Skillet Helper								
Stir-Fried Chicken as prep	1 cup	270	18	9	105	30	1	760
Hamburger Helper								
Reduced Sodium Cheddar Spirals Chicken Recipe as prep	1 cup	240	20	6	40	27	0	630
Reduced Sodium Italian Herb Chicken Recipe as prep	1 cup	200	19	2	35	29	2	630
Tyson								
Mandarin Wrap Kit	1½ wraps (14.6 oz)	630	30	15	50	92	5	1840
READY-TO-EAT								
salad low fat	⅓ cup	90	8	2	20	9	–	440
Shady Brook								
Chicken Breast w/ Rice Pilaf	1 serv (12 oz)	350	46	13	120	–	–	270
Teriyaki Breast	1 serv (12 oz)	490	34	3	15	–	–	1600
Wampler								
Cacciatore	1 cup	260	30	9	90	10	–	600
Fajitas	1 cup	210	23	7	70	13	–	1360
Salad	⅓ cup	200	9	14	30	9	–	420

FOOD	PORTION	CAL	PROT	FAT	CHOL	CARB	FIBER	SOD
Salad Lite	⅓ cup	130	9	7	25	9	–	370
Smokey Barbecue Chicken	1 cup	430	42	15	140	31	–	1020
Sweet-n-Sour	1 cup	250	20	4	55	35	–	510
SHELF-STABLE								
Dinty Moore								
Microwave Cup Chicken & Dumpling	1 pkg (7.5 oz)	200	15	6	35	21	1	890
Microwave Cup Stew	1 pkg (7.5 oz)	180	10	8	30	18	2	920
Lunch Bucket								
Chicken Fiesta	1 pkg (7.5 oz)	160	6	2	5	30	5	530
Dumplings'n Chicken	1 pkg (7.5 oz)	140	5	5	10	21	1	780
TAKE-OUT								
boneless breaded & fried w/ barbecue sauce	6 pieces (4.6 oz)	330	17	18	61	25	–	830
boneless breaded & fried w/ honey	6 pieces (4 oz)	339	17	18	61	27	–	537
boneless breaded & fried w/ mustard sauce	6 pieces (4.6 oz)	323	17	17	62	21	–	791
boneless breaded & fried w/ sweet & sour sauce	6 pieces (4.6 oz)	346	17	18	61	29	–	791
breast & wing breaded & fried	2 pieces (5.7 oz)	494	36	30	149	20	–	975
chicken & dumplings	¾ cup	256	23	12	109	12	tr	1283
chicken & noodles	1 cup	365	22	18	103	26	–	600
chicken a la king	1 cup	470	27	34	221	12	–	760
chicken cacciatore	¾ cup	394	33	24	99	9	2	671
chicken paprikash	1½ cups	296	–	10	90	–	–	–
chicken pie w/ top crust	1 slice (5.6 oz)	472	19	31	–	32	1	–
drumstick breaded & fried	2 pieces (5.2 oz)	430	30	27	165	16	–	756
groundnut stew hkatenkwan	1 serv (15.7 oz)	576	38	40	116	18	4	1009
jamaican jerk wings	4 wings (9.9 oz)	709	57	51	172	3	tr	1045

FOOD	PORTION	CAL	PROT	FAT	CHOL	CARB	FIBER	SOD
sancocho de pollo dominican chicken stew	1 serv	702	71	30	195	34	1	653
thigh breaded & fried	2 pieces (5.2 oz)	430	30	27	165	16	–	756

CHICKEN SUBSTITUTES
Health Is Wealth
Buffalo Wings	3 pieces (2.2 oz)	100	10	2	0	11	3	490
Chicken-Free Nuggets	3 pieces (2.25 oz)	90	10	1	0	11	2	330
Chicken-Free Patties	1 (3 oz)	120	14	2	0	15	2	440

Loma Linda
Chicken Supreme Mix not prep	⅓ cup (0.9 oz)	90	15	1	0	6	4	720
Chik Nuggets	5 pieces (3 oz)	240	12	16	0	13	5	710
Fried Chik'n w/ Gravy	2 pieces (2.8 oz)	160	12	10	0	4	2	440

Morningstar Farms
Chik Nuggets	4 pieces (3 oz)	160	13	4	0	17	5	670
Chik Patties	1 (2.5 oz)	150	9	6	0	15	2	570
Meatless Buffalo Wings	5 pieces (3 oz)	200	13	9	0	16	3	730

Quorn
Cutlets	1 (3.5 oz)	200	10	8	0	20	4	610
Nuggets	3–4 pieces (3 oz)	180	8	8	0	18	3	650
Patties	1 patty (2.6 oz)	160	8	7	0	12	3	525
Tenders	1 cup (3 oz)	90	12	2	0	8	3	350

Soy Is Us
Chicken Not!	½ cup (1.75 oz)	140	24	2	0	15	9	5

Worthington
Chic-Ketts	2 slices (1.9 oz)	120	13	7	0	2	2	390
Chicken Sliced or Roll	2 slices (2 oz)	80	9	5	0	1	tr	370
Chicken Sliced	2 slices (2 oz)	80	9	5	0	1	tr	270
ChikStiks	1 (1.6 oz)	110	9	7	0	3	2	360
CrispyChik Patties	1 (2.5 oz)	150	8	6	0	15	2	600
Cutlets	1 slice (2.1 oz)	70	11	1	0	3	2	340
Diced Chik	¼ cup (1.9 oz)	40	7	0	0	1	1	270
FriChik	2 pieces (3.2 oz)	120	10	8	0	1	1	430
FriChik Low Fat	2 pieces (3 oz)	80	10	3	0	2	1	430
Golden Croquettes	4 pieces (3 oz)	210	14	10	0	14	6	600

FOOD	PORTION	CAL	PROT	FAT	CHOL	CARB	FIBER	SOD
Yves								
Veggie Chicken Burgers	1 (3 oz)	120	17	3	0	6	3	390
CHICKPEAS								
CANNED								
chickpeas	1 cup	285	12	3	0	54	—	718
Green Giant								
Garbanzo	½ cup (4.4 oz)	110	6	2	0	18	5	380
Old El Paso								
Garbanzo	½ cup (4.6 oz)	120	5	3	0	20	7	280
Progresso								
Chick Peas	½ cup (4.6 oz)	120	5	3	0	20	5	280
Garbanzo	½ cup (4.4 oz)	110	6	2	0	18	5	380
DRIED								
cooked	1 cup	269	15	4	0	45	—	11
CHICORY								
greens raw chopped	½ cup	21	2	tr	0	4	—	41
root raw	1 (2.1 oz)	44	1	tr	0	11	—	30
roots raw cut up	½ cup (1.6 oz)	33	1	tr	0	8	—	23
witloof head raw	1 (1.9 oz)	9	tr	tr	0	2	—	1
witloof raw	½ cup (1.6 oz)	8	tr	tr	0	2	—	1
CHILI								
chile pepper paste	1 tbsp	6	tr	1	—	1	1	1445
chili w/ beans	1 cup	286	15	14	43	30	—	1330
dried ancho	1 tsp	3	tr	tr	0	1	tr	0
dried casabel	1 tsp	3	tr	tr	0	1	tr	—
dried guajillo	1 tsp	3	tr	tr	0	1	tr	—
dried mulato	1 tsp	3	tr	tr	0	1	tr	—
dried pasilla	1 tsp	3	tr	tr	0	1	tr	1
dried smoked chipotle	1 tsp	3	tr	tr	0	1	tr	—
powder	1 tsp	8	tr	tr	0	1	—	26
Amy's Organic								
Whole Meals Chili & Cornbread	1 pkg (10.5 oz)	320	11	6	10	59	8	780
Armour								
Chili No Beans	1 cup (8.7 oz)	390	14	29	70	18	0	1200
Chili w/ Beans Western Style	1 cup (8.8 oz)	370	14	22	60	29	9	1130

FOOD	PORTION	CAL	PROT	FAT	CHOL	CARB	FIBER	SOD
Chili w/ Beans	1 cup (8.9 oz)	370	13	21	50	33	10	1220
Chili w/ Beans Hot	1 cup (8.9 oz)	370	13	21	50	33	10	1220
Vienna Sausage & Chili	1 cup (8.7 oz)	410	14	27	80	27	15	1270
Carroll Shelby's								
Original Texas Chili Kit	2 tbsp	60	2	1	0	12	0	1320
Chef Boyardee								
Chili Mac	½ can (7 oz)	260	10	11	30	30	3	1480
Chili Man								
Seasoning Mix	1 tbsp (7 g)	25	1	1	–	4	2	330
Del Monte								
Sauce	1 tbsp (0.6 oz)	20	0	0	0	5	0	480
Dennison's								
Chili Beans In Chili Gravy	7.5 oz	180	–	1	–	–	–	–
Chili Con Carne w/ Beans	7.5 oz	310	–	15	–	–	–	–
Chili Con Carne w/ Beans	7.5 oz	300	–	19	–	–	–	–
Chunky Chili w/ Beans	7.5 oz	310	–	14	–	–	–	–
Cook-off Chili w/ Beans	7.5 oz	340	–	19	–	–	–	–
Hot Chili Con Carne w/ Beans	7.5 oz	310	–	16	–	–	–	–
Gebhardt								
Chili Powder	¼ tsp (0.3 g)	1	tr	tr	0	tr	tr	tr
Chili Quik Seasoning	1 tbsp (0.3 oz)	43	1	1	0	8	2	985
Plain	1 cup (9.4 oz)	232	7	19	0	11	3	737
With Beans	1 cup (9.4 oz)	322	15	15	29	32	15	673
Health Valley								
Burrito	1 cup	160	13	1	0	28	12	360
Enchilada	1 cup	160	13	1	0	28	12	320
Fajita	1 cup	80	7	0	0	15	7	160
In A Cup Black Bean Mild	¾ cup	120	10	1	0	21	6	290
In A Cup Texas Style Spicy	¾ cup	120	10	1	0	21	6	290

FOOD	PORTION	CAL	PROT	FAT	CHOL	CARB	FIBER	SOD
Vegetarian Lentil Mild	1 cup	160	13	1	0	28	12	200
Vegetarian Lentil No Salt	1 cup	80	7	0	0	14	6	50
Vegetarian Mild	1 cup	160	13	1	0	28	12	200
Vegetarian Mild No Salt	1 cup	160	13	1	0	28	12	65
Vegetarian Spicy	1 cup	160	13	1	0	28	12	200
Vegetarian Spicy No Salt	1 cup	160	13	1	0	28	12	65
Vegetarian w/ 3 Beans Mild	1 cup	160	13	1	0	28	12	320
Vegetarian w/ Black Beans Mild	1 cup	160	13	1	0	28	12	320
Vegetarian w/ Black Beans Spicy	1 cup	160	13	1	0	28	12	320
Healthy Choice								
Bowls Chili & Cornbread	1 meal (9.5 oz)	350	21	8	35	49	8	600
Hormel								
Chunky w/ Beans	1 cup (8.7 oz)	270	18	7	35	34	7	1240
Hot No Beans	1 cup (8.3 oz)	210	16	9	35	17	3	910
Hot w/ Beans	1 cup (8.7 oz)	270	18	7	35	33	7	1240
Microcup Meals Chili Mac	1 cup (7.5 oz)	200	11	9	25	17	2	980
Microcup Meals Hot w/ Beans	1 cup (7.3 oz)	220	15	6	30	27	6	1050
Microcup Meals No Beans	1 cup (7.3 oz)	190	14	8	30	15	2	800
Microcup Meals w/ Beans	1 cup (7.3 oz)	220	15	6	30	27	6	1050
No Beans	1 cup (8.3 oz)	210	16	9	35	17	3	910
Turkey No Beans	1 cup (8.3 oz)	190	24	3	75	17	3	1250
Turkey w/ Beans	1 cup (8.7 oz)	210	17	3	35	30	5	1180
Vegetarian	1 cup (8.7 oz)	200	12	1	0	38	7	780
With Beans	1 cup (8.7 oz)	270	18	7	35	33	7	1240
With Beans	1 cup (8.7 oz)	270	18	7	35	33	7	1240
Hunt's								
Chili Beans	½ cup (4.5 oz)	87	6	1	0	17	6	597
Chili Sauce	2 tbsp (1.2 oz)	35	1	tr	0	8	1	393

FOOD	PORTION	CAL	PROT	FAT	CHOL	CARB	FIBER	SOD
Hurst								
HamBeens Chili Beans	1 serv	130	8	1	0	22	10	170
Just Rite								
With Beans	1 cup (9 oz)	379	18	27	35	31	13	51
Lean Cuisine								
Everyday Favorites Three Bean Chili w/ Rice	1 pkg (10 oz)	250	11	6	10	37	9	590
Lunch Bucket								
Chili w/ Beans	1 pkg (7.5 oz)	260	12	12	25	25	8	1040
Manwich								
Homestyle Fixins	½ cup (4.6 oz)	84	6	1	0	19	6	858
Marie Callender's								
Chili & Cornbread	1 meal (16 oz)	560	27	21	60	67	7	2110
McCormick								
Original Chili Seasoning	1⅓ tbsp (9 g)	30	–	1	0	5	2	310
Natural Choice								
Organic Vegan Three Bean	½ cup (4.6 oz)	140	9	1	0	24	7	510
Natural Touch								
Vegetarian	1 cup (8.1 oz)	170	18	1	0	21	11	870
Nature's Entree								
Texas Chili	1 pkg (12 oz)	320	26	7	15	43	11	960
Old El Paso								
Chili Seasoning Mix	1 tbsp (0.3 oz)	25	tr	1	0	4	1	770
Chili w/ Beans	1 cup (8 oz)	200	19	7	30	15	6	420
Open Range								
Plain	1 cup (8.8 oz)	353	18	26	48	19	6	1216
With Beans	1 cup (9 oz)	281	17	16	26	25	10	1291
Stouffer's								
With Beans	1 pkg (8.75 oz)	270	15	10	35	29	8	1130
Ultimate								
No Beans Hot	1 cup (8.7 oz)	420	20	30	85	18	5	1420
Turkey w/ Beans	1 cup (8.7 oz)	260	17	9	50	28	9	930
W/ Beans	1 cup (8.7 oz)	320	18	16	50	25	9	920
W/ Beans Hot	1 cup (8.7 oz)	320	18	16	50	25	9	920

FOOD	PORTION	CAL	PROT	FAT	CHOL	CARB	FIBER	SOD
Van Camp								
Beanee Weenee Chilee	1 cup (7.7 oz)	240	14	12	35	27	9	1090
Chili w/ Beans	1 cup (8.9 oz)	350	19	21	45	28	7	1020
Mexican Style Chili Beans	½ cup (4.6 oz)	110	7	2	0	21	8	430
Wampler								
Turkey	1 cup	250	23	7	75	22	–	1840
Wick Fowler's								
2 Alarm Chili Kit	3 tbsp	60	2	2	0	10	0	980
False Alarm Chili Kit	2 tbsp	50	2	2	0	9	0	980
Wolf Brand								
Plain	7.5 oz	330	25	22	–	10	–	1165
Worthington								
Chili	1 cup (8.1 oz)	290	19	15	0	21	9	1130
Low Fat	1 cup (8.1 oz)	170	18	1	0	21	11	870
Yves								
Veggie Chili	1 pkg (10.5 oz)	230	21	1	0	37	14	850
TAKE-OUT								
con carne w/ beans	8.9 oz	254	25	8	133	22	–	1008

CHILI PEPPERS *(see* PEPPERS*)*

CHINESE CABBAGE *(see* CABBAGE*)*

CHINESE FOOD *(see* ASIAN FOOD*)*

CHINESE PRESERVING MELON

cooked	½ cup	11	tr	tr	0	3	–	93

CHIPS

corn	1 bag (7 oz)	1067	13	66	0	113	9	1248
potato	1 bag (8 oz)	1217	16	79	0	120	–	1347
potato light	1 bag (6 oz)	801	12	35	0	114	–	836
potato sour cream & onion	1 bag (7 oz)	1051	16	67	14	102	–	1237
potato sticks	½ cup (0.6 oz)	94	1	6	0	10	1	45
tortilla	1 bag (7.5 oz)	1067	15	56	0	134	14	1124
Barbara's Bakery								
Potato	1¼ cup (1 oz)	150	2	10	0	15	1	180
Potato No Salt Added	1¼ cups (1 oz)	150	2	10	0	15	1	20

FOOD	PORTION	CAL	PROT	FAT	CHOL	CARB	FIBER	SOD
Potato Ripple	1¼ cup (1 oz)	150	2	10	0	15	1	180
Potato Yogurt & Green Onion	1¼ cup (1 oz)	150	2	9	0	15	1	240
Tortilla Blue Corn	15 chips (1 oz)	140	3	7	0	16	1	40
Tortilla Blue Corn No Salt	15 chips (1 oz)	140	3	7	0	16	1	0
Tortilla Pinta Salsa	15 chips (1 oz)	130	2	6	0	19	2	210
Bruno & Luigi's								
Pasta Chips Garlic & Herb	1 oz	117	4	1	0	23	1	25
Cape Cod								
Potato Golden Russet	1 pkg (0.5 oz)	70	1	4	0	8	tr	75
Chester's								
Flamin'Hot	1 oz	140	2	8	0	17	tr	250
Salsa	1 oz	140	2	7	0	18	tr	290
Doritos								
3D's Cooler Ranch	27 (1 oz)	140	2	6	<5	18	1	350
3D's Nacho Cheesier	27 (1 oz)	140	2	7	<5	17	1	360
Cooler Ranch	12 (1 oz)	140	2	7	0	18	1	170
Flamin' Hot	11 (1 oz)	140	2	7	0	17	1	210
Nacho Cheesier	11 (1 oz)	140	2	7	0	17	1	200
Salsa Verde	12 (1 oz)	150	2	7	0	20	1	210
Smokey Red	12 (1 oz)	150	2	7	0	21	1	210
Spicy Nacho	12 (1 oz)	140	2	6	0	18	1	210
Toasted Corn	13 (1 oz)	140	2	7	0	18	1	120
Wow Nacho Cheesier	1 pkg (0.75 oz)	70	2	1	0	13	1	180
Durangos								
Tortilla	15 (1 oz)	150	2	7	0	20	2	105
Eden								
Brown Rice Chips	1 oz	150	2	7	0	19	0	100
Sea Vegetable Chips	1 oz	140	1	5	0	23	0	220
Fritos								
Chili Cheese	31 (1 oz)	160	2	10	0	16	1	240
Corn Chips BBQ	29 (1 oz)	150	2	9	0	16	1	290
Corn Chips King Size	12 (1 oz)	150	2	10	0	16	1	150
Corn Chips Sabrositas Flamin' Hot	30 (1 oz)	150	2	9	0	16	1	180

FOOD	PORTION	CAL	PROT	FAT	CHOL	CARB	FIBER	SOD
Corn Chips Sabrositas Lime'N Chile	28 (1 oz)	150	2	9	0	17	1	240
Corn Chips Wild N'Mild Ranch	28 (1 oz)	160	2	10	0	15	1	160
Original	32 (1 oz)	160	2	10	0	15	1	170
Scoops	11 (1 oz)	160	2	10	0	17	1	105
Texas Grill Honey BBQ	15 (1 oz)	150	2	9	0	16	1	200
Guiltless Gourmet								
Tortilla Baked Chili Lime	18 (1 oz)	110	2	2	0	22	2	200
Tortilla Baked Mucho Nacho	18 (1 oz)	110	2	2	0	22	2	200
Tortilla Baked Organic Blue Corn	18 (1 oz)	110	3	2	0	22	2	140
Tortilla Baked Picante Ranch	18 (1 oz)	110	2	2	0	22	2	200
Tortilla Baked Red Corn	18 (1 oz)	110	2	2	0	22	2	200
Tortilla Baked Spicy Black Bean	18 (1 oz)	110	3	2	0	22	2	200
Tortilla Baked Sweet White Corn	18 (1 oz)	110	3	2	0	22	2	140
Tortilla Baked Yellow Corn	18 (1 oz)	110	3	2	0	22	2	160
Tortilla Baked Yellow Corn Unsalted	18 (1 oz)	110	3	1	0	22	2	26
Herr's								
Potato	1 oz	140	2	8	0	16	1	180
Tortilla Restaurant Style White Corn	10 chips (1 oz)	140	3	6	0	18	2	90
Lance								
BBQ	22 (1 oz)	160	2	10	0	15	1	170
Cajun	15 (1 oz)	150	2	10	0	14	1	290
Corn Chips	39 (1.25 oz)	200	2	11	0	14	1	140

FOOD	PORTION	CAL	PROT	FAT	CHOL	CARB	FIBER	SOD
Corn Chips Hot BBQ	35 (1.25 oz)	210	2	13	0	20	1	210
Hot Fries	1 pkg (0.9 oz)	140	2	10	0	11	1	190
Mesquite BBQ	22 (1 oz)	150	2	10	0	15	1	280
Potato	23 (1 oz)	160	2	10	0	15	1	130
Ripple	15 (1 oz)	160	1	11	0	14	1	150
Salt & Vinegar	22 (1 oz)	160	2	10	0	14	2	340
Sour Cream & Onion	22 (1 oz)	160	2	10	0	15	1	170
Tortilla Fiesta Salsa Triangles	16 (1 oz)	140	2	7	0	18	2	200
Tortilla Nacho Mini Round	46 (½s oz)	180	3	9	0	21	2	240
Tortilla Nacho Triangles	15 (1 oz)	140	2	14	0	18	1	200
Lay's								
Adobadas	16 (1 oz)	170	2	10	0	18	1	240
Baked KC Masterpiece BBQ	11 (1 oz)	120	2	3	0	22	2	210
Baked Original	11 (1 oz)	110	2	2	0	23	2	150
Baked Roasted Herb	12 (1 oz)	130	2	3	0	25	2	190
Baked Sour Cream & Onion	12 (1 oz)	120	2	2	0	21	2	210
Classic	20 (1 oz)	150	2	10	0	15	1	180
Deli Style Hot N'Tangy BBQ	18 (1 oz)	150	2	10	0	16	1	220
Deli Style Jalapeno	17 (1 oz)	150	2	10	0	16	1	230
Deli Style Original	17 (1 oz)	140	1	10	0	16	1	180
Deli Style Salt & Vinegar	16 (1 oz)	90	1	10	0	16	1	380
Flamin' Hot	17 pieces (1 oz)	150	2	10	0	16	1	180
KC Masterpiece BBQ	15 (1 oz)	150	2	10	0	15	1	200
Onion & Garlic	19 (1 oz)	150	2	9	0	16	1	200
Salt & Vinegar	17 pieces (1 oz)	150	2	10	0	15	1	300
Sour Cream & Onion	17 pieces (1 oz)	160	2	11	<5	12	1	200
Toasted Onion & Cheese	17 pieces (1 oz)	160	2	10	0	14	1	240
Wavy Au Gratin	13 (1 oz)	150	2	10	<5	14	1	200
Wavy Original	11 pieces (1 oz)	160	2	10	0	15	1	210
Wavy Ranch	11 (1 oz)	160	2	11	0	14	1	150
Wow Mesquite BBQ	20 (1 oz)	75	2	0	0	17	1	250

FOOD	PORTION	CAL	PROT	FAT	CHOL	CARB	FIBER	SOD
Wow Mesquite BBQ	20 (1 oz)	75	2	0	0	17	1	250
Wow Original	20 (1 oz)	75	2	0	0	18	1	200
Wow Original	1 pkg (0.75 oz)	55	1	0	0	13	1	130
Wow Sour Cream & Chive	19 (1 oz)	80	2	0	0	17	1	230
Wow Sour Cream & Chive	19 (1 oz)	80	2	0	0	17	1	230
Old Dutch Foods								
Potato	12–15 chips (1 oz)	150	2	8	0	16	1	130
Potato BBQ	12–15 chips (1 oz)	150	2	9	0	15	1	300
Potato BBQ Ripple	12–15 chips (1 oz)	150	2	9	0	16	tr	180
Potato Cajun Ripple	12–15 chips (1 oz)	150	2	10	0	15	1	160
Potato Cheddar & Sour Cream Ripple	12–15 chips (1 oz)	160	2	9	0	16	1	190
Potato Cheddar & Sour Cream Ripples	12–15 chips (1 oz)	150	2	9	0	15	1	190
Potato Dill	12–15 chips (1 oz)	140	2	8	0	16	1	310
Potato Dutch Crunch	15–20 chips (1 oz)	130	2	6	0	18	2	140
Potato French Onion Ripple	12–15 chips (1 oz)	150	2	10	0	15	1	180
Potato Jalapeno & Cheddar Dutch Crunch	15–20 chips (1 oz)	130	2	6	0	17	1	190
Potato Jalapeno Cheese	12–15 chips (1 oz)	150	2	9	0	16	1	170
Potato Mesquite BBQ Dutch Crunch	15–20 chips (1 oz)	130	2	6	0	19	2	230
Potato Onion & Garlic	12–15 chips (1 oz)	140	2	8	0	16	1	210
Potato Outback Spicy BBQ	12–15 chips (1 oz)	150	2	10	0	15	1	170
Potato Ripples	12–15 chips (1 oz)	150	2	9	0	15	1	115
Potato Salt & Vinegar Dutch Crunch	15–20 chips (1 oz)	130	0	6	0	18	1	360
Potato Sour Cream & Onion	12–15 chips (1 oz)	150	2	9	0	15	1	230
Tortilla Bite Size White Corn	20 chips (1 oz)	150	2	8	0	18	1	105
Tortilla Nacho Cheese	15 chips (1 oz)	150	2	7	0	19	1	150
Tortilla Restaurant Style White	9 chips (1 oz)	140	2	7	0	20	2	95

FOOD	PORTION	CAL	PROT	FAT	CHOL	CARB	FIBER	SOD
Tostados White Corn	11 chips (1 oz)	140	2	7	0	20	2	115
Tostados Yellow	11 chips (1 oz)	140	2	6	0	21	1	90
Old El Paso								
Tortilla NACHIPS	9 chips (1 oz)	150	3	8	0	17	2	85
Tortilla White Corn	11 chips (1 oz)	140	2	8	0	18	1	60
Pita-Snax								
Cheddar Cheese	34 (1 oz)	110	3	2	0	21	tr	240
Chili & Lime	34 (1 oz)	120	3	2	0	20	tr	210
Cinnamon	34 (1 oz)	120	3	2	0	22	tr	60
Dill Ranch	34 (1 oz)	120	3	2	0	21	tr	170
Garlic	34 (1 oz)	120	3	2	0	22	tr	120
Lightly Salted	34 (1 oz)	110	3	1	0	22	tr	170
Planters								
Corn Chips	34 chips (1 oz)	170	2	10	0	17	2	180
Corn Chips King Size	17 chips (1 oz)	160	2	10	0	16	2	180
Corn Chips Snacks To Go	1 pkg (1.5 oz)	240	3	15	0	23	3	260
Pringles								
BBQ	14 chips (1 oz)	150	2	10	0	15	1	200
Cheese & Onion	14 chips (1 oz)	160	1	11	0	15	1	220
Cheez-ums	14 chips (1 oz)	150	2	10	0	14	1	190
Original	14 chips (1 oz)	160	2	11	0	15	1	170
Pizzalicious	14 chips (1 oz)	160	1	11	0	14	1	200
Ranch	14 chips (1 oz)	150	2	10	0	15	1	130
Salt & Vinegar	14 chips (1 oz)	160	1	11	0	15	1	200
Sour Cream & Onion	14 chips (1 oz)	160	2	10	0	15	1	135
Robert's American Gourmet								
Spirulina Spirals	1 oz	120	2	2	0	22	3	110
Ruffles								
Baked	10 (1 oz)	110	2	2	0	23	2	180
Baked Cheddar & Sour Cream	9 (1 oz)	120	2	3	0	21	2	270
Buffalo Style	11 chips (1 oz)	160	2	10	0	16	1	230
Cheddar & Sour Cream	11 chips (1 oz)	160	2	10	0	14	1	190
French Onion	11 (1 oz)	150	2	10	0	15	1	190
MC Masterpiece Mesquite BBQ	11 (1 oz)	150	1	10	0	15	1	190
Original	12 chips (1 oz)	150	2	10	0	14	1	180

FOOD	PORTION	CAL	PROT	FAT	CHOL	CARB	FIBER	SOD
Ranch	13 (1 oz)	150	2	9	0	15	1	280
Reduced Fat	16 (1 oz)	130	2	7	0	18	1	130
The Works	12 (1 oz)	160	2	11	0	14	1	210
Wow Cheddar & Sour Cream	15 (1 oz)	75	3	0	0	16	1	230
Wow Original	17 (1 oz)	75	2	0	0	17	1	200
Santitas								
100% White Corn	6 (1 oz)	130	2	6	0	19	1	110
Restaurant Style Chips	7 (1 oz)	130	2	6	0	19	1	110
Restaurant Style Strips	10 (1 oz)	130	2	6	0	19	1	110
Snyder's Of Hanover								
BBQ Rib	1 oz	140	2	7	0	17	tr	290
Barbeque Corn	1.5 oz	230	3	14	0	22	2	350
Cheddar Bacon	1 oz	150	2	6	0	20	3	270
Corn Chips	1.5 oz	230	3	15	0	22	2	220
Grilled Steak & Onion	1 oz	140	2	6	0	20	4	140
Hot Buffalo	1 oz	150	2	7	0	20	4	330
Kosher Dill	1 oz	140	2	6	0	20	3	360
No Salt	1 oz	140	2	6	0	19	3	0
Potato	1 oz	140	2	6	0	19	3	90
Ripple	1 oz	140	2	6	0	18	4	100
Salt & Vinegar	1 oz	140	2	6	0	19	4	150
Sausage Pizza	1 oz	150	2	6	0	20	4	250
Sour Cream & Onion	1 oz	150	2	7	0	19	4	150
Tasty Veggie Potato Chips	1 oz	150	3	6	0	20	4	260
Tortilla Nacho	1 oz	140	2	7	0	19	1	130
Tortilla No Salt Yellow Corn	1 oz	140	2	6	0	19	1	0
Tortilla White Corn	1 oz	140	2	6	0	20	1	130
Tortilla Yellow Corn	1 oz	140	2	6	0	19	1	130
Tortilla Yellow Corn Mini	1 oz	160	2	8	0	20	1	130
Soya King								
Soy Mongolian BBQ	23 chips (1 oz)	140	1	7	0	19	3	115
Soy Original	23 chips (1 oz)	140	1	7	0	19	3	115

FOOD	PORTION	CAL	PROT	FAT	CHOL	CARB	FIBER	SOD
Soy Sour Cream & Onion	23 chips (1 oz)	140	1	7	0	19	3	115
Soy Taco	23 chips (1 oz)	140	1	7	0	19	3	115
Sunchips								
French Onion	13 (1 oz)	140	2	7	0	18	2	115
Harvest Cheddar	13 (1 oz)	140	2	6	0	19	2	115
Original	14 (1 oz)	140	2	6	0	19	2	115
Torengos								
Chips	13 chips (1 oz)	140	2	9	0	15	1	150
Tostitos								
Baked Bite Size	20 (1 oz)	110	3	1	0	24	2	200
Baked Bite Size Salsa & Cream Cheese	16 (1 oz)	120	2	3	0	21	1	190
Baked Original	13 (1 oz)	110	3	1	3	21	1	200
Bite Size	15 (1 oz)	140	2	8	0	17	1	110
Crispy Rounds	13 (1 oz)	150	2	8	0	17	1	85
Nacho Style	6 (1 oz)	140	2	6	0	19	1	100
Restaurant Style	7 (1 oz)	140	2	6	0	19	1	110
Restaurant Style Hint Of Lime	6 (1 oz)	140	2	6	0	19	1	160
Santa Fe Gold	7 (1 oz)	140	2	6	0	19	1	80
Wow Original	6 (1 oz)	90	2	1	0	20	1	105
Tyson								
Tortilla Salted	13 (1 oz)	150	2	7	0	20	2	65
Tortilla Yellow Corn Salted	13 (1 oz)	150	2	7	0	20	2	65
Utz								
Baked Crisps	12 (1 oz)	110	2	2	0	23	2	180
Carolina Barbeque	20 (1 oz)	150	2	9	0	14	1	270
Cheddar & Sour Cream	20 (1 oz)	160	2	10	0	14	1	200
Corn Chips	24 (1 oz)	160	2	10	0	16	1	160
Corn Chips Barbecue	24 (1 oz)	160	2	10	0	16	1	180
Grandma	20 (1 oz)	140	2	8	5	14	1	120
Grandma BBQ	20 (1 oz)	140	2	8	5	15	1	240
Home Style Kettle	20 (1 oz)	140	2	8	0	14	1	120
Home Style Kettle BBQ	20 (1 oz)	140	2	8	0	15	1	240

FOOD	PORTION	CAL	PROT	FAT	CHOL	CARB	FIBER	SOD
Kettle Classics Crunchy	20 (1 oz)	150	2	9	0	15	1	95
Kettle Classics Crunchy Mesquite BBQ	20 (1 oz)	150	2	9	0	15	1	200
No Salt Added	20 (1 oz)	150	2	9	0	14	1	5
Onion & Garlic	20 (1 oz)	150	2	9	0	14	1	180
Potato	20 (1 oz)	150	2	9	0	14	1	95
Reduced Fat BBQ	22 (1 oz)	140	2	6	0	19	1	190
Reducted Fat Ripple	24 (1 oz)	140	2	7	0	18	1	120
Ripple	20 (1 oz)	150	2	10	0	14	1	95
Ripple Sour Cream & Onion	20 (1 oz)	160	2	10	0	14	1	140
Ripple Barbeque	20 (1 oz)	150	2	10	0	14	1	200
Salt'N Vinegar	20 (1 oz)	150	2	9	0	14	1	270
The Crab Chip	20 (1 oz)	150	2	9	0	14	1	300
Tortilla Black Bean & Salsa	13 (1 oz)	150	2	7	0	19	1	230
Tortilla Low Fat Baked	10 (1 oz)	120	2	2	0	24	2	200
Tortilla Nacho	13 (1 oz)	150	2	8	0	19	1	200
Tortilla Restaurant Style	6 (1 oz)	140	2	7	0	18	1	120
Tortilla Spicy Nacho	13 (1 oz)	150	2	8	0	19	1	220
Tortilla White Corn	12 (1 oz)	140	2	7	0	18	1	120
Wavy	20 chips (1 oz)	150	2	9	0	14	1	95
Yes! Fat Free	20 (1 oz)	75	2	0	0	17	1	180
Yes! Fat Free Barbeque	20 (1 oz)	75	2	0	0	16	1	210
Yes! Fat Free Ripple	20 (1 oz)	75	2	0	0	17	1	180
Wise								
Dipsy Doodles	1 pkg (1.5 oz)	240	2	15	0	24	1	270
Wow								
Tortilla Nacho Cheese	11 (1 oz)	90	2	1	0	18	1	240

CHITTERLINGS

FOOD	PORTION	CAL	PROT	FAT	CHOL	CARB	FIBER	SOD
pork cooked	3 oz	258	9	24	122	0	0	33

FOOD	PORTION	CAL	PROT	FAT	CHOL	CARB	FIBER	SOD
CHIVES								
freeze-dried	1 tbsp	1	tr	tr	0	tr	–	–
fresh chopped	1 tbsp	1	tr	tr	0	tr	–	0
fresh chopped	1 tsp	0	tr	tr	0	tr	–	0
CHOCOLATE *(see also* CANDY, CAROB, COCOA, ICE CREAM TOPPINGS, MILK DRINKS*)*								
BAKING								
baking	1 oz	145	3	15	0	8	–	1
grated unsweetened	1 cup (4.6 oz)	690	14	73	0	37	18	18
liquid unsweetened	1 oz	134	3	14	0	10	–	3
squares unsweetened	1 square (1 oz)	148	3	16	0	8	4	4
Baker's								
Bittersweet	½ square (0.5 oz)	70	1	6	0	7	1	0
German's Sweet	2 squares (0.5 oz)	60	1	4	0	8	tr	0
Semi-Sweet	½ square (0.5 oz)	70	1	5	0	8	1	0
Unsweetened	½ square (0.5 oz)	70	2	7	0	4	2	0
White	½ square (0.5 oz)	80	1	5	<5	8	0	15
Nestle								
Choco Bake	½ oz	80	1	8	0	5	2	0
Premier White Bar	½ oz	80	1	5	<5	8	0	15
Premier White Morsels	1 tbsp	80	tr	4	0	9	0	20
Semi-Sweet Bar	½ oz	70	<1	4	0	9	tr	0
Unsweetened Bar	½ oz	80	2	7	0	4	2	0
CHIPS								
milk chocolate	1 cup (6 oz)	862	12	52	38	100	–	138
semisweet	1 cup (6 oz)	804	7	50	0	106	–	19
semisweet	60 pieces (1 oz)	136	1	9	0	18	–	3
Baker's								
Real Milk Chocolate	½ oz	70	1	4	0	9	0	10
Real Semi-Sweet	½ oz	60	1	4	0	9	1	0
Semi-Sweet	½ oz	70	0	4	0	10	0	15
Hershey								
Almond Joy Bits	1 tbsp (0.5 oz)	60	tr	4	0	7	–	0
Chocolate & Peanut Butter Chips	1 tbsp (0.5 oz)	70	tr	3	0	10	–	40
Holiday Baking Bits	1 tbsp (0.5 oz)	70	tr	3	0	11	–	0
Milk Chocolate	1 tbsp (0.5 oz)	80	1	5	<5	9	–	10
Mini Kisses For Baking	11 pieces (0.5 oz)	80	1	5	<5	9	–	15

FOOD	PORTION	CAL	PROT	FAT	CHOL	CARB	FIBER	SOD
Mint Chocolate	1 tbsp (0.5 oz)	80	tr	4	0	10	–	0
Premier White Milk Chips	1 tbsp (0.5 oz)	80	1	4	0	9	–	30
Raspberry Chips	1 tbsp (0.5 oz)	80	tr	4	0	10	–	0
Semi-Sweet	1 tbsp (0.5 oz)	80	tr	4	0	10	–	0
Semi-Sweet Mini	1 tbsp (0.5 oz)	80	tr	4	0	10	–	0
Skor English Toffee Baking Bits	1 tbsp (0.5 oz)	70	0	5	10	7	–	60
M&M's								
Baking Bits Milk Chocolate	0.5 oz	70	7	3	5	10	0	0
Baking Bits Semi-Sweet	0.5 oz	70	1	4	0	9	1	0
Nestle								
Crunch Baking Pieces	1½ tbsp	80	tr	4	0	10	0	25
Milk Chocolate Morsels	1 tbsp	70	tr	4	<5	9	0	0
Mint Chocolate Morsels	1 tbsp	70	tr	4	0	9	tr	0
Morsels Semi-Sweet	1 tbsp	70	tr	4	0	9	tr	0
Semi-Sweet Mega Morsels	1 tbsp	70	tr	4	0	9	tr	0
Semi-Sweet Mini Morsels	1 tbsp	70	tr	4	0	9	tr	0
Toll House								
Mint-Chocolate	2 tbsp (1.5 oz)	130	1	3	0	25	1	30
Semi-Sweet	2 tbsp (1.5 oz)	130	1	4	0	24	1	30
MIX								
powder	2–3 heaping tsp	75	1	1	0	20	–	45
powder as prep w/ whole milk	9 oz	226	9	9	33	31	–	165
Quik								
Chocolate Powder	2 tbsp (0.8 oz)	90	1	1	0	19	1	30
Chocolate Powder No Sugar	2 tbsp (0.4 oz)	40	1	1	0	7	2	45

CHOCOLATE MILK *(see CHOCOLATE, COCOA, MILK DRINKS, MILKSHAKE)*

CHOCOLATE SYRUP

chocolate fudge	1 tbsp (0.7 oz)	73	1	3	–	12	–	27
chocolate fudge	1 cup (11.9 oz)	1176	15	46	–	200	–	442

FOOD	PORTION	CAL	PROT	FAT	CHOL	CARB	FIBER	SOD
syrup	1 cup	653	6	3	0	177	–	287
syrup	2 tbsp	82	1	tr	0	22	–	36
syrup as prep w/ whole milk	9 oz	232	9	9	33	34	–	156
Estee								
Chocolate	2 tbsp	15	tr	0	0	5	0	40
Hershey								
Chocolate Fudge	1 tbsp (0.7 oz)	70	tr	3	<5	10	–	25
Chocolate Malt	2 tbsp (1.4 oz)	100	tr	0	0	25	–	55
Lite	2 tbsp (1.2 oz)	50	0	0	0	12	–	35
Syrup	2 tbsp (1.4 oz)	100	1	0	0	24	–	25
Quik								
Chocolate	2 tbsp (1.3 oz)	100	1	1	0	23	tr	30
Smucker's								
Plate Scapers Chocolate	2 tbsp	100	1	5	–	23	1	20
Toll House								
Mint Chocolate	2 tbsp (1.5 oz)	130	1	3	0	25	1	30
Semi-Sweet	2 tbsp (1.5 oz)	130	1	4	0	24	1	30
CHUTNEY								
apple	1.2 oz	68	tr	0	–	18	1	–
apple cranberry	1 tbsp	16	tr	0	0	4	–	1
coconut	¼ cup	74	1	7	0	4	2	5
mango	1 tbsp	54	tr	2	0	10	tr	207
tomato	1 tbsp	32	tr	tr	0	8	tr	26
Sonoma								
Dried Tomato	1 tbsp (0.7 g)	35	0	0	0	9	0	0
CILANTRO								
fresh	1 tsp (2 g)	tr	tr	tr	0	tr	tr	1
fresh	1 cup (1.6 oz)	11	1	tr	0	2	1	25
CINNAMON								
ground	1 tsp	6	tr	tr	0	2	–	1
sticks	0.5 oz	39	1	tr	–	8	3	4
CISCO								
raw	3 oz	84	16	2	–	0	–	47
smoked	3 oz	151	14	10	27	0	–	409
smoked	1 oz	50	5	3	9	0	–	135

FOOD	PORTION	CAL	PROT	FAT	CHOL	CARB	FIBER	SOD
CLAMS								
CANNED								
liquid only	3 oz	2	tr	tr	—	tr	—	183
liquid only	1 cup	6	1	tr	—	tr	—	516
meat only	1 cup	236	41	3	107	8	—	179
meat only	3 oz	126	22	2	57	4	—	95
Bumble Bee								
Baby	2 oz	50	9	1	40	2	0	270
Progresso								
Creamy Clam Sauce	½ cup (4.2 oz)	110	5	6	10	8	0	440
Minced	¼ cup (2.1 oz)	25	4	0	10	2	0	250
Red Clam Sauce	½ cup (4.4 oz)	60	4	1	10	8	1	350
White Clam Sauce	½ cup (4.4 oz)	150	9	10	20	5	0	710
FRESH								
cooked	3 oz	126	22	2	57	4	—	95
cooked	20 sm	133	23	2	60	5	—	100
raw	3 oz	63	11	1	29	2	—	47
raw	9 lg (6.3 oz)	133	23	2	60	5	—	100
raw	20 sm (6.3 oz)	133	23	2	60	5	—	100
TAKE-OUT								
breaded & fried	20 sm	379	27	21	115	19	—	684
CLOVES								
ground	1 tsp	7	tr	tr	0	1	—	5
COCOA								
hot cocoa	1 cup	218	9	9	33	26	—	123
mix as prep w/ water	7 oz	103	3	1	—	23	—	149
mix w/ equal as prep w/ water	7 oz	48	4	tr	—	9	—	173
powder unsweetened	1 tbsp (5 g)	11	1	1	0	3	2	1
powder unsweetened	1 cup (3 oz)	197	17	12	0	47	29	18
Carnation								
Hot Cocoa 70 Calorie	1 pkg (0.7 oz)	70	3	0	0	15	tr	140
Hot Cocoa Double Chocolate Meltdown	1 pkg (1.2 oz)	150	2	4	0	27	1	170
Hot Cocoa Fat Free Raspberry	1 pkg (0.3 oz)	30	2	0	0	4	1	150
Hot Cocoa Fat Free w/ Marshmallows	1 pkg (0.4 oz)	45	7	0	0	10	tr	100

FOOD	PORTION	CAL	PROT	FAT	CHOL	CARB	FIBER	SOD
Hot Cocoa Lactose Free	1 pkg (1 oz)	120	1	2	0	25	1	115
Hot Cocoa Marshmallow Blizzard	1 pkg (1.5 oz)	180	2	2	<5	39	tr	140
Hot Cocoa Milk Chocolate	3 tbsp (1 oz)	110	2	1	<5	24	tr	95
Hot Cocoa Rich Chocolate	3 tbsp (1 oz)	110	1	1	<5	24	tr	100
Hot Cocoa Rich Chocolate Fat Free	1 pkg (0.3 oz)	25	2	0	0	4	1	135
Hot Cocoa Rich Chocolate No Sugar Added	3 tbsp (0.5 oz)	50	4	0	<5	8	tr	140
Hot Cocoa Rich Chocolate w/ Marshmallows	3 tbsp (1 oz)	110	1	1	<5	24	tr	95
Hershey								
Cocoa	1 tbsp (5 g)	20	1	1	0	3	–	0
European Cocoa	1 tbsp (5 g)	20	1	1	0	3	–	0
Nestle								
Cocoa	1 tbsp	15	1	1	0	3	1	0
Hot Cocoa Rich Chocolate	1 pkg (1 oz)	110	1	1	0	24	tr	60
Hot Cocoa Rich w/ Marshmallows	1 pkg (1 oz)	110	1	1	0	24	tr	60
Swiss Miss								
Hot Cocoa And Cream	1 serv	153	2	5	6	25	1	159
Hot Cocoa Chocolate Sensation	1 serv	148	2	4	tr	27	1	171
Hot Cocoa Diet	1 serv	22	2	tr	tr	4	1	185
Hot Cocoa Fat Free	1 serv	52	4	tr	0	9	1	185
Hot Cocoa Fat Free Marshmallow Lovers	1 serv	65	3	tr	0	13	1	155
Hot Cocoa Lite	1 serv	76	2	1	0	18	2	177
Hot Cocoa Marshmallow Lovers	1 serv	142	2	3	2	27	1	152

FOOD	PORTION	CAL	PROT	FAT	CHOL	CARB	FIBER	SOD
Hot Cocoa Milk Chocolate	1 serv	118	1	3	1	22	1	118
Hot Cocoa Milk Chocolate No Sugar Added	1 serv	55	2	1	1	10	1	164
Hot Cocoa Milk Chocolate w/ Marshmallows	1 serv	118	1	3	tr	22	1	123
Hot Cocoa Rich Chocolate	1 serv	110	2	2	1	23	1	140
Hot Cocoa White Chocolate	1 serv	109	3	1	1	21	tr	128
Hot Cocoa w/ Marshmallows No Sugar Added	1 serv	56	3	1	1	10	1	146
Premiere Hot Cocoa Almond Mocha	1 serv	144	2	3	1	28	1	207
Premiere Hot Cocoa English Toffee	1 serv	142	2	2	1	29	4	223
Premiere Hot Cocoa Raspberry Truffle	1 serv	144	2	3	1	28	1	220
Premiere Hot Cocoa Suisse Truffle	1 serv	142	2	2	1	28	1	225
Rich Hot Cocoa No Sugar Added	1 serv	54	2	1	1	10	1	165
Sidewalk Cafe Cappuccino	1 serv	119	3	4	1	18	1	35
Sidewalk Cafe Cinnamon	1 serv	126	3	4	1	21	1	46
Sidewalk Cafe French Vanilla	1 serv	121	3	4	1	19	tr	32
Sidewalk Cafe Mocha	1 serv	120	3	4	1	20	1	43
Weight Watchers								
Hot Cocoa Mix as prep	1 pkg	70	6	0	0	7	1	160

COCONUT

FOOD	PORTION	CAL	PROT	FAT	CHOL	CARB	FIBER	SOD
coconut water	1 tbsp	3	tr	tr	0	1	—	16
coconut water	1 cup	46	2	tr	0	9	—	252

FOOD	PORTION	CAL	PROT	FAT	CHOL	CARB	FIBER	SOD
cream canned	1 cup	568	8	52	0	25	–	149
cream canned	1 tbsp	36	1	3	0	2	–	10
dried sweetened flaked	7 oz pkg	944	7	64	0	95	–	509
dried sweetened flaked	1 cup	351	2	24	0	35	–	189
dried sweetened flaked canned	1 cup	341	3	24	0	32	–	15
dried sweetened shredded	7 oz pkg	997	6	71	0	95	–	522
dried sweetened shredded	1 cup	466	2	33	0	44	–	244
dried toasted	1 oz	168	2	13	0	13	–	11
dried unsweetened	1 oz	187	2	18	0	7	–	11
fresh	1 piece (1.5 oz)	159	2	15	0	7	4	9
fresh shredded	1 cup	283	3	27	0	12	7	16
milk canned	1 tbsp	30	tr	3	0	tr	–	2
milk canned	1 cup	445	5	48	0	6	–	29
milk frozen	1 tbsp	30	tr	3	0	1	–	2
milk frozen	1 cup	486	4	50	0	13	–	29
Baker's								
Angel Flake	1 tbsp (0.5 oz)	70	1	5	0	6	1	45
Angel Flake (canned)	2 tbsp (0.5 oz)	70	1	6	0	6	1	0
Premium Shred	2 tbsp (0.5 oz)	70	1	5	0	6	1	45

COD

FOOD	PORTION	CAL	PROT	FAT	CHOL	CARB	FIBER	SOD
atlantic canned	3 oz	89	19	1	47	0	–	185
atlantic canned	1 can (11 oz)	327	71	3	171	0	–	680
atlantic dried	3 oz	246	53	2	129	0	–	5973
atlantic fresh cooked	1 fillet (6.3 oz)	189	41	2	99	0	–	141
atlantic fresh cooked	3 oz	89	19	1	47	0	–	66
atlantic fresh raw	3 oz	70	15	1	37	0	–	46
pacific fresh baked	3 oz	95	21	1	43	0	–	82
roe canned	1 oz	34	6	1	–	tr	–	–
roe baked w/ butter & lemon juice	1 oz	36	6	1	–	tr	–	21
roe raw	1 oz	37	7	tr	103	tr	–	–
roe tarama	3.5 oz	547	8	55	–	6	–	600
Van De Kamp's								
Lightly Breaded Fillets	1 (4 oz)	220	14	10	35	19	0	410

FOOD	PORTION	CAL	PROT	FAT	CHOL	CARB	FIBER	SOD
COFFEE *(see also* COFFEE BEVERAGES, COFFEE SUBSTITUTES*)*								
INSTANT								
decaffeinated	1 rounded tsp (1.8 g)	4	tr	0	0	1	–	0
decaffeinated as prep	6 oz	4	tr	0	0	1	–	6
regular	1 rounded tsp	4	tr	0	0	1	–	1
regular as prep	6 oz	4	tr	0	0	1	–	6
regular w/ chicory	1 rounded tsp	6	tr	0	0	1	–	5
regular w/ chicory as prep	6 oz	6	tr	0	0	1	–	10
Nescafe								
Decafe	1 tsp (2 g)	0	tr	0	0	tr	0	0
Decafe w/ Chicory	1 tsp (2 g)	0	tr	0	0	tr	0	0
French Vanilla	1 tsp (2 g)	5	0	0	0	1	0	0
French Vanilla Decaf	1 tsp (2 g)	5	0	0	0	1	0	0
Hazelnut	1 tsp (2 g)	5	0	0	0	1	0	0
Irish Creme	1 tsp (2 g)	5	0	0	0	1	0	0
Regular	1 tsp (2 g)	0	tr	0	0	tr	0	0
With Chicory	1 tsp (2 g)	5	0	0	0	1	0	0
REGULAR								
brewed	6 oz	4	tr	0	0	1	–	4
roasted beans	1 oz	64	4	4	–	18	2	–
Folgers								
Colombian Supreme	1 tbsp	16	tr	tr	0	3	–	tr
Custom Roast	1 tbsp	16	tr	tr	0	3	–	tr
Decaffeinated	1 tbsp	17	1	tr	0	3	–	tr
French Roast	1 tbsp	16	tr	tr	0	3	–	tr
Gourmet Supreme	1 tbsp	16	tr	tr	0	3	–	tr
Instant	1 tsp	8	tr	tr	0	1	–	1
Instant Decaffeinated	1 tsp	8	tr	tr	0	2	–	2
Singles	1 bag	21	1	tr	0	4	–	1
Singles Decaffeinated	1 bag	21	1	tr	0	4	–	2
Special Roast	1 tbsp	16	tr	tr	0	3	–	tr
Vacuum Pack	1 tbsp	16	tr	tr	0	3	–	tr
Maryland Club								
Ground	1 tbsp	16	tr	tr	0	3	–	tr
Nescafe								
Cafe Mocha	1 can (10 oz)	140	3	3	10	27	1	115
Caffe Latte	1 can (10 oz)	130	3	3	15	22	1	130
Caffe Latte Decaffeinated	1 can (10 oz)	130	3	3	15	22	0	100

FOOD	PORTION	CAL	PROT	FAT	CHOL	CARB	FIBER	SOD
Espresso	1 tsp (2 g)	0	tr	0	0	tr	0	0
Espresso Cafe Latte	1 pkg (0.6 oz)	70	3	2	10	10	0	50
Espresso Cafe Mocha	1 pkg (1 oz)	110	3	3	10	20	1	35
Espresso Cappuccino	1 pkg (0.6 oz)	80	3	3	10	11	0	40
Espresso Roast	1 can (10 oz)	90	1	1	<5	21	0	75
French Vanilla	1 can (10 oz)	150	4	4	15	25	2	140
Hazelnut	1 can (10 oz)	130	3	3	15	22	0	100
Roasted Ground Decaffeinated as prep	1 cup (6 oz)	0	tr	0	0	tr	0	0
Roasted Ground as prep	1 cup (6 oz)	0	tr	0	0	tr	0	0
TAKE-OUT								
cafe au lait	1 cup (8 fl oz)	77	4	4	17	6	–	62
cafe brulot	1 cup (4.8 fl oz)	48	tr	0	0	3	–	2
cappuccino	1 cup (8 fl oz)	77	4	4	17	6	–	62
coffee con leche	1 cup (8 fl oz)	77	4	4	17	6	–	62
espresso	1 cup (3 fl oz)	2	tr	0	0	tr	–	2
irish coffee	1 serv (9 fl oz)	107	1	3	12	3	–	25
latte w/ skim milk	13 oz	88	8	tr	4	12	0	128
latte w/ whole milk	13 oz	152	8	8	33	12	0	122
mocha	1 mug (9.6 fl oz)	202	3	15	40	17	–	28

COFFEE BEVERAGES

FOOD	PORTION	CAL	PROT	FAT	CHOL	CARB	FIBER	SOD
cappuccino mix as prep	7 oz	62	tr	2	–	11	–	104
french mix as prep	7 oz	57	1	3	–	7	–	–
mocha mix as prep	7 oz	51	1	2	–	8	–	36
Arizona								
Iced Latte Supreme	8 oz	110	3	2	6	21	1	95
Iced Mocha Latte	8 oz	110	4	2	5	21	1	98
Chock full o'Nuts								
New York Cappuccino French Vanilla	1 pkg (0.9 oz)	90	2	2	0	19	0	115
New York Cappuccino Hazelnut	1 pkg. (0.9 oz)	90	2	2	0	19	0	115
Coffee House USA								
All Flavors	1 bottle (9.5 oz)	100	4	4	15	29	tr	160

FOOD	PORTION	CAL	PROT	FAT	CHOL	CARB	FIBER	SOD
Gehl's								
Iced Cappuccino	1 can (11 oz)	190	11	2	13	33	0	330
General Foods								
International Coffee Sugar Free Cafe Vienna as prep	1 serv (8 oz)	30	tr	2	0	3	0	75
International Coffees Cafe Francais as prep	1 serv (8 oz)	60	tr	4	0	7	0	95
International Coffees Cafe Vienna as prep	1 serv (8 oz)	70	tr	3	0	11	tr	110
International Coffees French Vanilla Cafe as prep	1 serv (8 oz)	60	tr	3	0	10	0	55
International Coffees Hazelnut Belgain Cafe as prep	1 serv (8 oz)	70	tr	2	0	12	0	60
International Coffees Irish Creme Cafe as prep	1 serv (8 oz)	60	tr	2	0	10	0	45
International Coffees Kahlua Cafe as prep	1 serv (8 oz)	60	tr	2	0	10	0	55
International Coffees Suisse Mocha as prep	1 serv (8 oz)	60	tr	2	0	8	0	35
Maxwell House								
Cafe Cappuccino Amaretto as prep	1 serv (8 oz)	90	1	1	0	19	0	65
Cafe Cappuccino Decaffeinated Mocha as prep	1 serv (8 oz)	100	2	3	0	17	0	70
Cafe Cappuccino Decaffeinated Vanilla as prep	1 serv (8 oz)	90	1	1	0	19	0	65
Cafe Cappuccino Irish Cream as prep	1 serv (8 oz)	90	1	1	0	19	0	65

FOOD	PORTION	CAL	PROT	FAT	CHOL	CARB	FIBER	SOD
Cafe Cappuccino Mocha as prep	1 serv (8 oz)	100	2	3	0	17	0	65
Cafe Cappuccino Sugar Free Mocha as prep	1 serv (8 oz)	60	1	3	0	7	tr	80
Cafe Cappuccino Sugar Free Vanilla as prep	1 serv (8 oz)	60	tr	3	0	7	0	85
Iced Cappuccino as prep w/ 2% milk	1 serv (8 oz)	180	8	5	20	27	tr	125
Starbucks								
Frappuccino	1 bottle (9.5 fl oz)	190	6	3	12	39	0	110

COFFEE SUBSTITUTES

powder	1 tsp	9	tr	tr	0	2	–	2
powder as prep	6 oz	9	tr	tr	0	2	–	7
powder as prep w/ milk	6 oz	121	6	6	25	10	–	91
Natural Touch								
Kaffree Roma	1 tsp (2 g)	10	0	0	0	2	0	0
Roma Cappuccino	3 tbsp (0.4 oz)	50	1	3	0	5	0	15
Pero								
Instant Grain Beverage	1 tsp (1.5 g)	5	0	0	0	1	–	0
Postum								
Instant Coffee Flavor as prep	1 serv (8 oz)	10	0	0	0	3	0	0
Instant as prep	1 serv (8 oz)	10	0	0	0	3	0	0

COFFEE WHITENERS *(see also* MILK SUBSTITUTES*)*

liquid nondairy frzn	1 tbsp (0.5 oz)	20	tr	2	0	2	–	12
powder nondairy	1 tsp	11	tr	tr	0	1	–	4
N-Rich								
Coffee Creamer	1 tsp (2 g)	10	tr	1	0	1	0	4

COLESLAW
TAKE-OUT

coleslaw w/ dressing	½ cup	42	1	2	5	7	–	14
vinegar & oil coleslaw	3.5 oz	150	1	9	0	16	–	480

FOOD	PORTION	CAL	PROT	FAT	CHOL	CARB	FIBER	SOD
COLLARDS								
fresh cooked	½ cup	17	1	tr	0	4	–	10
frzn chopped cooked	½ cup	31	3	tr	0	6	–	42
raw chopped	½ cup	6	tr	tr	0	1	–	4
Birds Eye								
Chopped Greens frzn	1 cup (3.1 oz)	30	2	0	0	2	2	20
COOKIES								
MIX								
chocolate chip	1 (0.56 oz)	79	1	4	7	10	–	47
Betty Crocker								
Chocolate Peanut Butter as prep	1 bar	180	2	9	18	25	–	150
Date Bar as prep	1 bar	150	1	6	0	23	1	30
Oatmeal as prep	2	150	2	6	12	22	1	100
GoldnBrown								
Fat Free	1 (1.1 oz)	120	2	0	0	27	0	135
READY-TO-EAT								
animal	11 crackers (1 oz)	126	2	4	–	21	–	112
animal crackers	1 (2.5 g)	11	tr	tr	–	2	–	10
australian anzac biscuit	1	98	1	3	0	17	1	59
cream cheese	1 (1.1 oz)	141	2	9	25	14	tr	53
digestive biscuits plain	2	141	2	7	–	21	1	–
fortune	1 (0.28 oz)	30	tr	tr	–	7	tr	22
graham	1 square (0.24 oz)	30	1	1	0	5	–	42
graham chocolate covered	1 (0.49 oz)	68	1	3	0	9	–	41
hermits	1 (1 oz)	117	2	5	23	18	1	54
jumbles coconut	1 (1 oz)	121	1	7	26	13	1	19
ladyfingers	1 (0.38 oz)	40	1	1	40	7	–	16
macaroons	1 (0.8 oz)	97	1	3	0	17	–	59
madeleines	1 (0.8 oz)	86	2	5	46	10	tr	34
marshmallow chocolate coated	1 (0.46 oz)	55	1	2	–	9	–	22
merinque	1 (0.3 oz)	20	tr	0	0	5	0	20
neapolitan tri-color cookie	1 (0.6 oz)	79	1	5	17	8	tr	10

FOOD	PORTION	CAL	PROT	FAT	CHOL	CARB	FIBER	SOD
pinenut cookies	1 (1.1 oz)	134	4	9	0	11	1	11
reginette queen'a biscuit	1 (0.8 oz)	86	2	3	tr	13	tr	83
spritz	1 (0.4 oz)	42	1	2	6	6	tr	9
toll house original	1 (0.8 oz)	105	2	6	15	13	tr	57
zeppole	1 (0.8 oz)	78	1	6	24	6	tr	14
Alternative Baking								
Vegan Chocolate Chip	1 serv (2.5 oz)	280	3	10	0	46	1	150
Vegan Expresso Chocolate Chip	1 serv (2 oz)	230	3	9	0	35	1	125
Vegan Lemon	1 serv (2.25 oz)	250	3	7	0	42	1	170
Vegan Oatmeal	1 serv (2.25 oz)	250	5	10	0	35	2	105
Vegan Peanut Butter	1 serv (2.25 oz)	270	5	10	0	40	1	115
Vegan Pumpkin	1 serv (2 oz)	200	2	6	0	35	1	120
Vegan Wheat Free Choco Cherry Chunk	1 serv (1.75 oz)	190	3	6	0	32	1	30
Vegan Wheat Free Hula Nut	1 serv (1.75 oz)	190	6	6	0	29	2	65
Vegan Wheat Free P-nut Fudge Fusion	1 serv (1.75 oz)	190	4	7	0	29	1	75
Vegan Wheat Free Snickerdoodle	1 serv (1.75 oz)	170	3	3	0	35	1	70
Amay's								
Chinese Style Almond	1 (0.5 oz)	80	1	4	4	10	0	13
Archway								
Alpine Fudge	1 (1.3 oz)	160	1	6	<5	24	tr	80
Carrot Cake	1 (1 oz)	130	1	5	5	19	0	200
Chocolate Chip	1 (0.9 oz)	120	tr	6	5	16	0	85
Chocolate Chip Sugar Free	1 (0.8 oz)	110	1	5	0	16	0	65
Coconut Macaroon	2 (1.4 oz)	180	1	11	0	21	1	500
Devils Food Chocolate Drop Fat Free	1 (0.7 oz)	60	1	0	0	15	0	70
Dutch Cocoa	1 (0.9 oz)	100	1	4	0	18	0	65
Frosty Lemon	1 (0.9 oz)	100	tr	4	0	16	0	100
Fruit & Honey Bar	1 (0.9 oz)	110	1	3	5	19	0	100
Fruit Bar Fat Free	1 (0.9 oz)	90	tr	0	0	21	0	90

FOOD	PORTION	CAL	PROT	FAT	CHOL	CARB	FIBER	SOD
Ginger Snaps	5 (1 oz)	120	1	5	0	20	0	150
Homestyle Chocolate Chip	3 (1 oz)	130	1	7	5	17	1	60
Iced Spice	1 (1 oz)	120	1	5	0	19	0	140
Oatmeal	1 (0.9 oz)	100	1	4	5	16	0	100
Oatmeal Apple Filled	1 (0.9 oz)	90	1	3	<5	16	0	70
Oatmeal Pecan	1 (0.9 oz)	110	1	4	5	16	1	120
Oatmeal Raisin Bran	1 (0.9 oz)	100	1	3	0	18	1	65
Oatmeal Raspberry Fat Free	1 (1.1 oz)	100	1	0	0	23	1	170
Oatmeal Sugar Free	1 (0.8 oz)	110	1	5	0	16	0	75
Oatmeal Raisin	1 (0.9 oz)	100	1	4	0	17	1	65
Oatmeal Raisin Fat Free	1 (1.1 oz)	100	1	0	0	24	1	60
Old Dutch Apple	1 (0.9 oz)	110	1	4	5	18	0	115
Peanut Butter	1 (1 oz)	150	2	9	5	16	0	110
Peanut Butter Fudge	1 (1.3 oz)	220	3	13	<5	23	1	135
Peanut Butter Sugar Free	1 (0.8 oz)	110	2	6	0	14	0	85
Pecan Crunch	3 (1.2 oz)	180	2	10	5	20	0	140
Raspberry Filled	1 (0.8 oz)	90	1	4	5	15	0	80
Rocky Road	1 (0.8 oz)	110	1	5	10	16	0	70
Rocky Road Sugar Free	1 (0.8 oz)	100	1	5	0	15	tr	65
Shortbread Sugar Free	1 (0.8 oz)	110	1	5	0	16	0	45
Strawberry Filled	1 (0.8 oz)	90	1	3	0	15	0	80
BP Gourmet								
Biscotti Fat Free Cinnamon Crunch	6 (1 oz)	110	2	0	0	24	0	75
Biscotti Fat Free Vanilla Crunch	4 (1 oz)	80	2	0	0	18	0	25
Chocolate Fudge Chip Sugar Free	5 (1 oz)	100	1	6	0	13	0	80
Dreams Chocolate	7 (1 oz)	120	2	3	0	21	0	35
Dreams Fat Free Chocolate Fudge	13 (1 oz)	100	2	0	0	25	0	35

FOOD	PORTION	CAL	PROT	FAT	CHOL	CARB	FIBER	SOD
Dreams Fat Free Vanilla	19 (1 oz)	100	2	0	0	25	0	35
Tangos Fat Free Chocolate Fudge Chip	4 (1 oz)	100	2	0	0	23	0	95
Bahlsen								
Afrika	8 (1.1 oz)	170	2	10	5	17	2	20
Butter Leaves	7 (1 oz)	140	2	7	15	19	tr	50
Choco Leibniz	2 (1 oz)	140	2	7	5	18	tr	50
Choco Star Dark Chocolate	3 (1.1 oz)	170	2	12	0	16	1	10
Choco Star Milk Chocolate	3 (1.1 oz)	180	2	12	<5	16	1	25
Chocolate Hearts	4 (1 oz)	160	2	9	5	18	1	25
Delice	6 (1 oz)	140	2	6	0	19	tr	100
Deloba	4 (0.9 oz)	130	2	5	0	19	tr	80
Hanover Waffelin	5 (1 oz)	160	1	10	0	16	0	35
Hit Chocolate Vanilla Filled	2 (1 oz)	140	2	8	0	18	tr	75
Hit Vanilla Chocolate Filled	2 (1 oz)	140	2	7	0	19	tr	65
Kipferl	4 (1 oz)	150	2	9	5	16	0	10
Leibniz	6 (1 oz)	130	2	4	10	23	1	125
Nuss Dessert	3 (1.1 oz)	180	2	11	10	19	tr	60
Probiers	6 (1.1 oz)	150	2	6	0	21	tr	60
Twingo	6 (1.1 oz)	170	2	11	0	18	1	15
Waffeletten	4 (1 oz)	160	2	9	<5	18	1	40
Baker's Harvest								
Animal	12 (0.9 oz)	130	2	3	–	22	–	80
Chocolate Graham	2 (0.9 oz)	130	2	3	–	24	1	120
Cinnamon Grahams	2 (0.9 oz)	130	1	5	–	19	tr	85
Cinnamon Grahams Low Fat	2 (0.9 oz)	110	2	2	0	22	1	120
Fig Bars	2 (1.2 oz)	120	tr	3	–	23	1	55
Graham	2 (0.9 oz)	120	1	4	–	21	tr	95
Graham Low Fat	2 (0.9 oz)	110	2	2	0	22	1	120
Iced Oatmeal	1 (0.6 oz)	70	1	3	0	11	0	65
Pecan Shortbread	1 (0.5 oz)	80	1	5	<5	10	0	55
Vanilla Wafers	7 (1.1 oz)	150	1	6	–	22	1	115

FOOD	PORTION	CAL	PROT	FAT	CHOL	CARB	FIBER	SOD
Barbara's Bakery								
Apple Cinnamon Bars Fat Free Whole Wheat	1 (0.7 oz)	60	1	0	0	14	2	20
Chocolate Chip	1 (0.6 oz)	80	1	4	5	10	1	60
Double Dutch Chocolate	1 (0.6 oz)	80	1	4	5	10	1	60
Fig Bars Fat Free Wheat Free	1 (0.7 oz)	60	tr	0	0	15	1	20
Fig Bars Fat Free Whole Wheat	1 (0.7 oz)	60	tr	0	0	16	2	20
Nature's Choice Coconut Almond	1 bar (1 oz)	120	2	5	0	20	1	10
Nature's Choice Expresso Bean	1 bar (1 oz)	120	2	3	0	22	1	10
Nature's Choice Lemon Yogurt	1 bar (1 oz)	120	2	4	0	22	1	10
Nature's Choice Roasted Peanut	1 bar (1 oz)	130	3	5	0	20	1	50
Old Fashioned Oatmeal	1 (0.6 oz)	70	1	3	5	11	1	65
Raspberry Bars Fat Free Wheat Free Raspberry	1 (0.7 oz)	60	1	0	0	15	1	25
Snackimals Chocolate Chip	8 (1 oz)	120	2	5	0	18	1	85
Snackimals Oatmeal Wheat Free	8 (1 oz)	120	2	5	0	19	2	75
Snackimals Vanilla	8 (1 oz)	120	2	5	0	19	1	55
Traditional Blueberry Low Fat	1 (0.7 oz)	60	1	1	0	14	1	25
Traditional Fig Low Fat	1 (0.7 oz)	60	1	1	0	14	1	25
Traditional Shortbread	1 (0.6 oz)	80	1	4	10	10	1	40
Bed & Breakfast								
Cranberry Orange Oatmeal	1 (0.8 oz)	110	1	5	10	17	1	75

FOOD	PORTION	CAL	PROT	FAT	CHOL	CARB	FIBER	SOD
Enrobed Shortbread	2 (1.4 oz)	190	2	9	15	24	1	125
Fruit Center Key Lime	2 (1.1 oz)	140	1	6	<5	22	0	55
Fruit Center Raspberry	2 (1.1 oz)	140	1	6	<5	22	0	55
Beigel's								
Black & White	1 (1 oz)	100	1	3	0	18	0	20
Breaktime								
Chocolate Chip	1 (0.3 oz)	37	tr	2	0	5	tr	37
Coconut	1 (0.3 oz)	35	1	1	0	5	tr	15
Ginger	1 (0.3 oz)	34	tr	1	0	6	—	<15
Oatmeal	1 (0.3 oz)	35	1	1	0	5	tr	27
Sprinkles	1 (0.3 oz)	36	tr	2	0	5	—	46
Brent & Sam's								
Chocolate Chip Pecan	2 (0.5 oz)	80	1	5	<5	9	0	60
Chocolate Chip Raspberry	2 (0.5 oz)	70	tr	4	<5	10	0	60
Chocolate Chips	2 (0.5 oz)	70	1	4	<5	10	0	65
Key Lime White Chocolate	2 (0.5 oz)	70	tr	4	<5	10	0	65
Oatmeal Raisin Pecan	2 (0.5 oz)	70	tr	7	<5	9	1	70
Toffee Pecan	2 (0.5 oz)	80	tr	5	5	9	0	75
White Chocolate Macadamia	2 (0.5 oz)	80	tr	5	<5	9	0	65
Bud's Best								
Caco Creme	7 (1 oz)	140	2	6	0	21	2	110
Chocolate Chip	6 (1 oz)	140	2	6	0	19	1	65
French Vanilla	7 (1 oz)	150	2	6	0	20	2	70
Oatmeal	6 (1 oz)	130	2	5	0	20	tr	65
Cadbury								
Fingers	3	85	1	4	2	11	tr	30
Cafe								
Cinnamony Twists Chocolate Chip	1 (0.5 oz)	40	0	2	0	7	0	25
Sugar Free California Almond	4 (1 oz)	110	2	4	0	17	0	60
Twists Cinnamony	1 (0.3 oz)	40	0	2	0	7	0	25

FOOD	PORTION	CAL	PROT	FAT	CHOL	CARB	FIBER	SOD
Carr's								
Ginger Lemon Cremes	2 (1 oz)	140	1	7	<5	19	tr	105
Carriage Trade								
Finnish Ginger Snaps	3	60	2	7	–	21	tr	135
Chortles								
Cookies	½ pkg. (1 oz)	125	2	3	0	23	1	109
Cookie Lover's								
Chocolate Chip	1 (0.8 oz)	90	1	4	10	16	0	90
Creme Supremes	2 (0.9 oz)	120	1	5	0	18	1	90
Creme Supremes Mint	2 (0.9 oz)	120	1	5	0	18	1	90
Grahams	2 (1 oz)	100	2	1	0	22	1	130
Grahams Cinnamon	2 (1 oz)	110	2	1	0	24	1	130
Peanut Butter	1 (0.8 oz)	100	2	4	15	16	0	55
Shortbread	1 (0.8 oz)	120	2	7	15	13	0	70
Dare								
Blueberry Cheesecake	1 (0.6 oz)	90	1	5	4	11	tr	56
Butter Shortbread	1 (0.5 oz)	63	1	4	6	7	tr	45
Butter Creme	1 (0.6 oz)	85	1	4	2	11	1	96
Carrot Cake	1 (0.6 oz)	92	1	5	3	11	tr	61
Chocolate Chip	1 (0.5 oz)	77	1	4	2	9	tr	42
Chocolate Fudge	1 (0.7 oz)	97	1	5	1	13	1	36
Cinnamon Danish	1 (0.4 oz)	47	1	2	2	7	tr	25
Coconut Creme	1 (0.7 oz)	99	1	5	1	12	tr	42
French Creme	1 (0.5 oz)	80	1	5	1	8	tr	21
Harvest From The Rain Forest	1 (0.5 oz)	70	1	4	2	7	tr	39
Key Lime Creme	1 (0.6 oz)	86	1	4	0	12	tr	69
Lemon Creme	1 (0.7 oz)	95	1	5	1	13	tr	66
Maple Leaf Creme	1 (0.6 oz)	83	1	4	0	12	tr	53
Maple Walnut Fudge	1 (0.7 oz)	99	1	5	0	13	tr	36
Milk Chocolate Fudge	1 (0.7 oz)	99	1	5	1	12	tr	32
Oatmeal Raisin	1 (0.4 oz)	59	1	3	4	8	tr	22
Social Tea	1 (0.2 oz)	26	tr	1	0	4	tr	25
Sun Maid Raisin Oatmeal	1 (0.5 oz)	52	1	3	5	8	tr	30

FOOD	PORTION	CAL	PROT	FAT	CHOL	CARB	FIBER	SOD
De Beukelaer								
Pirouline	8 (1 oz)	130	3	4	15	23	tr	50
Pirouline Viennese Wafers	1 (1 oz)	150	1	7	30	20	tr	25
Delarce								
Chocosprits	1 (0.6 oz)	90	1	5	9	11	tr	50
Marquisettes	3 (0.9 oz)	140	2	7	5	17	1	45
Roules d'Or	4 (1 oz)	180	1	8	0	19	0	35
Dunkaroos								
Chocolate Chip w/ Chocolate Frosting	1 pkg (1 oz)	120	1	5	0	20	tr	100
Cinnamon Graham w/ Vanilla Frosting & Sprinkles	1 pkg (1 oz)	130	1	5	0	21	—	75
Cookies'n Creme	1 pkg (1 oz)	120	1	5	0	20	—	120
Dutch Mill								
Chocolate Chip	3 (1.1 oz)	160	1	10	0	18	1	85
Coconut Macaroons	3 (1 oz)	120	1	7	0	14	0	115
Oatmeal Raisin	3 (1 oz)	130	2	6	0	18	1	75
Eddyleon								
Jelly Graham Raspberry	1 (0.9 oz)	134	1	8	2	15	tr	44
Pudding Cookies	1 (0.9 oz)	134	1	6	2	15	tr	44
Entenmann's								
Little Bites Chocolate Chip	8 (1.8 oz)	240	2	12	10	33	1	120
Soft Baked Chocolate Chip	1 (0.7 oz)	100	1	5	10	13	tr	60
Soft Baked Double Chocolate Chip	1 (0.7 oz)	100	1	5	10	14	tr	65
Soft Baked Milk Chocolate Chip	1 (0.7 oz)	100	1	5	10	13	tr	60
Soft Baked Original Chocolate Chip	3 (1 oz)	150	1	7	10	20	tr	90
Soft Baked White Chocolate Macadamia Nut	1 (0.7 oz)	100	1	6	10	12	tr	65
Soft Baked Light Chocolately Chip	2 (1 oz)	120	1	4	0	21	tr	80

FOOD	PORTION	CAL	PROT	FAT	CHOL	CARB	FIBER	SOD
Soft Baked Light Oatmeal Raisin	2 (1 oz)	100	2	0	0	23	1	150
Estee								
Chocolate Chip	4	150	2	7	0	21	tr	30
Coconut	4	140	2	6	0	19	tr	25
Fig Bars	2	100	1	1	0	23	3	20
Fudge	4	150	2	7	0	19	1	45
Lemon Thins	4	140	2	6	0	19	tr	25
Oatmeal Raisin	4	130	2	5	0	19	1	25
Sandwich Chocolate	3	160	2	6	0	24	1	60
Sandwich Original	3	160	2	6	0	24	1	45
Sandwich Peanut Butter	3	160	4	7	0	22	1	55
Sandwich Vanilla	3	160	2	5	0	25	tr	35
Shortbread	4	130	2	4	0	22	tr	150
Sugar Free Chocolate Chip	3	110	2	4	0	22	1	70
Sugar Free Chocolate Walnut	3	110	2	4	0	22	1	95
Sugar Free Coconut	3	110	2	4	0	22	1	110
Sugar Free Grahams Chocolate	2	110	3	2	0	27	3	110
Sugar Free Grahams Cinnamon	2	90	3	2	0	18	2	90
Sugar Free Grahams Old Fashion	2	90	3	2	0	17	2	115
Sugar Free Lemon	3	110	2	3	0	22	1	90
Sugar Free Wafer Banana Split	5	155	1	9	0	22	0	10
Sugar Free Wafer Chocolate	5	150	1	9	0	19	0	10
Sugar Free Wafer Chocolate Peanut Butter Caramel	5	150	1	8	0	22	0	45
Sugar Free Wafer Lemon Creme	5	150	1	8	0	22	0	10
Sugar Free Wafer Peanut Butter Creme	5	150	1	8	0	22	0	40

FOOD	PORTION	CAL	PROT	FAT	CHOL	CARB	FIBER	SOD
Sugar Free Wafer Vanilla	5	150	1	8	0	21	0	10
Sugar Free Wafer Vanilla Strawberry	5	150	1	8	0	22	0	10
Vanilla Thins	4	140	2	6	0	19	tr	25
Falcone's								
Sorrentini	1 (1 oz)	100	2	4	10	16	2	55
Famous Amos								
Butter Shortie	1 (0.5 oz)	80	1	5	10	9	tr	65
Chocolate Chip	4 (1 oz)	140	2	7	0	18	tr	105
Chocolate Chip & Pecan	4 (1 oz)	140	1	8	0	18	tr	100
Chocolate Chip Toffee	4 (1 oz)	130	1	6	0	18	0	115
Chocolate Creme Sandwich	3 (1.2 oz)	140	2	6	0	22	tr	90
Chunky Chocolate Chip	1 (0.5 oz)	70	1	4	0	9	0	80
Fat Free Fig Bar	2 (1 oz)	90	1	0	0	21	1	60
Fat Free Strawberry Fruit Bar	2 (1 oz)	90	1	0	0	22	0	50
Fig Bar	2 (1.1 oz)	120	1	3	0	22	tr	150
Oatmeal Chocolate Chip Walnut	4 (1 oz)	140	2	7	0	16	tr	120
Oatmeal Raisin	4 (1 oz)	130	2	6	5	20	tr	135
Oatmeal Macaroon Creme Sandwich	3 (1.2 oz)	160	2	7	0	23	1	–
Peanut Butter Chocolate Chunk	1 (0.5 oz)	80	1	5	0	9	tr	70
Peanut Butter Creme Sandwich	3 (1.2 oz)	160	4	8	0	19	1	115
Pecan Shortie	1 (0.5 oz)	80	1	5	0	9	tr	55
Vanilla Creme Sandwich	3 (1.2 oz)	160	2	7	0	24	0	85
Frookie								
Animal Frackers	14 (1 oz)	130	2	5	0	18	1	90
Chocolate Chip Wheat & Gluten Free	3 (1.1 oz)	140	1	5	0	23	1	100

FOOD	PORTION	CAL	PROT	FAT	CHOL	CARB	FIBER	SOD
Double Chocolate Wheat & Gluten Free	3 (1.1 oz)	130	1	4	0	23	1	105
Dream Creams Strawberry	4 (1 oz)	140	2	8	0	18	4	55
Dream Creams Vanilla	4 (1 oz)	140	2	8	0	18	4	55
Funky Monkeys Chocolate	16 (1 oz)	120	2	4	0	20	1	120
Funky Monkeys Vanilla	16 (1 oz)	120	2	4	0	20	1	120
Graham Cinnamon	2 (1 oz)	100	2	3	0	17	1	105
Graham Honey	2 (1 oz)	110	2	3	0	18	1	120
Lemon Wafers	8 (1 oz)	110	2	0	0	26	tr	130
Old Fashioned Ginger Snaps	8 (1 oz)	120	1	2	0	24	tr	110
Organic Chocolate Chip	3 (1.1 oz)	150	2	7	0	20	1	115
Organic Double Chocolate Chip	3 (1.1 oz)	140	2	6	0	20	1	95
Organic Iced Lemon	3 (1.3 oz)	165	2	6	0	27	0	115
Organic Oatmeal Raisin	3 (1.1 oz)	140	2	5	0	22	1	110
Peanut Butter Chunk Wheat & Gluten Free	3 (1.1 oz)	140	3	5	0	21	0	140
Sandwich Chocolate	2 (0.7 oz)	100	1	4	0	14	1	60
Sandwich Lemon	2 (0.7 oz)	100	1	4	0	14	1	60
Sandwich Peanut Butter	2 (0.7 oz)	100	1	4	0	14	1	60
Sandwich Vanilla	2 (0.7 oz)	100	1	4	0	14	1	60
Shortbread	5 (1 oz)	130	2	5	15	20	tr	95
Vanilla Wafers	8 (1 oz)	110	2	0	0	26	0	120
General Henry								
Fruit Bars Apple	1 (0.6 oz)	60	1	1	0	13	tr	70
Fruit Bars Blueberry	1 (0.6 oz)	60	1	1	0	12	tr	75
Fruit Bars Fig	1 (0.6 oz)	60	1	1	0	12	tr	70
Girl Scout								
Apple Cinnamon Reduced Fat	3 (1 oz)	120	2	5	0	18	tr	140

FOOD	PORTION	CAL	PROT	FAT	CHOL	CARB	FIBER	SOD
Do-si-dos	3 (1.2 oz)	170	3	8	0	22	1	105
Lemon Drops	3 (1.2 oz)	160	2	8	0	20	0	150
Samoas	2 (1 oz)	160	2	9	0	17	2	45
Striped Chocolate Chip	3 (1.2 oz)	180	2	10	0	20	tr	100
Tagalongs	2 (0.9 oz)	150	3	10	0	13	2	85
Thin Mints	4 (1 oz)	140	1	8	0	18	tr	80
Trefoils	5 (1.1 oz)	160	2	8	0	20	1	90
Godiva								
Biscotti Dipped In Milk Chocolate	1 (0.9 oz)	120	2	6	20	15	0	45
Golden Grahams Treats								
Chocolate Chunk	1 bar (0.8 oz)	90	1	3	0	17	0	110
Honey Graham	1 bar (0.8 oz)	90	1	2	0	17	0	120
King Size Chocolate Chunk	1 bar (1.6 oz)	190	2	5	0	35	1	220
King Size Honey Graham	1 bar (1.6 oz)	180	1	4	0	36	1	240
Gourmet								
Chocolate Chip	2 (1.1 oz)	160	2	9	15	19	1	85
Lemon Creme	2 (1.4 oz)	210	1	10	0	27	0	60
Oatmeal Raisin	2 (0.9 oz)	120	2	6	15	15	1	105
Peanut Butter Chip	2 (1 oz)	150	3	8	10	17	tr	135
Raspberry Center	2 (1.1 oz)	140	1	5	10	21	tr	60
Grandma's								
Chocolate Chip	1 (1.4 oz)	190	2	9	0	25	tr	135
Fudge Chocolate Chip	1 (1.4 oz)	170	1	7	<5	26	1	160
Fudge Sandwich	3	180	2	5	0	31	tr	200
Fudge Vanilla Sandwich	3	120	1	4	0	21	tr	130
Mini Fudge	9	150	2	7	0	21	1	180
Mini Peanut Butter	9	150	2	7	0	21	1	140
Mini Vanilla	9	150	2	7	<5	22	tr	85
Oatmeal Raisin	1 (1.4 oz)	160	1	6	5	26	1	250
Old Time Molasses	1 (1.4 oz)	160	2	4	<5	29	tr	230
Peanut Butter	1 (1.4 oz)	190	2	9	5	22	1	200
Peanut Butter Chocolate Chip	1 (1.4 oz)	190	4	9	<5	23	1	170
Peanut Butter Sandwich	5	210	3	10	0	28	1	200

FOOD	PORTION	CAL	PROT	FAT	CHOL	CARB	FIBER	SOD
Rich N'Chewy	1 pkg	270	2	12	10	39	1	130
Vanilla Sandwich	3	180	2	5	0	32	tr	160
Vanilla Sandwich	5	210	2	10	5	30	tr	125
Handi-Snack								
Cookie Jammers Cookies & Fruit Spread	1 pkg (1.3 oz)	130	1	3	0	26	tr	125
Health Valley								
Apple Spice	3	100	2	0	0	24	3	50
Apricot Delight	3	100	2	0	0	24	3	50
Biscotti Amaretto	2	120	3	3	0	23	3	50
Biscotti Chocolate	2	120	3	3	0	23	3	50
Biscotti Fruit & Nut	2	120	3	3	0	23	3	50
Cheesecake Bars Blueberry	1 bar	160	3	2	0	34	3	30
Cheesecake Bars Raspberry	1 bar	160	3	2	0	34	3	30
Cheesecake Bars Strawberry	1 bar	160	3	2	0	34	3	30
Chips Double Chocolate	3	100	3	0	0	24	4	40
Chips Old Fashioned	3	100	3	0	0	24	4	40
Chips Original	3	100	3	0	0	24	4	40
Chocolate Fudge Center	2	70	2	0	0	25	3	25
Chocolate Sandwich Bar Bavarian Creme	1 bar	150	3	0	0	35	3	30
Chocolate Sandwich Bars Caramel Creme	1 bar	150	3	0	0	35	3	30
Chocolate Sandwich Bars Vanilla Creme	1 bar	150	3	0	0	35	3	30
Date Delight	3	100	2	0	0	24	3	50
Graham Amaranth	8	100	4	0	0	23	3	30
Graham Oat Bran	8	100	4	0	0	30	3	30
Graham Original Amaranth	6	120	3	3	0	22	3	80
Hawaiian Fruit	3	100	2	0	0	24	3	50

FOOD	PORTION	CAL	PROT	FAT	CHOL	CARB	FIBER	SOD
Jumbo Apple Raisin	1	80	2	0	0	19	3	35
Jumbo Raisin Raisin	1	80	2	0	0	19	3	35
Jumbo Raspberry	1	80	2	0	0	19	3	35
Marshmallow Bars Chocolate Chip	1	90	1	0	0	22	1	20
Marshmallow Bars Old Fashioned	1	90	1	0	0	22	1	20
Marshmallow Bars Tropical Fruit	1	90	1	0	0	22	1	20
Oat Bran Fruit Bars Raisin Cinnamon	1 bar	160	3	1	0	34	2	10
Raisin Oatmeal	3	100	2	0	0	24	3	50
Raspberry Fruit Center	1	70	2	0	0	18	2	20
Tarts Baked Apple Cinnamon	1	150	3	0	0	35	3	40
Tarts California Strawberry	1	150	3	0	0	35	3	40
Tarts Chocolate Fudge	1	150	3	0	0	35	3	50
Tarts Cranberry Apple	1	150	3	0	0	35	3	40
Tarts Mountain Blueberry	1	150	3	0	0	35	3	40
Tarts Red Raspberry	1	150	3	0	0	35	3	40
Tarts Sweet Red Cherry	1	150	3	0	0	35	3	40
Hellema								
Almond	1 pkg (0.6 oz)	90	1	5	0	9	tr	35
Hershey								
Cripsy Rice Snacks Peanut Butter	1 (0.6 oz)	70	1	3	0	10	tr	130
Joseph's								
Almond Sugar Free	2 (0.9 oz)	100	1	5	0	14	0	20
Chocolate Chip Sugar Free	2 (0.9 oz)	100	1	5	0	15	0	40
Chocolate Walnut Sugar Free	2 (0.9 oz)	100	1	6	0	14	1	40
Coconut Sugar Free	2 (0.9 oz)	105	1	5	0	14	0	40

FOOD	PORTION	CAL	PROT	FAT	CHOL	CARB	FIBER	SOD
Lemon Sugar Free	2 (0.9 oz)	95	1	4	0	15	0	30
Oatmeal Raisin Sugar Free	2 (0.9 oz)	100	2	5	0	15	0	40
Peanut Butter Sugar Free	2 (0.9 oz)	95	2	5	0	13	1	40
Pecan Shortbread Sugar Free	2 (0.9 oz)	100	1	5	0	14	0	40
Keebler								
Animal Crackers Chocolate Chip	7 (1 oz)	130	2	5	0	22	0	120
Animal Crackers Ernie's	1 box	250	<4	9	0	41	1	290
Animal Crackers Iced	6 (1.1 oz)	150	2	5	0	24	0	110
Animal Crackers Sprinkled	6 (1.1 oz)	150	<2	5	0	24	0	105
Butter	5 (1.1 oz)	150	<2	6	10	22	tr	170
Chips Deluxe	1 (0.5 oz)	80	tr	5	0	9	0	60
Chips Deluxe Chocolate Lovers	1 (0.6 oz)	90	tr	5	5	11	0	80
Chips Deluxe Coconut	1 (0.5 oz)	80	tr	5	0	10	tr	50
Chips Deluxe Rainbow	1 (0.6 oz)	80	tr	4	<5	10	tr	45
Chips Deluxe Soft 'n Chewy	1 (0.6 oz)	80	tr	4	5	11	0	60
Chips Deluxe w/ Peanut Butter Cups	1 (0.6 oz)	90	tr	5	0	9	0	45
Classic Collection Chocolate Fudge Creme	1 (0.6 oz)	80	tr	4	0	12	0	75
Classic Collection French Vanllia Creme	1 (0.6 oz)	80	tr	4	0	12	0	65
Cookie Stix Butter	5 (1.2 oz)	160	<2	6	10	22	1	150
Cookie Stix Chocolate Chip	4 (0.9 oz)	130	<2	5	5	19	tr	100
Cookie Stix Rainbow	5 (1.2 oz)	150	<2	6	5	23	tr	110

FOOD	PORTION	CAL	PROT	FAT	CHOL	CARB	FIBER	SOD
Danish Wedding	4 (0.9 oz)	120	tr	5	0	20	tr	80
Droxies	3 (1.1 oz)	140	<2	6	0	21	tr	95
Droxies Reduced Fat	3 (1.1 oz)	140	<2	5	0	23	1	150
E.L. Fudge Butter w/ Fudge Filling	2 (0.9 oz)	120	tr	6	<5	17	tr	70
E.L. Fudge Fudge w/ Fudge Filling	2 (0.9 oz)	120	<2	6	0	17	tr	70
E.L. Fudge w/ Peanut Butter Filling	2 (0.9 oz)	120	<2	6	0	16	tr	150
Fudge Shoppe Deluxe Grahams	3 (1 oz)	140	tr	7	0	19	tr	105
Fudge Shoppe Double Fudge 'n Caramel	2 (1 oz)	140	tr	7	0	20	tr	65
Fudge Shoppe Fudge Sticks	3 (1 oz)	150	tr	8	0	20	tr	55
Fudge Shoppe Fudge Sticks Peanut Butter	3 (1 oz)	150	<2	8	0	18	tr	45
Fudge Shoppe Fudge Stripes	3 (1.1 oz)	160	tr	8	0	21	tr	140
Fudge Shoppe Fudge Stripes Reduced Fat	3 (1 oz)	140	tr	5	0	21	0	120
Fudge Shoppe Grasshoppers	4 (1 oz)	150	tr	7	0	20	tr	70
Fudge Shoppe S'mores	3 (1.2 oz)	160	tr	8	0	22	tr	95
Ginger Snaps	5 (1.1 oz)	150	<2	6	0	24	0	120
Golden Fruit Cranberry	1 (0.7 oz)	80	tr	2	0	14	tr	55
Golden Fruit Raisin	1 (0.7 oz)	80	tr	2	0	15	tr	50
Graham Cinnamon Crisp	8 (1 oz)	140	2	5	0	22	1	170
Graham Cinnamon Crisp Low Fat	8 (1 oz)	110	2	2	0	24	1	190
Graham Honey	8 (1.1 oz)	150	2	6	0	21	1	140
Graham Honey Low Fat	8 (1.1 oz)	120	2	2	0	26	1	210
Graham Original	8 (1 oz)	130	2	3	0	23	tr	135

FOOD	PORTION	CAL	PROT	FAT	CHOL	CARB	FIBER	SOD
Lemon Coolers	5 (1 oz)	140	tr	6	0	21	tr	100
Oatmeal Country Style	2 (0.8 oz)	120	<2	5	0	17	tr	115
Sandies Almond Shortbread	1 (0.5 oz)	80	tr	5	5	9	0	50
Sandies Pecan Shortbread	1 (0.5 oz)	80	tr	5	<5	9	tr	75
Sandies Simply Shortbread	1 (0.5 oz)	80	tr	5	10	9	0	70
Snack Size Chips Deluxe	1 pkg (2 oz)	300	3	16	5	36	tr	170
Snack Size Chips Deluxe Chocolate Lovers	1 pkg (2 oz)	280	3	15	20	36	1	170
Snack Size Mini Fudge Stripes	1 pkg (2 oz)	280	3	14	0	38	2	150
Snack Size Rainbow Chips Deluxe	1 pkg (2 oz)	290	3	16	5	36	1	170
Snack Size Sandies w/ Pecans	1 pkg (2 oz)	300	3	17	10	33	1	190
Snackin' Grahams Cinnamon	21 (1 oz)	130	<2	3	0	23	1	210
Snackin' Grahams Honey	23 (1 oz)	130	<2	4	0	22	tr	120
Soft Batch Chocolate Chip	1 (0.6 oz)	80	tr	4	0	10	tr	70
Soft Batch Homestyle Chocolate Chunk	1 (0.9 oz)	130	1	7	0	17	1	80
Soft Batch Homestyle Double Chocolate	1 (0.9 oz)	130	1	7	0	17	1	90
Soft Batch Homestyle Oatmeal Raisin	1 (0.9 oz)	130	1	5	0	20	tr	150
Soft Batch Oatmeal Raisin	1 (0.5 oz)	70	tr	3	0	10	tr	65
Sugar Wafers Creme	3 (0.9 oz)	130	tr	6	0	18	tr	20
Sugar Wafers Lemon	3 (0.9 oz)	130	tr	6	0	19	0	20
Sugar Wafers Peanut Butter	4 (1.1 oz)	170	<3	9	0	19	1	75
Vanilla Wafers	8 (1.1 oz)	150	tr	7	0	20	tr	120

FOOD	PORTION	CAL	PROT	FAT	CHOL	CARB	FIBER	SOD
Vanilla Wafers Reduced Fat	8 (1.1 oz)	130	<2	4	0	25	tr	140
Vienna Fingers	2 (1 oz)	140	2	6	0	21	tr	105
Vienna Fingers Lemon	2 (1 oz)	140	2	6	0	21	0	90
Knott's Berry Farm								
Shortbread Apricot	3 (1 oz)	120	2	5	4	17	0	70
Shortbread Boysenberry	3 (1 oz)	120	2	5	4	17	0	60
Shortbread Raspberry	3 (1 oz)	120	2	5	4	17	0	60
LU								
Le Bastogne	2 (0.8 oz)	120	1	5	0	18	0	50
Le Chocolatiers	3 (1 oz)	150	1	8	0	17	1	10
Le Dore	4 (1 oz)	140	2	6	<5	21	0	55
Le Fondant	4 (1.1 oz)	170	1	10	0	19	1	5
Le Palmier	4 (1.2 oz)	180	2	10	0	20	tr	140
Le Petit Beurre	4 (1.2 oz)	150	3	4	10	25	tr	180
Le Petit Ecolier Dark Chocolate	2 (0.9 oz)	130	2	6	5	17	1	55
Le Petit Ecolier Hazelnut Milk Chocolate	2 (0.9 oz)	130	2	7	5	16	0	55
Le Petit Ecolier Milk Chocolate	2 (0.9 oz)	130	1	6	5	17	tr	55
Le Pim's Orange	2 (0.9 oz)	90	1	3	5	17	tr	25
Le Pim's Raspberry	2 (0.9 oz)	90	1	3	5	17	tr	25
Le Raisin Dore	4 (1.2 oz)	160	2	7	20	23	tr	130
Le Truffe Coconut	4 (1.2 oz)	190	1	12	0	17	1	15
Le Truffe Praline Chocolate	4 (1.2 oz)	170	2	9	0	20	2	15
Les Varietes	3 (0.9 oz)	140	1	7	5	17	6	35
La Choy								
Fortune	4 (1 oz)	112	2	tr	0	26	1	11
Lance								
Apple Bar Fat Free	1 (1.75 oz)	160	1	0	0	38	tr	80
Apple Oatmeal Bar	1 (1.8 oz)	190	2	6	10	32	1	180
Big Town Banana	1 pkg (2 oz)	250	3	10	0	37	1	160
Big Town Chocolate	1 pkg (2 oz)	250	3	8	0	40	1	160
Big Town Vanilla	1 pkg (2 oz)	250	3	11	0	37	1	120

FOOD	PORTION	CAL	PROT	FAT	CHOL	CARB	FIBER	SOD
Choc-O-Lunch	1 pkg (1.5 oz)	200	3	8	0	31	1	190
Choc-O-Mint	1 pkg (1¼ oz)	190	2	9	0	24	1	100
Coated Graham	1 pkg (1.3 oz)	190	3	8	0	25	1	95
Fig Bar	1 (1.75 oz)	180	2	4	0	34	2	150
Fudge Chocolate Chip	1 (2 oz)	130	2	5	<5	19	1	75
Gourmet Chocolate Chip	1 (2 oz)	130	2	6	5	18	1	75
Lem-O-Lunch	1 pkg (3.4 oz)	240	3	11	0	32	1	150
Lemon Nekot	1 pkg (1.5 oz)	210	3	10	0	28	1	125
Nut-O-Lunch	1 pkg (3.3 oz)	240	6	11	0	29	3	150
Oatmeal	1 (2 oz)	130	2	6	0	18	1	90
Oatmeal Creme	1 (2 oz)	240	3	10	0	35	1	220
Peanut Butter	1 (2 oz)	140	4	8	<5	14	1	65
Peanut Butter Creme Wafer	1 pkg (1.5 oz)	230	4	12	0	26	2	80
Van-O-Lunch	1 pkg (1.5 oz)	210	2	8	0	31	0	130
Larzaroni								
Arancelli	8 (1 oz)	160	3	8	8	19	tr	36
Calypso	3 (1 oz)	150	2	8	0	18	1	30
Limonelli	5 (1 oz)	140	2	8	5	16	2	30
Malaika	5 (1 oz)	158	3	9	17	17	1	36
Nanette	4 (1.2 oz)	170	3	9	<5	20	tr	30
Okla	3 (1 oz)	186	3	10	6	21	1	43
Oskar	10 (1 oz)	150	2	9	0	18	tr	10
Samba	5 (1 oz)	160	3	10	0	14	2	150
Velieri	3 (0.9 oz)	120	2	5	10	17	tr	60
Linden's								
Lemon	1 (1 oz)	120	—	5	10	—	—	135
Little Debbie								
Apple Flips	1 (1.2 oz)	150	1	5	5	24	tr	115
Caramel Bars	1 (1.2 oz)	160	1	8	0	22	0	85
Cherry Cordials	1 (1.3 oz)	170	1	8	0	23	tr	95
Coconut Rounds	1 (1.2 oz)	150	1	7	0	23	tr	90
Cookie Wreaths	1 (0.6 oz)	100	1	5	0	12	0	60
Easter Puffs	1 (1.2 oz)	140	1	6	0	24	0	65
Fig Bars	1 (1.5 oz)	150	1	4	0	31	1	110
Fudge Delights	1 (1.1 oz)	110	1	2	0	24	tr	170
Fudge Rounds	1 (1.2 oz)	140	1	6	0	23	tr	85
German Chocolate Ring	1 (1 oz)	140	1	8	0	18	1	65

FOOD	PORTION	CAL	PROT	FAT	CHOL	CARB	FIBER	SOD
Ginger	1 (0.7 oz)	90	1	3	5	15	0	60
Jelly Creme Pies	1 (1.2 oz)	160	1	7	0	23	0	160
Marshmallow Crispy Bar	1 (1.3 oz)	140	2	4	0	26	0	170
Marshmallow Supremes	1 (1.1 oz)	130	1	5	0	22	tr	65
Marshmallow Pie Banana	1 pkg (1.5 oz)	180	2	6	0	30	0	110
Marshmallow Pie Chocolate	1 (1.4 oz)	160	1	6	0	27	1	95
Nutty Bar	1 (2 oz)	310	5	18	0	32	1	110
Oatmeal Raisin	1 (1.3 oz)	160	2	7	0	25	tr	170
Oatmeal Creme Pie	1 (1.3 oz)	170	1	7	0	26	tr	190
Oatmeal Delights	1 (1.1 oz)	110	2	2	0	24	tr	135
Oatmeal Lights	1 (1.3 oz)	130	2	3	0	29	tr	180
Peanut Butter Bars	1 (1.9 oz)	270	4	15	0	32	1	140
Peanut Butter & Jelly Oatmeal Pie	1 (1.1 oz)	130	2	5	0	22	tr	100
Peanut Clusters	1 (1.4 oz)	190	3	11	0	23	tr	120
Pumpkin Delights	1 (1.2 oz)	150	1	5	5	24	0	140
Raisin Creme Pie	1 (1.2 oz)	140	1	5	0	23	0	120
Star Crunch	1 (1.1 oz)	140	0	6	0	22	0	70
Sugar Free Chocolate Chip	3 (1.1 oz)	140	2	7	0	21	tr	100
Sugar Free Oatmeal	6 (1.1 oz)	120	2	4	0	23	1	130
Yo-Yo's	1 (1.2 oz)	130	1	6	0	21	tr	125
Milk Lunch Brand								
New England Biscuits	4 (1.1 oz)	140	2	5	<5	24	1	220
MoonPie								
Chocolate	1 (2.75 oz)	330	4	10	0	56	0	256
Mini Banana	1 (1.2 oz)	152	3	5	0	26	0	120
Mini Chocolate	1 (1.2 oz)	152	3	5	0	26	0	120
Mini Vanilla	1 (1.2 oz)	152	3	5	0	26	0	120
Mother's								
Almond Shortbread	3	180	2	11	0	19	1	115
Checkerboard Wafers	8	150	1	8	0	20	1	40
Chocolate Chip	2	160	2	8	10	20	0	105

FOOD	PORTION	CAL	PROT	FAT	CHOL	CARB	FIBER	SOD
Chocolate Chip Angel	3	180	2	9	0	21	1	70
Chocolate Chip Parade	4	130	1	5	0	19	1	100
Circus Animals	6	140	1	6	0	20	0	55
Classic Assortments	2	140	1	7	0	18	1	105
Cocadas	5	150	2	7	5	20	2	140
Cookie Parade	4	140	1	7	0	18	2	95
Dinosaur Grrrahams	2	130	2	3	0	24	2	130
Double Fudge	2	180	2	9	0	24	2	110
English Tea	2	180	2	7	0	26	1	100
Flaky Flix Fudge	2	140	1	7	0	17	2	50
Flaky Flix Vanilla	2	140	1	8	0	17	1	40
Gaucho Peanut Butter	2	190	3	10	0	22	2	200
Iced Oatmeal	2	130	2	4	0	22	1	160
Iced Raisin	2	180	1	8	0	24	1	110
MLB Double Header Duplex	3	170	2	8	5	23	1	130
Macaroon	2	150	1	8	0	18	2	80
Marias	3	170	2	6	5	28	1	150
Oatmeal	2	110	1	5	0	17	1	150
Oatmeal Chocolate Chip	2	120	2	5	0	19	1	140
Oatmeal Raisin	5	150	2	7	5	20	2	125
Oatmeal Walnut Chocolate Chip	2	130	2	6	0	17	1	135
Rainbow Wafers	8	150	1	8	0	20	1	40
Striped Shortbread	3	170	2	8	0	22	1	75
Sugar	2	140	1	6	0	19	1	75
Taffy	2	180	2	8	0	25	2	160
Triplet Assortment	2	140	1	7	0	18	1	112
Vanilla Wafers	6	150	2	6	4	24	1	85
Wallops Boysenberry	1	80	1	2	0	15	1	40
Wallops Honey Crust Fig	1	80	1	2	0	15	0	55
Wallops Honey Graham Fig	1	80	1	2	0	15	1	55

FOOD	PORTION	CAL	PROT	FAT	CHOL	CARB	FIBER	SOD
Wallops Mixed Berry	1	80	1	2	0	15	1	40
Wallops Peach Apricot	1	80	1	2	0	15	1	40
Wallops Raspberry	1	80	1	2	0	15	1	40
Wallops Strawberry	1	80	1	2	0	15	1	40
Walnut Fudge	2	130	1	7	0	16	1	90
Zoo Pals	14	140	2	5	0	23	1	120
Mrs. Alison's								
Coconut Bar	2 (1 oz)	130	2	6	0	19	0	85
Creme Wafers	5 (1.1 oz)	170	1	10	0	21	tr	35
Duplex Sandwich	3 (1 oz)	130	1	5	0	20	0	105
Fudge Fingers	3 (1 oz)	160	tr	10	0	19	0	20
Ginger Snaps	4 (1 oz)	130	2	3	<2	23	tr	170
Jelly Tops	5 (1 oz)	140	2	7	0	18	0	45
Lemon Creme	3 (1 oz)	130	1	5	0	21	0	115
Macaroons	2 (1 oz)	140	2	7	0	18	tr	95
Pecan	2 (1 oz)	140	2	7	0	19	0	75
Shortbread	5 (1 oz)	120	2	5	0	19	0	100
Vanilla Sandwich	3 (1 oz)	130	1	5	0	21	0	115
Murray's								
Sugar Free Double Fudge	3 (1.2 oz)	140	2	6	0	23	3	110
Sugar Free Ginger Snap	6 (1 oz)	110	2	4	0	21	tr	100
Sugar Free Peanut Butter	6 (1 oz)	130	3	7	0	17	1	85
Sugar Free Vanilla Sandwich Creme	3 (1 oz)	120	1	5	0	21	2	65
Sugar Free Vanilla Wafers	9 (1.1 oz)	120	2	4	0	23	tr	85
Nabisco								
Barnum's Animal Crackers	10 (1 oz)	130	2	4	0	23	tr	150
Barnum's Animal Crackers Chocolate	10 (1 oz)	130	2	4	0	23	1	160
Biscos Sugar Wafers	8 (1 oz)	140	tr	6	0	21	0	40
Cafe Cremes Cappuccino	2 (1.1 oz)	160	1	8	0	22	0	130

FOOD	PORTION	CAL	PROT	FAT	CHOL	CARB	FIBER	SOD
Cafe Cremes Vanilla	2 (1.1 oz)	160	1	7	0	22	0	130
Cafe Cremes Vanilla Fudge	2 (1.1 oz)	200	2	10	0	27	tr	140
Cameo	2 (1 oz)	130	1	5	0	21	0	105
Chips Ahoy!	3 (1.1 oz)	160	2	8	0	21	1	105
Chips Ahoy! Chewy	3 (1.3 oz)	170	1	8	0	24	tr	125
Chips Ahoy! Chunky	1 (0.5 oz)	80	tr	4	5	10	0	35
Chips Ahoy! Munch Size	6 (1.1 oz)	160	2	8	0	21	1	150
Chips Ahoy! Reduced Fat	3 (1.1 oz)	140	2	5	0	22	tr	150
Family Favorites Iced Oatmeal	1 (0.6 oz)	80	1	3	0	12	0	55
Family Favorites Oatmeal	1 (0.6 oz)	80	1	3	0	12	0	65
Famous Chocolate Wafers	5 (1.1 oz)	140	2	4	<5	24	1	230
Grahams	4 (1 oz)	120	2	3	0	22	1	180
Honey Maid Chocolate	8 (1 oz)	120	2	3	0	22	1	170
Honey Maid Cinnamon Grahams	8 (1 oz)	120	2	3	0	23	tr	180
Honey Maid Honey Grahams	8 (1 oz)	120	2	3	0	22	1	180
Honey Maid Low Fat Cinnamon Grahams	8 (1 oz)	110	2	2	0	23	tr	170
Honey Maid Low Fat Grahams	8 (1 oz)	110	2	2	0	23	tr	200
Honey Maid Oatmeal Crunch	8 (1 oz)	120	2	3	0	22	1	140
Lorna Doone	4 (1 oz)	140	2	7	5	19	tr	130
Mallomars	2 (0.9 oz)	120	1	5	0	17	tr	35
Marshmallow Twirls	1 (1 oz)	130	1	6	0	20	0	75
Mystic Mint	1 (0.5 oz)	90	1	5	0	11	0	65
National Arrowroot	1 (5 g)	20	0	1	—	4	0	15
Newton Fat Free Fig	2 (1 oz)	90	1	0	0	22	1	115
Newtons Fig	2 (1.1 oz)	110	1	3	0	22	1	125
Newtons Fat Free Apple	2 (1 oz)	90	1	0	0	21	tr	65

FOOD	PORTION	CAL	PROT	FAT	CHOL	CARB	FIBER	SOD
Newtons Fat Free Cobblers Apple Cinnamon	1 (0.8 oz)	70	1	0	0	17	tr	40
Newtons Fat Free Cobblers Peach Apricot	1 (0.8 oz)	70	1	0	0	17	0	55
Newtons Fat Free Cranberry	2 (1 oz)	100	1	0	0	22	tr	95
Newtons Fat Free Raspberry	2 (1 oz)	100	1	0	0	23	tr	115
Newtons Fat Free Strawberry	2 (1 oz)	90	1	0	0	21	0	95
Nilla Wafers	8 (1.1 oz)	140	1	5	<5	24	0	100
Nilla Wafers Chocolate Reduced Fat	8 (1 oz)	110	2	2	0	23	tr	120
Nilla Wafers Reduced Fat	8 (1 oz)	120	1	2	0	24	0	105
Nutter Butter Bites	10 (1 oz)	150	3	7	<5	20	1	125
Nutter Butter Chocolate Peanut Butter Sandwich	2 (1 oz)	130	2	5	0	19	1	140
Nutter Butter Peanut Butter Sandwich	2 (1 oz)	130	2	6	<5	19	tr	110
Old Fashioned Ginger Snaps	4 (1 oz)	120	1	3	0	22	tr	230
Oreo	3 (1.2 oz)	160	1	7	0	23	1	220
Oreo Double Stuff	2 (1 oz)	140	1	7	0	19	tr	150
Oreo Reduced Fat	3 (1.1 oz)	130	—	4	0	25	1	190
Oreo Halloween	2 (1 oz)	140	1	7	0	19	tr	115
Pecanz	1 (0.5 oz)	90	1	5	<5	9	0	50
Pinwheels Chocolate Marshmallow	1 (1 oz)	130	1	5	0	21	tr	35
Rugrats Chocolate Frosted	8 (1.1 oz)	150	1	5	0	24	tr	110
Rugrats Vanilla Frosted	8 (1.1 oz)	150	1	6	0	24	tr	105
Social Tea	6 (1 oz)	120	2	4	5	20	tr	115

FOOD	PORTION	CAL	PROT	FAT	CHOL	CARB	FIBER	SOD
Sweet Crispers Chocolate	18 (1.1 oz)	130	2	3	0	25	1	190
Sweet Crispers Chocolate Chip	18 (1.1 oz)	130	2	3	0	23	tr	160
Teddy Grahams Chocolate	24 (1 oz)	130	2	5	0	22	1	170
Teddy Grahams Chocolately Chip	24 (1 oz)	130	2	5	0	23	tr	135
Teddy Grahams Cinnamon	24 (1 oz)	130	2	4	0	23	1	150
Teddy Grahams Honey	24 (1 oz)	130	2	4	0	23	tr	150
Nestle								
Flipz Crunchy Graham White Fudge Chocolate	8 (1 oz)	140	2	6	0	19	0	85
Newman's Own								
Fig Newman's Organic	2 (1.3 oz)	120	2	0	0	28	1	140
Nonni's								
Biscotti Cioccalati	1 (1 oz)	130	2	5	5	19	1	50
Biscotti Decadence	1 (1.1 oz)	130	2	5	5	19	1	55
Biscotti Original	1 (1 oz)	100	2	4	25	15	1	65
Biscotti Paradiso	1 (1.1 oz)	130	2	6	5	19	0	60
NutraBalance								
Fibre Oatmeal Raisin	1 (0.7 oz)	80	1	4	0	13	3	85
Protein Fortified	1 (2 oz)	260	7	14	10	28	2	180
ReNeph Spice	1 (2 oz)	210	9	7	0	29	0	230
Old Brussels								
Ginger Crisps	2 (0.9 oz)	140	2	4	0	23	2	115
Old London								
Coffee Toppers Chocolate Creme	3 (0.5 oz)	70	1	3	0	9	0	75
Coffee Toppers Vanilla Creme	3 (0.5 oz)	70	1	4	0	9	0	80
Olde World								
Pizzelle Almond	3 (1 oz)	90	2	4	45	12	0	15
Pizzelle Anise	3 (1 oz)	90	2	4	45	12	0	15
Pizzelle Chocolate	3 (1 oz)	100	2	5	45	11	0	15

FOOD	PORTION	CAL	PROT	FAT	CHOL	CARB	FIBER	SOD
Pizzelle Lemon	3 (1 oz)	90	2	4	45	12	0	15
Pizzelle Vanilla	3 (1 oz)	90	2	4	45	12	0	15
Otis Spunkmeyer								
Butter Sugar	1 (2 oz)	250	3	12	20	35	1	210
Butter Sugar	1 med (1.3 oz)	160	2	8	15	23	tr	140
Carnival	1 med (1.3 oz)	170	2	7	10	25	0	80
Chocolate Chip	1 (2 oz)	250	3	11	15	36	tr	210
Chocolate Chip	1 med (1.3 oz)	170	2	8	10	24	0	120
Chocolate Chip	1 bite size (0.75 oz)	100	1	5	5	14	0	70
Chocolate Chip Pecan	1 med (1.3 oz)	170	2	9	10	22	tr	110
Chocolate Chip Walnut	1 bite size (0.75 oz)	100	1	5	5	13	0	60
Chocolate Chip Walnut	1 (2 oz)	270	3	14	15	34	tr	160
Chocolate Chip Walnut	1 med (1.3 oz)	180	2	9	10	22	tr	105
Double Chocolate Chip	1 med (1.3 oz)	180	2	9	10	23	tr	130
Double Chocolate Chip	1 bite size (0.75 oz)	100	1	5	5	13	1	75
Oatmeal Raisin	1 bite size (0.75 oz)	90	1	4	5	13	tr	75
Oatmeal Raisin	1 med (1.3 oz)	160	2	7	10	23	1	130
Otis Express Chocolate Chunk	1 (2 oz)	280	3	13	20	37	1	190
Otis Express Double Chocolate Chip	1 (2 oz)	270	3	14	15	35	1	200
Otis Express Oatmeal Raisin	1 (2 oz)	240	3	10	15	35	2	200
Otis Express Peanut Butter	1 (2 oz)	270	5	15	15	31	2	250
Peanut Butter	1 med (1.3 oz)	180	3	10	10	20	1	160
Pinnacle Checkpoint Chocolate Almond Coconut	1 (2.4 oz)	320	4	18	25	37	2	230
Pinnacle Mach One Mocha Chocolate Chunk	1 (2.4 oz)	300	3	13	20	43	1	230
Pinnacle Passport Peanut Butter Chocolate Chunk	1 (2.4 oz)	300	5	13	25	42	1	250

FOOD	PORTION	CAL	PROT	FAT	CHOL	CARB	FIBER	SOD
Pinnacle Ripcord Rocky Road	1 (2.4 oz)	310	3	15	15	41	2	230
Pinnacle Takeoff Triple Chocolate	1 (2.4 oz)	300	3	14	20	42	tr	180
Pinnacle Transatlantic Turtle	1 (2.4 oz)	310	3	16	20	39	2	250
Travel Lite Low Fat Apple Cinnamon	1 (1.3 oz)	130	2	2	0	26	tr	90
Travel Lite Low Fat Chocolate Chip	1 (1.3 oz)	130	2	2	0	27	tr	110
Travel Lite Low Fat Ginger Spice	1 (1.3 oz)	130	2	2	0	26	tr	90
Travel Lite Low Fat Oatmeal Rum Raisin	1 (1.3 oz)	130	2	2	0	26	1	90
White Chocolate Macadamia Nut	1 (2 oz)	280	3	15	20	33	tr	170
White Chocolate Macadamia Nut	1 med (1.3 oz)	180	2	10	10	21	tr	110
Pally								
Butter	5 (1 oz)	140	3	3	1	23	1	170
Carnival	5 (1 oz)	130	2	3	0	24	1	130
Cinnamon Biscuit	5 (1 oz)	130	2	3	0	23	0	130
Mariel Biscuit	6 (1 oz)	150	3	4	0	23	1	140
Tea Biscuits	5 (1 oz)	150	2	4	0	23	1	170
Pamela's								
Pecan Shortbread Rice Flour	1 (0.8 oz)	130	tr	8	20	15	tr	65
Parmalat								
Grisbi Lemon	1 (0.6 oz)	90	1	6	5	9	1	0
Grisbi Lemon	1 (0.6 oz)	90	1	6	<5	9	1	—
Peek Freans								
Arrowroot	4 (1.2 oz)	150	2	5	0	26	1	80
Assorted Creme	1 (1 oz)	130	1	6	<5	19	0	50
Dream Puffs	2 (0.9 oz)	110	tr	4	0	18	0	50
Fruit Creme	2 (0.9 oz)	130	1	5	0	20	0	35
Ginger Crisp	4 (1.2 oz)	150	2	4	0	28	tr	65
Nice	4 (1.2 oz)	160	2	6	0	25	1	100
Petit Beret Creme Caramel	2 (0.8 oz)	110	tr	5	0	15	tr	120

FOOD	PORTION	CAL	PROT	FAT	CHOL	CARB	FIBER	SOD
Petit Beret Fudge Truffle	2 (0.8 oz)	110	tr	5	0	15	tr	100
Petit Beurre	4 (1 oz)	130	2	4	tr	22	tr	115
Rich Tea	4 (1.2 oz)	160	2	5	0	25	tr	150
Shortcake	2 (0.9 oz)	140	1	7	20	18	0	70
Traditional Oatmeal	1 (0.7 oz)	90	1	3	0	15	tr	100
Tropical Cremes Calypso Lime	2 (0.9 oz)	130	1	5	0	20	0	15
Pepperidge Farm								
Biscotti Almond	1 (0.7 oz)	90	2	4	5	12	0	65
Biscotti Chocolate Hazelnut	1 (0.7 oz)	90	2	5	15	11	2	80
Biscotti Cranberry Pistachio	1 (0.7 oz)	90	2	3	5	13	0	65
Bordeaux	4	130	2	5	10	19	tr	95
Brussels	3	150	2	7	5	20	1	65
Chantilly Raspberry	2 (1 oz)	120	1	3	0	23	tr	115
Chessman	3	120	2	8	20	18	tr	80
Chocoate Chunk Soft Baked Double Chocolate	1 (0.9 oz)	130	2	7	0	15	1	60
Chocolate Chip	3	140	2	7	–	18	tr	70
Chocolate Chunk Chesapeake	1 (0.7 oz)	140	2	8	10	15	0	80
Chocolate Chunk Minis Nantauket	4 (1 oz)	150	0	8	10	20	0	70
Chocolate Chunk Minis Sausalito	4 (1 oz)	160	1	9	10	18	0	70
Chocolate Chunk Montauk	1 (0.9 oz)	130	1	7	10	17	0	90
Chocolate Chunk Nantucket	1 (0.9 oz)	140	2	7	10	16	0	80
Chocolate Chunk Sausalito	1 (0.7 oz)	140	2	8	10	16	0	80
Chocolate Chunk Soft Baked	1	130	2	6	10	16	0	80
Chocolate Chunk Soft Baked Milk Chocolate Macademia	1	130	2	7	10	16	0	75

FOOD	PORTION	CAL	PROT	FAT	CHOL	CARB	FIBER	SOD
Chocolate Chunk Soft Baked Reduced Fat	1	110	1	5	15	18	tr	85
Chocolate Chunk Soft Baked White Chocolate Pecan	1	120	1	5	5	16	1	65
Chocolate Chunk Tahoe	1 (0.9 oz)	130	2	8	10	15	0	90
Fruitful Apricot Raspberry Cup	3	140	2	6	–	22	tr	110
Fruitful Strawberry Cup	3	140	2	5	10	22	tr	105
Geneva	3	160	2	9	0	19	1	95
Ginger Man	4 (1 oz)	130	2	4	10	21	tr	100
Lemon Nut Crunch	3	170	2	9	15	18	2	60
Lido	1	90	tr	5	<5	10	0	40
Milano	3	180	2	10	–	21	tr	80
Milano Endless Chocolate	3	180	2	10	<5	21	1	85
Milano Milk Chocolate	3	170	2	9	10	21	tr	110
Milano Double Chocolate	2 (0.7 oz)	140	2	8	10	17	tr	70
Milano Mint	2	130	1	7	<5	16	1	65
Milano Orange	2	130	1	7	–	16	tr	65
Pirouettes Chocolate Laced	5 (1.1 oz)	180	2	10	5	20	tr	90
Pirouettes Traditional	5 (1.2 oz)	170	2	9	5	20	0	90
Shortbread	2	140	2	7	10	16	tr	105
Soft Baked Oatmeal Raisin	1 (0.9 oz)	130	2	7	10	16	0	75
Soft Baked Reduced Fat Oatmeal Raisin	1 (0.9 oz)	100	1	3	10	18	tr	85
Spritzers Cool Key Lime	6 (1.1 oz)	140	1	7	<5	21	0	60
Spritzers Ripe Red Raspberry	5 (1.1 oz)	140	1	7	<5	21	0	60

FOOD	PORTION	CAL	PROT	FAT	CHOL	CARB	FIBER	SOD
Spritzers Zesty Lemon	5 (1.1 oz)	140	1	7	<5	21	0	60
Sugar	3	140	2	6	—	20	tr	90
Verona Strawberry	3 (1.1 oz)	140	2	5	10	22	tr	105
Ralston								
Animal	12 (0.9 oz)	130	2	3	—	22	—	80
Chocolate Graham	2 (0.9 oz)	130	2	3	—	24	1	120
Cinnamon Grahams	2 (0.9 oz)	130	1	5	—	19	tr	85
Cinnamon Grahams Low Fat	2 (0.9 oz)	110	2	2	0	22	1	120
Fig Bars	2 (1.2 oz)	120	tr	3	—	23	1	55
Vanilla Wafers	7 (1.1 oz)	150	1	6	—	22	1	115
Real Torino								
Lady Fingers	3 (1 oz)	110	2	1	5	23	0	70
Reko								
Pizzelle Maple	5 (1 oz)	150	3	6	15	20	0	20
Pizzelle Vanilla	1 (6 g)	30	1	1	3	4	0	4
Royal								
Apple Bars	1 (1.1 oz)	100	1	2	0	21	1	65
Apple Cake	1 (1.1 oz)	110	1	3	0	19	1	50
Brownie Rounds	1 (1.1 oz)	130	1	6	0	19	0	135
Chocolate Chip	1 (1.1 oz)	140	1	6	0	20	1	120
Devilfood	1 (1 oz)	110	1	5	0	17	0	110
Fig Bars	1 (1.1 oz)	100	1	2	0	20	1	65
Oatmeal	1 (1.1 oz)	130	2	6	0	19	1	140
Raisin	1 (1 oz)	110	1	5	0	17	0	115
Strawberry Bars	1 (1.1 oz)	100	1	2	0	20	1	65
Salerno								
Mini Butter	25 (1 oz)	180	2	6	15	20	tr	125
Mini Dinosaur Chocolate Graham	16 (1.1 oz)	140	2	5	0	22	1	125
Scooter Pie	1 (1.2 oz)	140	1	5	0	23	0	80
Santa Fe Farms								
Chocolate Chocolate Chip Fat Free	2 (1 oz)	60	2	0	0	16	3	90
Chocolate Mint Fat Free	2 (1 oz)	60	2	0	0	16	3	90
Ginger Fat Free	2 (1 oz)	70	2	0	0	17	2	95

FOOD	PORTION	CAL	PROT	FAT	CHOL	CARB	FIBER	SOD
Sargento								
MooTown Snackers Vanilla Sticks & Chocolate Fudge Creme	1 pkg (1 oz)	130	1	6	0	18	tr	50
Savion								
Chocolate Biscuits	5 (1 oz)	120	2	3	0	22	0	45
Tea Biscuits	5 (1 oz)	120	2	3	0	22	0	80
Tea Biscuits Vanilla	5 (1 oz)	120	2	3	0	22	0	80
Scotto's								
Biscotti Fat Free French Vanilla	4 (1 oz)	80	2	0	0	18	0	25
Season								
Hamantashen Poppy	1 (1 oz)	150	1	7	7	20	1	60
Hamantasken Apricot	1 (1 oz)	150	1	7	7	20	1	60
Simple Pleasures								
Almond	1 (0.3 oz)	37	1	2	0	5	tr	9
Cinnamon Snaps	1 (0.2 oz)	31	1	1	0	6	tr	27
Digestive	1 (0.3 oz)	46	1	2	0	6	tr	34
Encore Tea Cookie	1 (0.2 oz)	29	tr	1	0	6	tr	32
Lemon Social Tea	1 (0.2 oz)	29	tr	1	0	6	tr	32
Oatmeal	1 (0.5 oz)	74	1	3	0	5	1	—
Spice Snaps	1 (0.3 oz)	34	1	1	0	6	tr	56
Sugar	1 (0.4 oz)	45	1	2	3	7	tr	—
SnackWell's								
Bite Size Chocolate Chip	13 (1 oz)	130	2	4	0	22	tr	160
Bite Size Double Chocolate Chip	13 (1 oz)	130	2	4	0	22	1	190
Bite Size Peanut Butter	13 (1 oz)	120	3	4	0	20	tr	210
Caramel Delights	1 (0.6 oz)	70	1	2	0	13	0	35
Chocolate Sandwich	2 (0.8 oz)	110	1	3	0	20	tr	210
Creme Sandwich	2 (0.9 oz)	110	1	3	0	20	0	130
Fat Free Devil's Food	1 (0.5 oz)	50	1	0	0	12	0	30
Golden Devil's Food	1 (0.5 oz)	50	1	1	0	11	0	25
Mint Creme	2 (0.9 oz)	110	1	4	0	19	tr	70
Oatmeal Raisin	2 (0.9 oz)	110	2	3	<5	20	tr	130

FOOD	PORTION	CAL	PROT	FAT	CHOL	CARB	FIBER	SOD
Stella D'Oro								
Almond Toast Mandel	2 (1 oz)	110	2	3	30	21	1	85
Angel Wings	2 (0.9 oz)	140	2	9	<5	13	tr	80
Angelica	1 (0.8 oz)	100	2	4	15	15	0	45
Anginetti	4 (1.1 oz)	140	2	4	40	23	tr	10
Anisette Sponge	2 (0.9 oz)	90	2	1	40	19	tr	80
Anisette Toast	3 (1.2 oz)	130	2	1	35	27	tr	150
Biscotti Almond	1 (0.8 oz)	100	2	3	10	15	tr	55
Biscotti Chocolate Almond	1 (0.8 oz)	90	2	3	10	15	1	55
Biscotti Chocolate Chunk	1 (0.8 oz)	90	2	3	10	16	0	60
Biscotti Hazelnut	1 (0.8 oz)	100	2	4	10	15	0	60
Biscottini Cashews	1 (0.7 oz)	110	1	6	5	13	0	50
Breakfast Treats	1 (0.8 oz)	100	1	3	10	16	tr	80
Breakfast Treats Chocolate	1 (0.8 oz)	100	2	4	10	15	tr	70
Breakfast Treats Viennese Cinnamon	1 (0.8 oz)	100	1	3	10	17	0	65
Chinese Dessert Cookies	1 (1.2 oz)	170	2	9	5	21	tr	90
Chocolate Castelets	2 (1 oz)	130	2	6	<5	19	1	55
Egg Jumbo	2 (0.8 oz)	90	2	1	30	18	tr	60
Fruit Slices Fat Free	1 (0.6 oz)	50	1	0	0	12	tr	45
Kichel Low Sodium	21 (1 oz)	150	4	9	80	13	0	25
Lady Stella Assortment	3 (1 oz)	130	1	5	5	19	0	55
Margherite Chocolate	2 (1.1 oz)	140	2	6	10	22	1	75
Margherite Vanilla	2 (1.1 oz)	140	2	5	15	22	tr	90
Roman Egg Biscuits	1 (1.2 oz)	140	2	5	20	21	1	125
Sesame Regina	3 (1.1 oz)	150	2	6	10	21	1	85
Swiss Fudge	2 (0.9 oz)	130	1	7	5	16	0	55
Stieffenhofer								
Choco Minis	4 (1 oz)	160	1	8	15	19	1	40
Snaky	3 (1 oz)	160	2	8	0	19	0	20
Streit's								
Wafers	3 (1 oz)	160	1	9	0	19	1	35

FOOD	PORTION	CAL	PROT	FAT	CHOL	CARB	FIBER	SOD
Suissette								
Swiss Chocolate Hearts	4 (1 oz)	170	2	10	5	17	—	40
Swiss Delight	4 (1 oz)	160	2	9	5	19	—	35
Swiss Praline	4 (1 oz)	150	1	9	15	17	1	15
Sunshine								
All American Butter	5 (1.1 oz)	140	2	6	<5	21	tr	135
All American Lemon Coolers	5 (1 oz)	140	1	6	0	21	tr	100
All American Mini Chip-A-Roos	5 (1.1 oz)	160	1	8	0	21	1	140
Animal Crackers	14 (1.1 oz)	140	2	4	0	24	tr	125
Ginger Snaps	7 (1 oz)	130	2	5	0	22	tr	150
Golden Fruit Cranberry	1 (0.7 oz)	80	1	2	0	14	tr	55
Golden Fruit Raisin	1 (0.7 oz)	80	1	2	0	15	tr	50
Hydrox	3 (1.1 oz)	150	2	7	0	21	1	125
Hydrox Reduced Fat	3 (1.1 oz)	140	2	5	0	23	1	150
Oatmeal Country Style	2 (0.8 oz)	120	2	5	0	17	tr	115
Sugar Wafers Peanut Butter Creme	4 (1.1 oz)	170	3	9	0	19	1	75
Sugar Wafers Vanilla Creme	3 (0.9 oz)	130	1	6	0	18	tr	30
Vanilla Wafers	7 (1.1 oz)	150	2	7	3	21	tr	110
Vienna Fingers	2 (1 oz)	140	2	6	0	21	tr	105
Vienna Fingers Lemon	2 (1 oz)	140	2	6	0	21	0	90
Vienna Fingers Reduced Fat	2 (1 oz)	130	1	5	0	22	tr	105
Sweet'N Low								
Sugar Free Amaretto Biscotti	4 (1 oz)	120	2	6	10	17	tr	180
Sugar Free Chocolate Chip	4 (1 oz)	135	2	8	10	17	tr	35
Sugar Free Cinnamon Graham	7 (1 oz)	120	2	6	15	19	tr	90

FOOD	PORTION	CAL	PROT	FAT	CHOL	CARB	FIBER	SOD
Sugar Free Morning Crunch Bars	2 (1 oz)	120	2	6	10	19	tr	150
Sugar Free Vanilla Wafers	7 (1 oz)	120	2	6	15	19	tr	80
Sweetzels								
Chocolate Chip	7 (1 oz)	160	1	9	5	18	0	70
Ginger Snaps	4 (1.2 oz)	140	2	3	0	25	tr	120
Vanilla Wafers	7 (1.1 oz)	137	2	5	0	22	0	94
Tastykake								
Chocolate Chip	1 (1.4 oz)	180	2	7	10	26	1	160
Chocolate Chip Bar	1 (2 oz)	270	2	12	10	39	tr	125
Chocolate Fudge Iced	1 (1.4 oz)	170	4	7	55	25	1	190
Fudge Bar	1 (2 oz)	250	3	10	5	37	1	140
Lemon Bar	1 (2 oz)	260	2	10	5	41	1	125
Oatmeal Raisin Bar	1 (2 oz)	260	4	10	15	40	2	230
Oatmeal Raisin Boxed	3 (0.4 oz)	130	1	6	5	14	tr	70
Oatmeal Raisin Iced	1 (1.4 oz)	170	3	6	25	27	1	150
Strawberry Bar	1 (2 oz)	260	2	10	5	41	1	125
Sugar Boxed	3 (0.4 oz)	120	1	6	10	18	0	85
The Source								
Barry's Raspberry Palmiers	1 (0.7 oz)	80	1	3	0	14	0	50
Tom's								
Animal Crackers	½ pkg (1 oz)	120	2	2	0	23	tr	140
Big Cookie Chocolate Chip	1 pkg (2.75 oz)	340	4	16	0	49	1	280
Big Cookie Peanut Butter Chocolate Chip	1 pkg (2 oz)	280	3	15	0	37	1	180
Chocolate Chip	1 pkg (2 oz)	280	3	15	0	37	1	180
Confetti Chip	1 pkg (2 oz)	300	3	13	0	40	tr	140
Fat Free Apple Bar	1 pkg (1.75 oz)	160	2	0	0	38	1	250
Fat Free Fig Bar	1 pkg (1.75 oz)	160	2	0	0	40	2	180
Vanilla Wafers	½ pkg (1 oz)	130	2	5	0	20	tr	100
Tree Of Life								
Fat Free Almond Butter	1 (0.8 oz)	60	1	0	0	14	1	50
Fat Free Carrot Cake	1 (0.8 oz)	60	1	0	0	14	1	50

FOOD	PORTION	CAL	PROT	FAT	CHOL	CARB	FIBER	SOD
Fat Free Devil's Food Chocolate	1 (0.8 oz)	70	2	0	0	15	1	80
Fat Free Oatmeal Raisin	1 (0.8 oz)	70	2	0	0	16	1	40
Fruit Bars Fat Free Fig	1 (0.8 oz)	70	1	0	0	16	2	100
Fruit Bars Fat Free Peach Apricot	1 (0.8 oz)	70	1	0	0	17	1	110
Fruit Bars Fat Free Wildberry	1 (0.8 oz)	70	1	0	0	16	2	170
Monster Carob Chip	1 (4.7 oz)	700	10	35	10	95	5	375
Monster Granola	1 (4.7 oz)	700	10	30	10	95	5	475
Monster Macaroon	1 (4.7 oz)	750	5	45	10	85	5	375
Monster Peanut Butter	1 (4.7 oz)	700	15	35	20	85	5	525
Monster Fat Free Carrot Cake	1 cookie (3.8 oz)	240	4	0	0	60	4	120
Monster Fat Free Devil's Food Chocolate	1 cookie (3.8 oz)	320	8	0	0	80	8	180
Monster Fat Free Gingerbread	1 cookie (3.8 oz)	320	8	0	0	76	8	200
Monster Fat Free Maple Pecan	1 cookie (3.8 oz)	360	8	0	0	80	8	200
Oatmeal	1 (0.8 oz)	100	2	4	15	16	0	55
Sandwich Royal Vanilla	2 (0.9 oz)	120	1	5	0	17	1	115
Wheat Free Carob	1 (0.8 oz)	100	1	5	0	14	6	75
Wheat Free Maple Walnut	1 (0.8 oz)	100	2	6	0	13	6	50
Wheat Free Oatmeal	1 (0.8 oz)	90	1	5	0	11	1	25
Wheat Free Peanut Butter	1 (0.8 oz)	109	2	6	0	8	1	100
Twix								
Bars Chocolate Caramel	1 (0.9 oz)	140	1	7	0	18	0	55
Voortman								
Almonette	2 (1 oz)	150	1	8	0	17	tr	65
Chocolate Chip	1 (0.7 oz)	100	tr	5	0	13	0	45

FOOD	PORTION	CAL	PROT	FAT	CHOL	CARB	FIBER	SOD
Chocolate Wafers Sugar Free	3 (1 oz)	160	tr	11	0	18	0	30
Coconut Delight	1 (0.6 oz)	90	tr	5	0	10	0	25
Peanut Delight	1 (0.9 oz)	130	2	7	<5	15	tr	90
Strawberry Wafers Sugar Free	3 (1 oz)	160	tr	11	0	18	0	30
Sugar	1 (0.6 oz)	80	tr	4	0	11	0	45
Turnovers Blueberry	1 (0.9 oz)	100	1	3	<5	16	0	50
Turnovers Cherry	1 (0.9 oz)	100	1	3	<5	16	0	50
Turnovers Strawberry	1 (0.9 oz)	100	1	3	<5	16	0	50
Vanilla Wafers Sugar Free	3 (1 oz)	160	tr	11	0	18	0	30
Windmill	1 (0.7 oz)	90	tr	4	0	13	0	100
Walkers								
Shortbread Triangles	2 (0.7 oz)	100	1	6	15	12	0	65
Weight Watchers								
Apple Raisin Bar	1 (0.75 oz)	70	1	2	0	14	2	60
Chocolate Chip	2 (1.06 oz)	140	2	5	0	22	1	90
Chocolate Sandwich	2 (1.06)	140	2	4	0	23	1	160
Fruit Filled Fig	1 (0.7 oz)	70	1	0	0	16	0	50
Fruit Filled Raspberry	1 (0.7 oz)	70	1	0	0	16	0	45
Oatmeal Raisin	2 (1.06 oz)	120	2	2	0	22	1	90
Vanilla Sandwich	2 (1.06 oz)	140	1	3	0	25	1	80
White Eagle Bakery								
Chruscik	2 (1 oz)	140	2	8	45	16	0	95
Wortz								
Animal	9 (1.1 oz)	140	2	5	—	22	1	140
Chocolate Graham	2 (0.9 oz)	130	2	3	—	24	1	120
Cinnamon Grahams	2 (0.9 oz)	130	1	5	—	19	tr	85
Vanilla Wafers	7 (1.1 oz)	150	1	6	—	22	1	115
REFRIGERATED								
chocolate chip	1 (0.42 oz)	59	1	3	3	8	—	28
chocolate chip unbaked	1 oz	126	1	6	7	17	—	59
oatmeal	1 (0.4 oz)	56	1	3	3	8	—	39
oatmeal raisin	1 (0.4 oz)	56	1	3	3	8	—	39
peanut butter	1 (0.4 oz)	60	1	3	4	7	—	52
peanut butter dough	1 oz	130	2	7	8	15	—	112
sugar	1 (0.42 oz)	58	1	3	4	8	—	56

FOOD	PORTION	CAL	PROT	FAT	CHOL	CARB	FIBER	SOD
sugar dough	1 oz	124	1	6	8	17	–	120
Pillsbury								
Bunny	2	130	1	7	<5	17	0	100
Chocolate Chip	1 (1 oz)	130	1	6	<5	17	tr	85
Chocolate Chip Reduced Fat	1 (1 oz)	110	1	3	<5	19	tr	85
Chocolate Chip w/ Walnuts	1 (1 oz)	140	1	7	<5	17	tr	90
Chocolate Chunk	1 (1 oz)	130	1	6	<5	17	tr	90
Christmas Tree	2	130	1	7	<5	17	0	100
Double Chocolate	1 (1 oz)	130	1	6	<5	17	tr	90
Flag	2	130	1	7	<5	17	0	100
Frosty	2	130	1	7	<5	17	0	100
M&M's	1 (1 oz)	130	1	6	<5	18	tr	75
Oatmeal Chocolate Chip	1 (1 oz)	120	1	6	<5	16	tr	95
One Step Pan Chocolate Chip	⅛ pan (1 oz)	130	1	6	<5	19	tr	100
One Step Pan M&M's	⅛ pan (1 oz)	130	1	6	<5	19	tr	85
Peanut Butter	1 (1 oz)	120	2	6	<5	15	tr	130
Pumpkin	2	130	1	7	<5	17	0	100
Reeses	1 (1 oz)	130	3	6	<5	15	tr	105
Shamrock	2	130	1	7	<5	17	0	100
Sugar	2	130	1	3	<5	19	0	125
Sugar Holiday Red & Green	2	130	1	6	<5	19	0	125
Valentine	2	130	1	7	<5	17	0	100
White Chocolate Chunk	1 (1 oz)	130	1	6	<5	17	0	100
TAKE-OUT								
biscotti w/ nuts chocolate dipped	1 (1.3 oz)	117	2	6	18	16	1	33
black & white	1 lg (3 oz)	302	4	9	58	52	1	72
finikia	1 (1.2 oz)	171	2	5	27	16	1	26
koulourakia butter cookie twist	1 (0.9 oz)	113	2	6	32	14	tr	59

CORIANDER

FOOD	PORTION	CAL	PROT	FAT	CHOL	CARB	FIBER	SOD
leaf dried	1 tsp	2	tr	tr	0	tr	–	1
leaf fresh	¼ cup	1	tr	tr	0	tr	–	1
seed	1 tsp	5	tr	tr	0	1	–	1

FOOD	PORTION	CAL	PROT	FAT	CHOL	CARB	FIBER	SOD

CORN (see also BRAN, CEREAL, CORNMEAL)

CANNED

FOOD	PORTION	CAL	PROT	FAT	CHOL	CARB	FIBER	SOD
cream style	½ cup	93	2	1	0	23	–	365
w/ red & green peppers	½ cup	86	3	1	0	21	–	396
white	½ cup	66	2	1	0	15	–	–
yellow	½ cup	66	2	1	0	15	1	–
Del Monte								
Cream Style Golden	½ cup (4.4 oz)	90	2	1	0	20	2	360
Cream Style Golden No Salt Added	½ cup (4.4 oz)	60	1	1	0	14	2	10
Cream Style White	½ cup (4.4 oz)	100	2	1	0	21	2	360
Fiesta	½ cup (4.4 oz)	50	2	1	0	12	2	310
Gold & White Supersweet	½ cup (4.4 oz)	80	2	1	0	18	2	360
Whole Kernel Golden	½ cup (4.4 oz)	90	2	1	0	18	3	360
Whole Kernel Golden Supersweet No Salt Added	½ cup (4.4 oz)	60	2	1	0	11	3	10
Whole Kernel Golden Supersweet No Salt Added	½ cup (4.4 oz)	70	2	1	0	13	3	10
Whole Kernel Golden Supersweet No Sugar	½ cup (4.4 oz)	60	2	1	0	11	3	360
Whole Kernel Golden Supersweet Vacuum Packed	½ cup (3.7 oz)	70	2	1	0	13	3	270
Whole Kernel White Sweet	½ cup (4.4 oz)	60	2	1	0	11	3	360
Green Giant								
Cream Style	½ cup (4.5 oz)	100	2	1	0	22	1	430
Mexicorn	⅓ cup (2.7 oz)	60	2	0	0	14	2	430
Niblets	⅓ cup (2.7 oz)	70	2	0	0	15	2	230

FOOD	PORTION	CAL	PROT	FAT	CHOL	CARB	FIBER	SOD
Niblets 50% Less Sodium	⅓ cup (2.7 oz)	60	2	0	0	14	1	115
Niblets Extra Sweet	⅓ cup (2.6 oz)	50	2	1	0	10	2	200
Niblets No Added Sugar or Salt	⅓ cup (2.7 oz)	60	2	0	0	13	2	0
White Shoepeg	⅓ cup	80	2	1	0	16	1	220
Whole Sweet	½ cup (4.3 oz)	80	2	1	0	18	2	360
Whole Sweet 50% Less Sodium	½ cup (4.2 oz)	80	2	1	0	17	2	180
Owatonna								
Cream Style	½ cup	100	–	1	0	–	–	–
Whole Kernel In Brine	½ cup	90	–	1	0	–	–	–
Whole Kernel Vacuum Pack	½ cup	100	–	1	0	–	–	–
S&W								
Cream Style	½ cup (4.4 oz)	60	1	1	0	14	2	360
Whole Kernel	⅓ cup (3 oz)	70	2	2	0	12	2	170
DRIED								
Goya								
Giant White	⅓ cup (1.6 oz)	160	2	2	0	35	4	10
FRESH								
on-the-cob w/ butter cooked	1 ear	155	4	3	6	32	–	30
white cooked	½ cup	89	3	1	0	21	–	14
white raw	½ cup	66	2	1	0	15	–	12
yellow cooked	1 ear (2.7 oz)	83	3	1	0	19	–	13
yellow cooked	½ cup	89	3	1	0	21	–	14
yellow raw	1 ear (3 oz)	77	3	1	0	17	–	14
yellow raw	½ cup	66	2	1	0	15	–	12
FROZEN								
cooked	½ cup	67	2	tr	0	17	–	4
on-the-cob cooked	1 ear (2.2 oz)	59	2	tr	0	14	–	3
Birds Eye								
Cob Big Ears	1 ear	120	–	1	0	–	3	0
Cut	⅓ cup	70	–	1	0	–	2	0
Gold & White Blend	½ cup (3.5 oz)	60	2	1	0	11	2	330

FOOD	PORTION	CAL	PROT	FAT	CHOL	CARB	FIBER	SOD
Green Giant								
Butter Sauce Niblets	⅔ cup (4.3 oz)	130	3	3	<5	23	3	350
Butter Sauce Shoepeg White	¾ cup (4 oz)	120	3	3	<5	21	3	320
Cream Corn	½ cup (4.1 oz)	110	2	1	0	23	2	330
Extra Sweet Niblets	⅔ cup (3.1 oz)	70	2	1	0	13	2	0
Harvest Fresh Niblets	⅔ cup (3.4 oz)	80	3	1	0	17	3	60
Harvest Fresh Shoepeg White	½ cup (2.6 oz)	70	2	1	0	14	2	45
Niblets	⅔ cup (2.9 oz)	80	2	1	0	17	2	5
On The Cob Extra Sweet	1 ear (4.4 oz)	120	4	2	0	22	3	0
On The Cob Nibblers	1 ear (2.1 oz)	70	2	1	0	14	1	0
On The Cob Niblets	1 ear (5 oz)	160	4	2	0	32	3	10
Select Extra Sweet White	⅔ cup (2.9 oz)	50	2	1	0	10	3	0
Select Shoepeg White	¾ cup (3.2 oz)	100	3	1	0	20	3	0
Stouffer's								
Souffle	½ cup (6 oz)	170	5	7	65	21	1	490
Tree Of Life								
Corn	⅔ cup (3.2 oz)	80	3	1	0	19	1	10
TAKE-OUT								
fritters	1 (1 oz)	62	2	2	12	9	1	126
scalloped	½ cup	258	7	7	47	43	–	246

CORN CHIPS (see CHIPS)

CORNISH HENS (see CHICKEN)

CORNMEAL (see also POLENTA)

FOOD	PORTION	CAL	PROT	FAT	CHOL	CARB	FIBER	SOD
corn grits cooked	1 cup	146	4	tr	0	31	–	0
corn grits uncooked	1 cup	579	14	2	0	124	–	1
white	1 cup (4.8 oz)	505	12	2	0	107	10	4
whole grain	1 cup (4.3 oz)	442	10	4	0	94	9	43
yellow	1 cup (4.8 oz)	505	12	2	0	107	10	4
yellow self-rising	1 cup (4.3 oz)	407	10	4	0	86	8	1521
Albers								
White	3 tbsp	110	2	0	0	24	tr	0
Yellow	3 tbsp	110	2	0	0	24	tr	0

FOOD	PORTION	CAL	PROT	FAT	CHOL	CARB	FIBER	SOD
MIX								
Hodgson Mill								
Cornbread Mix Jalapeno Mexican	¼ cup (1 oz)	100	4	1	0	21	1	310
Yellow Organic	¼ cup (1 oz)	100	3	1	0	22	3	0
Yellow Self Rising	¼ cup (1 oz)	90	3	1	0	21	3	260
Kentucky Kernal								
Sweet Cornbread Mix	¼ cup (1 oz)	120	2	2	0	24	0	310
TAKE-OUT								
hush puppies	1 (0.75 oz)	74	3	3	10	10	1	147
CORNSTARCH								
cornstarch	1 cup (4.5 oz)	488	tr	tr	0	117	1	12
Armour								
Cream Cornstarch	1 tbsp (0.4 oz)	40	0	0	0	9	0	0
COTTAGE CHEESE								
creamed	4 oz	117	14	5	17	3	—	457
creamed	1 cup (7.4 oz)	217	26	9	31	6	—	850
creamed w/ fruit	4 oz	140	11	4	13	15	—	457
dry curd	1 cup (5.1 oz)	123	25	1	10	3	—	19
dry curd	4 oz	96	20	tr	8	2	—	14
lowfat 1%	4 oz	82	14	1	5	3	—	459
lowfat 1%	1 cup (7.9 oz)	164	28	2	10	6	—	918
lowfat 2%	1 cup (7.9 oz)	203	31	4	19	8	—	918
lowfat 2%	4 oz	101	16	2	9	4	—	459
Breakstone's								
2% Fat Large Curd	½ cup (4.2 oz)	90	13	3	15	4	0	390
2% Fat Small Curd	½ cup (4.2 oz)	90	13	3	15	4	0	390
4% Fat Large Curd	½ cup (4.2 oz)	120	13	5	25	5	0	400
4% Fat Small Curd	½ cup (4.2 oz)	120	13	5	25	5	0	400
Cottage Doubles Peach	1 pkg (5.5 oz)	140	12	3	15	16	tr	390
Dry Curd	¼ cup (1.9 oz)	45	8	0	<5	3	0	30
Free	½ cup (4.4 oz)	80	13	0	5	6	0	440
Snack 2% Fat Small Curd	1 pkg (4 oz)	90	12	2	15	4	0	370
Snack 4% Fat Small Curd	1 pkg (4 oz)	110	12	5	25	4	0	380

FOOD	PORTION	CAL	PROT	FAT	CHOL	CARB	FIBER	SOD
Snack Free	1 pkg (4 oz)	70	12	0	5	6	0	400
Horizon Organic								
Cottage Cheese	½ cup (3.9 oz)	110	13	5	15	4	0	340
Knudsen								
1.5% Fat Small Curd Pineapple	½ cup (4.6 oz)	120	11	2	10	14	0	330
2% Fat Small Curd	½ cup (4.2 oz)	100	14	3	15	5	0	400
4% Fat Large Curd	½ cup (4.5 oz)	130	16	5	30	4	0	330
4% Fat Small Curd	½ cup (4.3 oz)	120	14	5	25	4	0	400
Free	½ cup (4.2 oz)	80	14	0	5	4	0	380
On The Go! 1.5% Fat Peach	1 pkg (4 oz)	110	10	2	10	13	0	300
On The Go! 1.5% Fat Pineapple	1 pkg (4 oz)	110	10	2	10	13	0	300
On The Go! 1.5% Fat Strawberry	1 pkg (4 oz)	110	10	2	10	13	0	290
On The Go! 1.5% Fat Tropical Fruit	1 pkg (4 oz)	110	10	2	10	13	0	300
On The Go! 2% Fat	1 pkg (4 oz)	90	13	2	15	5	0	370
On The Go! Free	1 pkg (4 oz)	70	13	0	5	4	0	350
Light N'Lively								
1% Fat	½ cup (4 oz)	80	12	1	10	5	0	370
1% Fat Garden Salad	½ cup (4.2 oz)	80	12	2	10	5	0	390
1% Fat Peach & Pineapple	½ cup (4.3 oz)	110	11	1	10	15	0	340
Fat Free	½ cup (4.4 oz)	80	13	0	5	6	0	440

COTTONSEED

kernels roasted	1 tbsp	51	3	4	0	2	–	3

COUGH DROPS

Lifesavers

Menthol	2 (0.5 oz)	60	0	0	0	14	–	0

COUSCOUS

cooked	1 cup (5.5 oz)	176	6	tr	0	36	2	8
dry	1 cup (6.1 oz)	650	22	1	0	134	9	17
Kitchen Del Sol								
Spicy Vegetable as prep	½ cup (1.1 oz)	120	3	3	0	20	1	290
Tomato & Olive	½ cup (1.1 oz)	120	3	4	0	19	1	290

FOOD	PORTION	CAL	PROT	FAT	CHOL	CARB	FIBER	SOD
Melting Pot								
Calypso Cranberry	1 cup	200	7	0	0	42	1	220
Lentil Curry	1 cup	170	7	0	0	35	1	290
Lucky Seven	1 cup	190	7	1	0	38	1	300
Mango Salsa	1 cup	190	6	0	0	40	1	270
Roasted Garlic	1 cup	170	7	0	0	34	1	370
Sesame Ginger	1 cup	180	7	1	0	36	0	350
Sun-Dried Tomatoes	1 cup	190	8	1	0	36	1	230
Wild Mushroom	1 cup	190	8	0	0	38	1	370
COWPEAS								
catjang dried cooked	1 cup (2.9 oz)	200	14	1	0	35	—	32
common canned	1 cup	184	11	1	0	33	—	718
frozen cooked	½ cup	112	7	tr	0	20	—	5
leafy tips chopped cooked	1 cup	12	2	tr	0	1	—	3
leafy tips raw chopped	1 cup	10	1	tr	0	2	—	2
CRAB								
CANNED								
blue	3 oz	84	17	1	76	0	—	283
blue	1 cup	133	28	2	120	0	—	5
Bumble Bee								
Fancy Lump Meat	½ can (1.9 oz)	40	8	1	50	0	0	300
Fancy White Meat	½ can (1.9 oz)	28	6	0	43	1	0	403
FRESH								
alaska king cooked	1 leg (4.7 oz)	129	26	2	72	0	—	1436
alaska king cooked	3 oz	82	16	1	45	0	—	911
alaska king raw	3 oz	71	16	1	35	0	—	711
alaska king raw	1 leg (6 oz)	144	32	1	72	0	—	1438
blue cooked	3 oz	87	17	2	85	0	—	237
blue cooked	1 cup	138	27	2	135	0	—	376
blue raw	1 crab (7 oz)	18	4	tr	16	tr	—	62
blue raw	3 oz	74	15	1	66	tr	—	249
dungeness raw	3 oz	73	15	1	50	1	—	251
dungeness raw	1 crab (5.7 oz)	140	28	2	97	1	—	481
queen steamed	3 oz	98	20	1	60	0	—	587
TAKE-OUT								
baked	1 (3.8 oz)	160	29	2	184	4	—	550
cake	1 (2 oz)	160	11	10	82	5	—	492

FOOD	PORTION	CAL	PROT	FAT	CHOL	CARB	FIBER	SOD
kenagi korean crab cooked	1 serv (3 oz)	71	16	tr	–	0	0	204
mousse	¼ cup	364	–	20	136	–	–	–
soft-shell fried	1 (4.4 oz)	334	11	18	45	31	–	1118

CRACKER CRUMBS

FOOD	PORTION	CAL	PROT	FAT	CHOL	CARB	FIBER	SOD
cracker meal	1 cup (4 oz)	440	11	2	0	93	–	32
graham cracker crumbs	½ cup (4.4 oz)	540	9	13	0	97	3	756
Baker's Harvest								
Graham	⅓ cup (1 oz)	130	2	4	0	23	1	110
Kellogg's								
Corn Flake Crumbs	2 tbsp (0.4 oz)	40	1	0	0	9	0	105

CRACKERS *(see also* CRACKER CRUMBS*)*

FOOD	PORTION	CAL	PROT	FAT	CHOL	CARB	FIBER	SOD
cheese	1 (1 in sq) (1 g)	5	tr	tr	0	1	–	10
cheese	14 (½ oz)	71	1	4	2	8	–	141
cheese low sodium	14 (½ oz)	71	1	4	2	8	–	68
cheese low sodium	1 (1 in sq) (1 g)	5	tr	tr	0	1	–	5
cheese w/ peanut butter filling	1 (0.24 oz)	34	1	2	0	4	tr	69
crispbread	3	61	1	2	–	9	1	–
crispbread rye	1 (0.35 oz)	37	1	tr	0	8	2	26
crispbread rye	3	77	2	1	–	17	3	–
melba toast plain	1 (5 g)	19	1	tr	0	4	tr	41
melba toast pumpernickel	1 (5 g)	19	1	tr	0	4	tr	45
melba toast rye	1 (5 g)	19	1	tr	0	4	tr	45
melba toast wheat	1 (5 g)	19	1	tr	0	4	tr	42
milk	1 (0.42 oz)	55	1	2	–	8	–	71
oyster cracker	1 (1 g)	4	tr	tr	0	1	tr	13
peanut butter sandwich	1 (7 g)	34	1	2	–	4	–	66
rusk toast	1 (0.35 oz)	41	1	1	–	7	–	25
rye w/ cheese filling	1 (0.24 oz)	34	1	2	1	4	–	73
rye wafers plain	1 (0.9 oz)	84	2	tr	0	20	–	199
rye wafers seasoned	1 (0.8 oz)	84	2	2	0	16	–	195
saltines	1 (3 g)	13	tr	tr	0	2	tr	38
saltines fat free low sodium	6 (1 oz)	118	3	tr	0	25	–	191

FOOD	PORTION	CAL	PROT	FAT	CHOL	CARB	FIBER	SOD
saltines fat free low sodium	3 (0.5 oz)	59	2	tr	0	12	–	95
saltines low salt	1 (3 g)	13	tr	tr	0	2	tr	19
snack cracker	1 (3 g)	15	tr	1	0	2	tr	25
snack cracker low salt	1 (3 g)	15	tr	1	0	2	tr	11
snack cracker w/ cheese filling	1 (7 g)	33	1	2	0	4	–	98
soup cracker	1 (1 g)	4	tr	tr	0	1	tr	13
water biscuits	3	92	2	3	–	16	1	–
wheat w/ cheese filling	1 (0.24 oz)	35	1	2	1	4	–	64
wheat w/ peanut butter filling	1 (0.24 oz)	35	1	2	0	4	–	57
wheat thins	1 (2 g)	9	tr	tr	0	1	–	16
wheat thins	7 (0.5 oz)	67	1	3	0	9	1	113
wheat thins low salt	7 (0.5 oz)	67	1	3	0	9	1	40
whole wheat	1 (4 g)	18	tr	1	0	3	–	26
whole wheat low salt	1 (4 g)	18	tr	1	0	3	–	10
zwieback	1 oz	107	3	1	–	21	1	75
Ak-mak								
100% Whole Wheat	5 (1 oz)	116	5	2	0	19	4	214
Armenian Cracker Bread	1 sheet (1 oz)	100	4	2	0	19	2	200
Armenian Cracker Bread Whole Wheat	1 sheet (1 oz)	116	5	2	0	19	4	214
Round Cracker Bread No Seeds	1 (1 oz)	100	4	1	0	20	1	170
Round Cracker Bread Seeded	1 (1 oz)	100	4	2	0	19	2	200
Round Cracker Bread Whole Wheat	1 (1 oz)	116	5	2	0	19	4	214
Austin								
Cracker Sandwich Cheese On Cheese	6 (1.3 oz)	170	3	7	0	25	tr	310
Cracker Sandwich Cheese Peanut Butter	6 (1.3 oz)	170	5	7	0	24	1	320

FOOD	PORTION	CAL	PROT	FAT	CHOL	CARB	FIBER	SOD
Cracker Sandwich Toasty Peanut Butter	6 (1.3 oz)	170	5	7	0	24	1	340
Cracker Sandwich Whole Wheat Cheese	6 (1.3 oz)	170	3	7	0	25	tr	280
Baker's Harvest								
Cheese	23 (1 oz)	150	3	6	0	18	tr	370
Cheese Reduced Fat	29 (1 oz)	130	3	4	0	21	tr	310
Oyster	35 (0.5 oz)	70	1	2	–	11	1	150
Saltines Unsalted	5 (0.5 oz)	70	1	2	–	11	–	110
Saltines Deluxe	5 (0.5 oz)	60	1	2	–	10	–	130
Snackers	9 (1.1 oz)	160	2	8	–	19	tr	250
Snackers Reduced Fat	10 (1.1 oz)	140	3	4	0	23	tr	260
Snackers Unsalted	9 (1.1 oz)	160	2	8	–	19	tr	80
Wheat Snacks	16 (1 oz)	140	3	6	–	20	2	120
Wheat Snacks Reduced Fat	16 (1.1 oz)	140	2	4	0	23	1	220
Woven Wheats	7 (1.1 oz)	140	3	5	0	21	4	170
Woven Wheats Reduced Fat	8 (1.1 oz)	130	3	3	0	24	4	180
Barbara's Bakery								
Cheese Bites	26 (1 oz)	120	3	2	0	24	1	290
Right Lite Rounds Original	5 (0.5 oz)	55	1	5	0	12	0	150
Rite Lite Rounds Savory Poppy	5 (0.5 oz)	70	tr	2	0	11	0	135
Rite Lite Rounds Tamari Sesame	5 (0.5 oz)	70	1	2	0	12	0	160
Wheatines All Flavors	1 lg sq (0.5 oz)	50	1	2	0	10	1	110
Blue Diamond								
Nut Thins Almond	16 (1 oz)	130	3	5	0	19	tr	75
Nut Thins Hazelnut	16 (1 oz)	120	2	4	0	20	1	75
Nut Thins Pecan	16 (1 oz)	130	2	5	0	20	tr	75
Cheetos								
Bacon Cheddar	1 pkg	190	3	9	<5	25	1	410
Cheddar Cheese	1 pkg	210	3	11	<5	23	1	340

FOOD	PORTION	CAL	PROT	FAT	CHOL	CARB	FIBER	SOD
Golden Toast	1 pkg	240	4	14	5	25	1	440
Cheez It								
Big	13 (1 oz)	150	4	8	0	16	tr	230
Big Reduced Fat	15 (1 oz)	140	4	5	0	20	tr	280
Heads & Tails	37 (1 oz)	140	1	6	0	18	1	330
Hot & Spicy	26 (1 oz)	150	4	8	0	17	tr	300
Low Sodium	27 (1 oz)	160	4	8	0	16	tr	70
Nacho	28 (1 oz)	150	3	7	0	18	tr	280
Original	27 (1 oz)	160	4	8	0	16	tr	240
Party Mix	½ cup (1 oz)	140	4	5	0	19	1	270
Party Mix Nacho	½ cup (1 oz)	130	3	5	0	20	1	330
Party Mix Reduced Fat	½ cup (1 oz)	130	4	3	0	21	1	300
Peanut Butter	1 pkg (1.3 oz)	190	4	10	0	22	1	400
Reduced Fat	29 (1 oz)	140	4	5	0	20	tr	280
Snack Mix	½ cup (1 oz)	130	3	5	0	21	2	330
Snack Mix Big Crunch	¾ cup (1 oz)	110	3	6	0	20	tr	360
Snack Mix Double Cheese	¾ cup (1 oz)	110	3	5	0	19	tr	450
White Cheddar	26 (1 oz)	150	3	7	<5	18	tr	280
Courtney's								
Sun-Dried Tomato Organic	4 (0.5 oz)	60	1	1	0	10	0	130
Dare								
Breton	1 (5 g)	21	1	1	0	3	tr	40
Breton Garden Vegetable	1 (5 g)	20	tr	1	0	3	tr	34
Breton Light	1 (5 g)	20	1	1	0	3	tr	39
Breton Reduced Fat & Sodium	3 (0.5 oz)	60	2	2	0	9	tr	75
Breton Sesame	1 (5 g)	22	tr	1	0	3	tr	40
Breton Minis	20 (0.6 oz)	89	2	4	0	11	tr	169
Breton Minis Cheddar Cheese	20 (0.6 oz)	87	3	4	3	11	–	211
Breton Minis Garden Vegetable	20 (0.6 oz)	87	2	4	0	12	1	144
Cabaret	1 (5 g)	23	tr	1	0	3	tr	45
Vinta	1 (6 g)	30	1	1	0	4	1	–
Vivant Italian Bruschetta	1 (5 g)	22	tr	1	0	3	tr	39

FOOD	PORTION	CAL	PROT	FAT	CHOL	CARB	FIBER	SOD
Doritos								
Jalapeno Cheese	1 pkg	230	3	14	<5	26	1	450
Nacho Cheddar	1 pkg	240	4	14	<5	25	1	340
Eden								
Nori Nori Rice	15 (1 oz)	110	3	0	0	24	2	160
Estee								
Sugar Free Cracked Pepper	18	120	3	2	0	24	1	200
Sugar Free Golden	10	130	3	2	0	28	1	200
Sugar Free Wheat	17	100	3	2	0	18	2	200
Frito Lay								
Cheddar Snacks	1 pkg	200	5	10	<5	27	1	530
Frookie								
Cheddar	17 (1 oz)	140	4	4	0	23	1	420
Cracked Pepper	8 (0.7 oz)	70	2	0	0	15	1	85
Garden Vegetable	13 (1 oz)	130	3	4	0	19	2	380
Garlic & Herb	8 (0.7 oz)	70	2	0	0	16	1	170
Pizza	17 (1 oz)	130	3	3	0	24	1	420
Snack & Party	10 (1 oz)	140	2	5	0	20	1	260
Water Crackers	8 (0.7 oz)	70	2	0	0	16	1	135
Wheat & Onion	12 (1 oz)	120	3	4	0	18	2	400
Wheat & Rye	13 (1 oz)	120	3	4	0	18	3	380
Gold'NKrackle								
Cheese	½ oz	65	2	2	2	9	0	85
Health Valley								
Healthy Pizza Garlic & Herb	6	50	2	0	0	11	2	140
Healthy Pizza Italiano	6	50	2	0	0	11	2	140
Healthy Pizza Zesty Cheese	6	50	2	0	0	11	2	140
Low Fat Mild Jalapeno	6	60	2	2	0	10	2	90
Low Fat Mild Ranch	6	60	2	2	0	10	2	90
Low Fat Roasted Garlic	6	60	2	2	0	10	2	90
Original Oat Bran	6	120	3	3	0	22	3	80
Original Rice Bran	6	110	3	3	0	19	3	70
Whole Wheat	5	50	2	0	0	11	2	80
Whole Wheat Cheese	5	50	2	0	0	11	2	100
Whole Wheat Herb	5	50	2	0	0	11	2	100

FOOD	PORTION	CAL	PROT	FAT	CHOL	CARB	FIBER	SOD
Whole Wheat No Salt Vegetable	5	50	2	0	0	11	2	15
Whole Wheat Onion	5	50	2	0	0	11	2	80
Whole Wheat Vegetable	5	50	3	0	0	11	2	80
Healthy Choice								
Bread Crisps Garlic Herb	11 (1 oz)	110	3	2	0	22	2	115
Keebler								
Club 33% Reduced Fat	5 (0.6 oz)	70	1	2	0	12	0	200
Club 50% Reduced Sodium	4 (0.5 oz)	70	1	3	0	9	tr	80
Club Orignal	4 (0.5 oz)	70	1	3	0	9	tr	160
Elfin	23 (1 oz)	130	2	2	0	24	tr	140
Export Soda	3 (0.5 oz)	60	1	2	0	10	tr	80
Harvest Bakery Multigrain	2 (0.6 oz)	70	1	3	0	10	tr	80
Munch'ems Cheddar	39 (1 oz)	140	3	5	0	20	1	320
Munch'ems Cheddar	30 (1 oz)	130	3	4	0	21	tr	320
Munch'ems Chili Cheese	28 (1.1 oz)	130	2	4	0	23	1	470
Munch'ems Mexquite BBQ	40 (1 oz)	140	2	5	0	22	1	290
Munch'ems Ranch	40 (1 oz)	140	3	5	0	20	1	260
Munch'ems Ranch	33 (1 oz)	130	3	4	0	21	tr	310
Munch'ems Salsa	28 (1.1 oz)	130	2	4	0	23	1	260
Munch'ems Seasoned Original	30 (1 oz)	130	3	5	0	20	tr	350
Munch'ems Sour Cream & Onion	39 (1 oz)	140	3	5	0	20	1	280
Munch'ems Sour Cream & Onion 55% Reduced Fat	33 (1 oz)	130	2	4	0	22	0	390
Paks Cheese & Peanut Butter	1 pkg	190	6	9	<5	22	tr	420
Paks Club & Cheddar	1 pkg	190	3	11	10	20	tr	320

FOOD	PORTION	CAL	PROT	FAT	CHOL	CARB	FIBER	SOD
Paks Toast & Peanut Butter	1 pkg	190	5	9	0	23	1	300
Paks Wheat & Cheddar	1 pkg (1.3 oz)	180	2	10	5	17	0	300
Toasteds Buttercrisp	5 (0.6 oz)	80	1	4	0	10	0	150
Toasteds Buttercrisp	9 (1 oz)	140	2	7	<5	19	tr	280
Toasteds Onion	9 (1 oz)	140	2	6	0	19	tr	310
Toasteds Sesame	5 (0.6 oz)	80	1	4	0	10	tr	135
Toasteds Sesame	9 (1 oz)	140	3	6	0	19	tr	320
Toasteds Sesame Reduced Fat	10 (1 oz)	120	3	3	0	21	2	310
Toasteds Wheat	5 (0.6 oz)	80	1	4	0	10	tr	150
Toasteds Wheat	9 (1 oz)	140	2	6	0	19	tr	270
Toasteds Wheat Reduced Fat	5 (0.5 oz)	60	1	2	0	10	tr	160
Toasteds Wheat Reduced Fat	10 (1 oz)	120	3	3	0	22	1	300
Town House	5 (0.6 oz)	80	1	5	0	9	tr	150
Town House 50% Reduced Sodium	5 (0.6 oz)	80	1	5	0	10	tr	75
Town House Reduced Fat	6 (0.6 oz)	70	1	2	0	11	tr	180
Town House Wheat	5 (0.6 oz)	80	1	4	0	10	tr	140
Wheatables Honey Wheat	12 (1 oz)	140	2	6	0	20	1	200
Wheatables Original	12 (1 oz)	140	2	6	0	10	1	210
Wheatables Seven Grain	12 (1 oz)	140	2	6	0	20	1	250
Zesta Saltine 50% Reduced Sodium	5 (0.5 oz)	60	1	2	0	11	tr	95
Zesta Saltine Fat Free	5 (0.5 oz)	50	1	0	0	11	0	150
Zesta Saltine Original	5 (0.5 oz)	60	1	2	0	10	tr	190
Zesta Saltine Unsalted Top	5 (0.5 oz)	70	1	2	0	10	tr	90
Zesta Soup & Oyster	42 (0.5 oz)	80	1	3	0	10	tr	160
Lance								
Bonnie	6 (1⅛ oz)	160	3	7	10	23	0	160

FOOD	PORTION	CAL	PROT	FAT	CHOL	CARB	FIBER	SOD
Captain Wafers w/ Cream Cheese & Chives	1 pkg (1.3 oz)	190	4	9	0	22	0	250
Cheese-On-Wheat	1 pkg (1.3 oz)	190	4	10	<5	21	2	280
Cranberry Bar Fat Free	1 (1.75 oz)	160	1	0	0	38	1	55
Lanchee	1 pkg (1¼ oz)	190	5	11	0	18	1	120
Malt	1 pkg (1¼ oz)	190	6	10	0	18	1	130
Nekot	1 pkg (1.5 oz)	210	6	10	0	25	1	130
Nip-Chee	1 pkg (1.3 oz)	190	4	10	<5	21	1	330
Peanut Butter Wheat	1 pkg (1.3 oz)	190	5	11	0	20	1	240
Rye-Chee	1 pkg (1.4 oz)	210	4	11	<5	22	1	340
Sour Dough w/ Cheddar & Sour Cream	1 pkg (1.6 oz)	240	4	15	5	23	1	430
Toastchee	1 pkg (1.4 oz)	200	7	12	0	19	1	260
Toasty	1 pkg (1¼ oz)	190	6	11	0	17	1	220
Wheat Italian	¾ cup (1.4 oz)	200	3	11	0	23	1	430
Wheat Pizza	¾ cup (1.4 oz)	200	3	10	0	23	1	390
Little Debbie								
Cheese Crackers w/ Peanut Butter	1 (0.9 oz)	140	3	8	0	16	tr	210
Cheese On Cheese Crackers	1 (0.9 oz)	140	2	8	<5	15	0	220
Cream Cheese & Chive	1 (0.9 oz)	140	2	7	0	17	0	220
Toasty Crackers w/ Peanut Butter	1 (0.9 oz)	140	3	7	0	16	tr	210
Wheat Crackers w/ Cheddar Cheese	1 (0.9 oz)	140	3	8	<5	15	0	230
Nabisco								
Royal Lunch	1 (0.4 oz)	60	tr	2	0	8	0	70
Zwieback	1 (8 g)	35	1	1	0	6	0	10
Partners								
Walla Walla Sweet Onion Perservative Free	0.5 oz	65	2	3	3	8	tr	60
Pepperidge Farm								
Butter Thins	4 (0.5 oz)	70	1	3	10	10	0	95

FOOD	PORTION	CAL	PROT	FAT	CHOL	CARB	FIBER	SOD
English Water Biscuits	4 (0.5 oz)	70	2	2	0	13	0	95
Goldfish Cheddar	55	140	4	6	10	19	tr	250
Goldfish Cheddar 30% Less Sodium	60 (1.1 oz)	150	3	6	10	18	tr	175
Goldfish Cheese Trio	58	140	4	6	<5	19	1	280
Goldfish Original	55	140	3	6	0	19	tr	230
Goldfish Parmesan Cheese	60	140	4	5	0	13	1	300
Goldfish Pizza Flavored	55 (1 oz)	140	3	6	0	19	1	160
Goldfish Pretzel	43 (1 oz)	120	3	3	0	22	tr	430
Goldfish Toasted Wheat	41	150	4	7	0	19	2	280
Hearty Wheat	3 (0.6 oz)	80	2	4	0	10	1	100
Sesame	3 (0.5 oz)	70	1	3	0	9	2	95
Snack Mix Fat Free Goldfish	⅔ cup (0.9 oz)	90	3	0	0	20	0	380
Peter Pan								
Cheese Peanut Butter	1 pkg	210	5	10	0	23	1	350
Toast Peanut Butter	1 pkg	210	5	11	0	23	tr	280
Planters								
Cheese Peanut Butter Sandwiches	1 pkg (1.4 oz)	190	4	10	0	24	1	390
Toast Peanut Butter Sandwiches	1 pkg (1.4 oz)	190	4	10	0	24	1	380
Premium								
Saltine Multigrain	5 (0.5 oz)	60	1	2	0	10	tr	150
Ralston								
Cheese	23 (1 oz)	150	3	6	0	18	tr	370
Cheese Reduced Fat	29 (1 oz)	130	3	4	0	21	tr	310
Oyster	35 (0.5 oz)	70	1	2	—	11	1	150
Rich & Crisp	1 (0.5 oz)	70	1	3	—	9	0	105
Saltines Fat Free	5 (0.5 oz)	60	1	0	0	13	—	135
Saltines Deluxe	5 (0.5 oz)	60	1	2	—	10	—	130
Snackers	9 (1.1 oz)	160	2	8	—	19	tr	250
Snackers Reduced Fat	10 (1.1 oz)	140	2	4	0	23	tr	260
Snackers Unsalted	9 (1.1 oz)	160	2	8	—	19	tr	80
Wheat Snacks	16 (1 oz)	140	3	6	—	20	2	120

FOOD	PORTION	CAL	PROT	FAT	CHOL	CARB	FIBER	SOD
Wheat Snacks Reduced Fat	16 (1.1 oz)	140	2	4	0	23	1	220
Woven Wheats	7 (1.1 oz)	140	3	5	0	21	4	170
Woven Wheats Reduced Fat	8 (1.1 oz)	130	3	3	0	24	4	180
RedOval Farms								
Stoned Wheat Thins Cracked Pepper	4 (0.6 oz)	70	1	3	0	10	tr	190
Savory Thins								
Toasted Onion & Garlic	15 (1 oz)	110	3	1	0	23	2	90
Smucker's								
Snackers Grape	1 pkg (3.3 oz)	410	11	20	0	47	3	480
Snackers Strawberry	1 pkg (3.3 oz)	410	11	20	0	47	3	480
SnackWell's								
Salsa Cheddar	32 (1 oz)	120	2	2	0	23	1	340
Sunshine								
Hi Ho	4 (0.5 oz)	70	1	4	0	8	tr	130
Hi Ho Reduced Fat	5 (0.5 oz)	70	1	3	0	10	tr	140
Krispy	5 (0.5 oz)	60	2	2	0	10	tr	180
Krispy Fat Free	5 (0.5 oz)	50	1	0	0	11	0	150
Krispy Mild Cheddar	5 (0.5 oz)	60	2	2	0	10	tr	180
Krispy Soup & Oyster	17 (0.5 oz)	60	2	2	0	11	tr	200
Krispy Unsalted Tops	5 (0.5 oz)	60	2	2	0	10	tr	120
Krispy Whole Wheat	5 (0.5 oz)	60	2	2	0	10	tr	130
Tree Of Life								
Bite Size Fat Free Cracked Pepper	12 (0.5)	55	1	0	0	12	0	80
Bite Size Fat Free Garden Vegetable	12 (0.5 oz)	55	2	0	0	12	0	80
Bite Size Fat Free Garlic & Herb	12 (0.5 oz)	55	2	0	0	12	0	80
Bite Size Fat Free Toasted Onion	12 (0.5 oz)	55	2	0	0	12	0	80
Oyster	40 (0.5 oz)	60	2	0	0	13	0	130
Saltine Cracked Pepper Fat Free	4 (0.5 oz)	60	2	0	0	13	1	130

FOOD	PORTION	CAL	PROT	FAT	CHOL	CARB	FIBER	SOD
Saltine Fat Free	4 (0.5 oz)	50	2	0	0	11	0	140
Venus								
Fat Free Cracked Pepper	11 (0.5 oz)	60	1	0	0	12	0	80
Fat Free Garden Vegetable	5 (0.5 oz)	60	2	0	0	12	0	80
Fat Free Garlic & Herb	11 (0.5 oz)	60	2	0	0	12	0	90
Fat Free Multi-Grain	5 (0.5 oz)	60	1	0	0	12	tr	100
Fat Free Spicy Chili	10 (0.5 oz)	60	1	0	0	12	tr	100
Fat Free Toasted Onion	5 (0.5 oz)	60	1	0	0	12	0	120
Fat Free Toasted Wheat	5 (0.5 oz)	60	2	0	0	12	tr	140
Fat Free Tomato & Basil	10 (0.5 oz)	60	1	0	0	12	tr	100
Fat Free Zesty Italian	10 (0.5 oz)	60	1	0	0	12	tr	120
Garden Vegetable	6 (1 oz)	150	2	8	0	20	1	230
Honey Wheat	1 oz	140	2	5	0	21	1	200
Low Fat Cracker Bread	5 (0.5 oz)	60	1	2	0	10	tr	105
Low Fat Water Crackers	4 (0.5 oz)	60	1	1	0	12	0	75
Sesame & Flaxseed	1 oz	130	3	3	0	23	1	240
Soup Original	0.5 oz	60	1	2	0	11	0	90
Toasted Wheat	6 (1 oz)	150	3	7	0	18	tr	240
Wine Cheese Caviar Original	0.5 oz	60	1	2	0	11	0	90
Wine Cheese Caviar Pepper & Poppy	0.5 oz	60	1	2	0	11	0	90
Wasa								
Crisp	3 (0.5 oz)	50	2	0	0	11	2	100
Crisp'N Light Sourdough Rye	3 (0.6 oz)	60	2	0	0	12	1	120
Crisp'N Light Wheat	2 (0.5 oz)	50	2	0	0	10	1	100
Crispbread Cinnamon Toast	1 (0.6 oz)	60	2	1	0	11	1	65
Crispbread Fiber Rye	1 (0.4 oz)	30	1	1	0	4	2	60
Crispbread Gluten & Wheat Free Corn	1 (0.4 oz)	40	tr	1	0	7	0	90

FOOD	PORTION	CAL	PROT	FAT	CHOL	CARB	FIBER	SOD
Crispbread Hearty Rye	1 (0.5 oz)	45	1	0	0	9	2	40
Crispbread Light Rye	1 (0.3 oz)	25	tr	0	0	5	1	40
Crispbread Multi Grain	1 (0.5 oz)	45	2	0	0	8	2	85
Crispbread Organic Rye	1 (0.3 oz)	25	tr	0	0	7	1	50
Crispbread Sodium Free Rye	1 (0.3 oz)	30	tr	0	0	7	2	0
Crispbread Sourdough Rye	1 (0.4 oz)	35	1	0	0	7	1	55
Crispbread Toasted Wheat	1 (0.5 oz)	50	2	2	0	8	1	85
Crispbread Whole Wheat	1 (0.5 oz)	50	2	1	0	11	1	55
Wisecrackers								
Low Fat Poblano Chili & Sweet Onion	4 (0.5 oz)	45	1	1	0	8	tr	89
Wortz								
Cheese	23 (1 oz)	150	3	6	0	18	tr	370
Oyster	35 (0.5 oz)	70	1	2	–	11	1	150
Rich & Crisp	1 (0.5 oz)	70	1	3	–	9	0	105
Saltines Fat Free	5 (0.5 oz)	60	1	0	0	13	–	135
Saltines Deluxe	5 (0.5 oz)	60	1	2	–	10	–	130
Wheat Snacks	16 (1 oz)	140	3	6	–	20	2	120
Wheat Snacks Reduced Fat	16 (1.1 oz)	140	2	4	0	23	1	220
Woven Wheats	7 (1.1 oz)	140	3	5	0	21	4	170

CRANBERRIES

FOOD	PORTION	CAL	PROT	FAT	CHOL	CARB	FIBER	SOD
cranberry sauce sweetened	½ cup	209	tr	tr	0	54	–	40
fresh chopped	1 cup	54	tr	tr	0	14	–	1
Ocean Spray								
Craisins	⅓ cup (1.4 oz)	130	0	0	0	33	2	0
Cran*Fruit Cranberry Orange	¼ cup	120	0	0	0	29	1	35

FOOD	PORTION	CAL	PROT	FAT	CHOL	CARB	FIBER	SOD
Cranberry Sauce Jellied	¼ cup	110	0	0	0	27	1	35
Fresh	2 oz	25	0	0	0	6	0	0
Whole Berry Sauce	¼ cup	110	0	0	0	28	1	35

CRANBERRY BEANS

canned	1 cup	216	14	1	0	39	–	863
dried cooked	1 cup	240	17	1	0	43	–	1

CRANBERRY JUICE

cocktail	1 cup	147	tr	tr	0	38	–	10
cranberry juice cocktail	6 oz	108	0	tr	0	27	–	4
cranberry juice cocktail low calorie	6 oz	33	0	0	0	9	–	6
cranberry juice cocktail frzn	12 oz can	821	tr	0	0	210	–	13
cranberry juice cocktail frzn as prep	6 oz	102	0	0	0	26	–	6

After The Fall

Cape Cod Cranberry	1 bottle (10 oz)	130	0	0	0	30	–	25
Cranberry Ginger Ale	1 can (12 oz)	140	1	0	0	35	0	65

Crystal Light

Cranberry Breeze Drink	1 serv (8 oz)	5	0	0	0	0	0	20
Cranberry Breeze Drink Mix as prep	1 serv (8 oz)	5	0	0	0	0	0	0

Everfresh

Cranberry Cocktail	1 can (8 oz)	140	0	0	0	36	0	0

Mott's

Cocktail	8 fl oz	150	0	0	0	37	–	5

Nantucket Nectars

Cocktail	8 oz	140	0	0	0	34	–	5

Ocean Spray

Cocktail	8 oz	140	0	0	0	34	0	35
Cocktail Reduced Calorie	8 oz	50	0	0	0	13	0	35

FOOD	PORTION	CAL	PROT	FAT	CHOL	CARB	FIBER	SOD
Lightstyle Cranberry Juice Cocktail	8 oz	40	0	0	0	10	0	75
White Cranberry	1 cup (8 oz)	120	0	0	0	29	–	35
White Cranberry Peach	1 cup (8 oz)	120	0	0	0	30	–	35
White Cranberry Strawberry	1 cup (8 oz)	120	0	0	0	31	–	35
Tropicana								
Twister Ruby Red	1 bottle (10 oz)	160	tr	0	0	42	–	40
Veryfine								
Cocktail	1 bottle (10 oz)	180	0	0	0	45	0	30
Wellfleet Farms								
Cranberry	8 oz	130	0	0	0	33	0	35
CRAYFISH								
cooked	3 oz	97	20	1	151	0	–	58
raw	3 oz	76	16	1	118	0	–	45
raw	8	24	5	tr	37	0	–	14
CREAM *(see also* SOUR CREAM, SOUR CREAM SUBSTITUTES, WHIPPED TOPPINGS*)*								
clotted cream	2 tbsp (1 oz)	164	tr	18	48	1	0	18
creme fraiche	2 tbsp (1 oz)	100	1	11	40	1	0	10
half & half	1 cup (8.5 oz)	315	7	28	89	10	–	98
half & half	1 tbsp (0.5 oz)	20	tr	2	6	1	–	6
heavy whipping	1 tbsp (0.5 oz)	52	tr	6	21	tr	–	6
heavy whipping whipped	1 cup (4.1 oz)	411	5	44	163	7	–	89
light coffee	1 tbsp (0.5 oz)	29	tr	3	10	1	–	6
light coffee	1 cup (8.4 oz)	496	6	46	159	9	–	95
light whipping	1 tbsp (0.5 oz)	44	tr	5	17	tr	–	5
light whipping cream whipped	1 cup (4.2 oz)	345	5	37	132	7	–	82
Land O Lakes								
Fat Free Half & Half	2 tbsp (1 oz)	20	tr	0	0	3	0	30
Half & Half	2 tbsp (1 oz)	40	1	4	15	1	0	20
Heavy Whipping	1 tbsp (0.5 oz)	50	0	6	20	0	0	10
Organic Valley								
Half & Half	2 tbsp (1 oz)	40	1	3	15	1	0	15
CREAM CHEESE								
cream cheese	1 oz	99	2	10	31	1	–	84
cream cheese	1 pkg (3 oz)	297	6	30	93	2	–	251

FOOD	PORTION	CAL	PROT	FAT	CHOL	CARB	FIBER	SOD
Alpine Lace								
Reduced Fat Roasted Garlic & Herbs	1 tsp (1 oz)	60	4	4	10	2	0	190
Reduced Fat Sundried Tomato & Basil	2 tsp (1 oz)	70	4	5	15	2	0	300
Boar's Head								
Cream Cheese	2 tbsp (1 oz)	100	2	10	30	2	0	100
Breakstone's								
Temp-Tee Whipped	2 tbsp (0.8 oz)	80	2	8	25	tr	0	70
Galaxy								
Slices	1 slice (1 oz)	50	4	3	10	2	0	190
Healthy Choice								
Herbs & Garlic	2 tbsp (1 oz)	25	4	0	<5	2	—	200
Plain	2 tbsp (1 oz)	25	4	0	<5	2	—	200
Strawberry	2 tbsp (1 oz)	30	4	0	<5	5	—	200
Horizon Organic								
Spreadable	2 tbsp	100	2	10	30	1	0	100
Organic Valley								
Cream Cheese	1 oz	100	2	9	30	1	0	100
Philadelphia								
Free	1 oz	30	4	0	<5	2	0	140
Regular	1 oz	100	2	10	30	tr	0	90
Soft	2 tbsp (1 oz)	100	2	10	30	1	0	100
Soft Apple Cinnamon	2 tbsp (1.1 oz)	100	1	8	25	5	0	100
Soft Cheesecake	2 tbsp (1 oz)	110	2	9	25	4	0	95
Soft Chives & Onions	2 tbsp (1.1 oz)	110	1	10	30	2	0	135
Soft Garden Vegetable	2 tbsp (1.1 oz)	110	1	11	30	1	0	170
Soft Honey Nut	2 tbsp (1.1 oz)	110	2	10	30	4	0	150
Soft Pineapple	2 tbsp (1.1 oz)	100	1	9	25	4	0	100
Soft Salmon	3 tbsp (1.1 oz)	100	2	9	30	2	0	200
Soft Strawberry	2 tbsp (1.1 oz)	100	1	9	25	5	0	100
Soft Free	2 tbsp (1.2 oz)	30	5	0	<5	2	0	200
Soft Free Garden Vegetable	2 tbsp (1.2 oz)	30	5	0	<5	2	0	220
Soft Free Strawberries	2 tbsp (1.2 oz)	45	4	0	<5	6	0	180

FOOD	PORTION	CAL	PROT	FAT	CHOL	CARB	FIBER	SOD
Soft Light	2 tbsp (1.1 oz)	70	3	5	15	2	0	150
Soft Light Jalapeno	2 tbsp (1.1 oz)	60	3	5	15	2	0	210
Soft Light Raspberry	2 tbsp (1.1 oz)	70	3	5	15	6	0	125
Soft Light Roasted Garlic	2 tbsp (1.1 oz)	70	3	5	15	2	0	180
Whipped	2 tbsp (0.7 oz)	70	1	7	25	tr	0	85
Whipped Chives	2 tbsp (0.7 oz)	70	1	6	20	tr	0	130
Whipped Smoked Salmon	2 tbsp (0.7 oz)	70	2	6	20	1	0	140
With Chives	1 oz	90	2	9	30	tr	0	135

CREAM OF TARTAR

FOOD	PORTION	CAL	PROT	FAT	CHOL	CARB	FIBER	SOD
cream of tartar	1 tsp	8	0	0	0	2	–	2

CREPES

FOOD	PORTION	CAL	PROT	FAT	CHOL	CARB	FIBER	SOD
basic crepe unfilled	1	75	–	2	55	–	–	–
Frieda's								
Ready-To-Use	2 (0.8 oz)	50	1	1	5	9	0	90

CRESS

FOOD	PORTION	CAL	PROT	FAT	CHOL	CARB	FIBER	SOD
garden cooked	½ cup	16	1	tr	0	3	–	5
garden raw	½ cup	8	tr	tr	0	1	–	4

CROAKER

FOOD	PORTION	CAL	PROT	FAT	CHOL	CARB	FIBER	SOD
atlantic breaded & fried	3 oz	188	15	11	71	6	–	296
atlantic raw	3 oz	89	15	3	52	0	–	47

CROCODILE

FOOD	PORTION	CAL	PROT	FAT	CHOL	CARB	FIBER	SOD
cooked	3 oz	78	17	1	–	0	0	–

CROISSANT

FOOD	PORTION	CAL	PROT	FAT	CHOL	CARB	FIBER	SOD
apple	1 (2 oz)	145	4	5	–	21	1	156
cheese	1 (2 oz)	236	5	12	–	27	2	316
plain	1 (2 oz)	232	5	12	–	26	2	424
plain	1 mini (1 oz)	115	2	6	–	13	1	211
Sara Lee								
Broccoli & Cheese	1 (3.7 oz)	280	11	13	30	30	2	430
French Style	1 (1.5 oz)	170	4	8	<5	20	1	200
Ham & Swiss	1 (3.7 oz)	300	12	16	45	27	2	570
Petite	2 (2 oz)	230	6	11	<5	26	1	260
TAKE-OUT								
w/ egg & cheese	1 (4.5 oz)	368	13	25	216	24	–	551

FOOD	PORTION	CAL	PROT	FAT	CHOL	CARB	FIBER	SOD
w/ egg cheese & bacon	1 (4.5 oz)	413	16	28	215	24	–	889
w/ egg cheese & ham	1 (5.3 oz)	474	19	34	213	24	–	1081
w/ egg cheese & sausage	1 (5.6 oz)	523	20	38	216	25	–	1115

CROUTONS

plain	1 cup (1 oz)	122	4	2	0	22	2	209
seasoned	1 cup (1.4 oz)	186	4	7	–	25	2	495
Pepperidge Farm								
Garlic	6 (0.2 oz)	30	1	1	0	5	0	80
Homestyle	6 (0.2 oz)	30	1	1	0	5	0	80
Sourdough	6 (0.2 oz)	35	1	2	0	4	0	70
Up Country Naturals								
Organic Whole Wheat Garlic & Herb	¼ cup (0.3 oz)	35	1	2	0	5	tr	110

CUCUMBER

fresh raw	1 (11 oz)	38	2	tr	0	8	3	6
fresh raw sliced	½ cup (1.8 oz)	7	tr	tr	0	1	1	1
FRESH								
Chiquita								
Cucumber	⅓ med (3.5 oz)	15	1	0	0	3	1	0
TAKE-OUT								
cucumber salad	3.5 oz	50	1	tr	0	11	–	480
kimchee	½ cup (1.8 oz)	36	tr	2	0	4	tr	173
tzatziki	½ cup (3.4 oz)	72	2	6	5	4	1	197

CUMIN

seed	1 tsp	8	tr	tr	0	1	–	4

CURRANT JUICE

black currant nectar	7 oz	110	tr	0	–	26	–	10
red currant nectar	7 oz	108	tr	tr	–	26	–	tr

CURRANTS

black fresh	½ cup	36	1	tr	0	9	–	1
zante dried	½ cup	204	3	tr	0	53	–	6

CUSK

fillet baked	3 oz	106	23	1	50	0	–	38

FOOD	PORTION	CAL	PROT	FAT	CHOL	CARB	FIBER	SOD
CUSTARD								
MIX								
as prep w/ 2% milk	½ cup (4.7 oz)	148	7	4	74	24	–	200
as prep w/ 2% milk	1 recipe 4 serv (18.7 oz)	595	22	15	297	95	–	801
as prep w/ whole milk	½ cup (4.7 oz)	163	6	5	–	23	–	–
as prep w/ whole milk	1 recipe 4 serv (18.7 oz)	652	22	22	–	94	–	–
flan as prep w/ 2% milk	½ cup (4.7 oz)	135	4	2	9	26	–	68
flan as prep w/ 2% milk	1 recipe 4 serv (18.7 oz)	542	16	9	57	102	–	265
flan as prep w/ whole milk	½ cup (4.7 oz)	150	4	4	17	25	–	65
flan as prep w/ whole milk	1 recipe 4 serv (18.7 oz)	600	16	16	66	102	–	291
Betty Crocker								
Flan w/ Caramel Sauce as prep	1 serv	330	0	7	24	60	–	25
Jell-O								
Americana Custard Dessert as prep w/ 2% milk	½ cup (5 oz)	140	5	3	10	25	0	190
Flan as prep w/ 2% milk	½ cup (5.1 oz)	140	4	3	10	26	0	65
READY-TO-EAT								
Kozy Shack								
Flan	1 pkg (4 oz)	150	4	4	40	25	0	90
Swiss Miss								
Egg Custard	1 pkg (4 oz)	153	5	5	4	22	0	138
TAKE-OUT								
baked	½ cup (5 oz)	148	7	7	123	15	–	109
flan	½ cup (5.4 oz)	220	7	6	140	35	–	86
zabaione	½ cup (57.2 g)	135	3	5	213	13	0	9
CUTTLEFISH								
steamed	3 oz	134	28	1	190	1	–	632

FOOD	PORTION	CAL	PROT	FAT	CHOL	CARB	FIBER	SOD
DANDELION GREENS								
fresh cooked	½ cup	17	1	tr	0	3	–	23
raw chopped	½ cup	13	1	tr	0	3	–	21
DANISH PASTRY								
FROZEN								
Morton								
Honey Buns	1 (2.28 oz)	270	3	13	0	35	1	160
Honey Buns Mini	1 (1.3 oz)	160	2	8	0	19	1	100
READY-TO-EAT								
plain ring	1 (12 oz)	1305	21	71	292	152	–	1302
Dolly Madison								
Danish Rollers	3 (2.8 oz)	290	3	10	0	46	1	130
Tastykake								
Cheese	1 (3 oz)	290	5	14	20	44	tr	290
Lemon	1 (3 oz)	290	5	14	20	44	1	280
Raspberry	1 (3 oz)	290	5	14	20	44	1	260
TAKE-OUT								
almond	1 (4¼ in)	280	5	16	30	30	2	236
apple	1 (4¼ in)	264	4	13	–	34	1	251
cheese	1 (3.2 oz)	353	6	25	20	29	–	319
cheese	1 (4¼ in)	266	6	16	–	26	–	319
cinnamon	1 (3.1 oz)	349	5	17	27	47	–	326
cinnamon	1 (4¼ in)	262	5	15	–	29	1	241
cinnimon nut	1 (4¼ in)	280	5	16	30	30	2	236
fruit	1 (3.3 oz)	335	5	16	19	45	–	333
lemon	1 (4¼ in)	264	4	13	–	34	1	251
raisin	1 (4¼ in)	264	4	13	–	34	1	251
raisin nut	1 (4¼ in)	280	5	16	30	30	2	236
raspberry	1 (4¼ in)	264	4	13	–	34	1	251
strawberry	1 (4¼ in)	264	4	13	–	34	1	251
DATES								
deglet noor dried	10	240	–	0	0	–	–	–
dried chopped	1 cup	489	4	1	0	131	–	5
dried whole	10	228	2	tr	0	61	–	2
jujube dried	1 oz	75	1	tr	–	19	2	2
jujube fresh	1 oz	30	tr	tr	0	7	–	1
jujube preserved in sugar	1 oz	91	tr	tr	–	22	–	2

FOOD	PORTION	CAL	PROT	FAT	CHOL	CARB	FIBER	SOD
Calavo								
Dried Pitted	5–6 (1.4 oz)	120	1	0	0	31	3	0
California Redi-Date								
Deglet Noor Dried	5–6 (1.4 oz)	120	1	0	0	31	3	0
Dromedary								
Chopped Dried	¼ cup	130	1	0	0	31	–	0
Sonoma								
Dried	5–6 (1.4 oz)	110	1	0	0	30	5	15

DEER (see VENISON)

DELI MEATS/COLD CUTS (see also BEEF, CHICKEN, HAM, MEAT SUBSTITUTES, TURKEY)

FOOD	PORTION	CAL	PROT	FAT	CHOL	CARB	FIBER	SOD
barbecue loaf pork & beef	1 oz	49	4	3	11	2	–	378
beerwurst beef	1 slice (2¾ in x ¹⁄₁₆ in)	20	1	2	4	tr	–	62
beerwurst beef	1 slice (4 in x ⅛ in)	75	3	7	13	tr	–	214
beerwurst pork	1 slice (2¾ in x ¹⁄₁₆ in)	14	1	1	4	tr	–	74
beerwurst pork	1 slice (4 in x ⅛ in)	55	4	4	13	tr	–	285
berliner pork & beef	1 oz	65	4	4	13	1	–	368
blood sausage	1 oz	95	4	9	30	tr	–	–
bologna beef	1 oz	88	4	8	16	tr	–	278
bologna beef & pork	1 oz	89	3	8	16	1	–	289
bologna pork	1 oz	70	4	6	17	tr	–	336
braunschweiger pork	1 slice (2½ in x ¼ in)	65	2	6	28	1	–	206
braunschweiger pork	1 oz	102	4	9	44	1	–	324
corned beef loaf	1 oz	43	7	2	13	0	–	270
dried beef	1 oz	47	–	1	–	tr	–	–
dutch brand loaf pork & beef	1 oz	68	4	5	13	2	–	354
headcheese pork	1 oz	60	5	5	23	tr	–	356
honey loaf pork & beef	1 oz	36	4	1	10	2	–	374
honey roll sausage beef	1 oz	42	4	2	12	1	–	304

FOOD	PORTION	CAL	PROT	FAT	CHOL	CARB	FIBER	SOD
lebanon bologna beef	1 oz	60	6	4	20	1	—	379
liver cheese pork	1 oz	86	4	7	49	1	—	347
liverwurst pork	1 oz	92	4	8	45	1	—	—
luncheon meat beef	1 oz	87	4	7	18	1	—	377
luncheon meat pork & beef	1 oz	100	4	9	15	1	—	367
luncheon meat pork canned	1 oz	95	4	9	18	1	—	365
luncheon sausage pork & beef	1 oz	74	4	6	18	tr	—	335
luxury loaf pork	1 oz	40	5	1	10	1	—	347
mortadella beef & pork	1 oz	88	5	7	16	1	—	353
mother's loaf pork	1 oz	80	3	6	13	2	—	320
new england sausage pork & beef	1 oz	46	5	2	14	1	—	346
olive loaf pork	1 oz	67	3	5	11	3	—	421
peppered loaf pork & beef	1 oz	42	5	2	13	1	—	432
pepperoni pork & beef	1 slice (0.2 oz)	27	1	2	—	tr	—	112
pepperoni pork & beef	1 (9 oz)	1248	53	110	—	7	—	5120
pickle & pimiento loaf pork	1 oz	74	3	6	10	2	—	394
picnic loaf pork & beef	1 oz	66	4	5	11	1	—	330
salami cooked beef & pork	1 oz	71	4	6	18	1	—	302
salami hard pork	1 slice (⅓ oz)	41	2	4	—	3	—	226
salami hard pork	1 pkg (4 oz)	460	26	38	—	2	—	2554
salami hard pork & beef	1 slice (⅓ oz)	42	2	3	8	tr	—	186
salami hard pork & beef	1 pkg (4 oz)	472	26	39	89	3	—	2101
sandwich spread pork & beef	1 oz	67	2	5	11	3	—	287

FOOD	PORTION	CAL	PROT	FAT	CHOL	CARB	FIBER	SOD
sandwich spread pork & beef	1 tbsp	35	1	3	6	2	–	152
summer sausage thuringer cervelat	1 oz	98	5	8	19	1	–	412
Boar's Head								
Bologna Beef	2 oz	150	7	13	35	0	0	520
Bologna Garlic	2 oz	150	7	13	35	1	0	530
Bologna Lowered Sodium	2 oz	150	8	13	30	0	0	410
Bologna Pork & Beef	2 oz	150	7	13	35	tr	0	530
Braunschweiger Lite	2 oz	120	9	8	50	1	0	450
Head Cheese	2 oz	90	10	5	65	tr	0	420
Liverwurst Strassburger	2 oz	170	8	15	85	1	0	560
Olive Loaf	2 oz	130	6	12	20	tr	0	630
Pastrami	2 oz	90	12	4	30	2	0	620
Prosciutto	1 oz	60	8	3	15	0	0	770
Red Pastrami	2 oz	90	12	4	30	2	0	620
Salami Beef	2 oz	120	10	9	25	0	0	470
Salami Cooked	2 oz	130	8	11	40	0	0	550
Salami Genoa	2 oz	180	12	14	55	1	0	970
Salami Hard	1 oz	110	6	9	25	tr	0	490
Spiced Ham	2 oz	120	7	10	30	1	0	570
Carl Buddig								
Beef	1 pkg (2.5 oz)	100	14	5	50	1	–	1020
Corned Beef	1 pkg (2.5 oz)	100	14	5	50	tr	–	980
Pastrami	1 pkg (2.5 oz)	100	14	5	50	1	–	750
Healthy Choice								
Bologna	1 slice (1 oz)	30	4	1	15	1	0	290
Bologna Beef	1 slice (1 oz)	35	4	1	10	3	0	280
Deli-Thin Bologna	4 slices (1.8 oz)	60	8	2	25	3	0	560
Well-Pack Bologna	1 slice (1 oz)	30	4	1	15	1	0	290
Hormel								
Liverwurst Spread	4 tbsp (2 oz)	130	8	10	70	2	0	650
Pepperoni Chunk	1 oz	140	5	13	35	0	0	470
Pepperoni Sliced	15 slices (1 oz)	140	5	13	35	0	0	470
Pepperoni Twin	1 oz	140	5	13	35	0	0	500
Pillow Pack Genoa Salami	2 oz	160	12	18	50	0	0	940

FOOD	PORTION	CAL	PROT	FAT	CHOL	CARB	FIBER	SOD
Pillow Pack Pepperoni	16 slices (1 oz)	140	5	13	35	0	0	470
Jordan's								
Healthy Trim 95% Fat Free Macaroni & Cheese Loaf	2 slices (1.6 oz)	50	6	2	15	3	0	290
Healthy Trim 95% Fat Free Olive Loaf	2 slices (1.6 oz)	50	6	2	15	2	0	290
Healthy Trim 95% Fat Free Pickle & Pepper Loaf	2 slices (1.6 oz)	50	6	2	15	2	0	290
Healthy Trim 97% Fat Free Corned Beef	2 slices (1.6 oz)	45	9	2	30	0	0	290
Healthy Trim Low Fat Cooked Salami	3 slices (2 oz)	70	8	3	25	2	0	360
Healthy Trim Low Fat German Brand Bologna	3 slices (2 oz)	70	6	3	25	3	0	360
Oscar Mayer								
Bologna	1 slice (1 oz)	90	3	8	30	1	0	290
Bologna Beef	1 slice (1 oz)	90	3	8	20	1	0	310
Bologna Garlic	1 slice (1.4 oz)	110	4	12	40	1	0	420
Bologna Wisconsin Made Ring	2 oz	180	6	16	35	2	0	460
Braunschweiger Spread	2 oz	190	8	17	90	2	0	630
Brunschweiger	1 slice (1 oz)	100	4	9	40	1	0	320
Free Bologna	1 slice (1 oz)	20	4	0	5	2	0	280
Light Bologna	1 slice (1 oz)	60	3	4	15	2	0	310
Light Bologna Beef	1 slice (1 oz)	60	3	4	15	2	0	310
Liver Cheese	1 slice (1.3 oz)	120	6	10	80	1	0	420
Luncheon Loaf Spiced	1 slice (1 oz)	70	4	5	20	2	0	340

FOOD	PORTION	CAL	PROT	FAT	CHOL	CARB	FIBER	SOD
Old Fashioned Loaf	1 slice (1 oz)	70	4	5	15	2	0	330
Olive Loaf	1 slice (1 oz)	70	3	6	20	2	0	370
Pepperoni	15 slices (1 oz)	140	6	13	25	0	0	550
Salami Cotto	1 slice (1 oz)	70	3	5	25	1	0	280
Salami Cotto Beef	1 slice (1 oz)	60	4	5	25	1	0	370
Salami For Beer	1 slice (1.6 oz)	110	6	9	30	1	0	580
Salami Hard	3 slices (1 oz)	100	6	9	25	0	0	510
Sandwich Spread	2 oz	130	4	10	25	8	0	460
Summer Sausage	2 slices (1.6 oz)	140	7	13	40	0	0	650
Summer Sausage Beef	2 slices (1.6 oz)	140	7	12	35	1	0	640
Spam								
Less Salt	2 oz	170	7	16	40	0	0	560
Lite	2 oz	110	9	8	45	0	0	560
Original	2 oz	170	7	16	40	0	0	750
Smoked	2 oz	170	7	16	40	0	0	750
TAKE-OUT								
corned beef	2 oz	70	12	2	40	0	–	390
corned beef brisket	2 oz	90	11	5	35	0	–	370
DILL								
seed	1 tsp	6	tr	tr	0	1	–	tr
sprigs fresh	5	0	tr	tr	0	tr	–	1
sprigs fresh	1 cup	4	tr	tr	0	1	–	5
weed dry	1 tsp	3	tr	tr	0	1	–	2

DIETING AIDS (see NUTRITION SUPPLEMENTS)

DINNER (see also ASIAN FOOD, PASTA DISHES, POT PIES, SPANISH FOOD)

FOOD	PORTION	CAL	PROT	FAT	CHOL	CARB	FIBER	SOD
Amy's Organic								
Whole Meals Country Dinner	1 pkg (11 oz)	380	11	12	15	60	9	570
Banquet								
Beef Patty w/ Country Style Vegetables	1 meal (9.5 oz)	310	11	20	40	22	2	1090
Boneless Pork Rib	1 meal (10 oz)	400	17	19	45	40	4	1070
Boneless White Fried Chicken	1 meal (8.25 oz)	540	16	34	60	41	3	1180

FOOD	PORTION	CAL	PROT	FAT	CHOL	CARB	FIBER	SOD
Chicken Parmigiana	1 meal (9.5 oz)	320	10	18	50	29	3	900
Chicken Fingers Meal	1 meal (7.1 oz)	740	22	43	70	67	6	1070
Chicken Fried Beef Steak	1 pkg (10 oz)	420	15	23	35	39	4	1200
Chicken Nuggets Meal	1 meal (6.75 oz)	430	14	23	50	42	4	650
Extra Helping Boneless Pork Riblet	1 meal (15.25 oz)	720	27	40	80	62	7	1590
Extra Helping Fried Beef Steak	1 meal (16 oz)	820	29	50	70	63	6	2260
Extra Helping Fried Chicken	1 meal (14.7 oz)	910	34	55	160	70	5	2400
Extra Helping Meatloaf	1 meal (16 oz)	610	29	40	110	34	6	1940
Extra Helping Salisbury Steak	1 meal (16.5 oz)	740	27	54	130	37	7	2200
Extra Helping Turkey & Gravy w/ Dressing	1 meal (17 oz)	620	28	32	80	54	10	2250
Extra Helping White Fried Chicken	1 meal (13 oz)	690	24	48	70	40	8	1900
Extra Helping Yankee Pot Roast	1 meal (14.5 oz)	410	25	20	50	33	3	1660
Family Size Brown Gravy & Salisbury Steak	1 serv	240	9	20	40	7	1	900
Family Size Brown Gravy & Sliced Beef	1 serv	140	13	8	40	5	tr	850
Family Size Chicken & Broccoli Alfredo	1 serv	270	11	12	40	28	3	540
Family Size Country Style Chicken & Dumplings	1 serv	290	12	14	40	30	7	1270

FOOD	PORTION	CAL	PROT	FAT	CHOL	CARB	FIBER	SOD
Family Size Creamy Broccoli Chicken Cheese & Rice	1 serv	280	14	14	45	25	2	980
Family Size Hearty Beef Stew	1 cup	170	10	7	30	18	4	1120
Family Size Homestyle Gravy & Sliced Turkey	2 slices	140	7	10	40	5	1	600
Family Size Mushroom Gravy & Charbroiled Beef Patties	1 patty	250	11	20	35	6	2	750
Family Size Potato Ham & Broccoli Au Gratin	⅔ cup	210	7	13	30	16	2	970
Family Size Savory Gravy & Meatloaf	1 slice	120	10	13	35	7	1	750
Fish Sticks	1 meal (6.6 oz)	290	11	13	30	33	4	820
Grilled Chicken	1 meal (9.9 oz)	330	16	13	50	37	2	1210
Honey Roast Turkey Breast	1 meal (9 oz)	270	11	12	30	29	4	1310
Meatloaf	1 meal (9.5 oz)	280	12	16	60	23	3	1020
Our Original Fried Chicken	1 meal (9 oz)	470	21	27	90	35	2	1500
Pork Cutlet Meal	1 meal (10.25 oz)	420	11	25	35	36	4	1060
Salisbury Steak	1 meal (9.5 oz)	380	12	24	60	28	4	1140
Sliced Beef	1 meal (9 oz)	270	26	10	70	19	4	740
Turkey	1 meal (9.25 oz)	270	14	11	55	30	3	1060
Veal Parmagiana	1 meal (8.75 oz)	330	13	14	20	37	2	860
Western Style Beef Patty	1 meal (9.5 oz)	360	14	21	40	28	3	1400
White Meat Fried Chicken	1 meal (8.75 oz)	460	18	28	100	40	2	1100
Yankee Pot Roast	1 meal (9.4 oz)	230	14	10	60	20	4	1130
Birds Eye								
Chicken Voila! Alfredo	1 cup (6.1 oz)	230	15	8	20	26	2	660
Chicken Voila! Garden Herb	1 cup	310	16	15	40	28	2	540

FOOD	PORTION	CAL	PROT	FAT	CHOL	CARB	FIBER	SOD
Chicken Voila! Grilled Salsa	1 cup	240	14	5	25	35	3	1180
Chicken Voila! Teriyaki	2 cups (6.4 oz)	240	13	9	25	26	2	700
Chicken Voila! Zesty Garlic Chicken	2 cups (6.2 oz)	260	15	11	25	28	1	550
Steak Voila! Beef Sirloin Steak And Garlic Potatoes	1 cup	240	13	9	25	26	3	650
Turkey Voila! Homestyle w/ Roasted Potatoes	1 cup	200	12	6	10	24	3	830
Green Giant								
Create A Meal Broccoli Stir Fry as prep	1⅓ cups (9.9 oz)	290	27	13	60	16	4	1160
Create A Meal Cheese & Herb Primavera as prep	1¼ cups (10 oz)	330	30	11	65	27	4	920
Create A Meal Garlic Herb as prep	1¼ cups (10 oz)	340	24	14	145	30	4	670
Create A Meal Hearty Vegetable Stew as prep	1¼ cups (10 oz)	280	23	9	55	25	3	1000
Create A Meal Lemon Herb as prep	1½ cups (10 oz)	360	28	11	65	37	3	830
Create A Meal Mushroom & Wine as prep	1¼ cups (10 oz)	390	28	16	75	31	4	910
Create A Meal Vegetable Almond Stir Fry as prep	1⅓ cups (10 oz)	320	32	11	65	22	6	1190
Healthy Choice								
Beef Pepper Steak Oriental	1 meal (9.5 oz)	260	19	5	35	34	2	520
Beef Pot Roast	1 meal (11 oz)	300	20	6	40	41	6	600
Beef Stoganoff	1 meal (11 oz)	320	22	8	60	40	7	600

FOOD	PORTION	CAL	PROT	FAT	CHOL	CARB	FIBER	SOD
Beef Tips Francais	1 meal (9.5 oz)	300	20	7	40	40	4	520
Beef Tips Portabello	1 meal (11.25 oz)	270	23	5	40	34	7	600
Bowls Chicken Teriyaki w/ Rice	1 meal (9.5 oz)	270	17	4	30	41	4	570
Bowls Country Chicken Bake	1 meal (9.5 oz)	230	18	8	50	22	4	600
Bowls Fiesta Chicken	1 meal (9.5 oz)	220	15	2	30	34	3	550
Bowls Garlic Lemon Chicken w/ Rice	1 meal (9.5 oz)	300	18	4	40	48	4	400
Bowls Roasted Potatoes w/ Ham	1 meal (8.5 oz)	210	17	4	30	26	6	600
Bowls Southwestern Chicken & Pasta	1 meal (9.5 oz)	320	31	4	40	39	6	350
Bowls Turkey Divan	1 meal (9.5 oz)	250	18	6	30	31	4	600
Charbroiled Beef Patty	1 meal (11 oz)	310	16	9	45	40	4	550
Chicken Cantonese	1 meal (10.75)	280	22	6	50	34	2	480
Chicken Parmigiana	1 meal (11.5 oz)	330	19	8	40	46	3	490
Chicken & Vegetables Marsala	1 meal (11.5 oz)	240	20	4	30	32	3	440
Chicken Broccoli Alfredo	1 meal (11.5 oz)	300	25	7	50	34	2	530
Chicken Dijon	1 meal (11 oz)	270	23	5	40	33	6	470
Chicken Teriyaki	1 meal (11 oz)	270	17	6	45	37	3	600
Country Breaded Chicken	1 meal (10.25 oz)	350	16	9	45	51	5	460
Country Glazed Chicken Breast	1 meal (8.5 oz)	250	19	5	30	31	3	600
Country Herb Chicken	1 meal (12.15 oz)	320	16	8	45	44	3	540
Country Inn Roast Turkey	1 meal (10 oz)	250	20	6	40	28	4	530
Garlic Chicken Milano	1 meal (9.5 oz)	260	18	6	35	34	3	510
Grilled Chicken Sonoma	1 meal (9 oz)	230	16	4	45	30	3	530
Grilled Chicken w/ Mashed Potatoes	1 meal (8 oz)	180	16	4	45	18	3	600

FOOD	PORTION	CAL	PROT	FAT	CHOL	CARB	FIBER	SOD
Herb Baked Fish	1 meal (10.9 oz)	340	16	7	35	54	5	480
Herb Breaded Pork Patty	1 meal (8 oz)	280	18	6	30	38	4	570
Homestyle Chicken & Pasta	1 meal (9 oz)	270	21	6	35	32	5	570
Honey Glazed Chicken	1 meal (10 oz)	270	21	7	45	32	4	600
Honey Mustard Chicken	1 meal (9.5 oz)	290	21	6	40	38	1	520
Lemon Pepper Fish	1 meal (10.7 oz)	320	14	7	30	50	5	480
Mandarin Chicken	1 meal (10 oz)	280	20	3	35	44	4	520
Mesquite Beef w. Barbecue Sauce	1 meal (11 oz)	320	21	9	55	36	5	490
Mesquite Chicken Barbecue	1 meal (10.5 oz)	310	18	5	55	48	6	480
Oriental Style Chicken & Vegetable Stir Fry	1 meal (11.9)	360	19	6	25	57	5	600
Oven Roasted Beef	1 meal (10.15 oz)	280	18	8	50	35	4	600
Roast Turkey Breast	1 meal (8.5 oz)	220	18	5	25	28	5	600
Roasted Chicken	1 meal (11 oz)	230	20	5	50	23	4	560
Sesame Chicken	1 meal (10.8 oz)	360	19	7	20	54	4	600
Shrimp & Vegetables	1 meal (11.8 oz)	270	15	6	50	39	6	560
Sweet & Sour Chicken	1 meal (11 oz)	360	20	7	45	53	5	360
Traditional Meatloaf	1 meal (12 oz)	330	15	7	35	52	6	460
Tradtional Breast Of Turkey	1 meal (10.5 oz)	290	22	5	45	40	5	460
Tradtional Salisbury Steak	1 meal (11.5 oz)	330	18	7	50	48	6	470
Tuna Casserole	1 meal (8 oz)	240	16	5	25	33	4	560
Kid Cuisine								
Circus Show Corn Dog	1 meal (8.8 oz)	490	8	20	30	70	5	800
Cosmic Chicken Nuggets	1 meal (9.1 oz)	500	18	25	45	50	5	1070
Futuristic Fish Sticks	1 meal (8.25 oz)	410	9	16	20	57	4	550
Game Time Taco Roll Up	1 meal (7.35 oz)	420	9	18	25	55	4	740
High Flying Fried Chicken	1 meal (10.1 oz)	440	18	20	70	48	3	940

FOOD	PORTION	CAL	PROT	FAT	CHOL	CARB	FIBER	SOD
Parachuting Pork Ribettes	1 meal (7.55 oz)	390	16	19	50	39	3	760
Lean Cuisine								
Cafe Classics Baked Chicken	1 pkg (8.6 oz)	240	17	5	30	33	3	550
Cafe Classics Baked Fish	1 pkg (9 oz)	290	20	6	40	40	2	590
Cafe Classics Beef Peppercorn	1 pkg (8.75 oz)	260	16	7	25	32	4	590
Cafe Classics Beef Portobello	1 pkg (9 oz)	220	14	7	35	24	2	590
Cafe Classics Beef Pot Roast	1 pkg (9 oz)	210	13	6	30	25	6	570
Cafe Classics Chicken Carbonara	1 pkg (9 oz)	280	17	7	30	36	4	560
Cafe Classics Chicken Mediterranean	1 pkg (10.5 oz)	260	17	4	20	38	4	690
Cafe Classics Chicken & Vegetables	1 pkg (10.5 oz)	240	19	5	30	30	4	690
Cafe Classics Chicken In Peanut Sauce	1 pkg (9 oz)	260	20	6	30	32	4	690
Cafe Classics Chicken In Wine Sauce	1 pkg (8.1 oz)	220	20	5	45	23	2	690
Cafe Classics Chicken L'Orange	1 pkg (9 oz)	230	20	2	40	33	2	300
Cafe Classics Chicken Parmesan	1 pkg (10.9 oz)	300	21	6	35	41	5	600
Cafe Classics Chicken Piccata	1 pkg (9 oz)	300	14	9	30	41	2	590
Cafe Classics Chicken w/ Basil Cream Sauce	1 pkg (8.5 oz)	260	17	7	35	33	2	650
Cafe Classics Country Vegetables & Beef	1 pkg (9 oz)	210	11	4	25	33	3	590

FOOD	PORTION	CAL	PROT	FAT	CHOL	CARB	FIBER	SOD
Cafe Classics Fiesta Chicken	1 pkg (9.25 oz)	270	17	5	30	40	3	690
Cafe Classics Glazed Chicken	1 pkg (8.5 oz)	240	22	6	55	25	0	480
Cafe Classics Glazed Turkey Tenderloins	1 pkg (9 oz)	260	14	5	25	41	4	640
Cafe Classics Grilled Chicken	1 pkg (9.4 oz)	250	22	5	40	29	3	690
Cafe Classics Grilled Chicken Salsa	1 pkg (8.9 oz)	270	15	7	45	36	4	570
Cafe Classics Herb Roasted Chicken	1 pkg (8 oz)	190	17	4	35	22	4	690
Cafe Classics Honey Mustard Chicken	1 pkg (8 oz)	270	19	4	35	40	1	690
Cafe Classics Honey Roasted Chicken	1 pkg (8.5 oz)	270	13	6	25	41	5	550
Cafe Classics Honey Roasted Pork	1 serv (9.5 oz)	250	17	6	45	32	3	590
Cafe Classics Meatloaf w/ Whipped Potatoes	1 pkg (9.4 oz)	260	20	7	45	28	4	600
Cafe Classics Oriental Beef	1 pkg (9.25 oz)	210	14	4	25	30	2	530
Cafe Classics Oven Roasted Beef	1 pkg (9.25 oz)	260	18	8	50	28	4	590
Cafe Classics Roasted Turkey Breast	1 pkg (9.75 oz)	270	13	2	25	49	3	590
Cafe Classics Salisbury Steak	1 pkg (9.5 oz)	280	24	8	60	29	4	590
Cafe Classics Sirlion Beef Peppercorn	1 pkg (8.75 oz)	220	15	7	35	23	2	580
Cafe Classics Southern Beef Beef Tips	1 pkg (8.75 oz)	270	16	6	35	37	4	480

FOOD	PORTION	CAL	PROT	FAT	CHOL	CARB	FIBER	SOD
Everday Favorites Vegetable Lasagna	1 pkg (10.5 oz)	260	15	7	20	36	5	590
Everyday Favorite Chicken Florentine	1 pkg (8 oz)	220	13	5	25	32	3	640
Everyday Favorites Chicken Chow Mein	1 pkg (9 oz)	240	14	4	35	37	3	590
Everyday Favorites Homestyle Turkey	1 pkg (9.4 oz)	240	22	5	40	27	3	590
Everyday Favorites Hunan Beef & Broccoli	1 pkg (8.5 oz)	240	11	4	20	40	2	690
Everyday Favorites Mandarin Chicken	1 pkg (9 oz)	260	15	5	35	38	2	570
Everyday Favorites Roasted Chicken	1 pkg (8.1 oz)	260	14	7	20	34	4	640
Everyday Favorites Stuffed Cabbage	1 pkg (9.5 oz)	210	9	8	20	25	5	590
Everyday Favorites Swedish Meatballs	1 pkg (9.1 oz)	290	22	7	45	35	4	590
Hearty Portions Cheese & Spinach Manicotti	1 serv	370	25	8	35	50	8	850
Hearty Portions Chicken & Barbecue Sauce	1 serv	370	20	6	40	60	6	840
Hearty Portions Homestyle Beef Stroganoff	1 serv	350	23	9	30	44	9	850
Hearty Portions Jumbo Rigatoni w/ Meatballs	1 serv	440	25	9	35	64	7	820
Hearty Portions Oriental Glazed Chicken	1 serv	370	21	2	35	66	4	850
Hearty Portions Roasted Chicken w/ Mushrooms	1 serv	330	23	4	40	49	4	740

FOOD	PORTION	CAL	PROT	FAT	CHOL	CARB	FIBER	SOD
Skillet Sensations Beef Teriyaki & Rice	1 serv	280	14	3	25	48	5	700
Skillet Sensations Chicken Primavera	1 serv	320	20	5	30	50	4	790
Skillet Sensations Chicken Oriental	1 serv	280	17	3	15	46	6	790
Skillet Sensations Fiesta Beef & Rice	1 serv	300	19	4	25	48	6	760
Skillet Sensations Garlic Chicken	1 serv	340	20	5	20	56	4	730
Skillet Sensations Herb Chicken & Roasted Potatoes	1 serv	270	18	5	40	39	5	790
Skillet Sensations Roasted Turkey	1 serv	220	14	2	25	37	6	790
Skillet Sensations Savory Beef & Vegetables	1 serv	290	18	7	35	38	9	1440
Skillet Sensations Three Cheese Chicken	1 serv	370	26	10	50	45	3	820
Luzianne								
Cajun Creole Dirty Rice	1 serv	160	4	1	0	35	0	680
Cajun Creole Etouffee	1 serv	200	5	1	0	42	1	1030
Cajun Creole Gumbo	1 serv	160	4	1	0	33	1	760
Cajun Creole Jambalaya	1 serv	200	5	1	0	43	1	690
Marie Callender's								
Beef Stroganoff w/ Noodles	1 meal (13 oz)	600	20	27	70	59	4	1140
Beef Tips In Mushroom Sauce	1 meal (13 oz)	430	25	19	50	39	6	1020
Breaded Chicken Parmigiana	1 meal (16 oz)	860	30	32	50	63	5	920
Breaded Fish w/ Mac & Cheese	1 meal (12 oz)	550	22	28	60	53	3	1400

FOOD	PORTION	CAL	PROT	FAT	CHOL	CARB	FIBER	SOD
Cheesy Rice w/ Chicken & Broccoli	1 meal (12 oz)	390	24	13	55	44	6	1220
Chicken & Dumplings	1 meal (14 oz)	390	17	20	130	34	4	1650
Chicken & Noodles	1 meal (13 oz)	520	21	30	80	42	5	1320
Chicken Cordon Bleu	1 meal (13 oz)	610	23	28	75	58	6	1920
Chicken Fried Beef Steak & Gravy	1 meal (15 oz)	650	20	37	50	50	7	2260
Chicken Teriyaki	1 meal (13 oz)	510	24	12	55	71	2	1510
Country Fried Chicken & Gravy	1 meal (16 oz)	620	24	30	75	63	6	2300
Country Fried Pork Chop	1 meal (15 oz)	540	23	28	65	50	8	2240
Escalloped Noodles & Chicken	1 meal (13 oz)	740	21	46	90	60	5	1600
Glazed Chicken	1 meal (13 oz)	490	25	25	90	40	1	2130
Grilled Southwestern Style Chicken	1 meal (14 oz)	410	24	11	80	43	6	2020
Grilled Chicken & Mashed Potatoes	1 meal (10 oz)	340	24	16	90	20	1	1090
Grilled Chicken Breast & Rice Pilaf	1 meal (11.75 oz)	360	20	14	40	36	4	1070
Grilled Chicken In Mushroom Sauce	1 meal (14 oz)	480	32	15	65	54	7	1030
Grilled Turkey Breast & Rice Pilaf	1 meal (11.75 oz)	310	22	10	40	34	4	940
Herb Roasted Chicken & Mashed Potatoes	1 meal (14 oz)	580	42	34	205	26	7	2100
Homestyle Turkey & Noodles	1 meal (12 oz)	600	18	35	90	52	5	1570
Honey Roasted Chicken	1 meal (14 oz)	440	45	17	140	27	7	1170
Honey Smoked Ham Steak w/ Macaroni & Cheese	1 meal (14 oz)	490	29	13	80	63	5	2310

FOOD	PORTION	CAL	PROT	FAT	CHOL	CARB	FIBER	SOD
Meatloaf & Gravy w/ Mashed Potatoes	1 meal (14 oz)	540	23	30	95	42	5	1570
Old Fashioned Beef Pot Roast & Gravy	1 meal (15 oz)	500	23	17	110	55	3	1460
Roast Beef	1 meal (14.5 oz)	390	24	19	70	30	11	1240
Sirloin Salisbury Steak & Gravy	1 meal (14 oz)	550	30	25	85	51	6	1660
Skillet Meal Au Gratin Potatoes	⅔ cup (5 oz)	190	7	10	30	19	2	400
Skillet Meal Beef Pot Roast	½ pkg	290	20	9	60	33	5	1200
Skillet Meal Beef Stroganoff	½ pkg	310	21	11	60	31	5	1290
Skillet Meal Chicken & Rice w/ Broccoli & Cheese	½ pkg	440	30	14	70	47	8	1450
Skillet Meal Chicken Teriyaki	½ pkg	340	21	1	30	61	5	1140
Skillet Meal Herb Chicken	½ pkg	290	22	4	35	42	5	1030
Skillet Meal Roasted Chicken & Vegetables	½ pkg	260	21	6	40	30	7	1020
Skillet Meal White & Wild Rice In Cheese Sauce	1 cup	300	11	13	35	35	2	750
Swedish Meatballs	1 meal (12.5 oz)	520	28	26	65	44	3	1020
Sweet & Sour Chicken	1 meal (14 oz)	570	23	15	40	66	7	700
Turkey w/ Gravy & Dressing	1 meal (14 oz)	500	31	19	80	52	4	2040
Morton								
Breaded Chicken Pattie	1 meal (6.75 oz)	290	10	17	35	24	4	840
Chicken Nuggets	1 meal (7 oz)	340	12	19	30	31	2	470

FOOD	PORTION	CAL	PROT	FAT	CHOL	CARB	FIBER	SOD
Chili Gravy w/ Beef Enchilada & Tamale	1 meal (10 oz)	270	7	9	10	40	7	1000
Fried Chicken	1 meal (9 oz)	470	20	30	90	30	3	1100
Gravy & Charbroiled Beef Patty	1 meal (9 oz)	310	10	18	20	26	5	1210
Gravy & Salisbury Steak	1 meal (9 oz)	310	7	20	30	24	3	1100
Gravy & Turkey w/ Stuffing	1 meal (9 oz)	240	10	10	40	27	4	1200
Tomato Sauce w/ Meat Loaf	1 meal (9 oz)	250	9	13	20	24	3	1200
Veal Parmagiana w/ Tomato Sauce	1 meal (8.75 oz)	290	8	15	25	30	4	950
Nature's Choice								
Broccoli Parmesan Alfredo	1 pkg (12 oz)	270	20	9	10	29	5	960
Nature's Entree								
Hearty Stew	1 pkg (12 oz)	290	18	9	10	34	3	960
Tuscany White Bean	1 pkg (12 oz)	330	21	8	5	42	4	920
Patio								
Ranchera	1 pkg (13 oz)	470	13	22	35	55	9	2470
Stouffer's								
Baked Chicken Breast w/ Mashed Potatoes	1 serv (12.2 oz)	330	25	14	60	25	3	1070
Beef Stroganoff	1 pkg (9.75 oz)	390	23	20	85	30	2	1100
Chicken A La King	1 pkg (9.5 oz)	350	17	13	40	41	2	800
Creamed Chicken	1 pkg (6.5 oz)	260	15	19	80	8	0	680
Creamed Chipped Beef	½ cup (5.5 oz)	160	10	11	40	6	1	690
Creamy Chicken & Broccoli	1 pkg (8.9 oz)	320	19	15	60	26	2	820
Escalloped Chicken & Noodles	1 pkg (10 oz)	430	17	27	50	30	3	1120
Fish w/ Macaroni & Cheese	1 serv (9.5 oz)	460	22	20	55	47	2	970
Glazed Chicken w/ Rice	1 serv (11.8 oz)	290	21	6	45	39	2	810
Green Pepper Steak	1 pkg (10.5 oz)	330	17	9	35	45	3	650

FOOD	PORTION	CAL	PROT	FAT	CHOL	CARB	FIBER	SOD
Homestyle Beef Pot Roast & Browned Potatoes	1 pkg (8.9 oz)	250	16	8	35	29	4	780
Homestyle Fish Filet w/ Macaroni & Cheese	1 pkg (9 oz)	430	24	21	70	37	2	930
Homestyle Fried Chicken & Whipped Potatoes	1 pkg (7.5 oz)	310	17	12	45	33	5	680
Homestyle Meatloaf & Whipped Potatoes	1 pkg (9.9 oz)	330	20	16	70	26	3	850
Homestyle Roast Turkey w/ Gravy Stuffing & Whipped Potatoes	1 pkg (9.6 oz)	320	19	13	50	31	3	950
Homestyle Baked Chicken & Gravy & Whipped Potatoes	1 pkg (8.9 oz)	270	22	12	75	19	2	750
Meatloaf	1 serv (5.5 oz)	210	16	12	60	9	1	520
Meatloaf w/ Whipped Potatoes	1 serv (11.5 oz)	380	22	18	70	33	4	950
Stuffed Pepper	1 pkg (10 oz)	200	11	5	20	27	3	820
Swedish Meatballs	1 pkg (10.25 oz)	480	24	24	60	43	3	960
Swanson								
Beef Pot Roast	1 pkg (14 oz)	320	19	8	35	44	4	1200
Chicken Parmigiana w/ Spaghetti	1 pkg (11 oz)	380	17	17	25	41	5	700
Chicken Duet Gourmet Nuggets Pizza Style	3 oz	210	—	12	—	—	—	—
Turkey	8¾ oz	270	—	11	—	—	—	—
Turkey Breast	1 pkg (11.7 oz)	330	18	6	40	50	4	1290
Tamarind Tree								
Alu Chole	1 pkg (9.2 oz)	350	12	6	0	63	9	620
Channa Dal Masala	1 pkg (9.2 oz)	340	13	5	0	62	10	700
Dal Makhini	1 pkg (9.2 oz)	330	14	6	5	55	14	670
Dhingri Mutter	1 pkg (9.2 oz)	290	8	5	0	53	7	680
Navratan Korma	1 pkg (9.2 oz)	430	12	15	5	60	7	700

FOOD	PORTION	CAL	PROT	FAT	CHOL	CARB	FIBER	SOD
Palak Paneer	1 pkg (9.2 oz)	380	14	15	35	46	6	640
Saag Chole	1 pkg (9.2 oz)	370	14	10	0	55	13	800
Vegetable Jalfrazi	1 pkg (9.2 oz)	310	8	6	0	57	7	600
Tyson								
BBQ Chicken Potato & Vegetable Medley	1 pkg (14.7 oz)	560	19	21	30	73	9	1190
Beef Stir Fry	1 pkg (14 oz)	430	26	5	45	70	4	1560
Blackened Chicken Spanish Rice & Corn	1 pkg (8.8 oz)	260	17	5	30	36	4	480
Chicken Primavera	1 pkg (11.3 oz)	350	25	6	30	48	5	610
Chicken Divan Candied Carrots & Pasta	1 pkg (9.8 oz)	370	20	15	50	38	2	530
Chicken Francais Sliced Potatoes & Green Beans	1 pkg (8.8 oz)	260	19	10	45	23	6	790
Chicken Kiev Rice Pilaf & Broccoli Carrots	1 pkg (9.1 oz)	440	18	25	85	36	2	900
Chicken Marsala Carrots & Red Potatoes	1 pkg (8.8 oz)	180	15	5	30	19	4	520
Chicken Mesquite Corn & Pea Medley & Au Gratin Potatoes	1 pkg (8.8 oz)	320	18	8	25	44	4	780
Chicken Picatta	1 pkg (8.8 oz)	190	17	6	35	18	5	500
Chicken Stir Fry Kit	2¾ cups (14 oz)	430	24	5	45	73	5	1700
Chicken w/ Broccoli & Cheese Carrots & Pasta	1 pkg (8.8 oz)	270	20	12	40	19	3	690
Chicken w/ Mushroom Sauce Rice Pilaf & Candied Carrots	1 pkg (8.8 oz)	220	15	6	30	27	2	510
Chicken w/ Tabasco BBQ Sauce	1 pkg (8.8 oz)	260	13	7	25	37	5	610

FOOD	PORTION	CAL	PROT	FAT	CHOL	CARB	FIBER	SOD
Fried Chicken & Gravy w/ Mashed Potatoes & Corn	1 pkg (10.8 oz)	360	16	15	30	39	4	840
Grilled Chicken Corn O'Brien & Ranch Beans	1 pkg (8.8 oz)	230	19	4	30	30	7	590
Grilled Italian Chicken Pasta & Vegetable Medley	1 pkg (8.8 oz)	190	21	4	30	19	3	440
Honey Dijon Chicken Pasta & Pea Medley	1 pkg (11.3 oz)	340	20	7	25	49	6	900
Roasted Chicken w/ Garlic Sauce Pasta & Vegetable Medley	1 pkg (8.8 oz)	210	17	7	25	20	3	460
Weight Watchers								
Smart One Grilled Salisbury Steak	1 pkg (8.5 oz)	250	18	9	40	24	3	620
Smart Ones Chicken Mirabella	1 pkg (9.2 oz)	180	11	2	20	30	4	480
Smart Ones Fiesta Chicken	1 pkg (8.5 oz)	210	13	2	25	35	5	570
Smart Ones Honey Mustard Chicken	1 pkg (8.5 oz)	200	11	2	30	35	3	370
Smart Ones Lemon Herb Chicken Piccata	1 pkg (8.5 oz)	190	11	2	25	33	3	460
Smart Ones Pepper Steak	1 pkg (10 oz)	240	18	5	35	32	4	690
Smart Ones Risotto w/ Cheese & Mushrooms	1 pkg (10 oz)	290	11	7	20	47	4	540
Smart Ones Roast Turkey Medallions & Mushrooms	1 pkg (8.5 oz)	180	11	2	20	30	2	530

FOOD	PORTION	CAL	PROT	FAT	CHOL	CARB	FIBER	SOD
Smart Ones Shrimp Marinara	1 pkg (9 oz)	180	9	2	40	31	4	570
Smart Ones Stuffed Turkey Breast	1 pkg (10 oz)	260	13	7	30	37	5	680
Smart Ones Swedish Meatballs	1 pkg (9 oz)	280	19	70	30	34	3	690
Yves								
Veggie Country Stew	1 pkg (10.5 oz)	170	17	0	0	24	7	1020

DIP

FOOD	PORTION	CAL	PROT	FAT	CHOL	CARB	FIBER	SOD
Breakstone's								
Bacon & Onion	2 tbsp (1.1 oz)	60	2	5	20	2	0	180
Chesapeake Clam	2 tbsp (1.1 oz)	50	1	4	20	1	0	180
Free Creamy Salsa	2 tbsp (1.1 oz)	20	1	0	<5	3	0	240
Free French Onion	2 tbsp (1.1 oz)	25	2	0	<5	4	0	260
Free Ranch	2 tbsp (1.1 oz)	25	2	0	<5	4	0	330
French Onion	2 tbsp (1.1 oz)	50	1	5	20	2	0	160
Toasted Onion	2 tbsp (1.1 oz)	50	1	5	20	2	0	170
Cheez Whiz								
Medium Cheese & Salsa	2 tbsp (1.2 oz)	100	3	8	20	3	0	490
Mild Cheese & Salsa	2 tbsp (1.2 oz)	100	3	8	20	3	0	490
Chi-Chi's								
Fiesta Bean	2 tbsp (0.9 oz)	35	1	2	0	4	1	140
Fiesta Cheese	2 tbsp (0.9 oz)	40	1	3	10	3	0	270
Fritos								
Bean	2 tbsp (1.2 oz)	40	2	1	0	6	0	140
Chili Cheese	1.2 oz	45	1	3	<5	3	0	310
French Onion	2 tbsp (1.1 oz)	60	1	5	15	4	0	230
Hot Bean	2 tbsp (1.2 oz)	40	2	1	0	5	1	170
Jalapeno & Cheddar Cheese	2 tbsp (1.2 oz)	50	1	4	5	4	0	300
Guiltless Gourmet								
Black Bean Mild	2 tbsp (1 oz)	30	2	0	0	5	1	100
Black Bean Spicy	2 tbsp (1 oz)	30	2	0	0	5	1	100
Knudsen								
Free Creamy Salsa	2 tbsp (1.1 oz)	20	1	0	<5	3	0	240
Free French Onion	2 tbsp (1.1 oz)	25	2	0	<5	4	0	260
Free Ranch	2 tbsp (1.1 oz)	25	2	0	<5	4	0	330

FOOD	PORTION	CAL	PROT	FAT	CHOL	CARB	FIBER	SOD
Kraft								
Avocado	2 tbsp (1.1 oz)	60	1	4	0	4	0	240
Bacon & Horseradish	2 tbsp (1.1 oz)	60	1	5	0	3	0	220
Clam	2 tbsp (1.1 oz)	60	1	4	0	3	0	250
Free French Onion	2 tbsp (1.1 oz)	25	2	0	<5	4	0	260
Free Ranch	2 tbsp (1.1 oz)	25	2	0	<5	4	0	330
Free Salsa	2 tbsp (1.1 oz)	20	1	0	<5	3	0	240
French Onion	2 tbsp (1.1 oz)	60	1	4	0	4	0	230
Green Onion	2 tbsp (1.1 oz)	60	1	4	0	4	0	190
Jalapeno Cheese	2 tbsp (1.1 oz)	60	1	4	0	3	0	260
Premium Sour Cream	2 tbsp (1.1 oz)	50	1	4	20	1	0	180
Premium Sour Cream Bacon & Horseradish	2 tbsp (1.1 oz)	60	2	5	15	2	0	240
Premium Sour Cream Bacon & Onion	2 tbsp (1.1 oz)	60	2	5	20	2	0	180
Premium Sour Cream Creamy Onion	2 tbsp (1.1 oz)	45	1	4	15	2	0	160
Premium Sour Cream French Onion	2 tbsp (1.1 oz)	45	tr	4	15	2	0	160
Premium Sour Cream Ranch	2 tbsp (1.1 oz)	50	tr	4	15	2	0	230
Ranch	2 tbsp (1.1 oz)	60	1	5	0	3	0	210
Old El Paso								
Black Bean	2 tbsp (1 oz)	20	1	0	0	4	1	150
Cheese 'n Salsa Medium	2 tbsp (1 oz)	40	tr	3	<5	3	0	300
Cheese 'n Salsa Mild	2 tbsp (1 oz)	40	tr	3	<5	3	0	300
Chunky Salsa Medium	2 tbsp (1 oz)	15	1	0	0	3	1	230
Chunky Salsa Mild	2 tbsp (1 oz)	15	1	0	0	3	1	230
Jalapeno	2 tbsp (1 oz)	30	1	1	<5	4	2	125

FOOD	PORTION	CAL	PROT	FAT	CHOL	CARB	FIBER	SOD
Ruffles								
French Onion	2 tbsp	70	1	5	0	4	1	240
Ranch	2 tbsp (1.2 oz)	70	1	6	0	4	0	300
Snyder's Of Hanover								
Microwavable Hot Nacho Cheese	2 tbsp	48	1	3	3	5	0	270
Microwavable Mild Cheese	2 tbsp	45	2	3	5	2	0	250
Mustard Pretzel	2 tbsp	60	1	2	0	12	0	0
Sour Cream & Onion	2 tbsp	60	1	5	15	2	0	220
Taco Bell								
Fat Free Black Bean	2 tbsp (1.2 oz)	30	2	0	0	6	2	220
Salsa Con Queso Medium	2 tbsp (1.2 oz)	45	tr	3	<5	5	tr	270
Salsa Con Queso Mild	2 tbsp (1.2 oz)	45	tr	3	<5	5	tr	270
Tyson								
Bleu Cheese For Dipping Wings	2 tbsp (1.4 oz)	140	1	14	25	3	1	370
Utz								
Fat Free Sour Cream & Onion	2 tbsp (1.1 oz)	30	1	0	0	7	0	210
Jalapeno & Cheddar	2 tbsp (1 oz)	30	0	3	0	2	0	250
Low Fat Desert Garden	2 tbsp (1.1 oz)	40	1	2	0	5	0	210
Low Fat Salsa Con Queso	2 tbsp (1 oz)	40	1	2	0	5	0	240
Mild Cheddar	2 tbsp (1 oz)	45	2	3	5	2	0	250
Sour Cream & Onion	2 tbsp (1 oz)	60	1	5	15	2	0	220
DOCK								
fresh cooked	3½ oz	20	2	1	0	3	–	3
raw chopped	½ cup	15	1	tr	0	2	–	3
DOLPHINFISH								
fresh baked	3 oz	93	20	1	80	0	–	96
fresh fillet baked	5.6 oz	174	38	1	149	0	–	179
DOUGHNUTS								
cake type unsugared	1 (1.6 oz)	198	2	11	18	23	1	257
chocolate glazed	1 (1.5 oz)	175	2	8	–	24	1	143

FOOD	PORTION	CAL	PROT	FAT	CHOL	CARB	FIBER	SOD
chocolate sugared	1 (1.5 oz)	175	2	8	—	24	1	143
chocolate coated	1 (1.5 oz)	204	2	13	—	21	1	185
creme filled	1 (3 oz)	307	6	21	20	26	—	262
french cruller glazed	1 (1.4 oz)	169	1	8	5	24	—	142
frosted	1 (1.5 oz)	204	2	13	—	21	1	185
honey bun	1 (2.1 oz)	242	4	14	4	27	1	205
jelly	1 (3 oz)	289	5	16	22	33	—	249
old fashioned	1 (1.6 oz)	198	2	11	18	23	1	257
sugared	1 (1.6 oz)	192	2	10	14	23	1	181
wheat glazed	1 (1.6 oz)	162	3	9	9	19	—	160
wheat sugared	1 (1.6 oz)	162	3	9	9	19	—	160
yeast glazed	1 (2.1 oz)	242	4	14	4	27	1	205
Dolly Madison								
Chocolate Frosted	1 (1.1 oz)	140	1	8	5	15	1	130
Donut Gems Chocolate	4 (2 oz)	260	3	15	10	28	1	230
Donut Gems Crunch	3 (2 oz)	220	3	10	10	31	0	250
Donut Gems Powdered	4 (2 oz)	230	3	11	15	30	0	260
English Cruller	1 (2 oz)	250	2	14	30	31	1	190
Glazed Whirl	1 (1.6 oz)	210	2	11	25	25	0	150
Glazed Yeast	1 (1.5 oz)	190	2	9	10	23	0	130
Old Fashioned	1 (2.1 oz)	280	4	16	20	28	0	360
Plain	1 (1.2 oz)	140	2	7	10	15	0	190
Powdered	1 (1 oz)	120	1	6	10	14	0	140
Dutch Mill								
Cider	1 (2.1 oz)	240	3	10	15	35	1	220
Cinnamon	1 (1.8 oz)	210	3	11	15	26	1	250
Donut Holes Double-Dipped Chocolate	3 (1.4 oz)	220	2	16	5	19	0	140
Donut Holes Shootin' Stars	3 (1.4 oz)	190	2	10	5	23	0	110
Double-Dipped Chocolate	1 (2.1 oz)	280	3	17	15	31	1	360
Glazed	1 (2.1 oz)	250	3	12	15	34	1	220
Glazed Chocolate	1 (2.4 oz)	270	3	11	15	40	1	380
Plain	1 (1.8 oz)	210	3	12	15	25	1	270
Sugared	1 (1.8 oz)	220	3	11	15	27	1	260

FOOD	PORTION	CAL	PROT	FAT	CHOL	CARB	FIBER	SOD
Hostess								
Blueberry	1 (1.7 oz)	210	2	13	10	21	0	120
Donettes Crumb	3 (1.5 oz)	170	2	8	10	23	0	190
Donettes Frosted	3 (1.5 oz)	200	2	12	10	21	0	170
Donettes Powdered	3 (1.5 oz)	180	2	9	10	23	0	190
Frosted	1 (1.4 oz)	180	2	11	5	19	0	170
O's Raspberry Filled	1 (2.2 oz)	230	3	10	5	34	1	230
Old Fashioned Glazed	1 (2.1 oz)	260	2	13	25	33	1	220
Plain	1 (1.1 oz)	140	2	7	10	15	0	190
Powdered	1 (1.3 oz)	150	2	8	10	19	0	180
Little Debbie								
Donut Sticks	1 (1.6 oz)	210	2	12	10	24	0	150
Mini Powdered	1 pkg (2.5 oz)	290	3	14	10	38	2	290
Tastykake								
Mini Plain Glaze	1 pkg (2.5 oz)	260	3	11	25	40	1	330
Mini Powdered Sugar	1 pkg (2.5 oz)	260	3	12	30	38	tr	360
Mini Rich Frosted	1 pkg (3 oz)	370	5	22	25	43	3	340
Tom's								
Chocolate Gem	1 pkg (2.5 oz)	320	4	18	10	37	1	430
Dunkin' Sticks	1 pkg (2.5 oz)	370	2	22	10	43	tr	300
Powdered Gems	1 pkg (2.5 oz)	320	3	18	10	41	1	430

DRESSING *(see STUFFING/DRESSING)*

DRINK MIXERS *(see also SODA, WATER)*

FOOD	PORTION	CAL	PROT	FAT	CHOL	CARB	FIBER	SOD
whiskey sour mix not prep	1 pkg (0.6 oz)	64	tr	0	0	16	—	46
whiskey sour mix	2 oz	55	0	0	0	14	—	66
whiskey sour mix as prep	3.6 oz	169	tr	0	0	16	—	48
Daily's								
Bloody Mary Original	1 serv (6 oz)	50	0	0	0	14	—	1040
Margarita Daiquiri Strawberry	1 serv (4 oz)	180	0	0	0	47	2	65
Margarita Green Demon	1 serv (3 oz)	80	0	0	0	19	—	45
Pina Colada	1 serv (3 oz)	160	0	2	0	37	1	115
Tabasco								
Bloody Mary Mix	1 serv (8.4 oz)	56	2	tr	0	11	1	1548

FOOD	PORTION	CAL	PROT	FAT	CHOL	CARB	FIBER	SOD
Bloody Mary Mix Extra Spicy	1 serv (8.4 oz)	58	3	tr	0	11	2	1645

DRUM

FOOD	PORTION	CAL	PROT	FAT	CHOL	CARB	FIBER	SOD
freshwater fillet baked	5.4 oz	236	35	10	126	0	–	148
freshwater baked	3 oz	130	19	5	70	0	–	82

DUCK

FOOD	PORTION	CAL	PROT	FAT	CHOL	CARB	FIBER	SOD
w/ skin roasted	1 cup (4.9 oz)	472	27	40	118	0	0	83
w/ skin w/ bone leg roasted	3 oz	184	23	10	97	0	–	94
w/ skin w/o bone breast roasted	3 oz	172	21	9	116	0	–	71
w/o skin roasted	1 cup (4.9 oz)	281	33	16	125	0	0	91
w/o skin w/ bone leg braised	1 cup (6.1 oz)	310	51	10	183	0	–	188
w/o skin w/o bone breast broiled	1 cup (6.1 oz)	244	48	4	249	0	–	183
wild w/ skin raw	½ duck (9.5 oz)	571	47	41	216	0	–	152
wild w/o skin breast raw	½ breast (2.9 oz)	102	16	4	–	0	–	47
Grimaud Farms								
Muscovy Duck Confit	1 serv (3 oz)	170	20	10	95	tr	–	140

DUMPLING

FOOD	PORTION	CAL	PROT	FAT	CHOL	CARB	FIBER	SOD
Health Is Wealth								
Potstickers Chicken Free	2 (1.6 oz)	80	4	4	0	11	1	300
Potstickers Pork Free	2 (1.6 oz)	80	4	4	0	11	1	300
Potstickers Vegetable	2 (1.6 oz)	90	7	3	0	11	5	190
Steamed Dumpling	2 (1.6 oz)	50	7	2	0	12	1	310
Pepperidge Farm								
Apple	1 (3 oz)	230	3	11	0	30	1	180
Peach	1 (3 oz)	320	3	11	0	50	4	150

DURIAN

FOOD	PORTION	CAL	PROT	FAT	CHOL	CARB	FIBER	SOD
fresh	3.5 oz	141	3	2	0	29	–	1

EDAMAME *(see SOYBEANS)*

FOOD	PORTION	CAL	PROT	FAT	CHOL	CARB	FIBER	SOD
EEL								
fresh cooked	1 fillet (5.6 oz)	375	38	24	257	0	—	104
fresh cooked	3 oz	200	20	13	137	0	—	55
raw	3 oz	156	16	10	107	0	—	43
smoked	3.5 oz	330	19	28	—	0	0	—
EGG *(see also* EGG DISHES, EGG SUBSTITUTES*)*								
CHICKEN								
fresh	1	75	6	5	213	1	—	63
frozen	1	75	6	5	213	1	—	63
frozen	1 cup	363	30	24	1033	3	—	307
hard cooked	1	77	6	5	213	1	—	62
hard cooked chopped	1 cup	210	17	14	578	2	—	169
poached	1	74	6	5	212	1	—	140
white only	1	17	4	0	0	tr	—	55
white only	1 cup	121	26	0	0	2	—	399
EggsPlus								
Fresh	1 (1.8 oz)	70	6	5	215	0	0	65
Horizon Organic								
Medium	1 (1.5 oz)	70	6	4	190	1	—	55
Organic Valley								
Brown Extra Large	1 (2.2 oz)	90	8	6	225	tr	—	330
Brown Large	1 (2 oz)	80	7	6	200	tr	—	380
Brown Medium	1 (1.8 oz)	70	6	5	175	tr	—	260
OTHER POULTRY								
duck	1 (2.5 oz)	130	9	10	619	1	0	102
duck 100 year old	1 (1 oz)	49	4	3	173	1	—	154
duck preserved hard core	1 (1.8 oz)	80	6	6	220	1	0	350
duck preserved soft core	1 (1.8 oz)	80	7	6	220	1	0	350
duck salted	1 (1 oz)	54	4	4	184	2	—	769
goose	1 (5 oz)	267	20	19	—	2	—	—
quail	1 (9 g)	14	1	1	76	tr	—	—
turkey	1 (2.7 oz)	135	9	9	737	1	—	—
EGG DISHES								
FROZEN								
Weight Watchers								
Handy Ham & Cheese Omelet	1 (4 oz)	220	13	5	30	30	2	440

FOOD	PORTION	CAL	PROT	FAT	CHOL	CARB	FIBER	SOD
TAKE-OUT								
deviled	2 halves	145	6	13	280	1	—	180
omelette plain	1 serv (3.5 oz)	172	15	13	350	tr	0	245
salad	½ cup	307	13	28	562	2	—	565
scotch egg	1 (4.2 oz)	301	14	21	—	16	2	—
scrambled plain	2 (3.3 oz)	199	13	15	400	2	0	211
scrambled w/ whole milk & margarine	1 serv	365	24	27	774	5	—	616
sunny side up	1	91	6	7	211	1	—	162
EGG ROLLS (see also ASIAN FOODS)								
egg roll wrapper fresh	1	83	3	tr	3	16	—	162
Chun King								
Chicken Mini	6	210	6	9	15	25	2	650
Chicken Restaurant Style	1 (3 oz)	190	6	9	20	22	2	550
Pork & Shrimp Mini	6	210	6	9	15	27	2	540
Shrimp Mini	6	190	5	6	10	28	2	730
Shrimp Restaurant Style	1 (3 oz)	180	5	7	15	25	2	490
Health Is Wealth								
Broccoli	1 (3 oz)	150	4	5	5	23	2	560
Oriental Vegetable	1 (3 oz)	160	4	4	0	23	2	390
Oriental Chicken Free	1 (3 oz)	120	8	4	0	21	2	390
Pizza	1 (3 oz)	200	7	9	0	23	3	470
Spinach	1 (3 oz)	180	7	8	0	20	3	300
Spring Rolls	1 (1.6 oz)	70	2	2	0	10	5	200
Veggie	1 (3 oz)	130	4	4	0	21	3	550
La Choy								
Chicken Mini	6	210	6	9	15	25	2	650
Chicken Restaurant Style	1 (3 oz)	210	6	9	15	25	2	550
Pork Restaurant Style	1 (3 oz)	220	5	11	10	24	2	390
Pork & Shrimp Bite Size	12	210	6	10	10	25	2	540
Pork & Shrimp Mini	6	210	6	9	15	27	2	540
Shrimp Mini	6	190	5	6	10	28	2	730
Shrimp Restaurant Style	1 (3 oz)	180	5	7	15	25	2	490

FOOD	PORTION	CAL	PROT	FAT	CHOL	CARB	FIBER	SOD
Sweet & Sour Chicken Restaurant Style	1 (3 oz)	220	6	9	15	29	2	550
Vegetable w/ Lobster Mini	6	190	5	7	5	27	2	440
Lo-An								
White Meat Chicken	1 (2.7 oz)	140	6	4r	10	20	1	400
Worthington								
Vegetarian Egg Rolls	1 (3 oz)	180	6	8	0	20	2	380
TAKE-OUT								
lobster	1 (4.8 oz)	270	8	7	0	43	6	460
lumpia vegetable & shrimp	2 (3 oz)	120	4	0	10	26	2	300
meat & shrimp	1 (4.8 oz)	320	10	12	10	41	4	470
pork & shrimp	1 (5 oz)	300	13	10	15	41	7	890
shrimp	1 (3 oz)	170	6	5	<5	24	5	420
spicy pork	1 (3 oz)	200	6	9	5	23	3	410
vegetable	1 (3 oz)	170	5	4	0	28	4	520
EGG SUBSTITUTES								
frozen	¼ cup	96	7	7	1	2	—	120
frozen	1 cup	384	27	27	5	8	—	479
liquid	1 cup (8.8 oz)	211	30	8	3	2	—	444
liquid	1½ oz	40	6	2	tr	tr	—	83
powder	0.35 oz	44	5	1	57	2	—	79
powder	0.7 oz	88	11	3	113	4	—	158
Better'n Eggs								
Fat Free Cholesterol Free	¼ cup (2 oz)	30	6	0	0	1	0	100
Egg Beaters								
Eggs Substitute	¼ cup	30	5	0	0	1	0	115
Omelette Cheese	½ cup	110	14	5	5	2	—	480
Omelette Vegetable	½ cup	50	7	0	0	5	—	170
Morningstar Farms								
Breakfast Sandwich Bagel Scramblers Pattie Cheese	1 (5.9 oz)	320	28	5	10	40	4	900
Scramblers	¼ cup (2 oz)	35	6	0	0	2	0	95
EGGNOG								
eggnog	1 cup	342	10	19	149	34	—	138
eggnog	1 qt	1368	39	76	596	138	—	553

FOOD	PORTION	CAL	PROT	FAT	CHOL	CARB	FIBER	SOD
eggnog flavor mix as prep w/ milk	9 oz	260	8	8	33	39	–	163
Oberweis								
Egg Nog	½ cup	240	3	15	40	25	0	70
EGGPLANT								
cubed cooked	½ cup	13	tr	tr	0	3	–	2
raw cut up	½ cup (1.4 oz)	11	tr	tr	0	2	–	1
slices grilled	4 (7 oz)	38	2	0	0	0	–	–
whole peeled raw	1 (1 lb)	117	5	1	0	28	–	14
Progresso								
Caponata	2 tbsp (1 oz)	25	0	2	0	2	2	130
TAKE-OUT								
baba ghannouj	¼ cup	55	2	4	0	5	–	95
caponata	2 tbsp (1 oz)	30	1	2	0	3	–	115
iman bayildi eggplant w/ onion & tomato	1 serv (15.6 oz)	345	3	28	0	25	2	552
indian eggplant runi	1 serv	180	2	14	0	13	1	228
papoutsakis little shoes	1 serv (15.5 oz)	245	12	16	40	15	1	751
ELDERBERRIES								
fresh	1 cup	105	1	1	0	27	–	–
ELDERBERRY JUICE								
elderberry	7 oz	76	4	0	0	16	–	2
ELK								
roasted	3 oz	124	26	2	62	0	–	52
EMU								
cooked	3 oz	130	–	–	111	–	–	97
ENDIVE								
fresh	3.5 oz	9	2	tr	0	tr	2	53
raw chopped	½ cup	4	tr	tr	0	1	–	6
ENERGY BARS *(see also* CEREAL BARS, ENERGY DRINKS, NUTRITION SUPPLEMENTS*)*								
AllGoode Organics								
Amazin' Peanut Raisin	1 bar	210	7	11	0	25	3	80
Banana Nut Nirvana	1 bar	190	5	8	0	30	3	5
Cashew Almond Passion	1 bar	210	7	9	0	25	3	50

FOOD	PORTION	CAL	PROT	FAT	CHOL	CARB	FIBER	SOD
Chocolate Peanut Pleasure	1 bar	200	5	9	5	29	3	15
Honey Nut Harvest	1 bar	210	7	9	0	29	3	50
Nutty Chocolate Apricot	1 bar	200	6	10	5	26	5	15
Atkins Advantage								
Praline Crunch	1 bar (2.11 oz)	221	21	13	–	–	–	–
Balance								
Chocolate Raspberry Fudge	1 bar (1.76 oz)	180	14	6	–	–	–	–
Oasis Strawberry Cheesecake	1 bar (1.69 oz)	180	8	3	0	28	tr	250
Benecol								
Chocolate Crisp	1 bar (1.2 oz)	130	3	3	5	23	2	60
Peanut Crisp	1 bar (1.2 oz)	140	3	4	5	23	1	105
Better Bar								
Chocolate Coated Caramel Pecan	1 bar (1.8 oz)	180	18	4	0	15	0	35
Chocolate Coated Peanut	1 bar (1.8 oz)	180	18	4	0	15	0	35
Yogurt Coated Raspberry	1 bar (1.8 oz)	180	18	3	0	15	0	35
Breakthru								
Organic Chocolate Fudge	1 bar (2.1 oz)	230	10	3	0	39	3	120
Organic Cinnamon Crunch	1 bar (2.1 oz)	220	12	3	0	37	3	160
Organic Honey Graham	1 bar (2.1 oz)	220	12	3	0	37	3	160
Organic Mocha Fudge	1 bar (2.1 oz)	230	10	3	0	39	3	120
Carbolite								
Chocolate Peanut Butter Sugar Free	1 bar (1 oz)	144	tr	12	4	2	0	28
Centrum								
Energy Chocolate Nougat	1 (1.98 oz)	220	8	5	0	34	tr	185
Energy Chocolate Peanut Butter	1 (1.98 oz)	220	8	5	0	34	tr	185

FOOD	PORTION	CAL	PROT	FAT	CHOL	CARB	FIBER	SOD
Clif Bar								
Apricot	1 bar (2.4 oz)	220	8	3	0	43	5	90
Carrot Cake	1 bar (2.4 oz)	240	10	4	0	43	5	150
Chocolate Brownie	1 bar (2.4 oz)	240	10	4	0	41	6	150
Chocolate Almond Fudge	1 bar (2.4 oz)	230	10	5	0	36	5	140
Chocolate Chip	1 bar (2.4 oz)	240	10	4	0	41	5	170
Chocolate Chip Peanut Crunch	1 bar (2.4 oz)	240	12	5	0	39	5	290
Cookies'N Cream	1 bar (2.4 oz)	230	10	4	0	39	5	180
Cranberry Apple Cherry	1 bar (2.4 oz)	220	8	2	0	44	5	135
Crunchy Peanut Butter	1 bar (2.4 oz)	240	12	5	0	39	5	290
GingerSnap	1 bar (2.4 oz)	230	10	4	0	42	6	140
Ensure								
All Flavors	1 bar (2.1 oz)	230	9	6	<5	35	1	135
Extend								
Chocolate Chip Crunch	1 bar (1.4 oz)	160	3	3	0	31	tr	80
Peanut Butter Crunch	1 bar (1.4 oz)	160	4	3	0	30	0	85
Gatorade								
GatorBar	1 bar (1.17 oz)	110	1	1	0	13	1	10
Peanut Butter Chocolate Chip	1 bar (2.3 oz)	260	8	5	–	–	–	–
GeniSoy								
Soy Protein Chocolate	1 bar (2.2 oz)	210	14	0	0	36	1	190
Soy Protein Chocolate Coated	1 bar (2.2 oz)	220	14	4	0	33	1	190
Glucerna								
All Flavors	1 bar (1.3 oz)	140	6	4	<5	24	4	75
HeartBar								
Cranberry	1 bar (1.8 oz)	190	13	3	0	27	3	95
Original	1 bar (1.76 oz)	180	14	3	0	26	3	140
Jenny Craig								
Meal Bar Chocolate Peanut	1 bar (2 oz)	220	10	5	0	33	1	240
Meal Bar Lemon Meringue	1 bar (2 oz)	210	10	5	0	31	0	130

FOOD	PORTION	CAL	PROT	FAT	CHOL	CARB	FIBER	SOD
Meal Bar Milk Chocolate	1 bar (2 oz)	210	10	5	0	33	1	180
Meal Bar Oatmeal Raisin	1 bar (1.97 oz)	210	10	3	0	35	3	75
Meal Bar Yogurt Peanut	1 bar (2 oz)	220	10	5	0	33	0	270
Kashi								
GoLean Chocolate Peanut Butter	1 (2.7 oz)	280	13	6	0	50	7	150
GoLean Honey Vanilla Yogurt	1 (2.7 oz)	280	11	4	0	53	7	70
GoLean Strawberry Vanilla Yogurt	1 (2.7 oz)	280	11	4	0	53	6	75
Lean Body For Her								
Chocolate Honey Peanut	1 bar (1.76 oz)	190	16	7	0	10	tr	135
Luna								
Chai Tea	1 bar (1.7 oz)	180	10	4	0	27	2	125
Chocolate Pecan Pie	1 bar (1.7 oz)	180	10	5	0	24	2	125
LemonZest	1 bar (1.7 oz)	180	10	4	0	24	2	50
Nutz Over Chocolate	1 bar (1.7 oz)	180	10	5	0	24	2	100
S'Mores	1 bar (1.7 oz)	180	10	4	0	26	2	125
Sesame Raisin Crunch	1 bar (1.7 oz)	170	10	3	0	26	2	125
Toasted Nuts 'n Cranberry	1 bar (1.7 oz)	170	10	3	0	26	2	130
Tropical Crisp	1 bar (1.7 oz)	180	10	5	0	24	2	135
Met-Rx								
Big 100 Gram Bar Peanut Butter	1 bar (3.5 oz)	340	26	4	15	52	2	135
Source/One Chocolate Cheesecake	1 bar (2.1 oz)	160	15	5	5	21	tr	50
NiteBite								
Chocolate Fudge	1 bar (0.9 oz)	100	3	4	5	15	0	40
Peanut Butter	1 bar (0.9 oz)	100	3	4	5	15	0	80
Nutiva								
Flaxseed & Raisin Organic	1 bar (1.4 oz)	280	14	19	0	12	6	10

FOOD	PORTION	CAL	PROT	FAT	CHOL	CARB	FIBER	SOD
Hempseed Bar Organic	1 bar (1.4 oz)	210	9	14	0	11	5	5
Nutribar								
Chocolate Covered Belgian Chocolate	1 bar (2.3 oz)	252	13	8	–	33	2	255
Chocolate Covered Chocolate Fudge	1 bar (2.3 oz)	267	14	8	5	35	2	300
Chocolate Covered Hazelnut	1 bar (2.3 oz)	261	13	8	–	34	1	295
Chocolate Covered Mocha Almond	1 bar (2.3 oz)	261	13	8	–	34	tr	280
Chocolate Covered Peanut	1 bar (2.3 oz)	262	13	9	–	34	1	255
Yogurt Covered Peach Apricot	1 bar (2.3 oz)	261	13	8	–	34	tr	260
Yogurt Covered Raspberry	1 bar (2.3 oz)	261	13	8	–	34	tr	260
Yogurt Covered Wildberry	1 bar (2.3 oz)	261	13	8	–	34	tr	260
Odwalla Bar!								
Peanut Crunch	1 bar (2.2 oz)	260	8	7	0	40	3	180
PermaLean								
Protein Crunch Chocoholic Chocolate	1 bar (1.8 oz)	170	21	3	0	10	tr	65
Protein Crunch Chocolate Raspberry	1 bar (1.8 oz)	180	21	2	10	9	0	35
Protein Crunch Stark Raving Peanutz	1 bar (1.8 oz)	180	21	4	0	9	0	75
PowerBar								
Apple Cinnamon	1 bar (2.3 oz)	230	10	3	0	45	3	90
Banana	1 bar (2.3 oz)	230	9	2	0	45	3	90
Chocolate	1 bar (2.3 oz)	230	10	2	0	45	3	90
Essentials Chocolate	1 bar (1.9 oz)	180	10	4	0	28	3	105
Harvest Apple Crisp	1 bar (2.3 oz)	240	7	4	–	–	–	–
Harvest Blueberry	1 bar (2.3 oz)	240	7	4	0	45	4	80
Harvest Strawberry	1 bar (2.3 oz)	240	7	4	0	45	4	80
Malt-Nut	1 bar (2.3 oz)	230	10	3	0	45	3	90

FOOD	PORTION	CAL	PROT	FAT	CHOL	CARB	FIBER	SOD
Mocha	1 bar (2.3 oz)	230	10	3	0	45	3	90
Oatmeal Raisin	1 bar (2.3 oz)	230	10	3	0	45	3	120
Peanut Butter	1 bar (2.3 oz)	230	10	3	0	45	3	110
Power Gel Strawberry Banana	1 pkg	110	0	0	0	28	–	50
Vanilla Crisp	1 bar (2.3 oz)	230	9	3	0	45	3	90
Wild Berry	1 bar (2.3 oz)	230	10	3	0	45	3	90
Revival								
Marshmallow Krunch	1 bar (2.1 oz)	220	17	3	0	30	tr	310
Protein Bars Chocolate Temptation	1 bar (2.1 oz)	220	15	4	0	31	tr	290
Protein Bars Peanut Butter Chocolate Pal	1 bar (2.1 oz)	240	16	6	0	30	1	310
Protein Bars Peanut Butter Pal	1 bar (2.1 oz)	240	17	5	0	29	tr	320
Slim-Fast								
Crispy Peanut Caramel	1 bar	120	1	4	<5	21	tr	80
Dutch Chocolate	1 bar	140	5	5	5	20	2	80
Meal On-The-Go Apple Cobbler	1 bar	220	8	5	<5	33	2	150
Meal On-The-Go Chocolate Cookie Dough	1 bar	220	8	5	<5	35	2	180
Meal On-The-Go Honey Peanut	1 bar	220	8	5	<5	34	2	160
Meal On-The-Go Milk Chocolate Peanut	1 bar	220	8	5	<5	36	2	120
Meal On-The-Go Oatmeal Raisin	1 bar	220	8	5	<5	36	2	100
Meal On-The-Go Rich Chocolate Brownie	1 bar	220	8	5	<5	34	2	150
Meal On-The-Go Toasted Oat & Spice	1 bar	220	8	5	<5	35	2	140

FOOD	PORTION	CAL	PROT	FAT	CHOL	CARB	FIBER	SOD
Peanut Butter	1 bar	150	6	5	5	19	2	80
Peanut Butter Crunch	1 bar	130	1	4	0	21	tr	80
Rich Chewy Caramel	1 bar	120	tr	4	5	22	2	65
Sweet Success								
Chewy Chocolate Brownie	1 bar (1.2 oz)	120	2	4	3	23	3	35
Think!								
Apple Spice	1 bar (2 oz)	205	5	3	62	40	7	36
Chocolate Almond Coconut Raisin	1 bar (2 oz)	243	6	7	9	39	2	160
Chocolate Fruit Harvest	1 bar (2 oz)	217	5	3	38	43	7	42
Zoe								
Flax & Soy Apple Crisp	1 bar (1.83 oz)	180	8	6	–	–	–	–
ZonePerfect								
Honey Peanut	1 bar (1.8 oz)	200	14	7	0	22	1	150

ENERGY DRINKS (*see also* ENERGY BARS, NUTRITION SUPPLEMENTS)

FOOD	PORTION	CAL	PROT	FAT	CHOL	CARB	FIBER	SOD
Boost								
Chocolate	1 can (8 oz)	240	10	4	5	40	0	130
Vanilla	8 oz	240	10	4	5	40	0	130
California Joe								
All Natural Protein Drink Mix as prep	1 serv (8 oz)	165	12	4	0	21	0	166
Calorie Shed								
Shake Fat Free No Sugar Caramel Ripple	½ cup (4 fl oz)	70	3	0	5	21	2	45
Shake Fat Free No Sugar Chocolate	½ cup (4 fl oz)	70	3	0	5	21	2	45
Fat Burner								
Diet Fruit Punch	8 fl oz	0	8	0	0	0	–	–
Gatorade								
Citrus Cooler	1 cup (8 oz)	50	0	0	0	14	–	110
Fruit Punch	1 cup (8 oz)	50	0	0	0	14	–	110
GatorLode	1 can (11.6 fl oz)	280	0	0	0	71	–	90
GatorPro	1 can (11 fl oz)	360	17	6	0	59	0	270

FOOD	PORTION	CAL	PROT	FAT	CHOL	CARB	FIBER	SOD
Grape	1 cup (8 oz)	50	0	0	0	14	–	110
Iced Tea Cooler	1 cup (8 oz)	50	0	0	0	14	–	110
Lemon-Lime	1 cup (8 oz)	50	0	0	0	14	–	110
Lemonade	1 cup (8 oz)	50	0	0	0	14	–	110
Orange	1 cup (8 oz)	50	0	0	0	14	–	110
Tropical Fruit	1 cup (8 oz)	50	0	0	0	14	–	110
GeniSoy								
Soy Protein Shake Chocolate	1 scoop (1.2 oz)	120	14	0	0	17	2	170
Soy Protein Shake Vanilla	1 scoop (1.2 oz)	130	14	0	0	18	–	180
Hansen's								
D-Stress	1 can (8.2 oz)	110	0	0	0	31	–	25
Energy	1 can (8.3 oz)	120	0	0	0	32	–	25
Healthy Pleasures								
Chocolate Irish Cream	1 bottle (10.5 oz)	260	12	2	6	45	0	320
Kashi								
GoLean Shake Man	1 pkg (2.5 oz)	260	30	1	0	34	7	135
GoLean Shake Woman	1 pkg (2.5 oz)	250	30	2	0	32	7	120
Nancy Grey's								
Shake Hi-Protein Black Raspberry	1 cup (8 fl oz)	340	10	16	65	40	0	160
Shake Hi-Protein Chocolate	1 cup (8 fl oz)	340	10	15	60	42	–	140
Shake Hi-Protein Vanilla	1 cup (8 fl oz)	340	10	16	65	40	0	160
Nantucket Nectars								
Super Nectars Ginkgo Mango	8 oz	150	0	0	0	38	–	15
Super Nectars Green Angel	8 oz	140	tr	0	0	35	–	15
Super Nectars Protein Smoothie	8 oz	170	2	1	0	38	–	45
Super Nectars Red Guarana Tea	8 oz	110	0	0	0	26	–	5
Super Nectars Vital C	8 oz	130	tr	0	0	32	–	10

FOOD	PORTION	CAL	PROT	FAT	CHOL	CARB	FIBER	SOD
NutraShake								
Citrus	1 pkg (4 oz)	200	6	0	0	44	–	30
Citrus Free	1 serv (4 oz)	200	6	0	0	44	0	110
Vanilla	1 serv (8 oz)	400	12	12	36	62	–	120
Vanilla No Added Sugar	1 serv (4 oz)	200	7	8	18	25	–	75
Pounds Off								
Dark Chocolate Ectasy	1 can (11 oz)	200	11	3	0	39	6	220
French Vanilla	1 can (11 oz)	220	12	3	0	41	5	460
Powerade								
Fruit Punch	8 fl oz	70	0	0	0	19	–	55
Lemon Lime	8 fl oz	70	0	0	0	19	–	55
Mountain Blast	8 fl oz	70	0	0	0	19	–	55
Red Bull								
Energy Drink	1 can (8.3 oz)	113	0	0	0	28	–	215
Resource								
Fruit Beverage	1 pkg (8 oz)	180	9	0	–	36	–	55
Slim-Fast								
Chocolate as prep w/ fat free milk	1 serv	190	14	1	9	32	2	240
Chocolate Malt as prep w/ fat free milk	1 serv	190	14	1	8	32	2	250
JumpStart Chocolate as prep w/ fat free milk	1 serv	240	18	2	14	39	5	280
JumpStart Vanilla as prep w/ fat free milk	1 serv	240	18	2	9	39	5	300
Strawberry as prep w/ fat free milk	1 serv	190	14	1	9	32	2	260
Vanilla as prep w/ fat free milk	1 serv	190	14	1	9	32	2	260
SoBe								
Adrenaline Rush	1 can (8.3 oz)	140	1	0	0	36	–	60
Drive	8 oz	120	0	0	0	32	–	15
Edge	8 fl oz	110	0	0	0	30	–	15
Elixir 3C Strawberry Carrot	8 fl oz	90	0	0	0	25	–	15

FOOD	PORTION	CAL	PROT	FAT	CHOL	CARB	FIBER	SOD
Jing Essentials	1 bottle (14 oz)	140	0	0	0	36	0	35
Jing Essentials Citrus Soy Blend	1 bottle (14 oz)	170	1	1	0	44	–	70
Karma	8 oz	120	0	0	0	33	–	5
Lean Sugar Free Metabolic Enhancer Diet Green Tea	8 fl oz	5	0	0	0	1	–	15
Lean Sugar Free Metabolic Enhancer Diet Orange Carrot	8 fl oz	10	0	0	0	2	6	15
Lizard Lightning Orange Mango	8 fl oz	130	0	0	0	33	–	20
Qi Essentials	1 bottle (14 oz)	140	0	0	0	36	0	35
Qi Essentials Berry Soy Blend	1 bottle (14 oz)	170	1	1	0	44	–	70
Shen Essentials	1 bottle (14 oz)	140	0	0	0	36	0	35
Shen Essentials Peach Soy Blend	1 bottle (14 oz)	170	1	1	0	44	–	70
Tsunami Orange Cream	8 fl oz	110	0	0	0	29	–	20
Sustacal								
Vanilla	8 oz	240	15	6	<5	33	tr	220
Sweet Success								
Creamy Milk Chocolate	1 can	200	10	3	4	36	3	230
Creamy Milk Chocolate as prep w/ skim milk	1 serv	180	11	1	6	36	6	240
The Pumper								
Body Building MilkShake Chocolate	1 serv (13.5 oz)	390	21	2	5	80	5	260
Body Building MilkShake Banana	1 serv (13.5 oz)	390	17	2	10	82	3	230
TwinLab								
Hydra Fuel	16 fl oz	132	0	0	0	33	–	50

FOOD	PORTION	CAL	PROT	FAT	CHOL	CARB	FIBER	SOD
Nitro Fuel	16 oz	460	15	0	0	100	–	–
Ultra Fuel	1 bottle (16 oz)	400	0	0	0	100	–	55
Ultra Slim-Fast								
Cafe Mocha as prep w/ fat free milk	1 serv	200	14	2	9	36	5	240
Chocolate Fudge as prep w/ fat free milk	1 serv	200	14	3	9	36	5	230
Chocolate Malt as prep w/ fat free milk	1 serv	200	14	2	9	36	5	230
Chocolate Royale as prep w/ fat free milk	1 serv	200	14	2	9	36	5	260
Fruit Juice Mixable as prep w/ juice	1 serv	200	12	1	5	44	5	210
Milk Chocolate as prep w/ fat free milk	1 serv	210	14	2	8	34	5	270
Ready-To-Drink Cappuccino Delight	1 serv	220	10	2	5	42	5	240
Ready-To-Drink Apple Cranberry Raspberry	1 serv	220	7	2	10	46	5	160
Ready-To-Drink Chocolate Royale	1 serv	220	10	3	5	38	5	220
Ready-To-Drink Creamy Milk Chocolate	1 serv	220	10	3	5	42	5	220
Ready-To-Drink Dark Chocolate Fudge	1 serv	220	10	3	5	42	5	300
Ready-To-Drink Orange Strawberry Banana	1 serv	220	7	2	10	46	5	160
Ready-To-Drink Orange Pineapple	1 serv	220	7	2	10	46	5	200

FOOD	PORTION	CAL	PROT	FAT	CHOL	CARB	FIBER	SOD
Ready-To-Drink Strawberries N' Cream	1 serv	220	10	3	5	40	5	220
Strawberry as prep w/ fat free milk	1 serv	200	14	1	9	37	4	250
Vanilla as prep w/ fat free milk	1 serv	200	14	1	9	37	5	260

ENGLISH MUFFIN
FROZEN
Weight Watchers

FOOD	PORTION	CAL	PROT	FAT	CHOL	CARB	FIBER	SOD
Sandwich	1 (4 oz)	210	13	5	20	28	2	420
READY-TO-EAT								
apple cinnamon	1	138	4	2	0	28	–	255
crumpets	1 (1.5 oz)	80	3	0	0	16	tr	270
granola	1	155	6	1	0	31	–	275
mixed grain	1	155	6	1	0	31	–	275
plain	1	134	4	1	0	26	–	265
plain toasted	1	133	4	1	0	26	–	262
raisin cinnamon	1	138	4	2	0	28	–	255
sourdough	1	134	4	1	0	26	–	265
wheat	1	127	5	1	0	26	–	218
whole wheat	1	134	6	1	0	27	4	420
Milton's								
Multi-Grain	1 (2 oz)	150	4	1	0	33	3	180
Wonder								
Cinnamon Raisin	1 (2.1 oz)	140	5	2	0	26	2	260
Original	1 (2 oz)	130	4	1	0	25	1	290
Sourdough	1 (2 oz)	130	4	1	0	25	1	290
TAKE-OUT								
w/ butter	1 (2.2 oz)	189	5	6	13	30	–	386
w/ cheese & sausage	1 (4 oz)	393	15	24	59	29	–	1036
w/ egg cheese & canadian bacon	1 (4.8 oz)	289	17	13	234	28	2	729
w/ egg cheese & sausage	1 (5.8 oz)	487	22	31	274	31	–	1135

EPAZOTE

FOOD	PORTION	CAL	PROT	FAT	CHOL	CARB	FIBER	SOD
fresh	1 tbsp (1 g)	tr	0	0	0	tr	tr	tr
fresh sprig	1 (2 g)	1	tr	tr	0	tr	tr	1

FOOD	PORTION	CAL	PROT	FAT	CHOL	CARB	FIBER	SOD
EPPAW								
raw	½ cup	75	2	1	0	16	–	6
FALAFEL								
TAKE-OUT								
falafel	1 (1.2 oz)	57	2	3	0	5	–	50
FAT (see also BUTTER, BUTTER BLENDS, BUTTER SUBSTITUTES, MARGARINE, OIL)								
beef cooked	1 oz	193	20	27	3	0	–	12
beef suet	1 oz	242	tr	27	19	0	–	–
beef tallow	1 tbsp (13 g)	115	0	13	14	0	–	0
chicken	1 cup	1846	0	205	174	0	–	–
chicken	1 tbsp	115	0	13	11	0	–	–
cocoa butter	1 tbsp	120	0	14	0	0	–	–
duck	1 tbsp (13 g)	115	0	13	13	0	0	0
goose	1 tbsp	115	0	13	13	0	–	–
goose	1 oz	257	0	29	–	0	–	–
lamb new zealand	1 oz	182	2	19	25	0	–	6
lard	1 tbsp (13 g)	115	0	13	12	0	–	0
lard	1 cup (205 g)	1849	0	205	195	0	–	tr
nutmeg butter	1 tbsp	120	0	14	–	0	–	–
pork backfat	1 oz	230	1	25	16	0	0	3
pork cooked	1 oz	178	3	18	26	0	0	10
salt pork	1 oz	212	23	23	25	0	–	404
shortening	1 tbsp	113	0	13	0	0	–	–
shortening	1 cup	1812	0	205	0	0	–	–
turkey	1 tbsp	115	0	13	13	0	–	–
ucuhuba butter	1 tbsp	120	0	14	–	0	–	–
Crisco								
Butter Flavor	1 tbsp	110	0	12	0	0	–	0
Shortening	1 tbsp (0.4 oz)	110	0	12	0	0	–	0
Sticks	1 tbsp (0.4 oz)	110	0	12	0	0	0	0
Sticks Butter Flavor	1 tbsp (0.4 oz)	110	0	12	0	0	0	0
FAT SUBSTITUTES								
Smucker's								
Baking Healthy 100% Fat Free	1 tbsp	30	0	0	0	7	0	7
Soy Is Us								
Fat Not! Organic	3 tbsp	66	11	1	0	7	4	3

FOOD	PORTION	CAL	PROT	FAT	CHOL	CARB	FIBER	SOD
FAVA BEANS								
Progresso								
Fava Beans	½ cup (4.6 oz)	110	6	1	0	20	5	250
FEIJOA								
fresh	1 (1.75 oz)	25	1	tr	0	5	–	2
puree	1 cup	119	3	2	0	26	–	7
FENNEL								
fresh bulb	1 (8.2 oz)	72	3	tr	0	17	–	122
fresh sliced	1 cup	27	1	tr	0	6	–	45
leaves	1 oz	7	tr	tr	–	1	1	25
seed	1 tsp	7	tr	tr	0	1	–	2
FENUGREEK								
seed	1 tsp	12	1	tr	0	2	–	2
FIBER								
Apple Fiber								
Pure	2 tbsp (7 g)	16	–	0	0	7	4	–
Benefiber								
Supplement	1 pkg (4 g)	20	0	0	0	4	3	20
Metamucil								
Fiber Wafers Apple Crisp	2	120	2	5	0	17	6	20
ND Labs								
Pure Apple Fiber	1 tbsp (7 g)	16	0	0	0	7	4	–
FIDDLEHEAD FERNS								
fresh	3.5 oz	34	5	tr	0	6	–	1
FIGS								
canned in heavy syrup	3	75	tr	tr	0	19	–	1
canned in light syrup	3	58	tr	tr	0	15	–	1
canned water pack	3	42	tr	tr	0	11	–	1
dried cooked	½ cup	140	2	1	0	16	–	6
dried whole	10	477	6	2	0	122	17	20
fresh	1 med	50	tr	tr	0	10	–	1
Sonoma								
Dried White Misson	3–4 (1.4 oz)	110	1	0	0	26	5	0

FOOD	PORTION	CAL	PROT	FAT	CHOL	CARB	FIBER	SOD
FIREWEED								
leaves chopped	1 cup (0.8 oz)	24	1	1	0	4	2	8
FISH *(see also individual names,* FISH SUBSTITUTES, SUSHI*)*								
FROZEN								
breaded fillet	1 (2 oz)	155	9	7	64	14	—	332
sticks	1 stick (1 oz)	76	4	3	31	7	—	163
Gorton's								
Baked Au Gratin	1 piece (4.6 oz)	130	14	5	50	7	—	400
Baked Broccoli Cheddar	1 piece (4.6 oz)	130	14	5	50	7	—	310
Baked Primavera	1 piece (4.6 oz)	120	15	5	50	4	—	340
Batter Dipped Portions	1 piece (2.5 oz)	170	6	11	20	12	—	390
Crunchy Golden Fillets Breaded	2 (3.8 oz)	250	10	14	35	21	—	480
Crunchy Golden Sticks	6 (3.8 oz)	250	12	13	30	21	—	340
Garlic & Herb	2 pieces (3.6 oz)	220	10	11	30	21	—	670
Garlic Butter Crumb	1 piece (4.6 oz)	170	17	9	55	5	—	350
Grilled Cajun Blackened	1 piece (3.8 oz)	120	16	6	60	1	—	240
Grilled Garlic Butter	1 piece (3.8 oz)	120	16	6	60	1	—	200
Grilled Italian Herb	1 piece (3.8 oz)	130	17	6	60	2	—	330
Grilled Lemon Butter	1 piece (3.8 oz)	120	16	6	60	1	—	380
Grilled Lemon Pepper	1 piece (3.8 oz)	120	16	6	60	1	—	160
Parmesan	2 pieces (3.6 oz)	260	10	15	30	20	—	650
Ranch	1 piece (3.6 oz)	240	9	13	30	22	—	650
Southern Fried Country Style	2 pieces (3.6 oz)	230	10	14	30	16	—	660
Tenders	3.5 pieces (4 oz)	250	11	14	30	20	—	530
Tenders Extra Crunchy	3.5 pieces (4 oz)	270	11	12	30	29	—	640
Van De Kamp's								
Battered Fish Fillets	1 (2.6 oz)	180	8	11	20	12	0	340
Battered Fish Nuggets	8 (4 oz)	280	11	18	25	20	0	600
Battered Fish Portions	2 pieces (5 oz)	350	13	22	35	26	0	710
Battered Fish Sticks	6 (4 oz)	260	11	16	30	18	0	540
Breaded Fillets	2 (3.5 oz)	280	11	19	35	17	0	270

FOOD	PORTION	CAL	PROT	FAT	CHOL	CARB	FIBER	SOD
Breaded Fish Portions	3 pieces (4.5 oz)	330	14	21	35	23	0	410
Breaded Fish Sticks	6 (4 oz)	290	13	17	35	23	0	390
Breaded Mini Fish Sticks	13 (3.3 oz)	250	11	14	30	19	0	330
Crisp & Healthy Breaded Fillets	2 (3.5 oz)	150	12	3	30	20	0	380
Crisp & Healthy Fish Sticks	6 (4 oz)	180	13	3	25	26	0	440
Fish 'n Fries	1 pkg (6.6 oz)	380	13	18	25	41	2	370
TAKE-OUT								
fish cake	1 (4.7 oz)	166	18	7	–	6	–	–
jamaican brown fish stew	1 serv	426	48	22	84	9	2	419
kedgeree	5.6 oz	242	21	11	–	15	1	–
mousse	1 serv (3.5 oz)	185	13	14	–	3	tr	540
stew	1 cup (7.9 oz)	157	19	4	–	10	–	–
taramasalata	2 tbsp	124	1	14	10	1	–	182
FISH OIL								
cod liver	1 tbsp	123	0	14	78	0	–	–
herring	1 tbsp	123	0	14	104	0	–	–
menhaden	1 tbsp	123	0	14	71	0	–	–
salmon	1 tbsp	123	0	14	66	0	–	–
sardine	1 tbsp	123	0	14	97	0	–	–
shark	1 oz	270	0	29	–	0	–	–
whale	1 oz	270	0	29	–	0	–	–
FISH PASTE								
fish paste	2 tsp	15	1	1	–	tr	0	–
FISH SUBSTITUTES								
Loma Linda								
Ocean Platter not prep	⅓ cup (0.9 oz)	90	14	1	0	8	4	450
Worthington								
Fillets	2 (3 oz)	180	16	10	0	8	4	750
Tuno	½ cup (1.9 oz)	80	6	6	0	2	1	290
FLAXSEED								
Bite Me								
Flax Bar	1 bar (1.8 oz)	242	7	11	0	30	12	79

FOOD	PORTION	CAL	PROT	FAT	CHOL	CARB	FIBER	SOD
FLOUNDER								
FRESH								
cooked	3 oz	99	21	1	58	0	–	89
cooked	1 fillet (4.5 oz)	148	31	2	86	0	–	133
FROZEN								
Van De Kamp's								
Lightly Breaded Fillets	1 (4 oz)	230	15	11	40	19	0	400
Natural Fillets	1 (4 oz)	110	22	2	45	0	0	105
TAKE-OUT								
battered & fried	3.2 oz	211	13	11	31	15	–	484
breaded & fried	3.2 oz	211	13	11	31	15	–	484
FLOUR								
buckwheat whole groat	1 cup (4.2 oz)	402	15	4	0	85	12	13
corn masa	1 cup (4 oz)	416	11	4	0	87	11	6
cottonseed lowfat	1 oz	94	14	tr	0	10	–	10
peanut defatted	1 cup	196	31	tr	0	21	–	108
peanut defatted	1 oz	92	15	tr	0	10	–	50
peanut lowfat	1 cup	257	20	13	0	19	–	0
potato	1 cup (6.3 oz)	628	14	1	0	143	–	61
rice brown	1 cup (5.5 oz)	574	11	4	0	121	7	13
rice white	1 cup (5.5 oz)	578	9	2	0	127	4	1
rye dark	1 cup (4.5 oz)	415	18	3	0	88	29	2
rye light	1 cup (3.6 oz)	374	9	1	0	82	15	2
rye medium	1 cup (3.6 oz)	361	10	2	0	79	15	3
sesame lowfat	1 oz	95	14	tr	0	10	–	11
triticale whole grain	1 cup (4.6 oz)	439	17	2	0	95	19	3
white all-purpose	1 cup (4.4 oz)	455	13	1	0	95	2	3
white bread	1 cup (4.8 oz)	495	16	2	0	99	3	3
white cake unsifted	1 cup (4.8 oz)	496	11	1	0	107	2	3
white self-rising	1 cup (4.4 oz)	443	12	1	0	93	3	1588
white unbleached	1 cup (4.4 oz)	455	13	1	0	95	3	3
whole wheat	1 cup (4.2 oz)	407	16	2	0	87	15	6
All Trump								
Flour	¼ cup (1 oz)	100	4	0	0	22	tr	0
Betty Crocker								
Softasilk Velvet Cake Flour	¼ cup (1 oz)	100	2	0	0	23	tr	0

FOOD	PORTION	CAL	PROT	FAT	CHOL	CARB	FIBER	SOD
Gold Medal								
All Purpose	¼ cup (1 oz)	100	3	0	0	22	tr	0
Better For Bread	¼ cup (1 oz)	100	4	0	0	22	tr	0
Organic All Purpose	¼ cup (1 oz)	100	3	0	0	22	tr	0
Self Rising	¼ cup (1 oz)	100	3	0	0	22	tr	400
Unbleached	¼ cup (1 oz)	100	3	0	0	22	tr	0
Wondra	¼ cup	100	3	0	0	23	tr	0
Hodgson Mill								
White Unbleached Organic	¼ cup (1 oz)	100	3	0	0	23	3	0
Whole Wheat Graham Organic	¼ cup (1 oz)	100	3	1	0	22	3	0
La Pina								
Flour	¼ cup (1 oz)	100	2	0	0	23	1	0
Red Band								
All Purpose	¼ cup (1 oz)	100	2	0	0	23	tr	0
Self-Rising	¼ cup (1 oz)	100	2	0	0	22	tr	400
Robin Hood								
All Purpose	¼ cup (1 oz)	100	3	0	0	22	tr	0
Self-Rising	¼ cup (1 oz)	100	3	0	0	22	tr	0
Unbleached	¼ cup (1 oz)	100	3	0	0	22	tr	0
Whole Wheat	¼ cup (1 oz)	90	4	1	0	21	3	0

FRANKFURTER (see HOT DOG)

FRENCH BEANS

dried cooked	1 cup	228	12	1	0	43	–	11

FRENCH FRIES (see POTATOES)

FRENCH TOAST

FROZEN

french toast	1 slice (2 oz)	126	4	4	48	19	2	292

TAKE-OUT

sticks	5 (4.9 oz)	513	8	29	75	58	3	499
w/ butter	2 slices (4.7 oz)	356	10	19	116	36	–	513

FROG'S LEGS

TAKE-OUT

as prep w/ seasoned flour & fried	1 (0.8)	70	4	5	12	15	–	–

FROSTING (see CAKE ICING)

FOOD	PORTION	CAL	PROT	FAT	CHOL	CARB	FIBER	SOD
FRUCTOSE								
Estee								
Fructose	1 tsp	15	0	0	0	4	0	0
Packet	1 pkg	10	0	0	0	3	0	0
FRUIT DRINKS *(see also individual names, LEMONADE)*								
FROZEN								
citrus juice drink as prep	1 cup	114	1	0	0	28	–	7
citrus juice drink not prep	1 can (12 fl oz)	684	5	tr	0	171	–	12
fruit punch as prep w/water	1 cup	113	tr	tr	0	29	–	11
fruit punch not prep	1 can (12 fl oz)	678	1	tr	0	173	–	34
limeade	1 can (6 oz)	408	tr	tr	0	108	–	–
limeade as prep w/ water	1 cup	102	tr	tr	0	27	–	6
Tree Of Life								
Organic Smoothie Banana Raspberry Strawberry	⅔ cup (5 oz)	90	1	0	0	23	3	0
Organic Smoothie Mango Strawberry Raspberry	⅔ cup (5 oz)	70	1	0	0	18	4	0
Organic Smoothie Strawberry Banana	⅔ cup (5 oz)	90	7	0	0	23	3	0
Organic Smoothie Strawberry Blueberry Banana	⅔ cup (5 oz)	90	1	0	0	22	3	0
MIX								
fruit punch as prep w/water	9 oz	97	tr	0	0	25	–	38
Crystal Light								
Fruit Punch as prep	1 serv (8 oz)	5	0	0	0	0	0	0
Lemon-Lime Drink as prep	1 serv (8 oz)	5	0	0	0	0	0	0
Passion Fruit Pineapple Drink as prep	1 serv (8 oz)	5	0	0	0	tr	0	0

FOOD	PORTION	CAL	PROT	FAT	CHOL	CARB	FIBER	SOD
Pineapple Orange Drink as prep	1 serv (8 oz)	5	0	0	0	0	0	0
Strawberry Orange Banana as prep	1 serv (8 oz)	5	0	0	0	0	0	0
Strawberry Kiwi as prep	1 serv (8 oz)	5	0	0	0	0	0	0
Watermelon Strawberry as prep	1 serv (8 oz)	5	0	0	0	0	0	0
Kool-Aid								
Cherry as prep	1 serv (8 oz)	60	0	0	0	16	0	0
Grape Berry Splash Drink as prep	1 serv (8 oz)	70	0	0	0	17	0	0
Grape Berry Splash Drink as prep w/ sugar	1 serv (8 oz)	100	0	0	0	25	0	0
Kickin' Kiwi Lime Drink as prep	1 serv (8 oz)	60	0	0	0	16	0	0
Kickin' Kiwi Lime Drink as prep w/ sugar	1 serv (8 oz)	100	0	0	0	25	0	10
Lemon-Lime Drink as prep w/ sugar	1 serv (8 oz)	100	0	0	0	25	0	5
Man-O-Mango Berry Drink as prep	1 serv (8 oz)	60	0	0	0	16	0	0
Man-O-Mango Berry Drink as prep w/ sugar	1 serv (8 oz)	100	0	0	0	25	0	0
Oh Yeah Orange Pineapple Drink as prep	1 serv (8 oz)	60	0	0	0	16	0	0
Oh Yeah Orange Pineapple Drink as prep w/ sugar	1 serv (8 oz)	100	0	0	0	25	0	0
Pina-Pineapple Drink as prep	1 serv (8 oz)	60	0	0	0	17	0	0
Pina-Pineapple Drink as prep w/ sugar	1 serv (8 oz)	100	0	0	0	25	0	0

FOOD	PORTION	CAL	PROT	FAT	CHOL	CARB	FIBER	SOD
Roarin' Raspberry Cranberry Drink as prep	1 serv (8 oz)	70	0	0	0	17	0	20
Roarin' Raspberry Cranberry Drink as prep w/ sugar	1 serv (8 oz)	100	0	0	0	25	0	10
Slammin' Strawberry Kiwi Drink as prep	1 serv (8 oz)	70	0	0	0	17	0	15
Slammin' Strawberry Kiwi Drink as prep w/ sugar	1 serv (8 oz)	100	0	0	0	25	0	15
Strawberry Raspberry Drink as prep	1 serv (8 oz)	60	0	0	0	16	0	0
Strawberry Raspberry Drink as prep w/ sugar	1 serv (8 oz)	100	0	0	0	25	0	0
Sugar Free Tropical Punch as prep	1 serv (8 oz)	5	0	0	0	0	0	10
Tropical Punch as prep	1 serv (8 oz)	60	0	0	0	16	0	0
Tropical Punch as prep w/ sugar	1 serv (8 oz)	100	0	0	0	25	0	15
Watermelon Cherry Drink as prep	1 serv (8 oz)	60	0	0	0	16	0	0
Watermelon Cherry Drink as prep w/ sugar	1 serv (8 oz)	100	0	0	0	25	0	10
Tang								
Orange Pineapple as prep	1 serv (8 oz)	100	0	0	0	24	0	45
READY-TO-DRINK								
cranberry apple drink	6 fl oz	123	tr	0	0	32	—	4
cranberry apricot drink	6 fl oz	118	0	0	0	30	—	4
fruit punch	6 fl oz	87	tr	tr	0	22	—	41
orange grapefruit juice	8 fl oz	107	1	tr	0	25	—	8
orange & apricot	8 fl oz	128	1	tr	0	32	—	—

FOOD	PORTION	CAL	PROT	FAT	CHOL	CARB	FIBER	SOD
pineapple & grapefruit	8 fl oz	117	1	tr	0	29	–	14
pineapple & orange drink	8 fl oz	125	3	0	0	29	–	9
After The Fall								
Amaretto Almond	1 can (12 oz)	170	tr	0	0	42	0	25
American Pie Cherry	1 can (12 oz)	190	tr	0	0	35	0	20
Apple Apricot	1 cup (8 oz)	100	1	0	0	26	0	20
Apple Raspberry	1 bottle (10 oz)	110	0	0	0	29	–	25
Apple Strawberry	1 bottle (10 oz)	120	1	0	0	30	–	23
Banana Casablanca	1 bottle (10 oz)	120	1	0	0	24	–	13
Berrymeister	1 can (12 oz)	160	1	0	0	40	0	25
Cranberry Meets Raspberry	1 bottle (10 oz)	120	0	0	0	29	–	25
Georgia Peach Blend	1 bottle (10 oz)	130	1	0	0	33	–	23
Mango Montage	1 bottle (10 oz)	140	1	0	0	33	–	15
Maui Grove	1 bottle (10 oz)	120	1	0	0	29	–	20
Nantucket Ginger Ale	1 can (12 oz)	140	1	0	0	35	0	25
Orange Icicle Cream	1 can (12 oz)	170	tr	0	0	42	0	25
Oregon Berry	1 bottle (10 oz)	130	0	0	0	31	–	30
Passion Of The Islands	1 bottle (10 oz)	125	1	0	0	32	–	15
Peach Vanilla	1 can (12 oz)	170	tr	0	0	42	0	35
Strawberry Vanilla	1 can (12 oz)	160	tr	0	0	42	0	25
Twist O' Strawberry	1 can (12 oz)	190	tr	0	0	37	0	25
Vanilla Bean Cream	1 can (12 oz)	170	tr	0	0	42	0	25
Apple & Eve								
Apple Cranberry	8 oz	120	1	0	0	30	–	20
Capri Sun								
Fruit Punch	1 pkg (7 oz)	100	0	0	0	26	0	20
Maui Punch	1 pkg (7 oz)	100	0	0	0	27	0	20
Mountain Cooler	1 pkg (7 oz)	90	0	0	0	24	0	25
Pacific Cooler	1 pkg (7 oz)	100	0	0	0	26	0	20
Red Berry	1 pkg (7 oz)	100	0	0	0	26	0	20
Safari Punch	1 pkg (7 oz)	100	0	0	0	25	0	20
Strawberry Kiwi Drink	1 pkg (7 oz)	100	0	0	0	26	0	20

FOOD	PORTION	CAL	PROT	FAT	CHOL	CARB	FIBER	SOD
Surfer Cooler Drink	1 pkg (7 oz)	100	0	0	0	27	0	20
Citrus Squeeze								
California Punch	8 oz	130	0	0	0	33	–	85
Florida Punch	8 oz	120	0	0	0	30	–	100
Coco Lopez								
Mango Kiwi	8 fl oz	130	0	0	0	33	–	0
Crystal Light								
Fruit Punch	1 serv (8 oz)	5	0	0	0	0	0	20
Kiwi Strawberry	1 serv (8 oz)	5	0	0	0	0	0	20
Orange Strawberry Banana Drink	1 serv (8 oz)	5	0	0	0	0	0	20
Del Monte								
Peach Raspberry	5.5 fl oz	160	1	0	0	40	3	10
Pineapple Banana Orange	5.5 fl oz	170	1	0	0	44	1	10
Strawberry Peach Banana	5.5 fl oz	150	1	0	0	39	1	10
Dole								
Apple Berry Burst	8 fl oz	120	0	0	0	31	–	20
Cranberry Apple	8 fl oz	120	0	0	0	30	–	35
Fruit Fiesta	8 fl oz	140	0	0	0	34	–	20
Fruit Punch	1 carton (10 oz)	160	0	0	0	39	–	25
Mountain Cherry	8 fl oz	150	0	0	0	30	–	30
Orange Peach Mango	8 oz	120	1	0	0	28	–	35
Orange Strawberry Banana	8 oz	120	1	0	0	28	–	30
Orchard Peach	8 oz	140	1	0	0	34	–	35
Pineapple Orange	8 oz	120	2	0	0	27	–	20
Pineapple Orange Strawberry	8 oz	130	0	0	0	32	–	20
Tropical Fruit	8 oz	160	0	0	0	38	0	30
Eden								
Organic Apple Cherry Juice	8 oz	120	0	0	0	30	1	15
Everfresh								
Cranberry-Apple Drink	1 can (8 oz)	120	0	0	0	31	0	0
Grape-Strawberry	1 can (8 oz)	120	0	0	0	31	0	0

FOOD	PORTION	CAL	PROT	FAT	CHOL	CARB	FIBER	SOD
Kiwi-Strawberry	1 can (8 oz)	120	0	0	0	30	0	0
Mandarin Orange Mango Drink	1 can (8 oz)	120	0	0	0	29	0	0
Orange Banana Strawberry Drink	1 can (8 oz)	120	0	0	0	30	0	19
Tropical Fruit Punch	1 can (8 oz)	120	0	0	0	30	0	0
Wild Blackberry Lime Drink	1 can (8 oz)	120	0	0	0	29	0	0
Fresh Samantha								
Banana Strawberry	1 cup (8 oz)	130	4	0	0	11	6	24
Carrot Orange	1 cup (8 oz)	100	4	0	0	8	4	24
Desperately Seeking C	1 cup (8 oz)	110	4	0	0	9	7	0
Protein Blast	1 cup (8 oz)	160	9	1	—	10	8	24
Super Juice	1 cup (8 oz)	140	4	1	—	11	8	0
The Big Bang	1 cup (8 oz)	100	2	0	0	8	8	0
Fruitopia								
Fruit Integration	8 fl oz	110	0	0	0	29	—	80
Guzzler								
Citrus Punch	8 fl oz	140	tr	0	0	25	—	10
Island Punch	8 fl oz	140	0	0	0	29	0	30
Juicy Juice								
Apple Grape	1 box (8.45 oz)	140	0	0	0	34	0	15
Berry	1 box (8.45 oz)	130	0	0	0	37	0	15
Punch	1 box (4.23 oz)	70	0	0	0	17	0	10
Punch	1 box (8.45 oz)	140	0	0	0	34	0	15
Tropical	1 box (8.45 oz)	140	0	0	0	34	0	15
Kool-Aid								
Bursts Great Bluedini	1 (7 oz)	100	0	0	0	24	0	30
Bursts Kickin' Kiwi Lime	1 (7 oz)	100	0	0	0	24	0	30
Bursts Oh Yeah Orange Pineapple	1 (7 oz)	100	0	0	0	24	0	30
Bursts Slammin' Strawberry Kiwi	1 (7 oz)	100	0	0	0	24	0	30
Bursts Tropical Punch	1 (7 oz)	100	0	0	0	24	0	30
Splash Grape Berry Punch	1 serv (8 oz)	120	0	0	0	31	0	35

FOOD	PORTION	CAL	PROT	FAT	CHOL	CARB	FIBER	SOD
Splash Kiwi Strawberry Drink	1 serv (8 oz)	110	0	0	0	29	0	35
Splash Tropical Punch	1 serv (8 oz)	120	0	0	0	31	0	35
Mauna La'i								
Island Guava	8 oz	130	0	0	0	32	0	35
Paradise Passion	8 oz	130	0	0	0	32	0	35
Mott's								
Berry	1 box (8 oz)	100	0	0	0	26	–	10
Fruit Punch	1 box (8 oz)	110	0	0	0	27	–	15
Fruit Punch	8 fl oz	130	0	0	0	32	–	0
Nantucket Nectars								
Apple Raspberry	8 oz	140	0	0	0	34	–	10
California Melonberry	8 oz	110	0	0	0	28	–	15
Cranberry Apple	8 oz	140	0	0	0	36	–	5
Fruit Punch	8 oz	130	0	0	0	32	–	5
Kiwi Berry	8 oz	120	0	0	0	30	–	5
Orange Passionfruit	8 oz	120	0	0	0	29	–	15
Orange Mango	8 oz	130	0	0	0	32	0	5
Pineapple Orange Banana	8 oz	140	tr	0	0	35	–	15
Pineapple Orange Guava	8 oz	120	0	0	0	31	–	0
Watermelon Strawberry	8 oz	120	0	0	0	30	–	5
Oberweis								
Fruit Punch	8 oz	120	0	0	0	30	0	5
Ocean Spray								
Cran*Blueberry	8 oz	160	0	0	0	41	0	35
Cran*Cherry	8 oz	160	0	0	0	39	0	35
Cran*Currant	8 oz	140	0	0	0	33	0	35
Cran*Grape	8 oz	170	0	0	0	41	0	35
Cran*Mango	8 oz	130	0	0	0	33	0	35
Cran*Raspberry	8 oz	140	0	0	0	36	0	35
Cran*Raspberry Reduced Calorie	8 oz	50	0	0	0	13	0	35

FOOD	PORTION	CAL	PROT	FAT	CHOL	CARB	FIBER	SOD
Cran*Strawberry	8 oz	140	0	0	0	36	1	35
Cran*Tangerine	8 oz	130	0	0	0	33	0	35
Cranapple	8 oz	160	0	0	0	41	1	35
Cranapple Reduced Calorie	8 oz	50	0	0	0	13	0	35
Cranicot	8 oz	160	0	0	0	40	0	35
Crazy Kiwi Passion	8 oz	130	0	0	0	32	0	35
Fruit Punch	8 oz	130	0	0	0	32	0	35
Kiwi Strawberry	8 oz	120	0	0	0	31	0	35
Lightstyle Cran*Grape	8 oz	40	0	0	0	9	0	75
Lightstyle Cran*Mango	8 oz	40	0	0	0	10	0	75
Lightstyle Cran*Raspberry	8 oz	40	0	0	0	10	0	35
Mandarin Magic	8 oz	120	0	0	0	31	0	35
Ruby Red & Tangerine Grapefruit	8 oz	130	0	0	0	32	0	35
Ruby Red & Mango	8 oz	130	0	0	0	33	0	35
Shasta Plus								
Apple-Strawberry	1 can (11.5 oz)	160	0	0	0	41	0	45
Fruit Punch	1 can (11.5 oz)	160	0	0	0	39	0	45
Pineapple-Cherry	1 can (11.5 oz)	160	0	0	0	40	0	45
Sipps								
Fruit Punch	8.45 oz	130	–	0	0	–	–	–
Snapple								
Cranberry Raspberry	8 fl oz	120	0	0	0	29	–	10
Diet Cranberry Raspberry	8 fl oz	10	0	0	0	2	–	10
Fruit Punch	8 fl oz	110	0	0	0	29	–	10
Kiwi Strawberry	8 fl oz	110	0	0	0	28	–	10
Squeezit								
Berry B. Wild	1 bottle (7 oz)	110	0	0	0	28	0	0
Blue Raspberry	1 bottle (7 oz)	110	0	0	0	28	0	0
Cherry Cola	1 bottle (7 oz)	110	0	0	0	27	0	0
Chucklin' Cherry	1 bottle (7 oz)	110	0	0	0	28	0	0
Green Apple	1 bottle (7 oz)	110	0	0	0	27	0	0
Grumpy Grape	1 bottle (7 oz)	110	0	0	0	28	0	0
Lemon Lime	1 bottle (7 oz)	110	0	0	0	28	0	0

FOOD	PORTION	CAL	PROT	FAT	CHOL	CARB	FIBER	SOD
Rockin' Red Puncher	1 bottle (7 oz)	110	0	0	0	24	0	0
Smarty Arty Orange	1 bottle (7 oz)	110	0	0	0	27	0	45
Strawberry	1 bottle (7 oz)	110	0	0	0	29	0	0
Tropical Punch	1 bottle (7 oz)	110	0	0	0	28	0	0
Watermelon	1 bottle (7 oz)	110	0	0	0	28	0	0
Sunny Delight								
Drink	6 fl oz	90	–	0	0	–	–	–
Tropicana								
Berry Punch	8 fl oz	130	0	0	0	32	–	15
Citrus Punch	8 fl oz	140	0	0	0	36	–	15
Fruit Punch	8 oz	130	0	0	0	32	–	15
Tangerine Orange Juice	8 fl oz	110	2	0	0	25	–	0
Tropics Orange Strawberry Banana	8 fl oz	110	tr	0	0	27	–	5
Tropics Orange Kiwi Passion	8 fl oz	100	tr	0	0	26	–	15
Tropics Orange Peach Mango	8 fl oz	110	tr	0	0	28	–	15
Tropics Orange Pineapple	8 fl oz	110	tr	0	0	27	–	15
Twister Apple Raspberry Blackberry	1 bottle (10 fl oz)	160	0	1	0	38	–	20
Twister Citrus Punch	1 bottle (10 oz)	180	0	0	0	45	–	15
Twister Cranberry Punch	1 bottle (10 oz)	170	0	0	0	43	–	20
Twister Fruit Punch	1 bottle (10 oz)	170	0	0	0	43	–	40
Twister Light Orange Strawberry Banana	1 bottle (10 oz)	45	tr	0	0	11	–	25
Twister Orange Cranberry	1 bottle (10 fl oz)	160	tr	0	0	40	–	60
Twister Orange Strawberry Banana	1 bottle (10 oz)	160	tr	0	0	40	–	60
Twister Ruby Red Tangerine	1 bottle (10 oz)	160	0	0	0	40	–	25

FOOD	PORTION	CAL	PROT	FAT	CHOL	CARB	FIBER	SOD
Twister Strawberry Kiwi	1 bottle (10 oz)	160	0	0	0	42	–	25
V8								
Splash Berry Blend	8 oz	110	0	0	0	28	–	40
Veryfine								
Apple Cranberry	1 bottle (10 oz)	190	0	0	0	48	0	10
Apple Quenchers Black Cherry White Grape	8 fl oz	120	0	0	0	30	0	10
Apple Quenchers Cranberry Tangerine	8 fl oz	120	0	0	0	31	0	10
Apple Quenchers Peach Kiwi	8 fl oz	130	0	0	0	33	0	25
Apple Quenchers Peach Plum	8 fl oz	130	0	0	0	32	0	25
Apple Quenchers Pear Passionfruit	8 fl oz	120	0	0	0	31	0	15
Apple Quenchers Raspberry Cherry	8 fl oz	120	0	0	0	31	0	25
Apple Quenchers Raspberry Lime	8 fl oz	120	0	0	0	30	0	25
Apple Quenchers Strawberry Banana	8 fl oz	120	0	0	0	30	0	20
Chillers Artic Mango Tangerine	8 fl oz	110	0	0	0	27	tr	5
Chillers Freezing Fruit Punch	8 fl oz	130	0	0	0	33	0	20
Chillers Lemon Lime Blizzard	8 fl oz	120	0	0	0	29	0	5
Chillers Shivering Strawberry Melon	1 can (11.5 oz)	160	0	0	0	41	0	10
Chillers Tropical Freeze	8 fl oz	120	0	0	0	30	0	10
Cranberry Raspberry	8 fl oz	160	0	0	0	41	0	10
Fruit Punch	1 bottle (10 oz)	170	0	0	0	42	0	25
Juice-Ups Berry	8 fl oz	140	0	0	0	34	0	15
Juice-Ups Fruit Punch	8 fl oz	140	0	0	0	34	0	15

FOOD	PORTION	CAL	PROT	FAT	CHOL	CARB	FIBER	SOD
Juice-Ups Orange Punch	8 fl oz	140	0	0	0	35	0	15
Orange Strawberry	8 fl oz	120	0	0	0	31	0	30
Papaya Punch	1 bottle (10 oz)	160	0	0	0	39	0	25
Pineapple Orange	1 bottle (10 oz)	160	0	0	0	39	0	20
Strawberry Banana	1 can (11.5 oz)	160	0	0	0	40	0	15
Strawberry Banana Punch	1 can (11.5 oz)	190	0	0	0	48	0	30
Wellfleet Farms								
Cranberry & Georgia Peach	8 oz	140	0	0	0	35	0	35
Cranberry & Granny Smith Apple	8 oz	130	0	0	0	33	0	35
Cranberry & Key Lime	8 oz	140	0	0	0	35	0	35

FRUIT MIXED (see also individual names)

CANNED

FOOD	PORTION	CAL	PROT	FAT	CHOL	CARB	FIBER	SOD
fruit cocktail in heavy syrup	½ cup	93	1	tr	0	24	–	7
fruit cocktail juice pack	½ cup	56	1	tr	0	15	–	4
fruit cocktail water pack	½ cup	40	1	tr	0	10	–	5
fruit salad in heavy syrup	½ cup	94	tr	tr	0	24	–	7
fruit salad in light syrup	½ cup	73	tr	tr	0	19	–	7
fruit salad juice pack	½ cup	62	1	tr	0	16	–	7
fruit salad water pack	½ cup	37	tr	tr	0	10	–	4
mixed fruit in heavy syrup	½ cup	92	tr	tr	0	24	–	5
tropical fruit salad in heavy syrup	½ cup	110	1	tr	0	29	–	3
Del Monte								
Cherry Mixed Light Syrup	½ cup (4.4 oz)	90	1	0	0	22	1	10
Chunk Mixed In Heavy Syrup	½ cup (4.5 oz)	100	0	0	0	24	1	10

FOOD	PORTION	CAL	PROT	FAT	CHOL	CARB	FIBER	SOD
Chunky Mixed Fruit Naturals	½ cup (4.4 oz)	60	0	0	0	15	1	10
Chunky Mixed In Extra Light Syrup	½ cup (4.4 oz)	60	0	0	0	15	1	10
Citrus Salad	½ cup (4.4 oz)	80	0	0	0	20	0	20
Fruit Cocktail Fruit Naturals	½ cup (4.4 oz)	60	0	0	0	15	1	10
Fruit Cocktail In Extra Light Syrup	½ cup (4.4 oz)	60	0	0	0	15	1	10
Fruit Cocktail In Heavy Syrup	½ cup (4.5 oz)	100	0	0	0	24	1	10
Fruit Cup Fruit Naturals Mixed	1 pkg (4 oz)	50	0	0	0	13	1	10
Fruit Cup Mixed In Extra Light Syrup	1 pkg (4 oz)	50	0	0	0	13	1	10
Fruit Salad In Extra Light Syrup	½ cup (4.5 oz)	70	1	0	0	22	2	5
Fruit To Go Fruity Combo	1 pkg (4 oz)	70	1	0	0	18	1	10
Fruit To Go Wild Berry Jumble	1 pkg (4 oz)	80	1	0	0	20	1	10
Fruitrageous Crazy Cherry Mixed	1 pkg (4 oz)	90	1	0	0	22	1	10
Orchard Select California Mixed	½ cup (4.5 oz)	80	1	0	0	19	1	10
Orchard Select Premium Mixed	½ cup (4.4 oz)	80	tr	0	0	20	tr	10
Snack Cups Mixed Fruit In Heavy Syrup	1 serv (4 oz)	80	0	0	0	20	1	10
SunFresh Ambrosia Salad	½ cup	70	0	0	0	16	1	25
Tropical Fruit Salad	½ cup (4.3 oz)	60	0	0	0	16	1	15
Tropical Fruit Salad In Light Syrup	½ cup (4.4 oz)	80	0	0	0	21	1	10
Very Cherry Mixed Fruit	½ cup (4.4 oz)	90	1	0	0	22	1	10

FOOD	PORTION	CAL	PROT	FAT	CHOL	CARB	FIBER	SOD
Dole								
FruitBowls Tropical Fruit	1 pkg (4 oz)	60	tr	0	0	16	2	10
Tropical Fruit Salad	½ cup (4.3 oz)	80	tr	0	0	20	1	10
Mott's								
Fruitsations Banana	1 pkg (4 oz)	90	0	0	0	23	—	0
Fruitsations Cherry	1 pkg (4 oz)	70	0	0	0	19	—	0
Fruitsations Mango Peach	1 pkg (4 oz)	70	0	0	0	22	—	0
Fruitsations Mixed Berry	1 pkg (4 oz)	90	0	0	0	22	1	0
Fruitsations Pear	1 pkg (4 oz)	90	0	0	0	23	—	0
Fruitsations Strawberry	1 pkg (4 oz)	80	0	0	0	19	—	10
Fruitsations Tropical Fruit	1 pkg (4 oz)	70	0	0	0	19	—	0
Hearlthy Harvest Peach Medley	1 pkg (3.9 oz)	50	0	0	0	13	1	0
Ocean Spray								
Cran*Fruit Cranberry Raspberry	¼ cup	120	0	0	0	29	2	35
Cran*Fruit Cranberry Strawberry	¼ cup	120	0	0	0	29	2	35
Sunfresh								
Ambrosia Salad	½ cup (4.5 oz)	70	0	0	0	16	1	25
Mixed Fruit In Light Syrup	½ cup (4.6 oz)	90	1	0	0	20	2	25
Tropical Salad In Extra Light Syrup	½ cup (4.5 oz)	80	1	0	0	20	0	10
White House								
Apple Banana Sauce	1 pkg (4 oz)	100	0	0	0	23	1	25
Apple Mixed Berry Sauce	1 pkg (4 oz)	110	0	0	0	23	1	25
Apple Peach Sauce	1 pkg (4 oz)	100	0	0	0	23	1	20
DRIED								
mixed	11 oz pkg	712	7	1	0	188	—	52
Paradise								
Old English Fruit & Peel Mix	1 tbsp (0.8 oz)	70	6	0	0	18	1	15

FOOD	PORTION	CAL	PROT	FAT	CHOL	CARB	FIBER	SOD
Planters								
Fruit'n Nut Mix	1 oz	140	4	9	0	13	2	105
Sonoma								
Diced	⅓ cup (1.4 oz)	120	1	0	0	31	3	0
Mixed Fruit	5-8 pieces (1.4 oz)	120	1	0	0	30	3	0
Sun-Maid								
Tropical Medley	¼ cup (1.4 oz)	130	1	0	0	32	1	10
FROZEN								
mixed fruit sweetened	1 cup	245	4	tr	0	61	–	8
Birds Eye								
Mixed Fruit	½ cup (4.4 oz)	90	1	0	0	23	–	5
Tree Of Life								
Organic Mixed Berries	¾ cup (5 oz)	60	0	0	0	16	3	0

FRUIT SNACKS

FOOD	PORTION	CAL	PROT	FAT	CHOL	CARB	FIBER	SOD
fruit leather	1 bar (0.8 oz)	81	tr	1	0	18	–	18
fruit leather pieces	1 pkg (0.9 oz)	92	tr	2	0	21	–	109
fruit leather pieces	1 oz	97	tr	2	0	22	–	114
fruit leather rolls	1 sm (0.5 oz)	49	tr	tr	0	12	–	8
fruit leather rolls	1 lg (0.7 oz)	73	tr	1	0	18	–	13
Betty Crocker								
Fruit Gushers All Flavors	1 pkg (0.9 oz)	90	0	1	0	20	0	40
Fruit String Thing All Flavors	1 pkg (0.7 oz)	80	0	1	0	17	0	45
Favorite Brands								
Cherry Fruit Snack	1 pkg (0.9 oz)	80	1	0	0	19	–	15
Creepy Crawler Fruit Snacks	1 pkg (0.9 oz)	80	1	0	0	19	–	15
Dinosaur Fruit Snack	1 pkg (0.9 oz)	80	1	0	0	19	–	15
Grape Fruit Snack	1 pkg (0.9 oz)	80	1	0	0	19	–	15
Space Alien Fruit Snack	1 pkg (0.9 oz)	80	1	0	0	19	–	15
Sports Fruit Snacks	1 pkg (0.9 oz)	80	1	0	0	19	–	15
Strawberry Fruit Snack	1 pkg (0.9 oz)	80	1	0	0	19	–	15
Teenage Mutant Ninja Turtle Fruit Snacks	1 pkg (0.9 oz)	80	1	0	0	19	–	15

FOOD	PORTION	CAL	PROT	FAT	CHOL	CARB	FIBER	SOD
The Mega Roll Strawberry	1 pkg (1 oz)	110	0	3	–	22	2	15
The Roll Cherry	1 pkg (0.75 oz)	80	0	2	–	16	1	10
The Roll Strawberry	1 pkg (0.75 oz)	80	0	2	–	16	1	10
Troll Fruit Snacks	1 pkg (0.9 oz)	80	1	0	0	19	0	15
Zoo Animal Fruit Snacks	1 pkg (0.9 oz)	80	1	0	0	19	–	15
General Mills								
Fruit Snacks All Flavors	1 pkg (0.9 oz)	80	0	0	0	21	0	50
Health Valley								
Bakes Apple	1 bar	70	2	0	0	19	2	30
Bakes Date	1 bar	70	2	0	0	19	2	30
Bakes Raisin	1 bar	70	2	0	0	19	2	30
Fruit Bars Apple	1	140	3	0	0	35	3	0
Fruit Bars Apricot	1	140	3	0	0	35	4	5
Fruit Bars Date	1	140	3	0	0	34	3	5
Fruit Bars Raisin	1	140	2	0	0	35	3	5
Seneca								
Apple Chips	12 chips (1 oz)	140	0	7	0	20	2	15
Sensible Foods								
Crackin' Fruit Cherry Berry	1 pkg (0.6 oz)	51	1	0	0	13	1	85
Crackin' Fruit Tropical Fruit	1 pkg (0.6 oz)	65	tr	1	0	16	1	61
Sonoma								
Trail Mix	¼ cup (1.4 oz)	160	3	7	0	24	2	5
Sunbelt								
Fruit Jammers	1 pkg (1 oz)	100	0	1	0	23	0	15
Sunkist								
100% Fruit Roll All Flavors	1 (0.5 oz)	50	0	0	0	12	1	10
Weight Watchers								
Apple & Cinnamon	1 pkg (0.5 oz)	50	0	0	0	13	2	125
Apple Chips	1 pkg (0.75 oz)	70	0	0	0	18	3	125
Peach & Strawberry	1 pkg (0.5 oz)	50	0	0	0	13	2	125

FOOD	PORTION	CAL	PROT	FAT	CHOL	CARB	FIBER	SOD
GARLIC								
clove	1	4	tr	tr	0	1	–	1
powder	1 tsp	9	tr	tr	0	2	–	1
Dorot								
Frozen Crushed Cubes	1 cube (4 g)	5	0	0	0	1	0	40
GEFILTE FISH								
sweet	1 piece (1.5 oz)	35	4	1	12	3	–	220
GELATIN								
MIX								
low calorie	½ cup	8	2	0	0	0	0	9
mix artifically sweetened as prep	½ cup (4.1 oz)	8	1	0	0	1	–	56
mix artifically sweetened as prep	1 pkg 4 serv (16.5 oz)	33	5	0	0	3	–	224
mix as prep	½ cup (4.7 oz)	80	2	0	0	19	–	57
mix as prep	1 pkg 4 serv (19 oz)	319	7	0	0	76	–	227
mix not prep	1 pkg (3 oz)	324	7	0	0	77	–	216
mix w/ fruit as prep	½ cup (3.7 oz)	73	1	tr	0	18	–	30
mix w/ fruit as prep	1 pkg 8 serv (19 oz)	588	10	2	0	144	–	242
powder unsweetened	1 pkg (7 g)	23	6	0	–	0	–	14
powder unsweetened	1 oz	94	24	0	–	0	–	55
Jell-O								
1-2-3-Brand Strawberry as prep	⅔ cup (5.2 oz)	130	2	2	0	26	0	50
Apricot as prep	½ cup (5 oz)	80	2	0	0	19	0	80
Berry Black as prep	½ cup (5 oz)	80	2	0	0	19	0	80
Berry Blue as prep	½ cup (5 oz)	80	2	0	0	19	0	80
Black Cherry as prep	½ cup (5 oz)	80	2	0	0	19	0	80
Cherry as prep	½ cup (5 oz)	80	2	0	0	19	0	100
Cranberry Raspberry as prep	½ cup (5 oz)	80	2	0	0	19	0	75

FOOD	PORTION	CAL	PROT	FAT	CHOL	CARB	FIBER	SOD
Cranberry Strawberry as prep	½ cup (5 oz)	80	2	0	0	19	0	75
Cranberry as prep	½ cup (5 oz)	80	0	0	0	19	0	75
Grape as prep	½ cup (5 oz)	80	2	0	0	19	0	80
Lemon as prep	½ cup (5 oz)	80	2	0	0	19	0	120
Lime as prep	½ cup (5 oz)	80	2	0	0	19	0	90
Mango as prep	½ cup (5 oz)	80	2	0	0	19	0	80
Mixed Fruit as prep	½ cup (5 oz)	80	2	0	0	19	tr	80
Orange as prep	½ cup (5 oz)	80	2	0	0	19	0	80
Peach as prep	½ cup (5 oz)	80	2	0	0	19	0	80
Peach Passion Fruit as prep	½ cup (5 oz)	80	2	0	0	19	0	80
Pineapple as prep	½ cup (5 oz)	80	2	0	0	19	0	80
Raspberry as prep	½ cup (5 oz)	80	2	0	0	19	0	80
Sparkling White Grape as prep	½ cup (5 oz)	80	2	0	0	19	0	80
Strawberry Banana as prep	½ cup (5 oz)	80	2	0	0	19	0	80
Strawberry Kiwi as prep	½ cup (5 oz)	80	2	0	0	19	0	80
Strawberry as prep	½ cup (5 oz)	80	2	0	0	19	0	90
Sugar Free Cherry as prep	½ cup (4.2 oz)	10	1	0	0	0	0	70
Sugar Free Cranberry as prep	½ cup (4.2 oz)	10	1	0	0	0	0	80
Sugar Free Lemon	½ cup (4.2 oz)	10	1	0	0	0	0	55
Sugar Free Lime as prep	½ cup (4.2 oz)	10	1	0	0	0	0	60
Sugar Free Mixed Fruit as prep	½ cup (4.2 oz)	10	1	0	0	0	0	50
Sugar Free Orange as prep	½ cup (4.2 oz)	10	1	0	0	0	0	65
Sugar Free Raspberry as prep	½ cup (4.2 oz)	10	1	0	0	0	0	55
Sugar Free Strawberry Banana as prep	½ cup (4.2 oz)	10	1	0	0	0	0	50
Sugar Free Strawberry as prep	½ cup (4.2 oz)	10	1	0	0	0	0	55
Sugar Free Strawberry Kiwi as prep	½ cup (4.2 oz)	10	1	0	0	0	0	60

FOOD	PORTION	CAL	PROT	FAT	CHOL	CARB	FIBER	SOD
Sugar Free Watermelon as prep	½ cup (4.2 oz)	10	1	0	0	0	0	55
Watermelon as prep	½ cup (5 oz)	80	2	0	0	19	0	80
Wild Strawberry as prep	½ cup (5 oz)	80	2	0	0	19	0	120
READY-TO-EAT								
Handi-Snacks								
Gels Blue Raspberry	1 serv (4 oz)	80	0	0	0	20	0	45
Gels Cherry	1 serv (4 oz)	80	0	0	0	20	0	45
Gels Orange	1 serv (3.5 oz)	80	0	0	0	20	0	45
Gels Strawberry	1 serv (3.5 oz)	80	0	0	0	20	0	40
Hunt's								
Snack Pack Juicy Gels Mixed Fruit	1 (4 oz)	100	0	0	0	25	0	42
Snack Pack Gels Cherry	1 serv (3.5 oz)	100	0	0	0	25	0	42
Snack Pack Gels Raspberry Berry	1 serv (3.5 oz)	100	0	0	0	25	0	42
Snack Pack Gels Strawberry	1 serv (3.5 oz)	100	0	0	0	25	0	42
Snack Pack Gels Strawberry Orange	1 serv (3.5 oz)	100	0	0	0	25	0	42
Jell-O								
Berry Black	1 serv (3.5 oz)	70	1	0	0	17	0	40
Berry Blue	1 serv (3.5 oz)	70	1	0	0	17	0	40
Cherry	1 serv (3.5 oz)	70	1	0	0	17	0	40
Orange	1 serv (3.5 oz)	70	1	0	0	17	0	40
Orange Strawberry Banana	1 serv (3.5 oz)	70	1	0	0	17	0	40
Raspberry	1 serv (3.5 oz)	70	1	0	0	17	0	40
Rhymin' Lymon	1 serv (3.5 oz)	70	1	0	0	17	0	40
Strawberry	1 serv (3.5 oz)	70	1	0	0	17	0	40
Strawberry Kiwi	1 serv (3.5 oz)	10	1	0	0	0	0	45
Sugar Free Orange	1 serv (3.2 oz)	10	1	0	0	0	0	45
Sugar Free Raspberry	1 serv (3.2 oz)	10	1	0	0	0	0	45

FOOD	PORTION	CAL	PROT	FAT	CHOL	CARB	FIBER	SOD
Sugar Free Strawberry	1 serv (3.2 oz)	10	1	0	0	0	0	45
Tropical Berry	1 serv (3.5 oz)	10	1	0	0	0	0	45
Tropical Fruit Punch	1 serv (3.5 oz)	70	1	0	0	17	0	40
Wild Watermelon	1 serv (3.5 oz)	70	1	0	0	17	0	40
Kozy Shack								
Gel Treat Cherry	1 pkg (4 oz)	100	0	0	0	25	1	25
Gel Treat Lemon Lime	1 pkg (4 oz)	100	0	0	0	25	1	25
Gel Treat Orange	1 pkg (4 oz)	100	0	0	0	25	1	25
Gel Treat Strawberry	1 pkg (4 oz)	100	0	0	0	25	1	25
Gel Treat Sugar Free Orange	1 pkg (4 oz)	10	0	0	0	2	1	25
Gel Treat Sugar Free Strawberry	1 pkg (4 oz)	10	0	0	0	2	1	25
Swiss Miss								
Gels Berry Strawberry	1 pkg (3.5 oz)	79	1	0	0	18	0	38
Gels Berry Lemon	1 pkg (3.5 oz)	79	1	0	0	18	0	38
Gels Raspberry Orange	1 pkg (3.5 oz)	79	1	0	0	18	0	38
Gels Strawberry Raspberry	1 pkg (3.5 oz)	79	1	0	0	18	0	38
GIBLETS								
capon simmered	1 cup (5 oz)	238	38	8	629	0	–	80
chicken floured & fried	1 cup (5 oz)	402	47	19	647	6	–	164
chicken simmered	1 cup (5 oz)	228	37	7	570	1	–	85
turkey simmered	1 cup (5 oz)	243	39	7	606	3	–	85
GINGER								
ground	1 tsp (1.8 g)	6	tr	tr	0	1	–	1
pickled	0.5 oz	5	tr	0	0	1	tr	52
root fresh	¼ cup	17	tr	tr	0	4	–	3
root fresh	5 slices	8	tr	tr	0	2	–	1
root fresh sliced	¼ cup	17	tr	tr	0	4	–	3
Eden								
Pickled w/ Shiso Leaves	1 tbsp	15	0	0	0	3	1	340

FOOD	PORTION	CAL	PROT	FAT	CHOL	CARB	FIBER	SOD
GINKGO NUTS								
canned	1 oz	32	1	tr	0	6	–	87
dried	1 oz	99	3	tr	0	21	–	4
raw	1 oz	52	1	tr	0	11	–	1
GINSENG								
dried	1 oz	90	5	tr	–	20	2	16
fresh	1 oz	28	1	tr	–	6	tr	5
GIZZARDS								
chicken simmered	1 cup (5 oz)	222	5	5	281	2	–	97
turkey simmered	1 cup (5 oz)	236	43	6	336	1	–	79
Shady Brook								
Turkey	4 oz	130	22	4	180	–	–	90
GOAT								
roasted	3 oz	122	23	3	64	0	–	73
GOOSE								
w/ skin roasted	½ goose (1.7 lbs)	2362	195	170	708	0	–	543
w/ skin roasted	6.6 oz	574	47	41	172	0	–	132
w/o skin roasted	5 oz	340	41	18	138	0	–	108
w/o skin roasted	½ goose (1.3 lbs)	1406	171	75	569	0	–	447
GOOSEBERRIES								
canned in light syrup	½ cup	93	1	tr	0	24	–	3
fresh	1 cup	67	1	1	0	15	–	1
GRANOLA (see CEREAL, CEREAL BARS)								
GRAPE JUICE								
bottled	1 cup	155	1	tr	0	38	–	7
frzn sweetened as prep	1 cup	128	tr	tr	0	32	–	5
frzn sweetened not prep	6 oz	386	1	1	0	96	–	15
grape drink	6 oz	84	0	0	0	22	–	12
Capri Sun								
Drink	1 pkg (7 oz)	100	0	0	0	25	0	20
Daily								
Drink	8 oz	110	0	0	0	27	–	30

FOOD	PORTION	CAL	PROT	FAT	CHOL	CARB	FIBER	SOD
Everfresh								
Juice	1 can (8 oz)	150	0	0	0	38	0	10
Juicy Juice								
Drink	1 box (8.45 oz)	140	0	0	0	34	0	15
Drink	1 box (4.23 oz)	70	0	0	0	17	—	10
Kool-Aid								
Bursts Grape Drink	1 (7 oz)	100	0	0	0	25	0	30
Drink as prep w/ sugar	1 serv (8 oz)	100	0	0	0	25	0	10
Drink Mix as prep	1 serv (8 oz)	60	0	0	0	16	0	0
Sugar Free Drink Mix as prep	1 serv (8 oz)	5	0	0	0	0	0	0
Mott's								
100% Juice	1 box (8 oz)	130	0	0	0	33	—	15
Grape Juice	8 fl oz	130	0	0	0	31	—	10
Nantucket Nectars								
100% Juice	8 oz	160	0	0	0	39	—	20
Grapeade	8 oz	130	0	0	0	33	—	5
Shasta Plus								
Grape Drink	1 can (11.5 oz)	160	0	0	0	39	0	45
Veryfine								
100% Juice	1 bottle (10 oz)	200	0	0	0	47	0	35
Chillers Glacial Grape	1 can (11.5 oz)	160	0	0	0	41	0	10
Grape Drink	1 bottle (10 oz)	160	0	0	0	41	0	10
Juice-Ups	8 fl oz	130	0	0	0	32	0	10
Welch's								
100% White	8 oz	160	0	0	0	39	—	20
GRAPE LEAVES								
canned	1 (4 g)	3	tr	tr	0	tr	0	114
fresh raw	1 (3 g)	3	tr	tr	0	1	tr	tr
TAKE-OUT								
dolmas	5 (4.2 oz)	200	2	11	0	23	2	570
GRAPEFRUIT								
CANNED								
juice pack	½ cup	46	1	tr	0	11	—	9
unsweetened	1 cup	93	1	tr	0	22	—	3
water pack	½ cup	44	1	tr	0	11	—	2

FOOD	PORTION	CAL	PROT	FAT	CHOL	CARB	FIBER	SOD
Sunfresh								
Red & White	½ cup (4.4 oz)	45	1	0	0	9	2	15
FRESH								
pink	½	37	1	tr	0	9	1	0
pink sections	1 cup	69	1	tr	0	18	1	1
red	½	37	1	tr	0	9	–	0
red sections	1 cup	69	1	tr	0	18	–	1
white	½	39	1	tr	0	10	1	0
white sections	1 cup	76	2	tr	0	19	1	0
Ocean Spray								
Fresh	2 oz	50	1	0	0	14	0	0
GRAPEFRUIT JUICE								
fresh	1 cup	96	1	tr	0	23	–	2
frzn as prep	1 cup	102	1	tr	0	24	–	2
frzn not prep	6 oz	302	4	1	0	72	–	6
sweetened	1 cup	116	1	tr	0	28	–	4
After The Fall								
Pink	1 bottle (10 oz)	100	1	0	0	23	–	10
Apple & Eve								
Made In The Shade Ruby Red	8 fl oz	130	0	0	0	32	–	35
Everfresh								
Juice	1 can (8 oz)	90	0	0	0	22	0	0
Ruby Red Cocktail	1 can (8 oz)	130	0	0	0	32	0	0
Fresh Samantha								
Juice	1 cup (8 oz)	90	1	0	0	7	0	0
Mott's								
100% Juice	8 fl oz	110	2	0	0	27	–	10
Nantucket Nectars								
100% Juice	8 oz	100	1	0	0	23	–	0
100% Ruby Red	8 oz	100	0	0	0	25	–	5
Ocean Spray								
100% Juice	8 oz	100	1	0	0	24	0	35
100% Juice Pink	8 oz	110	0	0	0	28	0	35
Ruby Red Drink	8 oz	130	0	0	0	33	0	35
Tropicana								
Golden	8 oz	90	1	0	0	22	–	0
Ruby Red	8 oz	90	1	0	0	22	–	0
Season's Best	8 oz	90	tr	0	0	22	–	15

FOOD	PORTION	CAL	PROT	FAT	CHOL	CARB	FIBER	SOD
Twister Pink	1 bottle (10 oz)	140	0	0	0	34	—	20
W/ Double Vitamin C	8 fl oz	110	1	0	0	27	—	15
Veryfine								
100% Juice	1 bottle (10 oz)	110	0	0	0	25	0	20
Pink	1 bottle (10 oz)	150	0	0	0	38	0	35
Ruby Red	8 fl oz	120	0	0	0	29	0	25

GRAPES

FOOD	PORTION	CAL	PROT	FAT	CHOL	CARB	FIBER	SOD
fresh	10	36	tr	tr	0	9	tr	1
thompson seedless in heavy syrup	½ cup	94	1	tr	0	25	—	7
thompson seedless water pack	½ cup	48	1	tr	0	13	—	7
Chiquita								
Grapes	1½ cups (4.8 oz)	90	1	1	0	24	1	0

GRAVY

CANNED

FOOD	PORTION	CAL	PROT	FAT	CHOL	CARB	FIBER	SOD
au jus	1 cup	38	3	tr	1	6	—	—
beef	1 cup	124	9	6	7	11	—	1305
beef	1 can (10 oz)	155	11	7	9	14	—	1630
chicken	1 cup	189	5	14	5	13	—	1375
mushroom	1 cup	120	3	6	0	13	—	1259
turkey	1 cup	122	6	5	5	12	—	—
Campbell								
Beef	¼ cup	29	1	1	1	4	tr	421
Brown	¼ cup	46	1	3	tr	4	1	350
Chicken	¼ cup	42	1	2	3	4	1	244
Turkey	¼ cup	29	1	1	2	3	tr	289
MIX								
au jus as prep w/ water	1 cup	32	1	1	1	4	—	964
brown as prep w/ water	1 cup	75	2	2	2	13	—	1076
chicken as prep	1 cup	83	3	2	3	14	—	1133
mushroom as prep	1 cup	70	2	1	1	14	—	1402
onion as prep w/ water	1 cup	77	2	1	tr	16	—	1013
pork as prep	1 cup	76	2	2	3	13	—	1235
turkey as prep	1 cup	87	3	2	3	15	—	1498

FOOD	PORTION	CAL	PROT	FAT	CHOL	CARB	FIBER	SOD
Bournvita								
Extract	2 heaping tsp	34	1	1	–	7	–	–
Bovril								
Extract	1 heaping tsp	9	2	0	–	tr	0	–
Durkee								
Au Jus as prep	¼ cup	5	0	0	0	1	0	320
Brown as prep	¼ cup	10	0	1	0	3	0	250
Brown Mushroom as prep	¼ cup	15	1	0	0	3	0	300
Brown Onion as prep	¼ cup	15	1	0	0	4	0	290
Chicken as prep	¼ cup	20	1	1	0	4	0	350
Country as prep	¼ cup	35	1	2	0	5	0	370
Homestyle as prep	¼ cup	15	1	1	0	3	0	240
Mushroom as prep	¼ cup	15	1	0	0	3	0	230
Onion as prep	¼ cup	10	1	0	0	3	0	310
Pork as prep	¼ cup	10	1	0	0	3	0	240
Sausage as prep	¼ cup	35	1	2	0	5	0	570
Swiss Steak as prep	¼ cup	15	0	0	0	4	0	370
Turkey as prep	¼ cup	20	1	0	0	4	0	270
French's								
Au Jus as prep	¼ cup	5	0	0	0	1	0	220
Brown as prep	¼ cup	10	0	1	0	3	0	250
Chicken as prep	¼ cup	25	1	1	0	4	0	250
Country as prep	¼ cup	35	1	2	0	5	0	370
Herb Brown as prep	¼ cup	15	1	1	0	3	0	350
Homestyle as prep	¼ cup	10	0	1	0	3	0	230
Mushroom as prep	¼ cup	10	0	1	0	3	0	250
Onion as prep	¼ cup	15	0	1	0	4	0	260
Pork as prep	¼ cup	10	0	1	0	3	0	250
Turkey as prep	¼ cup	20	1	0	0	4	0	270
Loma Linda								
Gravy Quik Brown	1 tbsp (5 g)	20	tr	0	0	4	0	370
Gravy Quik Chicken	1 tbsp (5 g)	20	1	0	0	3	0	410
Quik Gravy Country	1 tbsp (5 g)	25	tr	1	0	4	0	250
Quik Gravy Mushroom	1 tbsp (5 g)	15	tr	0	0	3	tr	300
Quik Gravy Onion	1 tbsp (5 g)	20	tr	0	0	3	tr	230
Marmite								
Extract	1 heaping tsp	9	2	0	–	tr	–	–

FOOD	PORTION	CAL	PROT	FAT	CHOL	CARB	FIBER	SOD
McCormick								
Au Jus Natural as prep	¼ cup	5	0	0	–	1	–	310
Beef & Herb as prep	¼ cup	30	1	1	<5	3	–	290
Brown as prep	¼ cup	20	tr	1	–	3	–	340
Chicken as prep	¼ cup	20	0	0	–	4	–	330
Onion as prep	¼ cup	20	tr	1	–	3	–	340
Pork as prep	¼ cup	20	0	–	–	4	–	320
Turkey as prep	¼ cup	20	0	0	–	3	–	350
GREAT NORTHERN BEANS								
CANNED								
great northern	1 cup	300	19	1	0	55	14	11
Eden								
Organic	½ cup (4.6 oz)	110	5	1	0	20	8	65
Green Giant								
Great Northern	½ cup (4.4 oz)	100	6	1	0	18	6	290
DRIED								
cooked	1 cup	210	15	1	0	37	–	4
Hurst								
HamBeens w/ Ham	3 tbsp (1.2 oz)	120	7	1	0	22	11	63
GREEN BEANS								
CANNED								
green beans	½ cup	13	1	tr	0	3	1	170
italian	½ cup	13	1	tr	0	3	1	170
italian low sodium	½ cup	13	1	tr	0	3	1	1
low sodium	½ cup	13	1	tr	0	3	1	1
Del Monte								
Cut	½ cup (4.2 oz)	20	1	0	0	4	2	390
Cut Italian	½ cup (4.2 oz)	30	1	0	0	6	3	390
Cut No Salt Added	½ cup (4.2 oz)	20	1	0	0	4	2	10
French Style	½ cup (4.2 oz)	20	1	0	0	4	2	390
French Style No Salt Added	½ cup (4.2 oz)	20	1	0	0	4	2	10
French Style Seasoned	½ cup (4.2 oz)	20	1	0	0	4	2	360
Whole	½ cup (4.2 oz)	20	1	0	0	4	2	390
Green Giant								
Cut	½ cup (4.2 oz)	20	tr	0	0	4	1	400

FOOD	PORTION	CAL	PROT	FAT	CHOL	CARB	FIBER	SOD
Cut 50% Less Sodium	½ cup (4.2 oz)	20	tr	0	0	4	1	200
French Style	½ cup (4.1 oz)	20	tr	0	0	4	1	390
Kitchen Sliced	½ cup (4.2 oz)	20	tr	0	0	4	1	400
Whole	½ cup (4.1 oz)	25	tr	0	0	5	2	330
Owatonna								
Cut	½ cup	20	–	0	0	–	–	–
French	½ cup	20	–	0	0	–	–	–
S&W								
Blue Lake Cut	½ cup (4.2 oz)	20	1	0	0	4	2	340
French Style	½ cup (4.2 oz)	20	1	0	0	4	2	340
Whole Small	½ cup (4.2 oz)	20	1	0	0	4	2	390
FRESH								
cooked	½ cup	22	1	tr	0	5	–	2
raw	½ cup	17	1	tr	0	4	1	3
FROZEN								
cooked	½ cup	18	1	tr	0	4	–	9
italian cooked	½ cup	18	1	tr	0	4	–	9
Birds Eye								
Cut	½ cup	25	–	0	0	–	2	0
Italian	½ cup	35	–	0	0	–	3	0
Green Giant								
Cut	¾ cup (2.8 oz)	25	1	0	0	5	2	0
Harvest Fresh & Almonds	⅔ cup (2.8 oz)	60	2	3	0	5	2	95
Harvest Fresh Cut	⅔ cup (2.9 oz)	25	tr	0	0	5	2	95
Stouffer's								
Green Bean Mushroom Casserole	1 serv (4 oz)	130	3	8	2	12	2	450
Tree Of Life								
Cut	⅔ cup (2.8 oz)	25	1	0	0	4	2	10
GROUNDCHERRIES								
fresh	½ cup	37	1	tr	0	8	–	–
GROUPER								
cooked	3 oz	100	21	1	40	0	–	45
cooked	1 fillet (7.1 oz)	238	50	3	95	0	–	107
raw	3 oz	78	16	1	31	0	–	45

FOOD	PORTION	CAL	PROT	FAT	CHOL	CARB	FIBER	SOD
GUAVA								
fresh	1	45	1	1	0	11	—	2
guava sauce	½ cup	43	tr	tr	0	11	—	4
GUAVA JUICE								
Nantucket Nectars								
Cocktail	8 oz	130	0	0	0	33	—	5
GUINEA HEN								
w/ skin raw	½ hen (12.1 oz)	545	81	22	—	0	—	—
w/o skin raw	½ hen (9.3 oz)	292	55	7	166	0	—	—
HADDOCK								
fresh cooked	1 fillet (5.3 oz)	168	36	1	110	0	—	131
fresh cooked	3 oz	95	21	1	63	0	—	74
fresh raw	3 oz	74	16	1	49	0	—	58
roe raw	1 oz	37	7	tr	103	tr	—	—
smoked	3 oz	99	21	1	65	0	—	649
smoked	1 oz	33	7	tr	21	0	—	214
Van De Kamp's								
Battered Fillets	2 (4 oz)	260	13	16	30	18	0	530
Breaded Fillets	2 (3.5 oz)	280	12	17	25	19	0	310
Lightly Breaded Fillets	1 (4 oz)	220	14	10	30	19	0	410
TAKE-OUT								
breaded & fried	1 piece (3.5 oz)	187	23	9	63	3	tr	350
HAKE								
raw	3.5 oz	84	17	1	—	0	—	101
HALIBUT								
atlantic & pacific cooked	½ fillet (5.6 oz)	223	42	5	65	0	—	110
atlantic & pacific cooked	3 oz	119	23	2	35	0	—	59
atlantic & pacific raw	3 oz	93	18	2	27	0	—	46
greenland baked	3 oz	203	16	15	50	0	—	87
Van De Kamp's								
Battered Fillets	3 (4 oz)	300	13	21	20	16	0	520
FRESH								
greenland baked	5.6 oz	380	29	28	94	0	—	163

FOOD	PORTION	CAL	PROT	FAT	CHOL	CARB	FIBER	SOD
HALVA (see SESAME)								
HAM								
boneless 11% fat roasted	3 oz	151	19	8	50	0	0	1275
canned extra lean roasted	3 oz	116	18	4	26	tr	0	965
canned extra lean roasted	1 cup	190	30	7	42	1	0	1589
canned extra lean 4% fat	3 oz	116	18	4	25	tr	–	965
center slice country style lean roasted	4 oz	220	31	9	80	tr	0	3045
chopped	1 oz	65	5	5	15	0	–	389
chopped canned	1 oz	68	5	5	14	tr	–	387
ham & cheese loaf	1 oz	73	9	6	16	1	–	762
ham & cheese spread	1 oz	69	5	5	17	1	–	339
ham & cheese spread	1 tbsp	37	2	3	9	tr	–	179
ham salad spread	1 oz	61	2	4	10	3	–	259
ham salad spread	1 tbsp	32	1	2	6	2	–	137
minced	1 oz	75	5	6	20	1	–	353
patty cooked	1 patty (2 oz)	203	8	18	43	1	0	632
prosciutto	1 oz	55	8	2	20	tr	0	765
sliced extra lean 5% fat	1 oz	37	5	1	13	tr	–	405
sliced regular 11% fat	1 oz	52	5	3	16	1	–	373
steak boneless extra lean	1 (2 oz)	69	11	2	26	0	0	720
westphalian smoked	1 oz	105	5	10	–	0	–	398
Alpine Lace								
Boneless Cooked 98% Fat Free	2 slices (2 oz)	60	9	1	25	2	0	530
Honey Ham 98% Fat Free	2 slices (2 oz)	60	9	1	25	2	0	530
Smoked Virginia 98% Fat Free	2 slices (2 oz)	60	9	1	25	2	0	400

FOOD	PORTION	CAL	PROT	FAT	CHOL	CARB	FIBER	SOD
Armour								
Chopped Ham canned	2 oz	130	8	11	35	1	0	880
Deviled Ham Spread	1 pkg (3 oz)	210	13	18	60	0	0	700
Lean Slices Brown Sugar	1 pkg (2.5 oz)	90	13	2	35	4	—	700
Star Canned	1 oz	34	—	1	11	—	—	—
Boar's Head								
Black Forest Smoked	2 oz	60	10	1	30	2	0	580
Cappy	2 oz	60	10	2	15	3	0	530
Deluxe	2 oz	60	9	1	25	2	0	590
Deluxe Lowered Sodium	2 oz	50	10	1	20	tr	0	460
Maple Glazed Honey	2 oz	60	10	1	20	3	0	570
Pepper	2 oz	60	10	1	20	2	0	610
Rosemary & Sundried Tomato	2 oz	70	10	3	10	2	0	590
Sweet Slice Smoked	3 oz	100	15	3	30	1	0	780
Virgina	2 oz	60	9	1	25	3	0	590
Virginia Smoked	2 oz	60	9	1	25	2	0	590
Carl Buddig								
Ham Sliced w/ Natural Juices	1 pkg (2.5 oz)	120	12	7	40	1	—	980
Honey Ham Sliced w/ Natural Juice	1 pkg (2.5 oz)	120	12	7	40	3	—	760
Lean Slices Oven Roasted Honey Ham	1 pkg (2.5 oz)	90	13	2	35	4	—	850
Lean Slices Smoked	1 pkg (2.5 oz)	80	14	2	35	1	—	850
Healthy Choice								
Baked Cooked	3 slices (2.2 oz)	70	12	2	30	1	0	560
Cooked	3 slices (2.2 oz)	70	12	2	30	1	0	580
Deli-Thin Baked Cooked w/ Natural Juices	6 slices (2 oz)	60	10	2	25	2	0	500
Deli-Thin Cooked	6 slices (2 oz)	60	10	2	30	1	0	510
Deli-Thin Honey w/ Natural Juices	6 slices (2 oz)	60	10	2	25	2	0	540

FOOD	PORTION	CAL	PROT	FAT	CHOL	CARB	FIBER	SOD
Deli-Thin Smoked w/ Natural Juices	6 slices (2 oz)	60	10	2	25	1	0	530
Fresh-Trak Cooked	1 slice (1 oz)	30	5	1	10	1	0	250
Fresh-Trak Honey	1 slice (1 oz)	30	5	1	15	1	0	250
Honey Boneless	3 oz	100	15	3	40	5	0	580
Smoked	3 slices (2.2 oz)	70	13	2	30	1	0	560
Hillshire								
Deli Select Honey Ham	6 slices (2 oz)	60	10	2	25	2	0	600
Hormel								
Black Label Canned (refrigerated)	3 oz	100	14	5	40	1	0	1020
Black Label Canned (self stable)	3 oz	110	14	5	45	0	0	970
Cure 81 Half Ham	3 oz	100	16	5	45	0	0	890
Curemaster	3 oz	80	14	3	40	0	0	940
Deviled Ham	4 tbsp (2 oz)	150	9	12	40	2	0	430
Ham & Cheese Patties	1 patty (2 oz)	190	7	17	45	0	0	470
Ham Patties	1 (2 oz)	180	7	17	35	1	0	550
Light & Lean 97 Sliced	1 slice (1 oz)	25	4	1	15	0	0	340
Primissimo Proscuitti	2 oz	120	15	7	50	0	0	1080
Spiral Cure 81	3 oz	150	15	9	50	1	0	1090
Jordan's								
Healthy Trim 97% Fat Free Cooked	1 slice (1 oz)	30	5	1	10	2	0	180
Healthy Trim 97% Fat Free EZ Serve	1 slice (1 oz)	30	5	1	15	2	0	180
Healthy Trim 97% Fat Free Virginia	1 slice (1 oz)	30	5	1	15	2	0	180
Louis Rich								
Carving Board Baked	2 slices (1.6 oz)	50	8	2	25	1	0	550
Carving Board Honey Glazed Thin	6 slices (2.1 oz)	70	11	2	30	2	0	750

FOOD	PORTION	CAL	PROT	FAT	CHOL	CARB	FIBER	SOD
Carving Board Honey Glazed Traditional	2 slices (1.6 oz)	50	8	2	25	1	0	560
Carving Board Smoked	1 slice (1.6 oz)	45	8	2	20	0	0	570
Dinner Slices Baked	1 slice (3.3 oz)	80	16	2	40	1	0	1150
Oscar Mayer								
Baked	3 slices (2.2 oz)	70	11	3	30	2	0	790
Boiled	3 slices (2.2 oz)	60	10	3	30	0	0	820
Chopped	1 slice (1 oz)	50	4	3	15	1	0	340
Dinner Slice	3 oz	80	14	3	40	0	0	1010
Dinner Steaks	1 (2 oz)	60	10	2	30	0	0	750
Free Baked	3 slices (1.6 oz)	35	7	0	15	1	0	520
Free Honey	3 slices (1.6 oz)	35	7	0	15	2	0	580
Free Smoked	3 slices (1.6 oz)	35	7	0	15	1	0	550
Honey	3 slices (2.2 oz)	70	10	3	30	2	0	760
Lower Sodium	3 slices (2.2 oz)	70	10	3	30	2	0	520
Smoked	3 slices (2.2 oz)	60	11	3	30	0	0	760
Spam								
Spread	4 tbsp (2 oz)	140	8	12	40	1	0	570
Spreadables								
Ham Salad	¼ can	100	–	6	24	–	–	–
Wampler								
Black Forest	2 oz	60	10	2	25	2	–	650

HAM DISHES
TAKE-OUT

FOOD	PORTION	CAL	PROT	FAT	CHOL	CARB	FIBER	SOD
croquettes	1 (3.1 oz)	217	12	14	77	11	tr	475
salad	½ cup	287	16	23	237	5	tr	671

HAM SUBSTITUTES
Yves

FOOD	PORTION	CAL	PROT	FAT	CHOL	CARB	FIBER	SOD
Veggie Ham Deli Slices	1 serv (2.2 oz)	80	14	0	0	6	1	480

HAMBURGER
Kid Cuisine

FOOD	PORTION	CAL	PROT	FAT	CHOL	CARB	FIBER	SOD
Buckaroo Beef Patty Sandwich w/ Cheese	1 meal (8.5 oz)	410	12	15	30	58	4	600

FOOD	PORTION	CAL	PROT	FAT	CHOL	CARB	FIBER	SOD
White Castle								
Cheeseburger	2 (3.6 oz)	310	15	17	30	23	6	480
Hamburger	2 (3.2 oz)	270	12	14	20	23	5	270
TAKE-OUT								
double patty w/ bun	1 reg	544	30	28	99	43	—	554
double patty w/ cheese & bun	1 reg	457	28	28	110	22	—	635
double patty w/ cheese & double bun	1 reg	461	22	22	80	44	—	892
double patty w/ ketchup mustard onion pickle & bun	1 reg	576	32	32	102	39	—	742
single patty w/ bun	1 reg	275	12	12	36	31	—	387
single patty w/ bun	1 lg	400	23	23	71	25	—	474
single patty w/ cheese & bun	1 reg	320	15	15	50	32	—	500
single patty w/ cheese & bun	1 lg	608	30	33	96	47	—	1589
triple patty w/ cheese & bun	1 lg	769	56	51	161	27	—	1211
triple patty w/ ketchup mustard pickle & bun	1 lg	693	50	41	142	29	—	713

HAMBURGER SUBSTITUTES *(see also MEAT SUBSTITUTES)*

FOOD	PORTION	CAL	PROT	FAT	CHOL	CARB	FIBER	SOD
Amy's Organic								
Veggie Burger California	1 (2.5 oz)	100	4	3	0	17	3	290
Veggie Burger Chicago	1 (2.5 oz)	100	6	4	5	9	2	190
Veggie Burger Texas	1 (2.5 oz)	130	12	3	0	15	3	270
Boca Burgers								
Hint of Garlic	1 patty (2.5 oz)	110	14	2	3	9	4	296
Vegan Original	1 patty (2.5 oz)	84	12	0	0	9	5	269
Franklin Farms								
Veggiburger Portabella	1 (3 oz)	120	15	2	0	11	4	460
GardenVegan								
Fat-Free Patty	1 patty (2.5 oz)	140	11	0	0	23	4	250

FOOD	PORTION	CAL	PROT	FAT	CHOL	CARB	FIBER	SOD
Gardenburger								
Classic Greek	1 (2.5 oz)	120	6	3	10	17	2	310
Fire Roasted Vegetable	1 (2.5 oz)	120	7	3	10	17	2	270
Hamburger Style	1 (2.5 oz)	90	16	0	0	7	3	370
Hamburger Style w/ Cheese	1 (2.5 oz)	110	16	3	5	7	3	380
Savory Mushroom	1 (2.5 oz)	120	6	3	10	18	4	270
Green Giant								
Southwestern Style	1 patty (3.2 oz)	140	18	4	0	9	5	370
Harmony Farms								
Soy Burgers Garlic	1 (2.5 oz)	110	12	3	0	10	23	240
Soy Burgers Mushroom	1 (2.5 oz)	110	11	3	0	9	3	320
Soy Burgers Onion	1 (2.5 oz)	90	10	3	0	7	3	230
Soy Burgers Original	1 (2.5 oz)	110	12	3	0	7	4	250
Lightlife								
Barbecue Grilles	1 patty (2.7 oz)	120	10	4	0	11	0	180
Lemon Grilles	1 patty (2.7 oz)	140	11	6	0	11	0	280
Light Burgers	1 (3 oz)	130	16	1	0	12	2	410
Tamari Grilles	1 patty (2.7 oz)	120	11	5	0	9	0	260
Loma Linda								
Patty Mix not prep	⅓ cup (0.9 oz)	90	14	1	0	7	5	480
Redi-Burger	⅝ in slice (3 oz)	120	18	3	0	7	4	450
Vege-Burger	¼ cup (1.9 oz)	70	11	2	0	2	2	115
Morningstar Farms								
Better'n Burger	1 (2.7 oz)	80	13	0	0	8	3	360
Garden Grille	1 patty (2.5 oz)	120	6	3	<5	18	4	280
Garden Veggie Patties	1 patty (2.4 oz)	100	10	3	0	9	4	350
Hard Rock Cafe Veggie Burger	1 (3 oz)	170	6	8	0	18	3	340
Harvest Burger Italian Style	1 patty (3.2 oz)	140	17	5	0	8	5	370
Harvest Burger Original	1 (3.2 oz)	140	18	4	0	8	5	370
Harvest Burger Southwestern	1 (3.2 oz)	140	16	4	0	9	5	370
Spicy Black Bean Burger	1 (2.7 oz)	110	11	1	0	16	5	470

FOOD	PORTION	CAL	PROT	FAT	CHOL	CARB	FIBER	SOD
Natural Touch								
Garden Veggie Pattie	1 (2.4 oz)	110	10	3	0	8	3	280
Okara Pattie	1 (2.2 oz)	110	11	5	0	4	3	360
Original Veggie Burger Kit not prep	¼ pkg (0.8 oz)	80	14	0	0	6	4	360
Southwestern Veggie Burger Kit not prep	¼ pkg (0.9 oz)	90	12	0	0	9	4	360
Spicy Black Bean Burger	1 (2.7 oz)	100	11	1	0	15	5	330
Vegan Burger	1 (2.7 oz)	70	11	0	0	6	3	370
NewMenu								
VegiBurger	1 patty (3 oz)	110	13	1	0	12	1	320
Superburgers								
Vegan Organic Original	1 (3 oz)	98	10	2	0	14	2	350
Vegan Organic Smoked	1 (3 oz)	98	10	2	0	14	2	350
Vegan Organic TexMex	1 (3 oz)	110	10	1	0	14	3	195
V'dora								
Vegetable BurgerLites	1 (3.3 oz)	58	4	0	0	4	0	98
Veggie Patch								
Burgeriffics	1 (2.5 oz)	110	14	3	0	8	4	410
Worthington								
Granburger not prep	3 tbsp (0.6 oz)	60	10	1	0	3	2	410
Prosage Patties	1 (1.3 oz)	80	9	3	0	3	2	300
Vegetarian Burger	¼ cup (1.9 oz)	60	9	2	0	2	1	270
Yves								
Black Bean & Mushroom Burgers	1 (3 oz)	100	12	0	0	13	7	450
Garden Vegetable Patties	1 (3 oz)	90	11	0	0	11	7	470
Veggie Burger	1 (3 oz)	119	16	2	0	9	4	480
HAZELNUTS								
dried blanched	1 oz	191	4	19	0	5	—	1
dried unblanched	1 oz	179	4	18	0	4	—	1
dry roasted unblanched	1 oz	188	3	19	0	5	—	1

FOOD	PORTION	CAL	PROT	FAT	CHOL	CARB	FIBER	SOD
oil roasted unblanched	1 oz	187	4	18	0	5	2	1

HEART

beef simmered	3 oz	148	24	5	164	tr	–	54
chicken simmered	1 cup (5 oz)	268	11	11	350	tr	–	69
lamb braised	3 oz	158	21	7	212	2	–	54
pork braised	1	191	30	7	285	1	0	45
pork braised	1 cup	215	34	7	320	1	0	51
turkey simmered	1 cup (5 oz)	257	39	9	327	3	–	79
veal braised	3 oz	158	25	6	150	tr	–	50

HEARTS OF PALM

canned	1 cup (5.1 oz)	41	4	1	0	7	–	622
canned	1 (1.2 oz)	9	1	tr	0	2	–	141

HEMP
HempNut

Shelled Hempseed	1 oz	162	9	13	0	3	2	3

Nutiva

Hempseed	1½ tbsp (0.5 oz)	70	4	5	0	3	2	0

HERBAL TEA *(see TEA/HERBAL TEA)*

HERBS/SPICES *(see also individual names)*

chinese five spice	1 tsp	7	0	tr	–	2	tr	1
curry powder	1 tsp	6	tr	tr	0	1	–	1
garam masala	1 tsp	8	tr	tr	0	1	–	2
poultry seasoning	1 tsp	5	tr	tr	0	1	–	tr
pumpkin pie spice	1 tsp	6	tr	tr	0	1	–	1

Chi-Chi's

Seasoning Mix	1 tsp (3 g)	10	0	0	0	1	0	290

Eden

Furikake Seasoning	½ tsp	5	0	0	0	1	1	25

McCormick

Big'n Season Buffalo Wings	1 tbsp (8 g)	30	0	0	–	5	–	710
Big'n Season Chicken	1 tbsp (6 g)	20	tr	0	–	3	–	460
Big'n Season Pot Roast	1 tsp	10	tr	0	–	1	–	390
Meat Loaf Seasoning	1 tsp (4 g)	15	0	0	–	2	–	350

FOOD	PORTION	CAL	PROT	FAT	CHOL	CARB	FIBER	SOD
Mrs. Dash								
Extra Spicy	⅛ tsp (0.02 oz)	2	tr	0	0	tr	–	1
Garlic & Herb	⅛ tsp (0.02 oz)	2	tr	tr	tr	tr	–	tr
Lemon & Herb	⅛ tsp (0.02 oz)	2	tr	0	0	tr	–	1
Low Pepper No Garlic	⅛ tsp (0.02 oz)	2	tr	0	0	tr	–	tr
Original Blend	⅛ tsp (0.02 oz)	2	tr	0	0	tr	–	1
Table Blend	⅛ tsp (0.02 oz)	2	tr	0	0	tr	–	1
HERRING								
atlantic cooked	1 fillet (5 oz)	290	33	17	110	0	–	165
atlantic cooked	3 oz	172	20	10	65	0	–	98
atlantic raw	3 oz	134	15	8	51	0	–	76
pacific baked	3 oz	213	18	15	84	0	–	81
pacific fillet baked	5.1 oz	360	30	26	142	0	–	137
roe canned	1 oz	34	6	1	–	tr	–	–
roe raw	1 oz	37	7	tr	103	tr	–	–
smoked	3.5 oz	210	22	14	70	0	0	550
TAKE-OUT								
atlantic kippered	1 fillet (1.4 oz)	87	10	5	33	0	–	367
atlantic pickled	½ oz	39	2	3	2	1	–	131
fried	1 serv (3.5 oz)	233	23	15	69	2	0	100
HICKORY NUTS								
dried	1 oz	187	4	18	0	5	–	0
HOMINY								
CANNED								
white	1 cup (5.6 oz)	482	2	1	0	23	4	336
Van Camp								
Golden	½ cup (4.3 oz)	80	4	1	0	17	1	540
White	½ cup (4.3 oz)	80	1	1	0	16	1	530
HONEY								
honey	1 cup (11.9 oz)	1031	1	0	0	279	–	12
honey	1 tbsp (0.7 oz)	64	tr	0	0	17	–	1
wild honey	1 tbsp	60	0	0	0	17	–	0
HONEYDEW								
FRESH								
cubed	1 cup	60	1	tr	0	16	–	17
wedge	⅒ melon	46	1	tr	0	12	–	13

FOOD	PORTION	CAL	PROT	FAT	CHOL	CARB	FIBER	SOD
Chiquita								
Wedge	1/10 melon (4.7 oz)	50	1	0	0	13	1	35
HORSE								
roasted	3 oz	149	24	5	58	0	–	47
HORSERADISH								
japanese wasabi	1/4 tsp	1	–	–	0	tr	0	0
wasabi root raw	1 (5.9 oz)	184	8	1	0	40	12	29
wasabi root raw sliced	1 cup (4.6 oz)	142	6	1	0	31	10	22
Boar's Head								
Horseradish	1 tsp (5 g)	5	0	0	0	0	0	30
Eden								
Wasabi Powder	1 tsp	10	0	0	0	1	1	0
Kraft								
Cream Style	1 tsp (5 g)	0	0	0	0	0	0	50
Horseradish Sauce	1 tsp (5 g)	20	0	2	<5	tr	0	35
Prepared	1 tsp (5 g)	0	0	0	0	0	0	50
HOT COCOA (see COCOA)								
HOT DOG								
beef	1 (2 oz)	180	7	16	35	1	–	585
beef	1 (1.5 oz)	142	5	13	27	1	–	462
beef & pork	1 (2 oz)	183	6	17	29	1	–	639
beef & pork	1 (1.5 oz)	144	5	13	22	1	–	504
chicken	1 (1.5 oz)	116	6	9	45	3	–	617
pork cheesefurter smokie	1 (1.5 oz)	141	6	12	29	1	–	465
turkey	1 (1.5 oz)	102	6	8	48	1	–	642
Applegate Farms								
Chicken Natural Uncured	1 (1.5 oz)	120	14	5	40	1	0	450
Natural Turkey	1 (1.5 oz)	120	14	5	40	1	0	450
Armour								
Star Jumbo Beef	1	190	6	18	30	–	–	590
Boar's Head								
Beef	1 (2 oz)	160	7	14	30	1	0	440
Beef Lite	1 (1.6 oz)	90	7	6	25	0	0	270
Pork & Beef	1 (2 oz)	150	7	14	25	0	0	460

FOOD	PORTION	CAL	PROT	FAT	CHOL	CARB	FIBER	SOD
Health Is Wealth								
Uncured Beef	1 (1.5 oz)	80	6	6	20	1	–	340
Uncured Chicken	1 (1.5 oz)	100	8	8	30	1	–	320
Healthy Choice								
Beef Low Fat	1 (1.8 oz)	70	6	3	15	7	0	440
Bunsize	1 (2 oz)	70	8	2	20	5	0	590
Jumbo	1 (2 oz)	70	8	2	20	5	0	570
Low Fat Turkey Pork Beef	1 (1.4 oz)	60	5	2	10	5	–	350
Hormel								
Fat Free	1 (1.8 oz)	45	5	0	15	5	0	580
Fat Free Beef	1 (1.8 oz)	45	6	0	10	5	0	590
Jordan's								
Healthy Trim Low Fat	1 (1.8 oz)	70	8	3	25	3	0	350
Healthy Trim Low Fat Skinless	1 (1.8 oz)	70	8	3	25	3	0	350
Kid Cuisine								
Mystical Mini Corn Dogs	4 pieces	230	8	14	35	18	0	600
Louis Rich								
Bun Length	1 (2 oz)	110	6	8	55	3	0	650
Cheese	1 (1.6 oz)	90	6	6	40	2	0	480
Franks	1 (1.6 oz)	80	5	6	40	2	0	510
Organic Vallely								
All-Natural Beef	1 (1.6 oz)	90	7	6	25	1	–	310
Oscar Mayer								
Beef	1 (1.6 oz)	140	5	13	30	1	0	460
Big & Juicy Franks Deli Style	1 (2.7 oz)	230	9	22	50	1	0	680
Big & Juicy Franks Original	1 (2.7 oz)	240	9	22	45	1	0	700
Big & Juicy Franks Quarter Pound	1 (4 oz)	350	13	32	65	2	0	1050
Big & Juicy Weiners Hot 'N Spicy	1 (2.7 oz)	220	10	20	45	1	0	750
Big & Juicy Weiners Smokie Links	1 (2.7 oz)	220	10	19	50	1	0	770
Big & Juicy Wieners Original	1 (2.7 oz)	240	9	22	45	1	0	690

FOOD	PORTION	CAL	PROT	FAT	CHOL	CARB	FIBER	SOD
Bun-Length Beef	1 (2 oz)	180	6	17	35	2	0	580
Cheese	1 (1.6 oz)	140	5	13	35	1	0	510
Fat Free Beef	1 (1.8 oz)	40	7	0	15	3	0	460
Fat Free Turkey & Beef	1 (1.8 oz)	40	6	0	15	3	0	490
Jumbo Beef	1 (2 oz)	180	6	17	35	2	0	580
Light Beef	1 (2 oz)	110	6	8	30	2	0	620
Wieners	1 (1.6 oz)	150	5	13	35	1	0	430
Wieners Bun-Length	1 (2 oz)	190	6	17	40	2	0	550
Wieners Jumbo	1 (2 oz)	180	6	17	40	2	0	550
Wieners Light	1 (2 oz)	110	7	8	35	2	0	590
Wieners Little	6 (2 oz)	180	6	17	35	2	0	570
Wampler								
Chicken	1 (2 oz)	120	7	11	60	0	1	480
TAKE-OUT								
corndog	1	460	17	19	79	56	–	972
w/ bun chili	1	297	14	13	51	31	–	480
w/ bun plain	1	242	10	15	44	18	–	671

HOT DOG SUBSTITUTES

FOOD	PORTION	CAL	PROT	FAT	CHOL	CARB	FIBER	SOD
Lightlife								
Smart Deli Jumbo's	1 link (2.7 oz)	80	16	0	0	4	1	590
Smart Dogs	1 (1.5 oz)	45	9	0	0	2	0	230
Tofu Pups	1 (1.4 oz)	60	8	3	0	2	0	140
Wonder Dogs	1 (1.5 oz)	60	9	2	0	2	0	320
Loma Linda								
Big Franks	1 (1.8 oz)	110	10	7	0	2	2	240
Big Franks Low Fat	1 (1.8 oz)	80	11	3	0	3	2	220
Corn Dogs	1 (2.5 oz)	150	7	4	0	22	3	500
Morningstar Farms								
America's Original Veggie Dog	1 (2 oz)	80	11	1	0	6	1	580
Meatfree Corn Dog	1 (2.5 oz)	150	7	4	0	22	3	500
Meatfree Mini Corn Dog	4 (2.7 oz)	170	11	5	0	21	1	580
Natural Touch								
Vege Frank	1 (1.6 oz)	100	10	6	0	2	2	470
NewMenu								
VegiDogs	1 (1.5 oz)	45	9	0	0	1	0	170

FOOD	PORTION	CAL	PROT	FAT	CHOL	CARB	FIBER	SOD
Veggie Patch								
Perfectly Franks	1 (1.7 oz)	70	10	2	0	2	1	340
Worthington								
Veja Links Low Fat	1 (1.1 oz)	40	5	2	0	1	0	190
Yves								
Good Dog	1 (1.8 oz)	70	13	2	0	2	1	460
Tofu Dogs	1 (1.3 oz)	45	9	1	0	2	0	240
Veggie Dogs	1 (1.6 oz)	60	11	0	0	1	1	400
Veggie Dogs Chili	1 (1.6 oz)	50	10	0	0	3	2	360
Veggie Dogs Jumbo	1 (2.7 oz)	100	16	2	0	7	2	480
Veggie Dogs Jumbo Hot N' Spicy	1 (2.7 oz)	106	19	2	0	4	2	480

HUMMUS

FOOD	PORTION	CAL	PROT	FAT	CHOL	CARB	FIBER	SOD
hummus	1 cup	420	12	21	0	50	—	599
Athenos								
Roasted Red Pepper	2 tbsp (1.1 oz)	60	2	4	0	6	1	210
TAKE-OUT								
hummus	⅓ cup	140	4	7	0	17	—	200

HYACINTH BEANS

FOOD	PORTION	CAL	PROT	FAT	CHOL	CARB	FIBER	SOD
dried cooked	1 cup	228	16	1	0	40	—	13

ICE CREAM AND FROZEN DESSERTS (see also ICES AND ICE POPS, PUDDING POPS, SHERBET, YOGURT FROZEN)

FOOD	PORTION	CAL	PROT	FAT	CHOL	CARB	FIBER	SOD
chocolate	½ cup (4 fl oz)	143	3	7	22	19	—	50
dixie cup chocolate	1 (3.5 fl oz)	125	2	6	20	16	—	44
dixie cup strawberry	1 (3.5 fl oz)	112	2	5	17	16	—	35
dixie cup vanilla	1 (3.5 fl oz)	116	2	6	25	14	—	46
freeze dried ice cream chocolate strawberry & vanilla	1 pkg (0.75 oz)	158	2	5	1	24	1	97
french vanilla soft serve	½ gal	3014	56	180	1226	306	—	1228
french vanilla soft serve	½ cup (4 fl oz)	185	4	11	78	19	—	52
strawberry	½ cup (4 fl oz)	127	2	6	19	18	—	40
vanilla	½ cup (4 fl oz)	132	2	7	29	16	—	53
vanilla light	½ cup (2.3 oz)	92	3	3	9	15	—	56

FOOD	PORTION	CAL	PROT	FAT	CHOL	CARB	FIBER	SOD
vanilla rich	½ cup (2.6 oz)	178	3	12	45	17	–	41
vanilla soft serve	½ cup	111	4	2	10	19	–	62
vanilla 10% fat	½ gal	2153	38	115	476	254	–	929
vanilla 16% fat	½ gal	2805	33	190	256	256	–	868
vanilla light	½ gal	1469	41	45	146	232	–	836
vanilla light	1 cup	184	5	6	18	29	–	105
vanilla light soft serve	1 cup	223	8	5	13	38	–	163
vanilla light soft serve	½ gal	1787	64	37	106	307	–	1303
Ben & Jerry's								
Bovinity Divinity	½ cup	290	4	18	40	30	1	65
Butter Pecan	½ cup	330	6	25	65	22	2	140
Cherry Garcia	½ cup	260	5	16	70	26	0	60
Chocolate Chip Cookie Dough	½ cup	300	5	16	65	34	0	95
Chocolate Fudge Brownie	½ cup	280	5	15	45	32	2	90
Chubby Hubby	½ cup	350	6	21	55	33	1	250
Chunky Monkey	½ cup	310	5	19	55	32	3	55
Coconut Almond Fudge Chip	½ cup	310	5	22	40	24	2	70
Coffee Heath Bar Crunch	½ cup	310	4	18	65	32	0	125
Dilbert's World Totally Nuts	½ cup	310	5	21	45	27	tr	105
Low Fat Blackberry Cobbler	½ cup	180	3	3	20	34	tr	70
Low Fat Coconut Cream Pie	½ cup	160	4	3	15	29	0	75
Low Fat Mocha Latte	½ cup	150	5	2	10	28	tr	70
Low Fat S'mores	½ cup	190	5	2	15	35	1	85
Mint Chocolate Cookie	½ cup	280	4	17	70	28	1	130
New York Super Fudge Chunk	½ cup	320	5	21	50	28	4	65
No Fat Chocolate Comfort	½ cup	150	4	2	10	29	tr	85
Orange & Cream	½ cup	230	3	14	40	23	0	50

FOOD	PORTION	CAL	PROT	FAT	CHOL	CARB	FIBER	SOD
Peanut Butter Cup	½ cup	380	7	25	65	32	2	130
Phish Food	½ cup	300	4	14	35	41	3	80
Phish Stick	1	330	4	20	25	38	2	85
Pistachio Pistachio	½ cup	240	5	15	50	20	0	20
Pop Cookie Dough	1	420	5	25	55	44	tr	130
Pop Totally Nuts	1	370	6	29	30	24	1	115
Pop Vanilla	1	330	4	23	75	29	tr	55
Pop Vanilla Heath Bar Crunch	1	330	4	22	65	33	tr	105
S'mores Bar	1	350	5	18	25	43	1	130
Smooth White Russian	½ cup (3.8 oz)	240	4	16	90	23	0	55
Triple Caramel Chunk	½ cup	290	4	17	40	32	0	105
Vanilla World's Best	½ cup	250	4	16	75	22	0	60
Vanilla Caramel Fudge	½ cup	300	4	17	70	33	1	115
Vanilla Heath Bar Crunch	½ cup	310	4	19	70	30	0	135
Wavy Gravy	½ cup	340	7	20	60	32	9	120
Better Than Ice Creme								
Soy Vanilla as prep	½ cup	110	1	3	0	21	0	83
Bon Bons								
Dark Chocolate	5 pieces	190	2	13	15	16	0	35
Milk Chocolate	5 pieces	200	2	14	10	17	0	35
Breyers								
Butter Pecan	½ cup (2.4 oz)	180	3	12	35	14	0	115
Caramel Praline Crunch	½ cup (2.6 oz)	180	3	9	30	22	0	30
Cherry Vanilla	½ cup (2.4 oz)	150	3	8	30	17	0	30
Chocolate	½ cup (2.4 oz)	160	2	9	30	18	tr	20
Chocolate Chip	½ cup (2.4 oz)	170	3	10	35	17	0	35
Chocolate Chip Cookie Dough	½ cup (2.5 oz)	180	3	10	35	20	0	50
Chocolate Rainbow	½ cup (2.4 oz)	120	3	10	25	16	0	40
Coffee	½ cup (2.4 oz)	150	3	9	35	15	0	35
Cookies N Cream	½ cup (2.4 oz)	170	3	9	30	19	0	45
Creamsicle	½ cup (2.8 oz)	130	2	4	15	22	0	30
Double Chocolate Fudge	½ cup (2.6 oz)	150	2	9	40	23	tr	50

FOOD	PORTION	CAL	PROT	FAT	CHOL	CARB	FIBER	SOD
Fat Free Caramel Praline	½ cup (2.5 oz)	120	3	0	<5	25	0	90
Fat Free Chocolate	½ cup (2.4 oz)	90	3	0	0	19	tr	55
Fat Free Mint Cookies N Cream	½ cup (2.4 oz)	100	3	0	<5	21	0	75
Fat Free Strawberry	½ cup (2.4 oz)	90	3	0	0	19	0	50
Fat Free Take Two Vanilla Strawberry	½ cup (2.4 oz)	80	3	0	<5	19	0	55
Fat Free Vanilla	½ cup (2.4 oz)	90	3	0	0	19	tr	65
Fat Free Vanilla Chocolate Strawberry	½ cup (2.4 oz)	90	3	0	0	19	0	55
Fat Free Vanilla Fudge Twirl	½ cup (2.5 oz)	100	3	0	0	22	tr	65
French Vanilla	½ cup (2.4 oz)	160	4	10	105	15	0	40
Fruit Rainbow	½ cup (2.4 oz)	140	2	8	30	16	0	35
Hershey w/ Almonds	½ cup (2.7 oz)	190	3	8	25	23	tr	20
Light Butter Pecan	½ cup (2.3 oz)	120	4	4	<5	19	0	130
Light Caramel Praline Pecan	½ cup (3 oz)	180	4	5	15	30	0	90
Light French Chocolate	½ cup (2.4 oz)	150	4	5	30	22	tr	55
Light Mint Chocolate Chip	½ cup (2.4 oz)	140	3	5	10	21	0	50
Light Vanilla	½ cup (2.4 oz)	130	3	5	35	18	0	45
Light Vanilla Chocolate Strawberry	½ cup (2.4 oz)	120	4	3	10	19	0	50
Light Low Fat Brown Marble Fudge	½ cup (2.6 oz)	130	4	2	5	26	tr	65
Light Low Fat French Vanilla	½ cup (2.3 oz)	110	3	2	30	20	0	45
Light Low Fat Swiss Almond Fudge	½ cup (2.5 oz)	130	4	3	5	24	tr	60
Low Fat Butter Pecan	½ cup (2.6 oz)	150	3	7	15	21	0	125
Low Fat Vanilla	½ cup (2.6 oz)	120	3	3	15	22	0	40
Low Fat Vanilla Chocolate Strawberry	½ cup (2.6 oz)	120	3	3	10	22	0	40

FOOD	PORTION	CAL	PROT	FAT	CHOL	CARB	FIBER	SOD
Mint Chocolate Chip	½ cup (2.4 oz)	170	3	10	35	17	0	35
No Sugar Added Fudge Twirl	½ cup (2.6 oz)	100	3	5	25	14	0	55
No Sugar Added Mint Chocolate Chip	½ cup (2.4 oz)	100	3	5	25	12	0	50
No Sugar Added Vanilla	½ cup (2.4 oz)	90	3	5	25	11	0	50
No Sugar Added Vanilla Chocolate Strawberry	½ cup (2.4 oz)	90	3	5	25	11	0	45
Peach	½ cup (2.4 oz)	130	2	6	25	17	0	25
Peanut Butter Cup	½ cup (2.7 oz)	210	4	12	30	24	tr	90
Rocky Road	½ cup (2.5 oz)	180	2	9	25	24	tr	25
Soft'N Creamy Vanilla	½ cup (2.3 oz)	150	2	7	30	19	0	35
Soft'N Creamy Vanilla Chocolate Strawberry	½ cup (2.3 oz)	150	2	7	30	19	0	35
Strawberry	½ cup (2.4 oz)	130	2	7	30	15	0	30
Take Two Vanilla Chocolate	½ cup (2.5 oz)	160	3	9	35	17	0	35
Take Two Vanilla Orange Sherbet	½ cup (2.7 oz)	130	2	5	20	21	0	30
Vanilla	½ cup (2.4 oz)	150	3	9	35	15	0	35
Vanilla Chocolate Strawberry	½ cup (2.4 oz)	150	2	8	30	16	0	30
Vanilla Fudge Twirl	½ cup (2.6 oz)	160	3	8	35	19	tr	35
Viennetta Cappuccino	½ cup (2.4 oz)	190	3	11	35	19	0	35
Viennetta Chocolate	½ cup (2.4 oz)	190	3	12	25	18	0	40
Viennetta Vanilla	½ cup (2.4 oz)	190	3	11	40	19	0	40
Butterfinger								
Bar	1 (2.5 oz)	190	2	13	15	16	0	35
California Joe								
Soft Serve Chocolate	½ cup (2.5 oz)	72	5	0	0	11	1	60
Soft Serve Vanilla	½ cup (2.5 oz)	70	5	0	0	11	1	60

FOOD	PORTION	CAL	PROT	FAT	CHOL	CARB	FIBER	SOD
Carnation								
Cup Chocolate	1 (3 oz)	140	2	8	25	16	0	40
Cup Chocolate Malt	1 (12 oz)	270	7	6	20	48	1	130
Cup Strawberry	1 (3 oz)	100	1	5	20	12	0	25
Cup Vanilla	1 (5 oz)	170	2	10	35	19	0	50
Cup Vanilla	1 (3 oz)	100	1	6	20	11	0	30
Cup Vanilla Malt	1 (12 oz)	260	6	6	20	48	0	130
Sundae Cup Strawberry	1 (5 oz)	200	2	8	30	29	0	55
Sunday Cup Chocolate	1 (5 oz)	210	2	9	30	30	1	55
Cool Creations								
Cookies & Cream Sandwich	1 (3.5 oz)	240	2	11	15	34	1	250
Mickey Mouse Bar	1 (2.5 oz)	120	2	8	15	10	0	25
Mini Sandwich	1 (2.3 oz)	110	1	5	10	16	0	70
Dippin' Dots								
Dipping Dots Chocolate	⅜ cup (3 oz)	190	4	9	40	22	0	70
Drumstick								
Cone Chocolate	1 (4.6 oz)	320	6	17	25	36	2	90
Cone Chocolate Dipped	1 (4.6 oz)	320	5	16	25	40	1	90
Cone Vanilla	1 (4.6 oz)	340	6	19	20	35	2	90
Cone Vanilla Caramel	1 (4.6 oz)	360	6	20	25	38	2	100
Cone Vanilla Fudge	1 (4.6 oz)	360	5	20	20	39	2	100
Flintstones								
Cool Cream	1 (2.75 oz)	90	1	2	5	18	0	30
Push-Up Pebbles Treats	1 (2.75 oz)	120	1	6	20	15	0	25
Haagen-Dazs								
Bars Chocolate & Almonds	1 (3.7 oz)	380	6	27	90	27	2	65
Bars Chocolate & Dark Chocolate	1 (3.6 oz)	350	5	24	65	28	2	45
Bars Chocolate Peanut Butter Swirl	1 (3 oz)	320	6	23	60	21	2	65
Bars Coffee & Almond Crunch	1 (3.7 oz)	370	5	27	90	27	tr	80

FOOD	PORTION	CAL	PROT	FAT	CHOL	CARB	FIBER	SOD
Bars Cookies & Cream Crunch	1 (3.6 oz)	370	5	26	85	30	tr	100
Bars Dulce De Leche Caramel	1 (3.7 oz)	370	4	24	75	34	0	90
Bars Tropical Coconut	1 (3.5 oz)	340	5	24	90	25	0	70
Bars Vanilla & Almonds	1 (3.7 oz)	380	6	28	90	26	1	70
Bars Vanilla & Dark Chocolate	1 (3.6 oz)	350	5	24	85	27	1	50
Bars Vanilla & Milk Chocolate	1 (3.5 oz)	340	5	24	90	25	tr	65
Butter Pecan	½ cup	310	5	23	110	21	tr	110
Cappuccino Commotion	½ cup	310	5	21	100	25	1	90
Cherry Vanilla	½ cup	240	4	15	100	23	0	60
Chocolate	½ cup	270	5	18	115	22	1	60
Chocolate Chocolate Fudge	½ cup	290	5	18	100	27	tr	90
Chocolate Chocolate Chip	½ cup	300	5	20	105	26	2	55
Chocolate Swiss Almond	½ cup	300	4	20	100	24	2	55
Cinnamon	½ cup	250	4	17	110	20	0	65
Coffee	½ cup	270	5	18	120	21	0	70
Coffee Mocha Chip	½ cup	290	5	19	110	25	tr	75
Cookie Dough Chip	½ cup	310	4	20	95	29	0	125
Cookies & Cream	½ cup	270	5	17	105	23	0	90
Creme Caramel Pecan	½ cup	320	5	20	95	29	0	120
Dulce De Leche Caramel	½ cup	290	5	17	100	28	0	95
Low Fat Chocolate	½ cup	170	7	3	30	29	tr	50
Low Fat Coffee Fudge	½ cup	170	5	3	25	32	0	95
Low Fat Strawberry	½ cup	150	5	2	15	28	0	40
Low Fat Vanilla	½ cup	170	7	3	20	29	0	50
Macadamia Brittle	½ cup	300	4	20	110	25	0	110
Mango	½ cup	250	4	14	85	28	tr	50
Mint Chip	½ cup	300	5	19	105	26	tr	85

FOOD	PORTION	CAL	PROT	FAT	CHOL	CARB	FIBER	SOD
Pineapple Coconut	½ cup	230	4	12	90	25	0	55
Pistachio	½ cup	290	5	20	110	22	tr	80
Rum Raisin	½ cup	270	4	17	110	22	0	60
Strawberry	½ cup	250	4	16	95	23	tr	65
Vanilla	½ cup	270	5	18	120	21	0	70
Vanilla Chocolate Chip	½ cup	310	5	20	105	26	tr	75
Vanilla Fudge	½ cup	290	5	18	100	25	0	95
Vanilla Swiss Almond	½ cup	300	5	20	105	24	tr	75
Healthy Choice								
Butter Pecan Crunch	½ cup	120	3	2	5	22	tr	60
Cappuccino Chocolate Chunk	½ cup	120	3	2	10	22	1	60
Cappuccino Mocha Crunch	½ cup	120	3	2	5	22	tr	55
Cherry Chocolate Chunk	½ cup	110	3	2	<5	19	tr	55
Chocolate Chocolate Chunk	½ cup	120	3	2	5	21	2	45
Coconut Cream Pie	½ cup	120	3	2	5	23	1	75
Cookies 'N Cream	½ cup	120	3	2	5	21	tr	90
Cookies Creme De Mint	½ cup	130	3	2	5	24	tr	60
Fudge Brownie	½ cup	120	3	2	5	22	tr	55
Mint Chocolate Chip	½ cup	120	3	2	5	21	tr	50
Old Fashioned Blueberry Hill	½ cup	120	2	2	<5	23	1	50
Old Fashioned Butterscotch Blonde	½ cup	140	3	2	10	26	tr	75
Old Fashioned Cherry Vanilla	½ cup	120	2	2	5	22	tr	50
Old Fashioned Strawberry	½ cup	110	2	2	0	20	1	35
Peanut Butter Cup	½ cup	110	3	2	5	19	tr	65
Praline & Caramel	½ cup	130	3	2	5	25	tr	70
Praline Caramel Cluster	½ cup	130	3	2	<5	25	tr	70
Rocky Road	½ cup	140	3	2	5	28	tr	60

FOOD	PORTION	CAL	PROT	FAT	CHOL	CARB	FIBER	SOD
Turtle Fudge Cake	½ cup	130	3	2	<5	25	2	60
Vanilla	½ cup	100	3	2	5	18	tr	50
Vanilla Bean	½ cup	110	3	2	5	19	tr	45
Wild Raspberry Truffle	½ cup	120	3	2	6	22	tr	55
Heaven								
Sundae Bars Chocolate Fudge	1 bar	150	–	9	7	–	–	–
Sundae Bars Vanilla Fudge	1 bar	150	–	9	7	–	–	–
Vanilla Caramel Nut	1 bar	225	–	15	9	–	–	–
Vanilla Nut Fudge	1 bar	222	–	15	9	–	–	–
Klondike								
Choco Taco Fudge Grande	1 bar (3.2 oz)	310	41	17	15	36	tr	160
Oreo Ice Cream Cookie Sandwich	1 (2.6 oz)	240	4	10	15	35	2	310
Original	1 (3.3 oz)	290	4	19	30	25	0	85
Nestle Crunch								
Chocolate	1 bar (3 oz)	200	2	14	15	17	0	40
Crunch King	1 (4 oz)	270	3	19	20	21	0	45
Nuggets	8 pieces	310	4	21	20	25	0	60
Reduced Fat	1 (2.5 oz)	130	3	7	5	14	0	40
Vanilla	1 bar (3 oz)	200	2	14	15	16	0	40
NutraShake								
High Calorie High Protein All Flavors	1 serv (4 oz)	200	6	10	60	24	–	217
Perry's								
No Fat No Sugar Added Caramel	½ cup (2.8 oz)	90	4	0	0	25	1	90
No Fat No Sugar Added Chocolate	½ cup (2.6 oz)	80	5	0	0	21	2	80
No Fat No Sugar Added Peach	½ cup (2.9 oz)	90	3	0	0	24	tr	70
No Fat No Sugar Added Strawberry	½ cup (2.8 oz)	90	4	0	0	23	tr	75
No Fat No Sugar Added Vanilla	½ cup (2.6 oz)	80	4	0	0	21	tr	80

FOOD	PORTION	CAL	PROT	FAT	CHOL	CARB	FIBER	SOD
Rice Dream								
Cappuccino	½ cup (3.2 oz)	150	tr	6	0	23	1	100
Carob	½ cup (3.2 oz)	150	1	6	0	24	2	100
Carob Almong	½ cup (3.2 oz)	170	1	8	0	24	2	95
Cherry Vanilla	½ cup (3.2 oz)	150	tr	6	0	24	1	90
Cocoa Marble Fudge	½ cup (3.2 oz)	150	1	6	0	25	2	100
Cookies N' Dream	½ cup (3.2 oz)	170	1	7	0	26	1	100
Mint Chocolate Chip	½ cup (3.2 oz)	170	1	8	0	26	1	95
Neapolitan	½ cup (3.2 oz)	150	1	6	0	24	2	100
Orange Vanilla Swirl	½ cup (3.2 oz)	250	tr	6	0	23	1	100
Strawberry	½ cup (3.2 oz)	140	tr	5	0	24	1	85
Vanilla Swiss Almond	½ cup (3.2 oz)	180	1	8	0	25	1	95
Rice Dream Supreme								
Cappuccino Almond Fudge	½ cup (3.2 oz)	170	1	8	0	24	2	95
Cherry Chocolate Chunk	½ cup (3.2 oz)	170	1	7	0	27	1	85
Chocolate Almond Chunk	½ cup (3.2 oz)	170	2	8	0	25	2	95
Chocolate Fudge Brownie	½ cup (3.2 oz)	170	1	7	0	28	2	95
Double Espresso Bean	½ cup (3.2 oz)	160	1	7	0	24	1	100
Mint Chocolate Cookie	½ cup (3.2 oz)	170	1	8	0	26	1	100
Peanut Butter Cup	½ cup (3.2 oz)	180	3	8	0	25	2	105
Pralines N' Dream	½ cup (3.2 oz)	180	1	9	0	25	1	95
Silhouette								
The Skinny Cow Low Fat Ice Cream Sandwich Vanilla	1	130	5	2	0	23	2	145
Starbucks								
Biscotti Bliss	½ cup	240	4	12	55	30	—	70
Caffe Almond Fudge	½ cup	260	5	13	55	30	—	80
Cafe Almond Roast	1 bar	280	4	18	3	26	—	45
Dark Roast Expresso Swirl	½ cup	220	4	10	55	29	—	60
Frappuccino	1 bar (2.8 oz)	110	4	2	10	20	0	45
Italian Roast Coffee	½ cup	230	5	12	65	26	—	50

FOOD	PORTION	CAL	PROT	FAT	CHOL	CARB	FIBER	SOD
Javachip	½ cup	250	4	13	60	29	–	55
Low Fat Latte	½ cup	170	5	3	10	31	–	65
Low Fat Mocha Mambo	½ cup	170	5	3	10	32	–	75
Vanilla Mochachip	½ cup	270	5	16	75	27	–	60
Tofutti								
Cuties Chocolate	1 (1.4 oz)	130	2	5	0	16	0	110
Cuties Vanilla	1 (1.4 oz)	121	2	5	0	17	0	121
Monkey Bars Peanut Butter	1 bar (2.5 oz)	220	3	13	0	22	tr	105
Turkey Hill								
Black Cherry	½ cup	140	2	7	25	18	0	30
Black Raspberry	½ cup	140	–	7	30	18	–	35
Butter Pecan	½ cup	170	2	11	30	16	0	50
Chocolate Marshmallow	½ cup	160	–	7	30	24	–	30
Chocolate Mint Chip	½ cup	180	–	11	30	18	–	40
Chocolate Peanut Butter Cup	½ cup	180	–	11	30	18	–	60
Colombian Coffee	½ cup	140	–	8	30	16	–	35
Cookies 'N Cream	½ cup	160	2	9	30	19	0	60
Death By Chocolate	½ cup	160	–	8	30	21	–	35
Dutch Chocolate	½ cup	150	–	8	30	19	–	30
Egg Nog	½ cup	150	–	8	45	17	–	35
Fat Free No Sugar Added Caramel Fudge Decadence	½ cup	100	–	0	0	23	–	75
Fat Free No Sugar Added Cherry Vanilla Fudge	½ cup	90	–	0	0	20	–	80
Fat Free No Sugar Added Dutch Chocolate	½ cup	90	–	0	0	20	–	70
Fat Free No Sugar Added Vanilla Bean	½ cup	90	–	0	0	20	–	60
Fudge Ripple	½ cup	140	–	7	30	20	–	70
Light Butter Pecan	½ cup	130	3	6	15	17	0	80
Light Choco Mint Chip	½ cup	140	3	5	15	19	0	75

FOOD	PORTION	CAL	PROT	FAT	CHOL	CARB	FIBER	SOD
Light Tin Lissie Sundae	½ cup	140	—	5	10	21	—	120
Light Vanilla & Chocolate	½ cup	110	3	3	15	18	0	60
Light Vanilla Bean	½ cup	110	3	3	15	18	0	65
Neapolitan	½ cup	150	2	8	30	18	0	30
Orange Swirl	½ cup	140	—	6	20	19	—	25
Original Vanilla	½ cup	140	—	8	30	16	—	35
Peanut Butter Ripple	½ cup	170	—	11	30	16	—	60
Philadelphia Style Butter Almond	½ cup	180	—	12	35	15	—	105
Philadelphia Style Chocolate	½ cup	170	—	10	35	18	—	40
Philadelphia Style Mint Chocolate Chip	½ cup	180	—	11	35	18	—	50
Philadelphia Style Sweet Cherry Vanilla	½ cup	160	—	8	30	18	—	50
Philadelphia Style Vanilla Bean	½ cup	170	—	10	35	16	—	50
Rocky Road	½ cup	170	3	8	30	23	0	40
Rum Raisin	½ cup	150	—	7	30	19	—	30
Sandwich Choco Mint Chip	1	200	—	8	25	27	—	180
Sandwiches Vanilla	1	190	—	8	25	26	—	180
Strawberries 'N Cream	½ cup	140	—	6	25	19	—	30
Sundae Cones Rocky Road	1	340	—	19	25	37	—	110
Sundae Cones Tin Roof Sundae	1	290	—	17	25	30	—	135
Tin Roof Sundae	½ cup	160	2	9	30	19	0	70
Vanilla & Chocolate	½ cup	150	2	8	30	17	0	35
Vanilla Bean	½ cup	140	2	8	30	16	0	35
Weight Watchers								
Chocolate Chip Cookie Dough Sundae	1 (2.64 oz)	190	3	5	5	35	1	120

FOOD	PORTION	CAL	PROT	FAT	CHOL	CARB	FIBER	SOD
Chocolate Mousse	1 bar	40	2	1	5	9	1	20
Chocolate Treat	1 bar	100	3	1	0	20	1	25
English Toffee Crunch	1 bar	110	2	6	5	12	1	30
Orange Vanilla Treat	1 bar	40	2	1	5	10	0	15
Vanilla Sandwich	1 bar	150	3	3	5	28	1	150
TAKE-OUT								
cone vanilla light soft serve	1 (4.6 oz)	164	4	6	28	24	—	92
gelato chocolate hazelnut	½ cup (5.3 oz)	370	9	29	92	26	2	49
gelato vanilla	½ cup (3 oz)	211	3	15	151	18	0	78
sundae caramel	1 (5.4 oz)	303	7	9	25	49	—	195
sundae hot fudge	1 (5.4 oz)	284	6	9	21	48	—	182
sundae strawberry	1 (5.4 oz)	269	6	8	21	45	—	92

ICE CREAM CONES AND CUPS

FOOD	PORTION	CAL	PROT	FAT	CHOL	CARB	FIBER	SOD
sugar cone	1	40	1	tr	0	8	tr	32
wafer cone	1	17	tr	tr	0	3	tr	6
Dutch Mill								
Chocolate Covered Wafer Cups	1 (0.5 oz)	80	1	5	0	8	0	—
Frookie								
Chocolate Crunch	1 (0.4 oz)	50	1	1	0	10	tr	10
Honey Crunch	1 (0.4 oz)	45	1	1	0	9	tr	20
Keebler								
Chocolatey Cone	1 (0.4 oz)	50	tr	1	0	10	0	40
Fudge Dipped Cup	1 (0.3 oz)	35	0	2	0	6	0	20
Ice Creme Cup	1 (0.2 oz)	15	0	0	0	4	0	20
Sugar Cone	1 (0.4 oz)	50	tr	1	0	10	0	15
Waffle Bowl	1 (0.4 oz)	50	tr	1	0	10	0	25
Waffle Cone	1 (0.4 oz)	50	tr	1	0	10	0	25

ICE CREAM TOPPINGS

FOOD	PORTION	CAL	PROT	FAT	CHOL	CARB	FIBER	SOD
butterscotch	2 tbsp (1.4 oz)	103	1	tr	—	27	—	143
caramel	2 tbsp (1.4 oz)	103	1	tr	—	27	—	143
marshmallow cream	1 oz	88	1	tr	0	23	—	13
marshmallow cream	1 jar (7 oz)	615	3	tr	0	157	—	90
pineapple	2 tbsp (1.5 oz)	106	tr	0	0	28	—	26
pineapple	1 cup (11.5 oz)	861	1	—	0	226	—	214
strawberry	2 tbsp (1.5 oz)	107	tr	tr	0	28	—	9

FOOD	PORTION	CAL	PROT	FAT	CHOL	CARB	FIBER	SOD
strawberry	1 cup (11.5 oz)	863	1	1	0	225	–	73
walnuts in syrup	2 tbsp (1.4 oz)	167	2	9	0	22	–	–
Ben & Jerry's								
Hot Fudge	(1.3 oz)	140	2	7	10	19	2	25
Hershey								
Chocolate Shop Double Chocolate	1 tbsp (0.7 oz)	50	0	0	0	13	–	15
Chocolate Shoppe Apple Pie A La Mode	2 tbsp (1.3 oz)	100	0	0	0	25	–	90
Chocolate Shoppe Butterscotch Caramel	1 tbsp (0.7 oz)	70	tr	1	<5	14	–	75
Chocolate Shoppe Caramel	2 tbsp (1.3 oz)	100	tr	0	0	25	–	95
Chocolate Shoppe Chocolate Mini	1 tbsp (0.7 oz)	50	0	0	0	13	–	15
Chocolate Shoppe Double Chocolate	1 tbsp (0.6 oz)	60	tr	1	0	12	–	30
Chocolate Shoppe Hot Fudge	1 tbsp (0.7 oz)	70	tr	3	<5	10	–	80
Chocolate Shoppe Hot Fudge Fat Free	2 tbsp (1.4 oz)	100	1	0	0	23	–	135
Chocolate Shoppe Sprinkles Milk Chocolate	1 tbsp (0.5 oz)	70	tr	3	<5	10	–	10
Chocolate Shoppe Sprinkles Reeses	1 tbsp (0.5 oz)	70	1	4	0	10	–	25
Chocolate Shoppe Sprinkles York	1 tbsp (0.6 oz)	80	4	0	tr	11	–	0
Kraft								
Butterscotch	2 tbsp (1.4 oz)	130	tr	2	<5	28	0	150
Caramel	2 tbsp (1.4 oz)	120	2	0	0	28	0	90
Chocolate	2 tbsp (1.4 oz)	110	2	0	0	26	1	30
Hot Fudge	2 tbsp (1.4 oz)	140	1	5	0	24	tr	100
Pineapple	2 tbsp (1.4 oz)	110	0	0	0	28	0	15
Strawberry	2 tbsp (1.4 oz)	110	0	0	0	29	0	15
Planters								
Nut	2 tbsp (0.5 oz)	100	3	9	0	3	1	0

FOOD	PORTION	CAL	PROT	FAT	CHOL	CARB	FIBER	SOD
Smucker's								
Plate Scapers Caramel	2 tbsp	100	1	0	0	25	–	105

ICED TEA
MIX
Crystal Light

Decaffeinated as prep	1 serv (8 oz)	5	0	0	0	tr	0	0
Iced Tea as prep	1 serv (8 oz)	5	0	0	0	0	0	0
Peach Tea as prep	1 serv (8 oz)	5	0	0	0	0	0	0
Raspberry Tea as prep	1 serv (8 oz)	5	0	0	0	0	0	0
Lipton								
100% Tea Decaffeinated as prep	1 serv	0	0	0	0	0	–	0
100% Tea Unsweetened as prep	1 serv	0	0	0	0	0	–	0
100% Tea as prep	1 serv	0	0	0	0	0	–	0
Calorie Free as prep	1 serv	0	0	0	0	0	–	0
Decaffeinated Ice Tea Brew as prep	1 serv (8 oz)	0	0	0	0	0	0	0
Decaffeinated Lemon as prep	1 serv	90	0	0	0	22	–	0
Diet Decaffeinated Lemon as prep	1 serv	5	0	0	0	1	–	0
Diet Lemon as prep	1 serv	5	0	0	0	1	–	0
Diet Peach as prep	1 serv	5	0	0	0	1	–	0
Diet Raspberry as prep	1 serv	5	0	0	0	1	–	0
Diet Tea & Lemonade as prep	1 serv	10	0	0	0	2	–	5
Herbal Iced Collection	1 tea bag	0	0	0	0	tr	–	0
Ice Tea Brew as prep	1 serv (8 oz)	0	0	0	0	0	0	0
Lemon as prep	1 serv	90	0	0	0	22	–	0
Lemon as prep	1 pkg (0.5 oz)	50	0	0	0	13	–	0

FOOD	PORTION	CAL	PROT	FAT	CHOL	CARB	FIBER	SOD
Natural Brew 100% Tea Decaffeinated as prep	1 serv	0	0	0	0	0	—	0
Natural Brew 100% Tea as prep	1 serv	0	0	0	0	0	—	0
Natural Brew Diet Lemon as prep	1 serv	5	0	0	0	1	—	0
Natural Brew Diet Peach as prep	1 serv	5	0	0	0	1	—	0
Natural Brew Diet Tropical as prep	1 serv	5	0	0	0	1	—	0
Natural Brew Tropical as prep	1 serv	90	0	0	0	22	—	0
Natural Brew Unsweetened Lemon as prep	1 serv	0	0	0	0	tr	—	0
Peach as prep	1 serv	90	0	0	0	22	—	0
Rasberry as prep	1 serv	90	0	0	0	22	—	0
Tea & Lemonade as prep	1 serv	90	0	0	0	22	—	0
Nestea								
100% Tea	2 tsp (1 g)	0	0	0	0	tr	0	0
100% Tea Decafe	2 tsp (1 g)	0	0	0	0	tr	0	0
Ice Teasers Lemon	1 serv (0.5 oz)	5	0	0	0	1	0	0
Ice Teasers Orange	1 serv (0.5 oz)	5	0	0	0	1	0	0
Ice Teasers Wild Cherry	1 serv (0.5 oz)	5	0	0	0	1	0	0
Lemon	2 tsp (1 g)	5	0	0	0	1	0	0
Lemon & Sugar	2 tbsp (0.7 oz)	80	0	0	0	19	0	0
Lemonade Tea	2 tbsp (0.7 oz)	80	0	0	0	19	0	0
Sugar Free	2 tbsp (0.7 oz)	5	0	0	0	1	0	0
Sugar Free Decafe	1 tbsp (0.7 oz)	5	0	0	0	1	0	0
Sun Tea	1 tsp (1 g)	0	0	0	0	tr	0	0
READY-TO-DRINK								
Arizona								
Lemon	1 bottle (16 oz)	180	0	0	0	50	—	40
Crystal Light								
Lemon	1 serv (8 oz)	5	0	0	0	0	0	40
Peach Tea	1 serv (8 oz)	5	0	0	0	0	0	40
Raspberry Tea	1 serv (8 oz)	5	0	0	0	0	0	40

FOOD	PORTION	CAL	PROT	FAT	CHOL	CARB	FIBER	SOD
Honest Tea								
Gold Rush Herbal Cinnamon	8 fl oz	9	0	0	0	3	–	10
Lipton								
Carribean Cooler	1 can (12 oz)	130	0	0	0	34	–	75
Diet Lemon	8 oz	0	0	0	0	0	–	10
Diet Lemon	1 bottle (16 oz)	10	0	0	0	0	–	10
Green Tea & Passion Fruit	1 bottle (16 oz)	160	0	0	0	38	–	10
Lemon	8 oz	80	0	0	0	20	–	15
Lemon	1 can (12 oz)	120	0	0	0	33	–	75
Lemon	1 bottle (16 oz)	180	0	0	0	42	–	10
Natural Lemon	1 box (8 oz)	100	0	0	0	25	–	10
Peach	8 oz	80	0	0	0	20	–	15
Peach	1 bottle (16 oz)	220	0	0	0	52	–	10
Raspberry	8 oz	80	0	0	0	20	–	15
Raspberry	1 bottle (16 oz)	220	0	0	0	52	–	10
Raspberry Blast	1 can (12 oz)	130	0	0	0	35	–	75
Southern Style Extra Sweet No Lemon	1 bottle (16 oz)	240	0	0	0	58	–	10
Southern Style Lemon	1 bottle (16 oz)	200	0	0	0	50	–	10
Southern Style Sweetened No Lemon	1 bottle (16 oz)	200	0	0	0	48	–	10
Sweet	8 oz	80	0	0	0	20	–	15
Sweetened No Lemon	1 bottle (16 oz)	140	0	0	0	36	–	10
Sweetened Lemon	8 oz	80	0	0	0	20	–	15
Tangerine Twist	1 can (12 oz)	120	0	0	0	33	–	75
Tea & Lemonade	1 bottle (16 oz)	220	0	0	0	52	–	10
Unsweetened No Lemon	1 bottle (16 oz)	0	0	0	0	0	–	10
Mad River								
Red Tea w/ Guarana	8 oz	90	0	0	0	24	–	10
Nantucket Nectars								
Diet	8 oz	5	0	0	0	1	–	25
Diet Green Tea	8 oz	5	0	0	0	1	–	5

FOOD	PORTION	CAL	PROT	FAT	CHOL	CARB	FIBER	SOD
Half & Half	8 oz	90	0	0	0	23	–	0
Iced Tea	8 oz	80	0	0	0	20	–	0
Matt Fee	8 oz	80	0	0	0	20	–	0
Raspberry	8 oz	90	0	0	0	23	–	20
Savannah	8 oz	80	0	0	0	20	–	0
Snapple								
Diet Lemon	8 fl oz	0	0	0	0	1	–	10
Diet Peach	8 fl oz	0	0	0	0	1	–	10
Diet Raspberry	8 fl oz	0	0	0	0	1	–	10
Ginseng Tea	8 fl oz	80	0	0	0	20	–	10
Green Tea w/ Lemon	8 fl oz	100	0	0	0	25	–	10
Lemon	8 fl oz	100	0	0	0	25	–	10
Lemonade Ice Tea	8 fl oz	110	0	0	0	28	–	10
Peach	8 fl oz	100	0	0	0	26	–	10
Raspberry	8 fl oz	100	0	0	0	26	–	10
Turkey Hill								
Blueberry Oolong w/ Vitamins C & E	1 cup	100	–	0	0	24	–	–
Decaffeinated	1 cup	80	–	0	0	20	–	–
Decaffeinated Orange	1 cup	10	–	0	0	2	–	–
Diet	1 cup	0	0	0	0	0	–	–
Diet Decaffeinated	1 cup	0	0	0	0	0	–	0
Diet Green Tea w/ Ginseng & Honey	1 cup	5	–	0	0	tr	–	–
Green Tea w/ Ginseng & Honey	1 cup	70	17	0	0	17	–	–
Lemon	1 cup	100	–	0	0	24	–	–
Mint Tea w/ Chamomile	1 cup	90	–	0	0	21	–	–
Oolong w/ Ginkgo Biloba & Ginseng	1 cup	100	–	0	0	25	–	–
Orange	1 cup	100	–	0	0	25	–	–
Peach	1 cup	110	–	0	0	28	–	–
Raspberry Tea	1 cup	110	0	0	0	28	–	0
Regular	1 cup	90	0	0	0	22	–	0

FOOD	PORTION	CAL	PROT	FAT	CHOL	CARB	FIBER	SOD
ICES AND ICE POPS *(see also* SHERBET*)*								
fruit & juice bar	1 (3 fl oz)	75	tr	0	1	19	—	3
gelatin pop	1 (1.5 oz)	31	1	0	0	7	—	20
ice coconut pineapple	½ cup (4 fl oz)	109	0	3	0	23	—	34
ice fruit w/ Equal	1 bar (1.7 oz)	12	tr	0	0	3	—	3
ice lime	½ cup (4 fl oz)	75	tr	0	0	31	—	—
ice pop	1 (2 fl oz)	42	0	0	0	11	—	7
Ben & Jerry's								
Sorbet Devil's Food Chocolate	½ cup	170	2	3	0	36	2	60
Sorbet Doonesberry	½ cup	140	0	0	0	33	0	15
Sorbet Lemon Swirl	½ cup	120	0	0	0	30	0	15
Sorbet Purple Passion Fruit	½ cup	140	0	0	0	29	0	25
Carnation								
Cup Orange Sherbet	1 (5 oz)	150	1	2	5	32	0	30
Cup Orange Sherbet	1 (3 oz)	90	1	1	5	19	0	20
Cold Fusion								
Protein Juice Bar All Flavors	1 bar (3.8 oz)	130	11	0	0	23	0	0
Cool Creations								
Ice Pop	1 pop (2 oz)	50	0	0	0	13	0	5
Mickey Mouse Bar	1 (4 oz)	170	2	11	15	17	0	40
Surprise Pops	1 (2 oz)	60	0	0	0	14	0	5
Dole								
Fruit'n Juice Coconut	1 bar (4 oz)	210	3	7	10	33	0	50
Fruit'n Juice Lemonade	1 bar (4 oz)	120	1	0	0	28	0	55
Fruit'n Juice Lime	1 bar (4 oz)	110	0	0	0	28	0	55
Fruit'n Juice Peach Passion	1 bar (2.5 oz)	70	0	0	0	17	0	5
Fruit'n Juice Pineapple Coconut	1 bar (4 oz)	150	1	4	0	27	0	5
Fruit'n Juice Pineapple Orange Banana	1 bar (2.5 oz)	70	0	0	0	16	0	5

FOOD	PORTION	CAL	PROT	FAT	CHOL	CARB	FIBER	SOD
Fruit'n Juice Pineapple Orange Banana	1 bar (4 oz)	110	0	0	0	26	0	5
Fruit'n Juice Raspberry	1 bar (2.5 oz)	70	0	0	0	16	0	5
Fruit'n Juice Strawberry	1 bar (2.5 oz)	70	0	0	0	17	0	5
Fruit'n Juice Strawberry	1 bar (4 oz)	110	0	0	0	26	0	5
Grape No Sugar Added	1 bar (1.75 oz)	25	0	0	0	6	0	5
Raspberry	1 bar (1.75 oz)	45	0	0	0	11	0	5
Raspberry No Sugar Added	1 bar (1.75 oz)	25	0	0	0	6	0	5
Strawberry	1 bar (1.75 oz)	45	0	0	0	11	0	5
Strawberry No Sugar Added	1 bar (1.75 oz)	25	0	0	0	6	0	5
Edy's								
Fruit Bars Strawberry	1 (3 oz)	80	0	0	0	21	0	0
Sorbet Coconut	½ cup	140	1	3	5	28	0	20
Sorbet Lemon	½ cup	140	0	0	0	35	0	20
Sorbet Mandarin Orange	½ cup	130	0	0	0	32	0	25
Sorbet Peach	½ cup	130	0	0	0	32	1	10
Sorbet Raspberry	½ cup	130	0	0	0	33	1	15
Sorbet Strawberry	½ cup	120	0	0	0	31	0	10
Flinstones								
Push-Up Sherbet Treats	1 (2.75 oz)	100	1	2	5	20	0	25
Frozfruit								
Banana Cream	1 bar (4 oz)	150	1	7	25	20	1	20
Cantaloupe	1 bar (4 oz)	60	0	0	0	35	0	5
Cappuccino Cream	1 bar (3 oz)	140	1	6	25	18	0	20
Cherry	1 bar (4 oz)	70	1	0	0	18	1	0
Coconut Cream	1 bar (4 oz)	170	2	11	20	17	2	25
Kiwi Strawberry	1 bar (4 oz)	90	0	0	0	23	2	0
Lemon	1 bar (4 oz)	90	0	0	0	22	0	10
Lemon Iced Tea	1 bar (4 oz)	80	0	0	0	19	0	10
Lime	1 bar (4 oz)	90	0	0	0	21	0	10

FOOD	PORTION	CAL	PROT	FAT	CHOL	CARB	FIBER	SOD
Orange	1 bar (4 oz)	90	0	0	0	21	0	15
Pina Colada Cream	1 bar (4 oz)	170	2	8	20	23	1	20
Pineapple	1 bar (4 oz)	80	0	0	0	19	0	0
Raspberry	1 bar (4 oz)	80	0	0	0	20	1	5
Strawberry	1 bar (4 oz)	80	0	0	0	20	1	20
Strawberry Banana Cream	1 bar (4 oz)	140	1	6	20	22	1	20
Strawberry Cream	1 bar (4 oz)	130	1	5	20	21	1	20
Tropical	1 bar (4 oz)	90	0	0	0	23	1	0
Watermelon	1 bar (4 oz)	50	0	0	0	13	0	0
Haagen-Dazs								
Sorbet Chocolate	½ cup	120	2	0	0	28	2	70
Sorbet Manago	½ cup	120	0	0	0	31	tr	0
Sorbet Orange	½ cup	120	0	0	0	30	tr	0
Sorbet Orchard Peach	½ cup	130	0	0	0	33	tr	0
Sorbet Raspberry	½ cup	120	0	0	0	30	2	0
Sorbet Strawberry	½ cup	120	0	0	0	30	1	0
Sorbet Zesty Lemon	½ cup	120	0	0	0	31	tr	0
Sorbet Bar Chocolate	1 (2.7 oz)	80	1	0	0	20	1	50
Sorbet Bars Raspberry & Vanilla Yogurt	1 (2.5 oz)	90	2	0	0	21	tr	15
Sorbet Bars Strawberry & Vanilla Ice Cream	1 (2.5 oz)	110	1	5	35	15	0	20
Lifesavers								
Ice Pops	1 (1.75 oz)	35	0	0	0	9	0	0
Mr. Freeze								
Assorted	2 bars (3 oz)	45	0	0	0	11	0	20
Tropical	2 bars (3 oz)	45	0	0	0	11	0	20
Natural Choice								
Organic Banana	½ cup (3.6 oz)	110	0	0	0	28	tr	0
Organic Blueberry	½ cup (3.6 oz)	100	0	0	0	27	tr	0
Organic Kiwi	½ cup (3.6 oz)	110	0	0	0	28	tr	10
Organic Lemon	½ cup (3.6 oz)	110	0	0	0	28	tr	10
Organic Mango	½ cup (3.6 oz)	110	0	0	0	28	tr	10

FOOD	PORTION	CAL	PROT	FAT	CHOL	CARB	FIBER	SOD
Organic Strawberry	½ cup (3.6 oz)	110	0	0	0	28	tr	10
Organic Strawberry Kiwi	½ cup (3.6 oz)	110	0	0	0	28	tr	10

INSTANT BREAKFAST (see BREAKFAST DRINKS)

JACKFRUIT

FOOD	PORTION	CAL	PROT	FAT	CHOL	CARB	FIBER	SOD
fresh	3.5 oz	70	1	tr	0	4	–	2

JALAPENO (see PEPPERS)

JAM/JELLY/PRESERVES

FOOD	PORTION	CAL	PROT	FAT	CHOL	CARB	FIBER	SOD
all flavors jam	1 tbsp (0.7 oz)	48	tr	0	0	13	tr	–
all flavors jam	1 pkg (0.5 oz)	34	tr	0	0	9	tr	–
all flavors jelly	1 tbsp (0.7 oz)	52	tr	0	0	14	tr	–
all flavors jelly	1 pkg (0.5 oz)	38	tr	0	0	10	tr	–
all flavors preserve	1 pkg (0.5 oz)	34	tr	0	0	9	tr	–
all flavors preserve	1 tbsp (0.7 oz)	48	tr	0	0	13	tr	–
apple butter	1 tbsp (0.6 oz)	33	0	0	0	9	–	0
apple butter	1 cup (9.9 oz)	519	tr	1	0	135	–	1
apple jelly	1 tbsp (0.7 oz)	52	tr	0	0	14	tr	7
apple jelly	1 pkg (0.5 oz)	38	tr	0	0	10	tr	5
apricot jam	0.5 oz	36	tr	0	0	9	–	–
blackberry jam	0.5 oz	34	tr	0	0	8	–	–
cherry jam	0.5 oz	36	tr	0	0	9	–	–
linganberry jam	0.5 oz	23	tr	tr	–	6	tr	–
orange jam	0.5 oz	35	tr	0	0	9	–	2
orange marmalade	1 pkg (0.5 oz)	34	0	0	0	9	–	8
orange marmalade	1 tbsp (0.7 oz)	49	tr	0	0	13	–	11
plum jam	0.5 oz	34	tr	0	0	9	–	–
quince jam	0.5 oz	43	0	0	0	8	–	–
raspberry jam	0.5 oz	35	tr	0	0	9	–	–
raspberry jelly	0.5 oz	37	0	0	0	9	–	–
red currant jam	0.5 oz	34	1	0	0	8	–	–
red currant jelly	0.5 oz	38	0	0	0	9	–	1
rose hip jam	0.5 oz	36	tr	0	0	9	–	1
strawberry jam	1 pkg (0.5 oz)	34	tr	0	0	9	tr	6
strawberry jam	1 tbsp (0.7 oz)	48	tr	0	0	13	tr	8
strawberry preserve	1 pkg (0.5 oz)	34	tr	0	0	9	tr	6
strawberry preserve	1 tbsp (0.7 oz)	48	tr	0	0	13	tr	8

FOOD	PORTION	CAL	PROT	FAT	CHOL	CARB	FIBER	SOD
Eden								
Cherry Butter	1 tbsp	35	0	0	0	9	1	0
Organic Apple Butter	1 tbsp	20	0	0	0	5	0	0
Estee								
Fruit Spread Apple Spice	1 tbsp	16	0	0	0	4	0	20
Fruit Spread Apricot	1 tbsp	16	0	0	0	4	0	20
Fruit Spread Grape	1 tbsp	16	0	0	0	4	0	20
Fruit Spread Peach	1 tbsp	16	0	0	0	4	0	20
Fruit Spread Red Raspberry	1 tbsp	16	0	0	0	4	0	25
Fruit Spread Strawberry	1 tbsp	16	0	0	0	4	0	–
Polaner								
All Fruit Peach	1 tbsp	40	0	0	0	8	–	0
All Fruit Raspberry	1 tbsp	40	0	0	0	10	–	0
Smucker's								
Concord Grape Jelly	1 tbsp	50	0	0	0	13	–	5
Peach Preserves	1 tbsp	50	0	0	0	13	–	0
Simply Fruit Red Raspberry	1 tbsp	40	0	0	0	10	–	0
Tabasco								
Spicy Pepper Jelly	1 tbsp (0.6 oz)	50	0	0	0	12	0	40
White House								
Apple Butter	1 tbsp (0.6 oz)	35	0	0	0	9	–	5

JAPANESE FOOD *(see ASIAN FOOD, SUSHI)*

JAVA PLUM

fresh	1 cup	82	1	tr	0	21	–	18
fresh	3	5	tr	tr	0	1	–	1

JELLY *(see JAM/JELLY/PRESERVES)*

KALE

chopped cooked	½ cup	21	1	tr	0	4	–	15
frzn chopped cooked	½ cup	20	2	tr	0	4	–	10
raw chopped	½ cup	21	1	tr	0	3	–	15
scotch chopped cooked	½ cup	18	1	tr	0	4	–	29

FOOD	PORTION	CAL	PROT	FAT	CHOL	CARB	FIBER	SOD
KEFIR								
kefir	7 oz	132	6	8	–	10	–	92
KETCHUP								
ketchup	1 tbsp	16	tr	tr	0	4	tr	178
ketchup	1 pkg (0.2 oz)	6	tr	tr	0	2	tr	71
low sodium	1 tbsp	16	tr	tr	0	4	tr	3
Del Monte								
Ketchup	1 tbsp (0.5 oz)	15	0	0	0	4	0	190
Estee								
Ketchup	1 tbsp	15	0	0	0	5	0	190
Healthy Choice								
Ketchup	1 tbsp (0.5 oz)	9	tr	tr	0	2	tr	97
Heinz								
Ketchup	1 tbsp (0.6 oz)	15	0	0	0	4	0	190
Hunt's								
Ketchup	1 tbsp (0.6 oz)	16	tr	tr	0	3	0	198
No Salt Added	1 tbsp (0.6 oz)	16	tr	tr	0	3	0	6
McIlhenny								
Spicy	1 tbsp (0.6 oz)	20	0	0	0	5	0	160
Muir Glen								
Organic	1 tbsp (0.6 oz)	15	0	0	0	3	0	190
Smucker's								
Tomato	1 tbsp	25	0	0	0	7	–	110
Tree Of Life								
Ketchup	1 tbsp (0.5 oz)	10	0	0	0	3	–	25
KIDNEY								
beef simmered	3 oz	122	22	3	329	0	–	114
lamb braised	3 oz	117	20	3	481	1	–	128
pork cooked	1 cup	211	36	7	672	0	0	112
pork cooked	3 oz	128	22	4	408	0	0	68
veal braised	3 oz	139	22	5	672	0	–	93
KIDNEY BEANS								
CANNED								
kidney beans	1 cup	208	13	1	0	38	–	889
red	1 cup	216	13	1	0	40	–	873
B&M								
Red Baked Beans	½ cup (4.6 oz)	170	7	2	<5	32	6	440

FOOD	PORTION	CAL	PROT	FAT	CHOL	CARB	FIBER	SOD
Eden								
Organic Cannellini	½ cup (4.6 oz)	100	6	1	–	17	5	40
Friend's								
Red Baked Beans	½ cup (4.6 oz)	160	7	1	<5	32	6	510
Green Giant								
Dark Red	½ cup (4.5 oz)	110	6	0	0	18	5	400
Light Red	½ cup (4.5 oz)	110	8	0	0	20	6	340
Hunt's								
Kidney	½ cup (4.5 oz)	94	6	1	0	20	5	484
Progresso								
Dark Red	½ cup (4.5 oz)	110	8	0	0	20	6	340
Red	½ cup (4.6 oz)	110	7	1	0	20	8	280
S&W								
Dark Red Premium	½ cup (4.6 oz)	100	7	1	0	23	6	460
Van Camp								
Dark Red	½ cup (4.6 oz)	90	6	0	0	20	6	760
Light Red	½ cup (4.6 oz)	90	6	0	0	20	6	390
DRIED								
california red cooked	1 cup	219	16	tr	0	40	–	7
cooked	1 cup	225	15	1	0	40	–	4
red cooked	1 cup	225	15	1	0	40	–	4
royal red cooked	1 cup	218	17	tr	0	39	–	8

KIWI JUICE
After The Fall

Kiwi Bear	1 cup (8 oz)	100	1	0	0	24	0	15

KIWIS

fresh	1 med	46	1	tr	0	11	3	4
Chiquita								
Fresh	2 med (5.2 oz)	100	2	1	0	24	4	0
Sonoma								
Dried	7–8 pieces (1 oz)	90	2	1	0	19	2	0

KNISH
TAKE-OUT

cheese & blueberry	1 (7 oz)	378	24	13	40	40	–	–
cheese & cherry	1 (7 oz)	378	24	13	40	40	–	–
everything	1 (7 oz)	221	7	8	0	34	–	–
kashe	1 (7 oz)	270	7	8	0	45	–	–
potato	1 lg (7 oz)	332	8	12	72	49	1	470

FOOD	PORTION	CAL	PROT	FAT	CHOL	CARB	FIBER	SOD
potato	1 med (3.5 oz)	166	4	6	36	25	tr	235
potato w/ broccoli & cheese	1 (7 oz)	312	12	15	24	33	–	–
potato w/ spinach & mushroom	1 (7 oz)	214	6	8	0	32	–	–
KOHLRABI								
raw sliced	½ cup	19	1	tr	0	4	–	14
sliced cooked	½ cup	24	1	tr	0	5	–	17
KRILL								
fresh	1 oz	22	3	1	–	tr	0	119
KUMQUATS								
fresh	1	12	tr	tr	0	3	–	1
LAMB								
cubed lean only braised	3 oz	190	29	7	92	0	–	60
cubed lean only broiled	3 oz	158	24	6	77	0	–	65
ground broiled	3 oz	240	21	17	82	0	–	69
leg lean & fat Choice roasted	3 oz	219	22	14	79	14	–	56
loin chop w/ bone lean & fat Choice broiled	1 chop (2.3 oz)	201	16	15	64	0	–	49
new zealand lean & fat cooked	3 oz	259	21	19	93	0	–	39
new zealand lean only cooked	3 oz	175	25	8	93	0	–	43
rib chop lean & fat Choice broiled	3 oz	307	19	25	84	0	–	64
rib chop lean only Choice broiled	3 oz	200	24	11	78	0	–	73
shank lean & fat Choice braised	3 oz	206	24	11	90	0	–	61
shank lean & fat Choice roasted	3 oz	191	22	11	77	0	–	55
shoulder chop w/ bone lean & fat Choice braised	1 chop (2.5 oz)	244	21	17	84	0	–	51

FOOD	PORTION	CAL	PROT	FAT	CHOL	CARB	FIBER	SOD
sirloin lean & fat Choice roasted	3 oz	248	21	21	82	0	–	58

LAMB DISHES
TAKE-OUT

FOOD	PORTION	CAL	PROT	FAT	CHOL	CARB	FIBER	SOD
curry	¾ cup	345	26	17	89	22	–	258
moussaka	5.6 oz	312	15	21	–	16	1	–
stew	¾ cup	124	10	5	29	11	2	140

LAMBSQUARTERS

FOOD	PORTION	CAL	PROT	FAT	CHOL	CARB	FIBER	SOD
chopped cooked	½ cup	29	3	1	0	5	–	–

LEEKS

FOOD	PORTION	CAL	PROT	FAT	CHOL	CARB	FIBER	SOD
chopped cooked	¼ cup	8	tr	tr	0	2	–	3
cooked	1 (4.4 oz)	38	1	tr	0	9	–	13
freeze dried	1 tbsp	1	tr	0	0	tr	–	0
raw	1 (4.4 oz)	76	2	tr	0	18	–	25
raw chopped	¼ cup	16	tr	tr	0	4	–	5

LEMON

FOOD	PORTION	CAL	PROT	FAT	CHOL	CARB	FIBER	SOD
fresh	1 med	22	1	tr	0	12	–	3
peel	1 tbsp	0	tr	tr	0	1	–	0
wedge	1	5	tr	tr	0	3	–	1

LEMON CURD

FOOD	PORTION	CAL	PROT	FAT	CHOL	CARB	FIBER	SOD
lemon curd made w/ egg	2 tsp	29	tr	1	–	4	0	–
lemon curd made w/ starch	2 tsp	28	tr	–	–	6	0	–

LEMON EXTRACT
Virginia Dare

FOOD	PORTION	CAL	PROT	FAT	CHOL	CARB	FIBER	SOD
Extract	1 tsp	22	–	0	0	–	–	–

LEMON GRASS

FOOD	PORTION	CAL	PROT	FAT	CHOL	CARB	FIBER	SOD
fresh	1 tbsp (5 g)	5	tr	tr	0	1	0	tr
fresh	1 cup (2.4 oz)	66	1	tr	0	17	0	4

LEMON JUICE

FOOD	PORTION	CAL	PROT	FAT	CHOL	CARB	FIBER	SOD
bottled	1 tbsp	3	tr	tr	0	1	–	3
fresh	1 tbsp	4	tr	0	0	1	–	0
frzn	1 tbsp	3	tr	tr	0	1	–	0
After The Fall								
Spicy Lemon	1 can (12 oz)	150	tr	0	0	37	0	35

FOOD	PORTION	CAL	PROT	FAT	CHOL	CARB	FIBER	SOD
Canarino								
Italian Hot Lemon Beverage	1 cup	0	0	0	0	0	0	0
Realemon								
Juice	1 tsp (5 ml)	0	0	0	0	0	–	0
LEMONADE								
FROZEN								
as prep w/ water	1 cup	100	tr	tr	0	26	–	8
not prep	1 can (6 oz)	397	1	tr	0	103	–	8
MIX								
powder as prep w/ water	9 fl oz	113	0	tr	0	29	–	19
powder w/ equal	1 pitcher (67 oz)	40	tr	0	0	10	–	58
Country Time								
Lem'n Berry Sippers Raspberry Lemonade as prep	1 serv (8 oz)	90	0	0	0	21	0	0
Lem'n Berry Sippers Strawberry Lemonade as prep	1 serv (8 oz)	90	0	0	0	21	0	0
Lem'n Berry Sippers Wildberry Lemonade as prep	1 serv (8 oz)	90	0	0	0	21	0	0
Lemonade as prep	1 serv (8 oz)	70	0	0	0	17	0	15
Pink as prep	1 serv (8 oz)	70	0	0	0	17	0	15
Sugar Free Pink as prep	1 serv (8 oz)	5	0	0	0	0	0	0
Sugar Free as prep	1 serv (8 oz)	5	0	0	0	0	0	0
Crystal Light								
Lemonade as prep	1 serv (8 oz)	5	0	0	0	0	0	0
Pink as prep	1 serv (8 oz)	5	0	0	0	0	0	0
Kool-Aid								
Lemonade as prep	1 serv (8 oz)	70	0	0	0	17	0	0
Mix as prep w/ sugar	1 serv (8 oz)	100	0	0	0	25	0	10
Pink as prep w/ sugar	1 serv (8 oz)	100	0	0	0	25	0	10
Soarin' Strawberry Lemonade as prep	1 serv (8 oz)	70	0	0	0	17	0	15
Soarin' Strawberry Lemonade as prep w/ sugar	1 serv (8 oz)	100	0	0	0	25	0	0

FOOD	PORTION	CAL	PROT	FAT	CHOL	CARB	FIBER	SOD
Sugar Free Soarin' Strawberry Lemonade as prep	1 serv (8 oz)	5	0	0	0	0	0	0
Sugar Free Mix as prep	1 serv (8 oz)	5	0	0	0	0	0	0
READY-TO-DRINK								
After The Fall								
Apple Raspberry	1 bottle (10 oz)	120	1	0	0	29	—	15
Crystal Light								
Lemonade	1 serv (8 oz)	5	0	0	0	0	0	20
Pink	1 serv (8 oz)	5	0	0	0	0	0	20
Everfresh								
Lemonade	1 can (8 oz)	120	0	0	0	29	0	0
Ruby Red	1 can (8 oz)	110	0	0	0	27	0	0
Nantucket Nectars								
Authentic	8 oz	120	0	0	0	30	—	0
Pink	8 oz	120	0	0	0	30	—	0
Newman's Own								
Lemonade	1 bottle (10 oz)	140	0	0	0	34	0	45
Roadside Virginia	8 fl oz	110	0	0	0	27	0	40
Santa Cruz								
Organic	8 oz	100	0	0	0	24	—	0
Shasta Plus								
Lemonade	1 can (11.5 oz)	160	0	0	0	40	0	45
Snapple								
Diet Pink	8 fl oz	20	0	0	0	4	—	10
Lemonade	8 fl oz	120	0	0	0	30	—	10
Pink	8 fl oz	120	0	0	0	29	—	10
Turkey Hill								
Lemonade	1 cup	120	0	0	0	29	—	0
Raspberry	1 cup	120	—	0	0	29	—	—
Strawberry Kiwi	1 cup	120	—	0	0	29	—	—
Veryfine								
Chillers	1 can (11.5 oz)	190	0	0	0	48	0	15
Chillers Cherry	8 fl oz	120	0	0	0	29	0	15
Chillers Peach	8 fl oz	120	0	0	0	31	0	15
Chillers Pink	1 can (11.5 oz)	180	0	0	0	45	0	15
Chillers Strawberry	1 can (11.5 oz)	170	0	0	0	43	0	20

FOOD	PORTION	CAL	PROT	FAT	CHOL	CARB	FIBER	SOD
LENTILS								
dried cooked	1 cup	231	18	1	0	40	–	4
Natural Touch								
Lentil Rice Loaf	1 in slice (3.2 oz)	170	8	9	0	14	4	370
Shiloh Farms								
Organic Green not prep	¼ cup (1.6 oz)	150	11	0	0	27	7	15
TAKE-OUT								
indian sambar	1 serv	236	15	5	10	37	9	189
yemiser selatta eithopian lentil salad	1 serv (3 oz)	115	4	7	0	11	2	536
LETTUCE (*see also* SALAD)								
arugula	½ cup (0.4 oz)	3	tr	0	tr	tr	tr	3
bibb	1 head (6 oz)	21	2	tr	0	4	2	8
boston	2 leaves	2	tr	tr	0	tr	tr	1
boston	1 head (6 oz)	21	2	tr	0	4	2	8
cornsalad field salad	1 cup (1.9 oz)	7	1	tr	0	1	1	2
iceberg	1 leaf	3	tr	0	tr	tr	tr	2
iceberg	1 head (19 oz)	70	5	1	0	11	5	48
looseleaf shredded	½ cup	5	tr	tr	0	1	–	3
romaine shredded	½ cup	4	tr	tr	0	1	tr	2
Dole								
Iceberg	1 cup (3 oz)	15	1	0	0	3	1	10
Romaine	1½ cups (3 oz)	15	1	0	0	2	2	5
Shredded	1½ cup (3 oz)	15	1	0	0	3	1	10
Earthbound Farm								
Romaine Salad Organic	1½ cups (2.9 oz)	15	3	0	0	3	1	5
LILY ROOT								
dried	1 oz	89	2	1	–	21	tr	25
fresh	1 oz	32	1	tr	–	8	tr	3
LIMA BEANS								
CANNED								
large	1 cup	191	12	tr	0	36	–	809
lima beans	½ cup	93	6	tr	0	17	–	309
Del Monte								
Green	½ cup (4.4 oz)	80	4	0	0	15	4	390

FOOD	PORTION	CAL	PROT	FAT	CHOL	CARB	FIBER	SOD
Dennison's								
With Ham	7.5 oz	250	–	7	–	–	–	–
Eden								
Organic Baby	½ cup (4.6 oz)	100	6	1	0	17	4	35
S&W								
Small Green	½ cup (4.4 oz)	80	4	0	0	15	4	390
DRIED								
baby cooked	1 cup	229	15	1	0	42	17	5
cooked	½ cup	104	6	tr	0	20	–	14
large cooked	1 cup	217	15	1	0	39	14	4
Hurst								
HamBeens Baby Limas w/ Ham	1 serv	120	7	1	0	22	9	63
HamBeens Large Limas w/ Ham	1 serv	120	7	1	0	22	9	63
FROZEN								
cooked	½ cup	94	6	tr	0	18	–	26
fordhook cooked	½ cup	85	5	tr	0	16	–	45
Birds Eye								
Baby	½ cup	130	7	0	0	24	6	115
Fordhook	½ cup	100	6	0	0	19	5	10
Green Giant								
Butter Sauce	⅔ cup (3.6 oz)	120	6	3	<5	18	6	330
Harvest Fresh Baby	½ cup (2.7 oz)	80	4	0	0	15	4	130
LIME								
fresh	1	20	tr	tr	0	7	–	1
LIME JUICE								
bottled	1 tbsp	3	tr	tr	0	1	–	2
fresh	1 tbsp	4	tr	tr	0	1	–	0
After The Fall								
Caribbean Lime	1 can (12 oz)	170	2	0	0	42	0	25
Key West	1 cup (8 oz)	100	1	0	0	25	0	10
Realime								
Juice	1 tsp (5 ml)	0	0	0	0	0	–	0
LING								
blue raw	3.5 oz	83	17	1	–	0	–	–
fresh baked	3 oz	95	21	1	–	0	–	147
fresh fillet baked	5.3 oz	168	37	1	–	0	–	261

FOOD	PORTION	CAL	PROT	FAT	CHOL	CARB	FIBER	SOD
LINGCOD								
baked	3 oz	93	19	1	57	0	–	64
fillet baked	5.3 oz	164	34	2	101	0	–	114
LIQUOR/LIQUEUR *(see also* BEER AND ALE, CHAMPAGNE, DRINK MIXERS, MALT, WINE*)*								
anisette	⅔ oz	74	0	0	–	7	0	–
apricot brandy	⅔ oz	64	–	0	0	6	0	–
aquavit	1 oz	65	0	0	–	0	0	–
benedictine	⅔ oz	69	–	0	0	7	0	–
bloody mary	5 oz	116	1	tr	0	5	–	332
bourbon & soda	4 oz	105	0	0	0	0	–	16
coffee liqueur	1½ oz	174	0	tr	0	24	–	4
coffee w/ cream liqueur	1½ oz	154	1	7	–	10	–	43
cognac	1 oz	67	0	0	0	tr	0	–
cosmopolitan	1 (4 oz)	213	tr	tr	0	17	0	3
creme de menthe	1½ oz	186	0	tr	0	21	–	3
curacao liqueur	⅔ oz	54	–	0	0	6	0	–
daiquiri	2 oz	111	0	0	0	4	–	1
gin	1½ oz	110	0	0	0	0	–	1
gin & tonic	7.5 oz	171	0	0	0	16	–	10
gin ricky	4 oz	150	–	0	0	–	–	–
long island ice tea	1 serv (7.5 oz)	159	tr	0	0	14	0	12
manhattan	2 oz	128	0	0	0	2	–	2
martini	2½ oz	156	0	0	0	tr	–	2
mint julep	10 oz	210	–	0	0	3	0	–
old-fashioned	2½ oz	127	–	0	0	3	0	–
pina colada	4½ oz	262	1	3	0	40	–	9
planter's punch	3½ oz	175	–	0	0	–	–	–
rum	1½ oz	97	0	0	0	0	–	0
screwdriver	7 oz	174	1	tr	0	18	–	2
sloe gin fizz	2½ oz	132	0	0	0	4	0	1
tequila sunrise	5½ oz	189	1	tr	0	15	–	7
tom collins	7½ oz	121	tr	0	0	3	–	39
vodka	1½ oz	97	0	0	0	0	–	0
whiskey	1½ oz	105	0	0	0	tr	–	0
whiskey sour	3 oz	123	tr	tr	0	5	–	10
LIVER *(see also* PATÉ*)*								
beef braised	3 oz	137	21	4	331	3	–	59
beef pan-fried	3 oz	184	23	7	410	7	–	90

FOOD	PORTION	CAL	PROT	FAT	CHOL	CARB	FIBER	SOD
chicken stewed	1 cup (5 oz)	219	34	8	883	1	—	71
duck raw	1 (1.5 oz)	60	8	2	227	2	—	—
goose raw	1 (3.3 oz)	125	15	4	—	6	—	132
lamb braised	3 oz	187	26	7	426	2	—	48
lamb fried	3 oz	202	22	11	419	3	—	105
pork braised	3 oz	140	22	4	302	3	0	42
sheep raw	3.5 oz	131	21	4	—	0	—	95
turkey simmered	1 cup (5 oz)	237	34	8	876	5	—	89
veal braised	3 oz	140	18	6	477	2	—	45
veal fried	3 oz	208	25	10	280	3	—	112
Shady Brook								
Turkey	4 oz	160	23	5	530	—	—	110

LOBSTER

FOOD	PORTION	CAL	PROT	FAT	CHOL	CARB	FIBER	SOD
northern cooked	1 cup	142	30	1	104	2	—	551
northern cooked	3 oz	83	17	1	61	1	—	323
northern raw	3 oz	77	77	1	81	tr	—	—
northern raw	1 lobster (5.3 oz)	136	28	1	143	1	—	—
spiny steamed	3 oz	122	22	2	76	3	—	193
spiny steamed	1 (5.7 oz)	233	43	3	146	5	—	370
Progresso								
Lobster Sauce	½ cup (4.3 oz)	100	3	7	5	6	2	430
TAKE-OUT								
newburg	1 cup	485	46	27	455	13	—	127

LOGANBERRIES

FOOD	PORTION	CAL	PROT	FAT	CHOL	CARB	FIBER	SOD
frzn	1 cup	80	2	tr	0	19	—	1

LONGANS

FOOD	PORTION	CAL	PROT	FAT	CHOL	CARB	FIBER	SOD
fresh	1	2	tr	0	0	tr	—	0

LOQUATS

FOOD	PORTION	CAL	PROT	FAT	CHOL	CARB	FIBER	SOD
fresh	1	5	tr	tr	0	1	—	0

LOTUS

FOOD	PORTION	CAL	PROT	FAT	CHOL	CARB	FIBER	SOD
root raw sliced	10 slices	45	2	tr	0	14	—	33
root sliced cooked	10 slices	59	1	tr	0	14	—	40
seeds dried	1 oz	94	4	1	0	18	—	1
Eden								
Root	1 serv (0.3 oz)	35	1	0	0	8	2	25

LOX *(see SALMON)*

FOOD	PORTION	CAL	PROT	FAT	CHOL	CARB	FIBER	SOD
LUPINES								
dried cooked	1 cup	197	26	5	0	16	–	7
LYCHEES								
fresh	1	6	tr	tr	0	2	–	0
MACADAMIA NUTS								
dry roasted w/ salt	10–12 nuts (1 oz)	200	2	22	0	4	1	80
oil roasted	1 oz	204	2	22	0	4	–	3
Hawaiian Host								
Chocolate Covered	1 piece (0.5 oz)	53	1	6	2	8	tr	15
MacFarms of Hawaii								
Chocolate Covered	¼ cup (1.3 oz)	210	3	16	5	18	2	25
Dry Roasted Salted	¼ cup (1.3 oz)	220	3	23	0	4	3	65
Kona Coffee Dark Chocolate Covered	¼ cup (1.3 oz)	210	3	16	5	18	2	25
MACE								
ground	1 tsp	8	tr	1	0	1	–	1
MACKEREL								
CANNED								
jack	1 can (12.7 oz)	563	84	23	285	0	–	1368
jack	1 cup	296	44	12	150	0	–	720
DRIED								
Eden								
Bonito Flakes	2 tbsp	4	1	0	1	0	0	4
FRESH								
atlantic cooked	3 oz	223	20	15	64	0	–	71
atlantic raw	3 oz	174	16	12	60	0	–	76
jack baked	3 oz	171	22	9	51	0	–	94
jack fillet baked	6.2 oz	354	45	18	106	0	–	194
king baked	3 oz	114	22	2	58	0	–	172
king fillet baked	5.4 oz	207	40	4	105	0	–	312
pacific baked	3 oz	171	22	9	51	0	–	94
pacific fillet baked	6.2 oz	354	45	18	106	0	–	194
spanish cooked	3 oz	134	20	5	62	0	–	56
spanish cooked	1 fillet (5.1 oz)	230	34	9	107	0	–	96
spanish raw	3 oz	118	16	5	65	0	–	50

FOOD	PORTION	CAL	PROT	FAT	CHOL	CARB	FIBER	SOD
SMOKED								
atlantic	3.5 oz	296	19	24	93	0	–	384
MALANGA								
fresh	½ cup	137	2	tr	–	32	–	–
MALT								
nonalcoholic	12 fl oz	32	1	0	0	5	–	–
MALTED MILK								
chocolate as prep w/ milk	1 cup	229	9	9	34	30	–	172
chocolate flavor powder	3 heaping tsp (¾ oz)	79	1	1	1	18	–	53
natural flavor as prep w/ milk	1 cup	237	10	10	37	27	–	223
natural flavor powder	3 heaping tsp (¾ oz)	87	2	2	4	19	–	103
Carnation								
Chocolate	3 tbsp (0.7 oz)	90	1	1	0	18	tr	40
Original	3 tbsp (0.7 oz)	90	3	2	5	15	tr	40
MAMMY-APPLE								
fresh	1	431	4	4	0	106	–	127
MANGO								
fresh	1	135	1	1	0	35	–	4
Del Monte								
In Extra Light Syrup	½ cup (4.4 oz)	100	0	1	0	25	0	5
Rainforest Farms								
Slices Dried	6 slices (1.3 oz)	140	1	1	0	33	2	108
Sonoma								
Pieces Dried	8 pieces (2 oz)	180	0	1	0	44	0	50
MANGO JUICE								
After The Fall								
Hawaiian Mango	1 can (12 oz)	180	0	0	0	45	0	20
Mango Ginger	1 can (12 oz)	150	tr	0	0	35	0	25
Fresh Samantha								
Mango Mama	1 cup (8 oz)	120	2	0	0	10	8	0
Guzzler								
Mango Passion	8 fl oz	140	0	0	0	22	–	30

FOOD	PORTION	CAL	PROT	FAT	CHOL	CARB	FIBER	SOD
Ocean Spray								
Mango Mango	8 oz	130	0	0	0	33	0	35
Snapple								
Mango Madness	8 fl oz	110	0	0	0	29	–	10
Tang								
Drink Mix as prep	1 serv (8 oz)	100	0	0	0	25	0	0
MARGARINE								
Benecol								
Single Serve Light	1 pkg (0.3 oz)	30	–	3	0	–	–	65
Tub Light	1 tbsp (0.5 oz)	45	–	5	0	–	–	110
Tub Regular	1 tbsp (0.5 oz)	80	–	9	0	–	–	110
I Can't Believe Its Not Butter								
Tub	1 tbsp	90	–	10	0	–	–	–
Krona								
Stick	1 tbsp	100	–	11	15	–	–	–
Mother's								
Stick Unsalted	1 tbsp	100	–	11	0	–	–	–
Sticks	1 tbsp	100	–	11	0	–	–	–
Tub Salted	1 tbsp	100	–	11	0	–	–	–
Tub Unsalted	1 tbsp	100	–	11	0	–	–	–
Promise								
Spread Soft	1 tbsp	80	–	8	0	–	–	–
Spread Stick	1 tbsp	90	–	10	0	–	–	–
Spread Light Soft	1 tbsp	50	–	6	0	–	–	–
Spread Light Stick	1 tbsp	50	–	6	0	–	–	–
Ultra Soft	1 tbsp	30	–	4	0	–	–	–
Ultra Spread Fat Free	1 tbsp	5	–	0	0	–	–	–
Smart Balance								
No Trans Fat	1 tbsp (0.5 oz)	120	0	14	0	0	–	0
No Trans Fat Light	1 tbsp (0.5 oz)	45	0	5	0	0	–	100
No Trans Fat Spread	1 tbsp (0.5 oz)	80	0	9	0	0	–	90
Smart Beat								
Light Unsalted	1 tbsp (0.5 oz)	25	0	3	0	0	–	0
Squeeze Fat Free	1 tbsp (0.5 oz)	5	0	0	0	1	–	100
Super Light Trans Fat Free	1 tbsp (0.5 oz)	20	0	2	0	0	–	105
Take Control								
Spread	1 tbsp (0.5 oz)	50	0	6	<5	0	0	110

FOOD	PORTION	CAL	PROT	FAT	CHOL	CARB	FIBER	SOD
Weight Watchers								
Light	1 tbsp	45	0	4	0	2	0	70
Light Sodium Free	1 tbsp	45	0	4	0	2	0	0
MARINADE *(see SAUCE)*								
MARJORAM								
dried	1 tsp	2	tr	tr	0	tr	–	tr
MARLIN								
raw	3 oz	110	20	3	–	0	0	–
MARSHMALLOW								
marshmallow	1 reg (0.3 oz)	23	tr	0	0	6	–	3
marshmallow	1 cup (1.6 oz)	146	1	tr	0	37	–	22
Just Born								
Peeps	5 (1.5 oz)	160	1	0	0	40	–	15
MATZO								
egg	1 (1 oz)	111	4	1	–	22	1	6
egg & onion	1 (1 oz)	111	3	1	–	22	1	81
plain	1 (1 oz)	112	3	tr	0	24	1	0
whole wheat	1 (1 oz)	99	4	tr	0	22	3	1
Manischewitz								
Matzo Meal	¼ cup (1 oz)	130	3	0	0	23	1	0
MAYONNAISE								
mayonnaise	1 tbsp	99	tr	11	8	tr	–	78
mayonnaise	1 cup	1577	2	175	130	6	–	1250
reduced calorie	1 cup	556	1	46	58	38	–	1193
reduced calorie	1 tbsp	34	0	3	4	2	–	75
sandwich spread	1 tbsp	60	tr	5	12	3	–	–
Blue Plate								
Squeeze	1 tbsp	100	0	11	10	0	0	80
Hellman's								
Mayonnaise	1 tbsp	100	0	11	5	0	–	80
Kraft								
Fat Free	1 tbsp (0.6 oz)	10	0	0	0	2	0	120
Light	1 tbsp (0.5 oz)	50	0	5	5	2	0	90
Real	1 tbsp (0.5 oz)	100	0	11	5	0	0	75
Mother's								
Mayonnaise	1 tbsp	100	–	11	10	–	–	–

FOOD	PORTION	CAL	PROT	FAT	CHOL	CARB	FIBER	SOD
Smart Beat								
Fat Free	1 tbsp	10	0	0	0	3	–	135
Weight Watchers								
Fat Free	1 tbsp	10	0	0	0	3	0	105
Light	1 tbsp	25	0	2	5	1	0	130
Light Low Sodium	1 tbsp	25	0	2	5	1	0	40

MAYONNAISE TYPE SALAD DRESSING

FOOD	PORTION	CAL	PROT	FAT	CHOL	CARB	FIBER	SOD
home recipe	1 tbsp	25	1	2	–	2	–	117
home recipe	1 cup	400	11	24	–	38	–	1872
mayonnaise type salad dressing	1 cup	916	2	78	60	56	–	1670
mayonnaise type salad dressing	1 tbsp	57	tr	5	4	4	–	–
reduced calorie w/o cholesterol	1 tbsp	68	7	7	0	2	–	49
reduced calorie w/o cholesterol	1 cup	1084	tr	107	0	36	–	794
Miracle Whip								
Free	1 tbsp (0.5 oz)	15	0	0	0	2	0	125
Light	1 tbsp (0.5 oz)	35	0	3	<5	2	0	130
Salad Dressing	1 tbsp (0.6 oz)	70	0	7	5	2	0	95
Nasoya								
Nayonaise	1 tbsp	35	0	4	0	1	0	115
Nayonaise Dijon	1 tbsp	30	0	3	0	1	0	140
Weight Watchers								
Fat Free Whipped Dressing	1 tbsp	15	0	0	0	3	0	95

MEAT STICKS

FOOD	PORTION	CAL	PROT	FAT	CHOL	CARB	FIBER	SOD
jerky beef	1 lg piece (0.7 oz)	67	8	3	22	3	–	569
jerky beef	1 oz	96	11	4	32	4	–	815
smoked	1 oz	156	6	14	38	2	–	420
smoked	1 (0.7 oz)	109	4	10	26	1	–	293
Big Ones								
BBQ	1 (1 oz)	130	5	12	35	1	0	680
Hot n'Spicy	1 (1 oz)	130	6	12	35	1	0	580
Original	1 (1 oz)	130	5	12	35	1	0	620
Teriyaki	1 (1 oz)	130	6	12	35	2	0	440

FOOD	PORTION	CAL	PROT	FAT	CHOL	CARB	FIBER	SOD
Jack Link's								
Kippered Beefsteak Teriyaki	1 oz	80	13	1	25	5	0	440
Lance								
Beef & Cheese	1 pkg (1.5 oz)	150	9	11	45	3	0	630
Beef Jerky	1 piece (0.25 oz)	30	2	2	<5	tr	0	160
Beef Snack	1 piece (0.63 oz)	100	4	8	10	1	0	290
Hot Sausage	1 piece (0.9 oz)	60	4	5	15	1	0	540
Lowrey's								
Smokehouse Tender Hickory Smoked	1 pkg (1 oz)	80	10	2	25	5	0	710
Smokehouse Tender Original	1 pkg (1 oz)	60	11	1	25	2	1	750
Smokehouse Tender Peppered	1 pkg (1 oz)	60	11	1	25	2	1	720
Oberto								
Beef Jerky	1 pkg (1.3 oz)	100	15	1	25	8	–	780
Pemmican								
Original Tender Kippered Beef Steak	1	110	12	5	35	3	0	1100
Peppered Tender Kippered Beef Steak	1	110	12	5	35	3	0	1170
Rough Cut								
Beef Steak Hot	1 pkg (1 oz)	70	10	1	25	2	0	710
Beef Steak Original	1 pkg (1 oz)	60	10	1	25	2	0	730
Beef Steak Peppered	1 pkg (1 oz)	60	10	1	25	2	0	740
Rustlers Roundup								
Beef Jerky	1 serv (5 g)	20	2	2	5	tr	tr	115
Flamin' Hot	1 serv (8 g)	40	2	3	10	1	tr	140
Smoky Steak	1 serv (0.8 oz)	60	8	2	20	1	0	580
Spicy	1 serv (0.5 oz)	70	3	6	20	1	tr	250
Slim Jim								
Spicy	1 (4½ in) (0.3 oz)	50	2	4	5	0	0	125
Spicy Big	1 (.44 oz)	70	1	6	10	1	0	190
Spicy Giant	1 (0.97 oz)	150	6	14	15	2	1	410
Spicy Super	1 (0.64 oz)	100	4	9	10	1	0	260

FOOD	PORTION	CAL	PROT	FAT	CHOL	CARB	FIBER	SOD

MEAT SUBSTITUTES *(see also* BACON SUBSTITUTES, CANADIAN BACON SUBSTITUTES, CHICKEN SUBSTITUTES, HAMBURGER SUBSTITUTES, SAUSAGE SUBSTITUTES, TURKEY SUBSTITUTES*)*

FOOD	PORTION	CAL	PROT	FAT	CHOL	CARB	FIBER	SOD
simulated meat product	1 oz	88	11	1	0	11	–	3
Amy's Organic								
Whole Meals Veggie Loaf	1 pkg (10 oz)	260	8	5	0	47	7	690
Boca Burgers								
Chef Max's Original	1 patty (2.5 oz)	110	14	2	3	9	4	296
Frieda's								
SoyTaco	1 oz	50	4	3	0	3	2	180
Soyrizo	4 tbsp (1.9 oz)	120	7	9	0	5	3	440
Ken & Robert's								
Veggie Pockets	1 (4.5 oz)	250	8	8	0	40	5	490
Veggie Pockets Bar B Que	1 (4.5 oz)	290	10	8	0	45	5	450
Veggie Pockets Broccoli & Cheddar	1 (4.5 oz)	250	9	8	0	38	4	490
Veggie Pockets Greek	1 (4.5 oz)	250	10	8	0	37	4	450
Veggie Pockets Indian	1 (4.5 oz)	260	8	8	0	40	5	490
Veggie Pockets Pizza	1 (4.5 oz)	270	9	8	0	41	4	490
Veggie Pockets Pot Pie	1 (4.5 oz)	250	8	9	0	38	2	410
Veggie Pockets Potato & Cheddar	1 (4.5 oz)	260	6	8	0	42	2	370
Veggie Pockets Santa Fe	1 (4.5 oz)	250	8	8	0	39	5	550
Veggie Pockets Tex Mex	1 (4.5 oz)	260	9	8	0	46	6	490
Lightlife								
Foney Baloney	3 slices (1.5 oz)	60	8	3	0	2	0	240
Gimme Lean Beef	2 oz	70	9	0	0	8	1	240
Smart Deli Bologna	3 slices (1.5 oz)	50	10	0	0	2	0	300
Smart Deli Ham	3 slices (1.5 oz)	50	10	0	0	2	0	300
Smart Deli Peppercorn	3 slices (1.5 oz)	45	10	0	0	1	0	300
Smart Deli Sticks Pepperoni	1 oz	45	9	0	0	2	0	300

FOOD	PORTION	CAL	PROT	FAT	CHOL	CARB	FIBER	SOD
Smart Deli Sticks Soylami	1 oz	40	9	0	0	1	0	280
Smart Ground Original	⅓ cup (1.9 oz)	70	12	0	0	5	3	180
Smart Ground Taco	⅓ cup (2 oz)	60	10	0	0	6	3	170
Loma Linda								
Dinner Cuts	2 slices (3.2 oz)	90	17	2	0	3	2	500
Nuteena	⅜ in slice (1.9 oz)	160	6	13	0	6	2	120
Sandwich Spread	¼ cup (1.9 oz)	80	4	5	0	7	3	260
Savory Dinner Loaf Mix not prep	⅓ cup (0.9 oz)	90	14	2	0	7	5	560
Swiss Stake	1 piece (3.2 oz)	120	9	6	0	8	4	430
Tender Bits	6 pieces (3 oz)	110	11	5	0	7	3	440
Tender Rounds	6 pieces (2.8 oz)	120	14	5	0	5	3	330
Vita Burger Chunks not prep	¼ cup (0.7 oz)	70	10	1	0	6	3	350
Vita Burger Granules	3 tbsp (0.7 oz)	70	10	1	0	6	3	350
Morningstar Farms								
Burger Style Recipe Crumbles	⅔ cup (1.9 oz)	80	10	3	0	4	2	210
Ground Meatless	½ cup (1.9 oz)	60	10	0	0	4	2	260
Harvest Burger Recipe Crumbles	½ cup (2 oz)	70	12	0	0	5	3	200
Quarter Prime	1 patty (3.4 oz)	140	24	2	0	6	3	370
Natural Touch								
Dinner Entree	1 patty (3 oz)	220	19	15	0	2	2	380
Loaf Mix not prep	4 tbsp (1 oz)	100	14	1	0	10	7	700
Stroganoff Mix not prep	4 tbsp (0.8 oz)	90	5	4	10	10	3	610
Taco Mix not prep	3 tbsp (0.6 oz)	60	8	1	0	5	3	590
Vegan Burger Crumbles	½ cup (1.9 oz)	60	10	0	0	4	2	260
Quorn								
Grounds	⅔ cup (3 oz)	80	13	3	0	5	4	220
Soy Is Us								
Beef Not!	½ cup (1.75 oz)	140	25	2	0	15	9	5
Veggie Patch								
Veggie Rounds	1 (2.5 oz)	120	12	3	0	15	4	250
Veggitinos Meatballs	5 (2.8 oz)	120	13	4	0	10	3	470

FOOD	PORTION	CAL	PROT	FAT	CHOL	CARB	FIBER	SOD
Worthington								
Beef Style Meatless	⅜ in slice (1.9 oz)	110	9	7	0	4	3	620
Bolono	3 slices (2 oz)	80	10	4	0	2	2	720
Choplets	2 slices (3.2 oz)	90	17	2	0	3	2	500
Corned Beef Meatless	4 slices (2 oz)	140	10	9	0	5	2	520
Country Stew	1 cup (8.4 oz)	210	13	9	0	20	5	830
Dinner Roast	¾ in slice (3 oz)	180	12	12	<5	5	3	580
FriPats	1 patty (2.2 oz)	130	14	6	0	4	3	320
Multigrain Cutlets	2 slices (3.2 oz)	100	15	2	0	5	4	390
Numete	⅜ in slice (1.9 oz)	130	6	10	0	5	3	270
Prime Stakes	1 piece (3.2 oz)	120	10	7	0	4	4	440
Prosage Roll	⅝ in slice (1.9 oz)	140	10	10	0	2	2	390
Protose	⅜ in slice (1.9 oz)	130	13	7	0	5	3	280
Salami Meatless	3 slices (2 oz)	130	12	8	0	2	2	930
Savory Slices	3 slices (2.9 oz)	150	10	9	0	6	3	540
Smoked Beef Meatless	6 slices (2 oz)	120	11	6	0	6	3	730
Stakelets	1 piece (2.5 oz)	140	12	8	0	6	2	480
Veelets	1 patty (2.5 oz)	180	14	9	0	10	5	390
Vegetable Skallops	½ cup (3 oz)	90	15	2	0	3	2	410
Vegetable Steaks	2 pieces (2.5 oz)	80	15	2	0	3	3	300
Wham	2 slices (1.6 oz)	80	7	5	0	1	0	430
Yves								
Veggie Bologna	4 slices (2.2 oz)	70	15	0	0	2	0	460
Veggie Ground Italian	⅓ cup (2 oz)	60	10	0	0	4	3	270
Veggie Ground Round Italian	⅓ cup (1.9 oz)	60	10	0	0	4	3	270
Veggie Ground Round Original	2 oz	60	10	0	0	4	3	270
Veggie Pizza Pepperoni Slices	1 serv (1.7 oz)	70	14	0	0	4	3	480
Veggie Salami Deli Slices	1 serv (2.2 oz)	90	17	0	0	5	1	390
MELON								
melon balls frzn	1 cup	55	1	tr	0	14	—	53

FOOD	PORTION	CAL	PROT	FAT	CHOL	CARB	FIBER	SOD
Sunfresh								
Melon Salad In Extra Light Syrup	½ cup (4.5 oz)	45	0	0	0	10	2	15

MELON JUICE
Ocean Spray

Mega Melon	8 oz	130	0	0	0	33	0	35

MEXICAN FOOD *(see SALSA, SAUCE, SPANISH FOODS, TORTILLA)*

MILK
CANNED

FOOD	PORTION	CAL	PROT	FAT	CHOL	CARB	FIBER	SOD
condensed sweetened	1 oz	123	3	3	13	21	—	49
condensed sweetened	1 cup	982	24	27	104	166	—	389
evaporated	½ cup	169	9	10	37	13	—	122
evaporated skim	½ cup	99	10	tr	5	14	—	147
Carnation								
Evaporated	½ cup	150	2	8	10	3	—	30
Evaporated Fat Free	½ cup (4 fl oz)	100	9	0	0	4	—	40
Evaporated Lowfat	½ cup	110	2	2	5	3	—	35
Sweetened Condensed	⅓ cup	330	3	8	10	22	0	45
DRIED								
buttermilk	1 tbsp	25	2	tr	5	3	—	34
nonfat instantized	1 pkg (3.2 oz)	244	32	tr	12	47	—	499
Carnation								
Nonfat	⅓ cup	80	8	0	<5	12	0	125
Saco								
Cultured Buttermilk	4 tbsp (0.8 oz)	80	5	tr	4	13	0	166
Sanalac								
Powder	¼ cup (0.8 oz)	85	8	tr	6	13	0	117
REFRIGERATED								
1%	1 cup	102	8	3	10	12	—	123
1%	1 qt	409	32	10	39	47	—	493
1% protein fortified	1 qt	477	39	12	39	54	—	574
1% protein fortified	1 cup	119	10	3	10	14	—	143
2%	1 cup	121	8	5	18	12	—	122
2%	1 qt	485	33	19	73	47	—	487
buffalo	7 oz	224	8	16	—	10	—	80

FOOD	PORTION	CAL	PROT	FAT	CHOL	CARB	FIBER	SOD
buttermilk	1 cup	99	8	2	9	12	–	257
buttermilk	1 qt	396	32	9	34	47	–	1028
camel	7 oz	160	10	8	–	10	–	60
donkey	7 oz	86	4	2	–	12	–	–
goat	1 cup	168	9	10	28	11	–	122
goat	1 qt	672	35	40	111	43	–	486
human	1 cup	171	3	11	34	17	–	42
indian buffalo	1 cup	236	9	17	46	13	–	127
low sodium	1 cup	149	8	8	33	11	–	6
mare	7 oz	98	4	4	–	12	–	–
nonfat	1 cup	86	8	tr	4	12	–	125
nonfat	1 qt	342	33	2	18	48	–	505
nonfat protein fortified	1 qt	400	39	2	20	55	–	578
nonfat protein fortified	1 cup	100	10	1	5	14	–	144
sheep	1 cup	264	15	17	–	13	–	108
whole	1 cup	150	8	8	33	11	–	120
Cool Cow								
Low Fat	1 cup (8 oz)	110	9	3	<5	12	0	125
Farmland								
Skim Plus	1 cup (8 oz)	110	11	0	<5	17	0	170
Horizon Organic								
Fat Free	1 cup (8 oz)	80	8	0	4	12	0	125
Land O Lakes								
1% Lowfat	1 carton (10 oz)	120	10	3	15	13	–	135
Fat Free	1 carton (10 oz)	100	10	5	5	13	–	140
Whole	1 carton (10 oz)	180	10	10	45	13	–	135
NutraBalance								
LactaCare	1 pkg (8 oz)	500	18	18	0	64	–	240
Organic Valley								
Low Fat	1 cup	100	8	3	10	12	0	120
Nonfat	1 cup	80	8	0	5	13	0	125
Reduced Fat	1 cup	130	8	5	20	12	0	120
Whole	1 cup	150	8	8	30	12	0	120
Stonyfield Farm								
Organic Whole Milk	1 cup (8 oz)	180	9	10	40	12	0	125
Organic Whole Milk Vanilla	1 cup (8 oz)	230	8	8	30	30	0	130

FOOD	PORTION	CAL	PROT	FAT	CHOL	CARB	FIBER	SOD
Turkey Hill								
Cool Moos 2% Reduced Fat	1 cup	130	8	5	20	12	–	120
Cool Moos Whole Milk	1 cup	160	8	8	35	12	–	120
MILK DRINKS								
chocolate milk	1 cup	208	8	8	30	26	–	149
chocolate milk	1 qt	833	32	34	122	103	–	596
chocolate milk 1%	1 cup	158	8	3	7	26	–	152
chocolate milk 1%	1 qt	630	32	10	29	104	–	607
chocolate milk 2%	1 cup	179	8	5	17	26	–	150
strawberry flavor mix as prep w/ whole milk	9 oz	234	8	8	33	33	–	128
Horizon Organic								
Lowfat Chocolate Milk	1 cup (8 oz)	160	9	3	10	26	1	200
Land O Lakes								
Chocolate	1 cup (8.4 oz)	200	8	7	30	27	0	180
Organic Valley								
Chocolate Milk Reduced Fat	1 cup	180	8	5	10	26	0	190
Quik								
Banana Lowfat	1 cup (8.4 oz)	200	7	5	20	31	0	95
Banana Powder	2 tbsp (0.8 oz)	90	0	0	0	27	0	0
Chocolate	1 cup (8.4 oz)	230	7	8	30	33	1	130
Chocolate Lowfat	1 carton (8.4 oz)	200	8	5	20	30	0	130
Cookies n Cream Powder	2 tbsp (0.8 oz)	100	1	1	0	21	1	190
Strawberry	1 cup (8.4 oz)	230	7	8	30	33	0	100
Strawberry Lowfat	1 carton (8.4 oz)	210	8	5	20	35	0	100
Strawberry Powder	2 tbsp (0.8 oz)	90	0	0	0	22	0	0
Turkey Hill								
Cool Moos Chocolate 1% Lowfat	1 cup	180	8	3	10	32	–	180
Cool Moos Orange Cream 1% Lowfat	1 cup	190	8	3	10	33	–	135
Cool Moos Strawberry 1% Lowfat	1 cup	160	8	3	10	27	–	125
Cool Moos Vanilla 1% Lowfat	1 cup	160	8	3	10	26	–	125

FOOD	PORTION	CAL	PROT	FAT	CHOL	CARB	FIBER	SOD
MILK SUBSTITUTES *(see also* COFFEE WHITENERS*)*								
imitation milk	1 cup	150	4	8	tr	15	–	191
imitation milk	1 qt	600	17	33	2	60	–	764
8th Continent								
Soymilk Low Fat Chocolate	1 bottle (8 oz)	140	7	3	0	23	1	190
Soymilk Low Fat Original	1 bottle (8 oz)	80	7	3	0	8	tr	170
Soymilk Low Fat Vanilla	1 bottle (8 oz)	90	7	3	0	11	tr	170
Better Than Milk								
Rice Original	2 tbsp (0.66 oz)	78	0	2	0	15	1	150
Rice Original Light	2 tbsp (0.66 oz)	66	0	0	0	17	1	144
Rice Vanilla	2 tbsp (0.66 oz)	78	0	2	0	15	1	118
Rice Vanilla Light	2 tbsp (0.66 oz)	66	0	0	0	17	1	141
Soy Carob	2 tbsp (1 oz)	90	3	2	0	18	2	165
Soy Chocolate	2 tbsp (1.1 oz)	112	3	2	0	21	1	146
Soy Light	2 tbsp (0.66 oz)	73	6	2	0	8	1	139
Soy Original	2 tbsp (0.8 oz)	100	2	3	0	16	0	100
Soy Vanilla	2 tbsp (0.7 oz)	77	6	2	0	8	1	178
Blue Diamond								
Almond Breeze Chocolate	8 oz	120	1	3	0	21	1	160
Almond Breeze Original	8 oz	60	1	2	0	8	1	150
Almond Breeze Vanilla	8 oz	90	1	3	0	15	1	150
EdenBlend								
Organic	8 oz	120	7	3	0	18	0	85
Edensoy								
Organic Light	8 oz	93	5	2	0	14	0	84
Organic Light Vanilla	8 oz	120	4	2	0	21	0	87
Galaxy								
Veggi Milk Chocolate	1 cup (8 oz)	150	9	2	0	26	1	130
Veggie Milk Original	1 cup (8 oz)	110	9	3	0	13	2	130
Harmony Farms								
Original Rice Beverage	1 cup (8 oz)	90	13	0	0	21	0	100

FOOD	PORTION	CAL	PROT	FAT	CHOL	CARB	FIBER	SOD
Harmony House								
Enriched Rice Beverage	1 cup (8 oz)	90	1	0	0	21	0	100
Enriched Soy Beverage	1 cup (8 oz)	90	13	0	0	21	0	100
Original Soy Beverage	1 cup (8 oz)	90	13	0	0	21	0	100
Health Valley								
Soo Moo	1 cup	110	6	0	0	22	1	60
NutraBalance								
NuTaste	1 pkg (8 oz)	80	8	2	0	7	8	210
Rice Dream								
Carob	1 box (8 oz)	150	1	3	0	32	0	100
Chocolate	1 box (8 oz)	170	1	3	0	36	2	115
Chocolate Enriched	1 box (8 oz)	170	1	3	0	36	0	115
Organic Original	1 box (8 oz)	120	1	2	0	25	0	90
Organic Original Enriched	1 box (8 oz)	120	1	2	0	25	0	90
Vanilla	1 box (8 oz)	130	1	2	0	28	0	90
Vanilla Enriched	1 box (8 oz)	130	1	2	0	28	0	90
Silk								
Organic Chocolate	1 cup (8.3 oz)	108	5	3	0	17	1	95
Organic Plain	1 cup	100	7	4	0	8	0	75
Soy Dream								
Carob	8 oz	210	7	5	–	36	–	150
Chocolate Enriched	8 oz	210	7	5	–	35	–	150
Original	8 oz	140	8	5	–	14	–	140
Original Enriched	8 oz	140	8	5	–	14	–	140
Vanilla	8 oz	170	8	5	–	23	–	140
Vanilla Enriched	8 oz	140	8	5	–	23	–	160
Tree Of Life								
Original Rice Beverage	1 cup	90	13	0	0	21	0	100
Vitamite								
Non-Dairy 2% Fat	1 cup (8 oz)	110	3	5	0	14	0	120
Non-Diary Nonfat	1 cup (8 oz)	90	1	0	0	21	0	70
Vitasoy								
1% Low Fat Vanilla Delight	8 oz	90	4	2	0	13	0	120

FOOD	PORTION	CAL	PROT	FAT	CHOL	CARB	FIBER	SOD
Carob Supreme	8 fl oz	150	8	5	0	20	tr	180
Creamy Unsweetened	8 oz	80	6	4	0	5	0	150
Creamy Original	8 fl oz	110	9	5	0	9	1	150
Enriched Light Original	8 fl oz	60	4	2	0	7	0	115
Enriched Light Vanilla	8 fl oz	90	4	2	0	13	0	105
Green Tea Soymilk	8 oz	130	7	4	0	16	1	180
Original Creamy	8 fl oz	110	7	4	0	12	1	140
Original Light	8 fl oz	60	4	2	0	7	0	115
Rich Chocolate	8 fl oz	160	7	4	0	24	1	180
Rich Cocoa	8 fl oz	150	8	5	0	21	1	180
Vanilla Light	8 fl oz	90	4	2	0	14	0	110
Vanilla Delite	8 fl oz	120	7	4	0	14	1	115

MILKFISH

FOOD	PORTION	CAL	PROT	FAT	CHOL	CARB	FIBER	SOD
baked	3 oz	162	22	7	57	0	–	–

MILKSHAKE

FOOD	PORTION	CAL	PROT	FAT	CHOL	CARB	FIBER	SOD
chocolate	10 oz	360	10	11	37	58	–	273
strawberry	10 oz	319	10	8	31	53	–	234
thick shake chocolate	10.6 oz	356	9	8	32	63	–	333
thick shake vanilla	11 oz	350	12	10	37	56	–	299
vanilla	10 oz	314	10	8	32	51	–	232

D'Frosta Shake

FOOD	PORTION	CAL	PROT	FAT	CHOL	CARB	FIBER	SOD
Vanilla	1 serv (13.5 oz)	340	11	9	40	57	1	200

Freeze Flip

FOOD	PORTION	CAL	PROT	FAT	CHOL	CARB	FIBER	SOD
Fruit Shake No Fat Lactose Free Black Raspberry	1 serv (6 oz)	150	1	0	0	37	1	25

MILLET

FOOD	PORTION	CAL	PROT	FAT	CHOL	CARB	FIBER	SOD
cooked	1 cup (6.1 oz)	207	6	2	0	41	2	3

MINERAL WATER (see WATER)

MISO

FOOD	PORTION	CAL	PROT	FAT	CHOL	CARB	FIBER	SOD
dried	1 oz	86	7	3	–	10	1	2130
miso	½ cup	284	16	8	0	39	7	5036

Eden

FOOD	PORTION	CAL	PROT	FAT	CHOL	CARB	FIBER	SOD
Organic Genmai	1 tbsp	25	2	1	0	3	tr	810
Tekka	1 tsp	5	tr	0	0	tr	0	70

FOOD	PORTION	CAL	PROT	FAT	CHOL	CARB	FIBER	SOD
MOLASSES								
blackstrap	1 tbsp (0.7 oz)	47	0	0	0	12	–	11
blackstrap	1 cup (11.5 oz)	771	0	tr	0	199	–	180
molasses	1 tbsp (0.7 oz)	53	0	0	0	14	–	7
molasses	1 cup (11.5 oz)	873	0	1	0	226	–	120
Brer Rabbit								
Dark	1 tbsp	60	0	0	0	16	–	30
Mott's								
Sulphured	1 tbsp	50	0	0	0	12	–	10
Unsulphured	1 tbsp	50	0	0	0	14	–	0
MONKFISH								
baked	3 oz	82	16	2	27	0	–	20
MOOSE								
roasted	3 oz	114	25	1	66	0	–	58
MOTH BEANS								
dried cooked	1 cup	207	14	1	0	37	–	17
MOUSSE								
FROZEN								
Sara Lee								
Chocolate	⅓ pkg (4.3 oz)	400	5	25	30	37	2	190
Weight Watchers								
Chocolate Mousse	1 (2.75 oz)	190	6	5	5	31	3	150
TAKE-OUT								
chocolate	½ cup (7.1 oz)	447	9	33	299	33	–	87
orange	½ cup	87	3	5	1	19	–	24
MUFFIN								
FROZEN								
Pepperidge Farm								
Blueberry	1 (2 oz)	180	2	7	30	28	0	260
Bran w/ Raisins	1 (2 oz)	180	4	6	25	30	0	310
Corn	1 (2 oz)	190	3	7	30	28	0	270
Orange Cranberry	1 (2 oz)	180	2	6	36	29	0	190
Sara Lee								
Blueberry	1 (2.2 oz)	220	3	11	15	27	tr	170
Blueberry	1 (2.2 oz)	220	3	11	15	27	tr	170
Corn	1 (2.2 oz)	260	3	14	25	30	1	220

FOOD	PORTION	CAL	PROT	FAT	CHOL	CARB	FIBER	SOD
Weight Watchers								
Chocolate Chocolate Chip	1 (2.5 oz)	190	3	2	0	39	4	350
Fat Free Banana	1 (2.5 oz)	170	3	0	0	41	3	310
Fat Free Blueberry	1 (2.5 oz)	160	3	0	0	38	2	290
MIX								
blueberry	1 (1¾ oz)	149	3	4	23	24	—	219
corn	1 (1.75 oz)	160	4	5	31	25	—	397
wheat bran as prep	1 (1¾ oz)	138	5	5	34	23	—	233
Betty Crocker								
Apple Cinnamon as prep	1	170	1	7	36	23	—	200
Apple Streusel as prep	1	210	2	8	18	33	—	210
Banana Nut as prep	1	170	2	6	18	27	1	240
Cranberry Orange as prep	1	150	2	5	18	25	—	150
Double Chocolate as prep	1	220	2	11	27	30	—	210
Golden Corn as prep	1	160	2	5	36	24	—	210
Lemon Poppyseed as prep	1	180	1	8	36	24	—	180
Sunkist Lemon Poppyseed as prep	1	190	2	7	18	29	—	230
Twice The Blueberries as prep	1	140	2	3	18	25	1	180
Wild Blueberry as prep	1	170	2	5	18	28	tr	270
Gold Medal								
Corn	1	160	3	6	35	25	0	270
Hodgson Mill								
Bran	¼ cup (1.3 oz)	130	4	1	0	27	3	150
Cornbread	¼ cup (1.3 oz)	130	4	1	0	28	3	240
Whole Wheat	¼ cup (1.3 oz)	130	4	1	0	27	3	560
Robin Hood								
Apple Cinnamon	1	170	3	8	35	23	0	220
Banana Nut	1	170	3	8	35	21	0	190
Blueberry	1	160	3	6	35	24	0	220
Caramel Nut	1	170	3	7	35	24	0	230

FOOD	PORTION	CAL	PROT	FAT	CHOL	CARB	FIBER	SOD
Sweet Rewards								
Low Fat Apple Cinnamon as prep	1	140	2	2	16	26	—	180
READY-TO-EAT								
blueberry	1 (2 oz)	158	3	4	17	27	2	255
corn	1 (2 oz)	174	3	5	—	29	—	297
oat bran wheat free	1 (2 oz)	154	4	4	0	28	4	224
toaster type blueberry	1	103	2	3	—	18	—	158
toaster type corn	1	114	2	4	—	19	—	142
toaster type wheat bran w/ raisins	1 (1.3 oz)	106	2	3	—	19	—	178
Dolly Madison								
Blueberry	1 (1.75 oz)	170	2	7	0	26	0	280
Mega Banana Nut	1 (5.9 oz)	620	8	31	75	78	2	540
Mega Blueberry	1 (5.9 oz)	590	8	28	80	78	1	590
Mega Chocolate Chip	1 (5.9 oz)	620	8	29	80	78	2	580
Mega Cranberry Orange	1 (5.9 oz)	590	6	28	90	79	1	580
Mega Cream Cheese	1 (5.9 oz)	620	7	33	90	73	1	630
Dutch Mill								
Apple Oat Bran	1 (2 oz)	180	3	5	0	31	1	210
Banana Walnut	1 (2 oz)	220	3	6	5	33	1	210
Carrot	1 (2 oz)	190	3	7	30	31	1	230
Corn	1 (2 oz)	190	4	6	40	31	1	280
Cranberry Orange	1 (2 oz)	170	3	6	55	26	1	290
Raisin Bran	1 (2 oz)	230	2	5	30	37	3	330
Hostess								
Banana Bran Low Fat	1 (2.7 oz)	240	4	3	0	47	2	270
Blueberry Low Fat	1 (2.7 oz)	230	4	3	0	47	1	350
Hearty Banana Nut	1 (5.9 oz)	620	8	31	75	78	2	540
Hearty Blueberry	1 (5.9 oz)	590	8	28	80	78	1	590
Hearty Chocolate Chip	1 (5.9 oz)	620	8	29	80	78	2	580
Hearty Cranberry Orange	1 (5.9 oz)	590	6	28	90	79	1	580
Hearty Cream Cheese	1 (5.9 oz)	620	7	33	90	73	1	630

FOOD	PORTION	CAL	PROT	FAT	CHOL	CARB	FIBER	SOD
Mini Banana Walnut	3 (1.2 oz)	160	2	9	25	16	0	100
Mini Blueberry	3 (1.2 oz)	150	1	8	25	18	0	110
Mini Chocolate Chip	3 (1.2 oz)	160	2	9	20	17	0	100
Mini Cinnamon Apple	3 (1.2 oz)	160	1	9	25	16	0	110
Mini Cinnamon Bites	3 (1.1 oz)	130	1	6	15	18	0	110
Mini Rocky Road	3 (1.2 oz)	160	2	9	20	17	0	140
Muffin Loaf Apple Spice	1 (3.7 oz)	430	3	18	80	61	1	350
Muffin Loaf Banana Nut	1 (3.8 oz)	460	4	20	60	63	0	300
Muffin Loaf Blueberry	1 (3.8 oz)	440	5	19	80	62	2	460
Muffin Loaf Chocolate Chocolate Chip	1 (3.8 oz)	400	5	17	45	58	2	330
Muffin Loaf Raspberry	1 (3.8 oz)	440	5	19	80	62	2	460
Oat Bran	1 (1.5 oz)	160	8	0	2	21	1	150
Otis Spunkmeyer								
Apple Cinnamon	1 (2 oz)	220	3	11	36	27	tr	210
Low Fat Wild Blueberry	1 (2.25 oz)	200	3	4	35	38	tr	160
Mayport Almond Poppy Seed	½ muffin (2 oz)	210	3	12	40	23	tr	230
Mayport Banana Nut	1 (2.25 oz)	270	3	14	30	33	tr	210
Mayport Cheese Streusel	½ muffin (2 oz)	220	3	10	25	30	tr	170
Mayport Chocolate Chocolate Chip	1 (2.25 oz)	260	4	13	40	33	1	190
Mayport Chocolate Chip	½ muffin (2 oz)	240	3	13	35	28	tr	210
Mayport Cinnamon Spice	½ muffin (2 oz)	230	3	13	40	26	1	250
Mayport Corn	½ muffin (2 oz)	230	3	13	50	26	0	240
Mayport Harvest Bran	1 (2.25 oz)	240	4	10	35	34	3	240
Mayport Lemon	½ muffin (2 oz)	230	3	13	40	27	1	280
Mayport Orange	½ muffin (2 oz)	230	3	13	40	27	tr	230
Mayport Pineapple	½ muffin (2 oz)	210	3	12	40	25	1	270

FOOD	PORTION	CAL	PROT	FAT	CHOL	CARB	FIBER	SOD
Mayport Wild Blueberry	1 (2.25 oz)	230	3	13	45	27	1	230
Mayport Low Fat Apple Cinnamon	1 (4 oz)	380	5	6	65	75	1	300
Mayport Low Fat Banana Nut	1 (4 oz)	350	6	6	65	70	1	400
Mayport Low Fat Chocolate Chocolate Chip	1 (4 oz)	370	7	6	65	73	2	290
Uncle Wally's								
Fat Free Apple Cinnamon Delight	1 (1.9 oz)	110	3	0	0	28	1	280
Weight Watchers								
Fat Free Apple Crisp	1 (2.5 oz)	160	3	0	0	37	1	290
Fat Free Cranberry Orange	1 (2.5 oz)	160	3	0	0	38	1	290
Fat Free Double Chocolate	1 (2.5 oz)	180	3	0	0	40	2	300
Fat Free Wild Blueberry	1 (2.5 oz)	160	3	0	0	36	1	280
Low Fat Apple Cinnamon	1 (2.5 oz)	170	4	3	0	35	2	200
Low Fat Blueberry	1 (2.5 oz)	180	4	3	0	37	2	200
Low Fat Carrot	1 (2.5 oz)	160	4	3	0	34	2	200
Low Fat Chocolate Chip	1 (2.5 oz)	180	4	3	0	38	2	200
Low Fat Cranberry Orange	1 (2.5 oz)	180	4	3	0	38	2	190
Low Fat Lemon Poppy	1 (2.5 oz)	190	4	3	0	38	2	200
TAKE-OUT								
raisin bran lowfat	1 (4 oz)	270	5	1	0	61	5	560

MULBERRIES

fresh	1 cup	61	2	1	0	14	—	14

MULLET

striped cooked	3 oz	127	21	4	54	0	—	61
striped raw	3 oz	99	16	3	42	0	—	55

MUNG BEANS

dried cooked	1 cup	213	14	1	0	39	—	4

FOOD	PORTION	CAL	PROT	FAT	CHOL	CARB	FIBER	SOD
MUNGO BEANS								
dried cooked	1 cup	190	14	1	1	33	–	13
MUSHROOMS								
CANNED								
chanterelle	3.5 oz	12	1	1	0	tr	6	165
pieces	½ cup	19	1	tr	0	4	–	–
straw	1 cup (6.4 oz)	58	7	1	0	8	5	699
whole	1 (0.4 oz)	3	tr	tr	0	1	–	–
BinB								
Pieces & Stems	1 can (4.2 oz)	30	3	0	0	4	2	460
Sliced	1 can (4.2 oz)	30	3	0	0	4	2	460
Sliced w/ Garlic	1 can (4.2 oz)	35	3	1	0	4	1	410
Whole	1 can (4.2 oz)	30	3	0	0	4	2	460
Green Giant								
Pieces & Stems	½ cup (4.2 oz)	30	3	0	0	4	2	440
Sliced	½ cup (4.2 oz)	30	2	0	0	3	2	440
Whole	½ cup (4.2 oz)	30	3	0	0	4	2	440
DRIED								
chanterelle	1 oz	25	5	tr	0	tr	17	9
cloud ear	1 (5 g)	13	tr	tr	0	3	3	2
cloud ears	1 cup (1 oz)	80	3	tr	0	20	20	10
shiitake	4 (½ oz)	44	1	tr	0	11	–	2
straw	1 piece (6 g)	2	tr	tr	0	tr	tr	21
tree ear	½ cup (0.4 oz)	36	1	tr	0	10	–	8
wood ear mok yee	½ cup (0.4 oz)	25	2	tr	–	8	4	6
Eden								
Shitake	6 (0.4 oz)	35	2	0	0	7	5	0
FRESH								
chanterelle	3.5 oz	11	2	tr	0	tr	6	3
enoki raw	1 (4 in)	2	tr	tr	0	tr	–	0
morel	3.5 oz	9	2	tr	0	0	7	2
oyster raw	1 sm (0.5 oz)	6	1	tr	0	1	tr	5
oyster raw	1 lg (5.2 oz)	55	6	1	0	9	4	46
portabella	1 serv (2 oz)	14	1	tr	0	3	–	2
raw	1 (½ oz)	5	tr	tr	0	1	tr	1
raw sliced	½ cup	9	1	tr	0	2	tr	1
shitake cooked	4 (2.5 oz)	40	1	tr	0	10	–	3
sliced cooked	½ cup	21	2	tr	0	4	1	2
whole cooked	1 (0.4 oz)	3	tr	tr	0	1	–	0

FOOD	PORTION	CAL	PROT	FAT	CHOL	CARB	FIBER	SOD
Mother Earth								
Organic	4 oz	35	3	1	0	5	tr	0
MUSKRAT								
roasted	3 oz	199	26	10	–	0	–	81
MUSSELS								
blue raw	3 oz	73	10	2	24	3	–	243
blue raw	1 cup	129	18	3	42	6	–	429
fresh blue cooked	3 oz	147	20	4	48	6	–	313
MUSTARD								
dry mustard	1 tsp	15	1	1	0	1	–	tr
yellow ready-to-use	1 tsp	5	tr	tr	0	tr	–	63
Boar's Head								
Delicatessen Style	1 tsp (5 g)	0	0	0	0	0	0	40
Honey	1 tsp (5 g)	10	0	0	0	2	0	25
Eden								
Organic Stone Ground	1 tsp	0	0	0	0	1	0	65
Gulden's								
Diablo	1 tsp	8	–	0	–	–	–	–
Mild	1 tsp	6	–	0	–	–	–	–
Spicy Brown	1 tsp	8	–	0	–	–	–	–
Hunt's								
Mustard	1 tsp (5 g)	3	tr	tr	0	tr	tr	64
Kraft								
Horseradish Mustard	1 tsp (5 g)	0	0	0	0	0	0	55
Mustard	1 tsp (5 g)	0	0	0	0	0	0	60
Luzianne								
Creole Mustard	1 tbsp	10	1	0	0	2	0	320
Tree Of Life								
Dijon	1 tsp (5 g)	0	0	0	0	0	–	66
Dijon Imported	1 tsp (5 g)	5	tr	0	0	tr	–	120
Stone Ground	1 tsp (5 g)	0	0	0	0	0	–	55
Yellow	1 tsp (5 g)	0	0	0	0	0	–	55
MUSTARD GREENS								
fresh chopped cooked	½ cup	11	2	tr	0	1	–	11
fresh raw chopped	½ cup	7	1	tr	0	1	–	7

FOOD	PORTION	CAL	PROT	FAT	CHOL	CARB	FIBER	SOD
frozen chopped cooked	½ cup	14	2	tr	0	2	–	19
Birds Eye								
Chopped	1 cup (3 oz)	30	2	0	0	2	2	20
NATTO								
natto	½ cup	187	16	10	0	13	–	6
NAVY BEANS								
CANNED								
navy	1 cup	296	20	1	0	54	–	1173
DRIED								
cooked	1 cup	259	16	1	0	48	–	2
Hurst								
HamBeens w/ Ham	3 tbsp (1.2 oz)	120	8	1	0	20	11	63
NECTARINE								
fresh	1	67	1	1	0	16	2	0
Chiquita								
Fresh	1 med (4.9 oz)	70	1	1	0	16	2	0
NEUFCHATEL								
neufchatel	1 oz	74	3	7	22	1	–	113
neufchatel	1 pkg (3 oz)	221	8	20	65	3	–	339
Horizon Organic								
Neufchatel	2 tbsp	70	3	6	20	tr	0	120
Organic Valley								
Neufchatel	1 oz	70	2	6	20	1	0	115
Philadelphia								
Neufchatel	1 oz	70	3	6	20	tr	0	120
NOODLE DISHES (see also PASTA DINNERS)								
Hormel								
Microcup Meals Noodles & Chicken	1 cup (7.5 oz)	200	8	9	40	20	1	1140
Hunt's								
Noodles & Chicken	1 cup (8.7 oz)	176	12	6	37	21	2	1282
Noodles & Beef	1 cup (8.7 oz)	151	10	4	17	22	5	1241
Kraft								
Noodle Classics Cheddar Cheese as prep	1 cup (7.4 oz)	400	13	19	70	47	1	760

FOOD	PORTION	CAL	PROT	FAT	CHOL	CARB	FIBER	SOD
Noodle Classics Savory Chicken as prep	1 cup (8.5 oz)	340	10	13	55	46	2	1370
Lipton								
Noodles & Sauce Alfredo Broccoli as prep	1 cup (2.2 oz)	340	12	14	80	43	2	970
Noodles & Sauce Alfredo as prep	1 cup (2.2 oz)	330	15	14	80	42	2	1040
Noodles & Sauce Beef as prep	1 cup (2.1 oz)	280	8	10	60	43	2	910
Noodles & Sauce Butter as prep	1 cup (2.2 oz)	310	8	14	70	41	2	870
Noodles & Sauce Butter & Herb as prep	1 cup (2.2 oz)	300	9	13	65	42	2	780
Noodles & Sauce Chicken Broccoli as prep	1 cup (2.1 oz)	310	11	11	70	44	2	840
Noodles & Sauce Chicken Tetrazzini as prep	1 cup (2 oz)	300	10	12	70	41	2	950
Noodles & Sauce Chicken as prep	1 cup (2.1 oz)	290	8	11	65	42	2	830
Noodles & Sauce Creamy Chicken as prep	1 cup (2.1 oz)	320	11	13	75	42	2	810
Noodles & Sauce Parmesan as prep	1 cup (2.1 oz)	330	14	15	75	40	2	850
Noodles & Sauce Sour Cream & Chives as prep	1 cup (2.2 oz)	310	10	14	70	41	2	870
Noodles & Sauce Stroganoff as prep	1 cup (2 oz)	300	11	11	70	40	2	950
TAKE-OUT								
noodle pudding	½ cup	132	6	7	27	11	–	222

NOODLES

cellophane	1 cup	492	tr	tr	0	121	–	14
chow mein	1 cup (1.6 oz)	237	4	14	0	25	2	189

FOOD	PORTION	CAL	PROT	FAT	CHOL	CARB	FIBER	SOD
egg	1 cup (38 g)	145	5	2	36	27	–	8
egg cooked	1 cup (5.6 oz)	213	8	2	53	40	2	11
japanese soba cooked	1 cup (4 oz)	113	6	tr	0	24	–	68
japanese somen cooked	1 cup (6.2 oz)	231	7	tr	0	48	–	283
korean acorn noodles not prep	2 oz	195	7	tr	–	41	tr	–
rice cooked	1 cup (6.2 oz)	192	2	tr	0	44	–	33
spinach/egg cooked	1 cup (5.6 oz)	211	8	3	53	39	4	19
Azumaya								
Spinach	1 cup	210	8	1	0	42	2	370
Thin Cut	1 cup	210	8	1	0	43	2	400
Wide Cut	1 cup	210	8	1	0	43	2	410
Chun King								
Chow Mein	½ cup (1 oz)	137	3	6	0	19	1	217
Creamette								
Egg	2 oz	221	–	3	70	–	–	–
Eden								
Kudzu	2 oz	200	0	0	0	48	2	0
Hodgson Mill								
Four Color Veggie Egg	2 oz	200	9	2	35	37	2	25
Whole Wheat Egg	2 oz	190	10	2	30	34	4	20
La Choy								
Chow Mein	½ cup (1 oz)	137	3	6	0	19	1	217
Chow Mein Crispy Wide	½ cup (1 oz)	148	3	8	0	16	1	289
Rice	½ cup (1 oz)	121	2	3	0	21	tr	378
Manischewitz								
Fine Yolk Free	1 ½ cups	210	8	1	0	40	2	20
Nasoya								
Chinese	1 cup	210	8	1	0	43	2	400
Japanese	1 cup	210	8	1	0	43	2	410
Spinach	1 cup	210	8	1	0	42	2	0
NOPALES								
cooked	1 cup (5.2 oz)	23	2	tr	0	5	–	30
raw sliced	1 cup (3 oz)	14	1	tr	0	3	–	19
NUTMEG								
ground	1 tsp	12	tr	1	0	1	–	tr

FOOD	PORTION	CAL	PROT	FAT	CHOL	CARB	FIBER	SOD

NUTRITION SUPPLEMENTS *(see also* BREAKFAST DRINKS, CEREAL BARS, ENERGY BARS, ENERGY DRINKS*)*

FOOD	PORTION	CAL	PROT	FAT	CHOL	CARB	FIBER	SOD
Enlive!								
Drink All Flavors	1 box (8.1 oz)	300	10	0	<5	65	0	65
Ensure								
Supplement All Flavors	1 can (8 fl oz)	250	9	6	<5	40	0	200
Essential								
Protein Powder	1 serv (0.6 oz)	70	16	tr	0	6	tr	5
Gatorade								
ReLode	1 pkt (0.75 oz)	80	0	0	0	17	–	25
GeniSoy								
Soy Protein Powder	1 scoop (0.6 oz)	60	14	0	0	0	–	180
Glucerna								
Shakes All Flavors	1 can (8 oz)	220	10	9	<5	29	3	210
Juven								
Grape w/ Arginine, Glutamine, HMB	1 pkg (0.8 oz)	90	–	–	–	2	–	–
Orange w/ HMB	1 pkg (0.8 oz)	90	–	0	–	–	–	–
Met-Rx								
Lite	1 pkg (1.6 oz)	170	25	1	30	16	1	125
Mass Action	1 scoop (0.9 oz)	60	–	4	–	15	–	270
Original	1 pkg (2.5 oz)	250	37	2	15	22	tr	370
Protein Shake	1 can	200	25	3	10	20	2	110
Ultra	1 pkg (2.6 oz)	250	40	2	50	19	2	230
Nature Made								
CalBurst	1 piece	15	–	–	–	–	–	–
Nestle								
Additions	2⅓ tsp (0.7 oz)	100	6	5	0	9	0	90
NutraBalance								
EggPro	1 tbsp (7.5 g)	30	6	0	0	1	0	96
Nutribar								
Shake Chocolate Supreme as prep w/ 2% milk	1 serv (10 oz) (4.6 oz)	262	14	8	–	34	2	290
Shake Vanilla as prep w/ 2% milk	1 (10 oz)	259	14	7	–	35	2	285
PermaLean								
Protein Powder Bodacious Berry	1 scoop (1 oz)	104	20	tr	0	1	–	tr

FOOD	PORTION	CAL	PROT	FAT	CHOL	CARB	FIBER	SOD
Protein Powder Chocoholic Chocolate	1 scoop (1 oz)	104	20	tr	0	5	–	tr
Pounds Off								
All Flavors	1 bar (2.1 oz)	210	11	5	0	32	2	25
Resource								
Fructose Sweetened	1 pkg (8 oz)	250	15	11	–	23	3	230
Liquid Food	1 pkg (8 oz)	250	8	9	–	34	–	210
Plus Liquid Food	1 pkg (8 oz)	355	13	13	–	47	–	300
Viactiv								
Calcium Chews	1	20	–	1	–	–	–	–

NUTS MIXED *(see also individual names)*

FOOD	PORTION	CAL	PROT	FAT	CHOL	CARB	FIBER	SOD
dry roasted w/ peanuts	1 oz	169	15	0	5	7	–	3
dry roasted w/ peanuts salted	1 oz	169	5	15	0	7	–	223
mixed nuts chocolate covered	¼ cup (1.5 oz)	240	4	17	5	20	2	25
oil roasted w/ peanuts	1 oz	175	5	16	0	6	–	3
oil roasted w/ peanuts salted	1 oz	175	5	16	0	6	–	217
oil roasted w/o peanuts	1 oz	175	4	16	0	6	–	3
oil roasted w/o peanuts salted	1 oz	175	4	16	0	6	–	233
Estee								
Fruit & Nut Mix	¼ cup	210	6	12	<5	19	2	45
Planters								
Cashews & Peanuts Honey Roasted	1 oz	150	5	12	0	10	2	125
Deluxe Oil Roasted	1 oz	170	5	16	0	6	2	110
Dry Roasted	1 oz	170	6	14	0	7	2	250
Honey Roasted	1 oz	140	5	13	0	9	2	85
Lightly Salted Oil Roasted	1 oz	170	6	15	0	6	2	55
No Brazils Lightly Salted Oil Roasted	1 oz	170	6	15	0	6	2	55
No Brazils Oil Roasted	1 oz	170	5	15	0	6	2	110

FOOD	PORTION	CAL	PROT	FAT	CHOL	CARB	FIBER	SOD
Oil Roasted	1 oz	170	6	15	0	5	2	115
Select Mix Cashews Almonds & Macadamias Oil Roasted	1 oz	170	4	16	0	6	2	90
Select Mix Cashews Almonds & Pecans Oil Roasted	1 oz	170	4	15	0	7	2	95
Unsalted Oil Roasted	1 oz	170	6	15	0	6	3	0

OCTOPUS

fresh steamed	3 oz	140	25	2	82	4	–	–

OHELOBERRIES

fresh	1 cup	39	1	tr	0	10	–	2

OIL (see also FAT)

almond	1 cup	1927	0	218	0	0	–	–
almond	1 tbsp	120	0	14	0	0	–	–
apricot kernel	1 cup	1927	0	218	0	0	–	–
apricot kernel	1 tbsp	120	0	14	0	0	–	–
avocado	1 tbsp	124	0	14	0	0	–	–
avocado	1 cup	1927	0	218	0	0	–	–
babassu palm	1 tbsp	120	0	14	0	0	–	–
butter oil	1 tbsp	112	tr	13	33	0	–	–
butter oil	1 cup	1795	1	204	524	0	–	–
canola	1 cup	1927	0	218	0	0	–	–
canola	1 tbsp	124	0	14	0	0	–	–
coconut	1 tbsp	117	0	14	0	0	–	–
corn	1 tbsp	120	0	14	0	0	–	–
corn	1 cup	1927	0	218	0	0	–	–
cottonseed	1 cup	1927	0	218	0	0	–	–
cottonseed	1 tbsp	120	0	14	0	0	–	–
cupu assu	1 tbsp	120	0	14	0	0	–	–
grapeseed	1 tbsp	120	0	14	0	0	–	–
hazelnut	1 cup	1927	0	218	0	0	–	–
hazelnut	1 tbsp	120	0	14	0	0	–	–
mustard	1 cup	1927	0	218	0	0	–	–
mustard	1 tbsp	124	0	14	0	0	–	–
oat	1 tbsp	120	0	14	0	0	–	–

FOOD	PORTION	CAL	PROT	FAT	CHOL	CARB	FIBER	SOD
olive	1 tbsp	119	0	14	0	0	–	0
olive	1 cup	1909	0	216	0	0	–	tr
palm	1 tbsp	120	0	14	0	0	–	–
palm	1 cup	1927	0	218	0	0	–	–
palm kernel	1 cup	1879	0	218	0	0	–	–
palm kernel	1 tbsp	117	0	14	0	0	–	–
peanut	1 tbsp	119	0	14	0	0	–	tr
peanut	1 cup	1909	0	216	0	0	–	tr
poppyseed	1 tbsp	120	0	14	0	0	–	–
pumpkin seed	1 oz	217	0	29	–	0	–	–
rice bran	1 tbsp	120	0	14	0	0	–	–
safflower	1 tbsp	120	0	14	0	0	–	–
safflower	1 cup	1927	0	218	0	0	–	–
sesame	1 tbsp	120	0	14	0	0	–	–
sheanut	1 tbsp	120	0	14	0	0	–	–
soybean	1 tbsp	120	0	14	0	0	–	0
soybean	1 cup	1927	0	218	0	0	–	tr
sunflower	1 cup	1927	0	218	0	0	–	–
sunflower	1 tbsp	120	0	14	0	0	–	–
teaseed	1 tbsp	120	0	14	0	0	–	–
tomatoseed	1 tbsp	120	0	14	0	0	–	–
vegetable soybean & cottonseed	1 cup	1927	0	218	0	0	–	–
vegetable soybean & cottonseed	1 tbsp	120	0	14	0	0	–	–
walnut	1 cup	1927	0	218	0	0	1	–
walnut	1 tbsp	120	0	14	0	0	–	–
wheat germ	1 tbsp	120	0	14	0	0	–	–
Bertolli								
Classico	1 tbsp	120	–	14	0	–	–	–
Extra Light	1 tbsp	120	–	14	0	–	–	–
Extra Virgin	1 tbsp	120	–	14	0	–	–	–
Crisco								
Corn Canola	1 tbsp (0.5 fl oz)	120	0	14	0	0	–	0
Oil	1 tbsp (0.5 fl oz)	120	0	14	0	0	–	0
Puritan Canola	1 tbsp (0.5 fl oz)	120	0	14	0	0	0	0
Eden								
Olive Spanish Extra Virgin	1 tbsp	120	0	14	0	0	0	0
Safflower	1 tbsp (0.5 oz)	120	0	14	0	0	–	0

FOOD	PORTION	CAL	PROT	FAT	CHOL	CARB	FIBER	SOD
House Of Tsang								
Hot Chili Sesame	1 tsp (5 g)	45	0	5	0	0	0	0
Mongolian Fire	1 tsp (5 g)	45	0	5	0	0	0	0
Pure Sesame	1 tsp (5 g)	45	0	5	0	0	0	0
Singapore Curry	1 tsp (5 g)	45	0	5	0	0	0	0
Wok Oil	1 tbsp (0.5 oz)	130	0	14	0	0	0	0
Italica								
Olive Oil	1 tbsp	120	0	9	0	0	–	–
Orville Redenbacher's								
Popping	1 tbsp (0.5 oz)	120	0	14	0	0	0	0
Pam								
Butter	⅓ sec spray (0.3 g)	0	0	0	0	0	–	0
Cooking Spray	⅓ sec spray (0.3 g)	0	0	0	0	0	–	0
Olive Oil	⅓ sec spray (0.3 g)	0	0	0	0	0	–	0
Planters								
Peanut	1 tbsp (0.5 oz)	120	0	14	0	0	–	0
Popcorn	1 tbsp (0.5 oz)	120	0	14	0	0	–	0
Pompeian								
Olive	1 tbsp	130	–	14	0	–	–	–
Progresso								
Olive Extra Mild	1 tbsp (0.5 oz)	120	0	14	0	0	0	0
Olive Extra Virgin	1 tbsp (0.5 oz)	120	0	14	0	0	0	0
Olive Riviera Blend	1 tbsp (0.5 oz)	120	0	14	0	0	0	0
Smart Beat								
Canola	1 tbsp	120	0	14	0	0	–	0
Tree Of Life								
Olive Extra Virgin Organic	1 tbsp (0.5 g)	130	0	14	0	0	–	0
Weight Watchers								
Butter Spray	⅓ sec spray	0	0	0	0	0	0	0
Cooking Spray	⅓ sec spray	0	0	0	0	0	0	0
OKRA								
FRESH								
raw	8 pods	36	2	tr	0	7	–	8
raw sliced	½ cup	19	1	tr	0	4	–	4
sliced cooked	½ cup	25	1	tr	0	6	–	4
sliced cooked	8 pods	27	2	tr	0	6	–	5
FROZEN								
sliced cooked	1 pkg (10 oz)	94	5	1	0	21	–	8
sliced cooked	½ cup	34	2	tr	0	8	–	3

FOOD	PORTION	CAL	PROT	FAT	CHOL	CARB	FIBER	SOD
Birds Eye								
Cut	¾ cup (2.9 oz)	25	1	0	0	5	3	35
Whole	9 pods (3 oz)	25	1	0	0	5	3	35
OLIVES								
green	3 extra lg	15	tr	2	0	tr	tr	312
green	4 med	15	tr	2	0	tr	tr	312
ripe	1 sm	4	tr	tr	0	tr	tr	28
ripe	1 lg	5	tr	tr	0	tr	tr	38
ripe	1 colossal	12	tr	1	0	1	–	136
ripe	1 jumbo	7	tr	1	0	tr	–	75
spanish stuffed	5 (0.5 oz)	15	0	1	0	1	0	320
Italia In Tavola								
Black Olives Paste	1 tbsp (0.5 oz)	20	0	2	0	tr	–	470
Progresso								
Olive Salad (drained)	2 tbsp (0.8 oz)	25	0	3	0	1	tr	360
Tee Pee								
Spanish Green	2 oz	98	1	10	0	1	–	–
Vlasic								
Ripe Colossal Pitted	2 (0.6 oz)	20	0	2	0	1	0	110
Ripe Jumbo Pitted	3 (0.6 oz)	25	0	2	0	1	0	135
Ripe Large Pitted	4 (0.5 oz)	25	0	3	0	1	0	115
Ripe Medium Pitted	5 (0.5 oz)	25	0	3	0	1	0	115
Ripe Sliced	¼ cup (0.5 oz)	25	0	3	0	1	0	115
Ripe Small Pitted	6 (0.5 oz)	25	0	3	0	1	0	115
ONION								
CANNED								
chopped	½ cup	21	1	tr	0	5	–	416
whole	1 (2.2 oz)	12	1	tr	0	3	–	234
Boar's Head								
Sweet Vidalia In Sauce	1 tbsp	10	0	0	0	2	0	15
DRIED								
flakes	1 tbsp	16	tr	tr	0	4	–	1
powder	1 tsp	7	tr	tr	0	2	–	1
shallots	1 tbsp	3	tr	0	0	1	–	1
FRESH								
chopped cooked	½ cup	47	1	tr	0	11	–	3
raw chopped	1 tbsp	4	tr	tr	0	1	tr	0
raw chopped	½ cup	30	1	tr	0	7	–	2
scallions raw chopped	1 tbsp	2	tr	tr	0	tr	tr	1

FOOD	PORTION	CAL	PROT	FAT	CHOL	CARB	FIBER	SOD
scallions raw sliced	½ cup	16	1	tr	0	4	1	8
shallots raw chopped	1 tbsp	7	tr	tr	0	2	–	1
welsh raw	3½ oz	34	2	tr	0	7	–	–
Antioch Farms								
Vidalia	1 med	60	1	0	0	14	3	10
FROZEN								
chopped cooked	½ cup	30	tr	tr	0	7	–	12
chopped cooked	1 tbsp	4	tr	tr	0	1	–	2
rings	7 (2.5 oz)	285	4	19	0	27	–	263
rings cooked	2 (0.7 oz)	81	1	5	0	8	–	75
whole cooked	3½ oz	28	tr	tr	0	7	–	8
Birds Eye								
Diced	⅔ cup (3 oz)	30	tr	0	0	6	1	30
Pearl Onions In Cream Sauce	½ cup (4.4 oz)	60	2	2	10	8	1	280
Small Whole	17	30	–	0	0	–	1	10
TAKE-OUT								
fried	½ cup (7.5 oz)	176	3	11	–	17	–	–
rings breaded & fried	8 to 9	275	4	16	14	31	–	430

OPOSSUM

FOOD	PORTION	CAL	PROT	FAT	CHOL	CARB	FIBER	SOD
roasted	3 oz	188	26	9	–	0	–	–

ORANGE
CANNED
Del Monte

FOOD	PORTION	CAL	PROT	FAT	CHOL	CARB	FIBER	SOD
Mandarin In Light Syrup	½ cup (4.5 oz)	80	0	0	0	19	1	10
Dole								
FruitBowls Mandarin Oranges	1 pkg (4 oz)	70	0	0	0	18	0	10
FRESH								
california navel	1	65	1	tr	0	16	3	1
california valencia	1	59	1	tr	0	14	3	0
florida	1	69	1	tr	0	17	4	1
peel	1 tbsp	6	tr	tr	0	2	–	0
sections	1 cup	85	2	tr	0	21	4	0

ORANGE EXTRACT
Virginia Dare

FOOD	PORTION	CAL	PROT	FAT	CHOL	CARB	FIBER	SOD
Virginia Dare	1 tsp	22	–	0	0	–	–	–

FOOD	PORTION	CAL	PROT	FAT	CHOL	CARB	FIBER	SOD
ORANGE JUICE								
canned	1 cup	104	1	tr	0	25	–	6
chilled	1 cup	110	2	1	0	25	–	2
fresh	1 cup	111	2	tr	0	26	–	2
frzn as prep	1 cup	112	2	tr	0	27	1	2
frzn not prep	6 oz	339	5	tr	0	81	2	7
mandarin orange	7 oz	94	2	tr	–	20	–	–
orange drink	6 oz	94	0	0	0	24	–	31
After The Fall								
Juice	1 bottle (10 oz)	110	2	0	0	26	–	10
Big Juicy								
Drink	8 oz	110	0	0	0	28	–	55
Capri Sun								
Drink	1 pkg (7 oz)	100	0	0	0	25	0	20
Everfresh								
Juice	1 can (8 oz)	100	0	0	0	24	0	0
Ruby Red Orange Drink	1 can (8 oz)	130	0	0	0	33	0	0
Fresh Samantha								
Juice	1 cup (8 oz)	100	1	0	0	8	0	0
Horizon Organic								
Juice Pulp Free	8 fl oz	110	2	0	0	26	–	0
Juicy Juice								
Punch	1 box (8.45 oz)	130	0	0	0	33	0	15
Punch	1 box (4.23 oz)	60	0	0	0	15	0	5
Kool-Aid								
Drink Mix Orange as prep	1 serv (8 oz)	60	0	0	0	16	0	5
Orange Drink as prep w/ sugar	1 serv (8 oz)	100	0	0	0	25	0	10
Minute Maid								
Simply Orange 100%	8 fl oz	110	2	0	0	26	–	0
Simply Orange Calcium Fortified	8 fl oz	110	2	0	0	26	–	0
Simply Orange Grove Made	8 fl oz	110	2	0	0	26	–	0
Mott's								
100% Juice	1 box (8 oz)	130	2	0	0	31	–	10
100% Juice	8 fl oz	130	2	0	0	31	–	10

FOOD	PORTION	CAL	PROT	FAT	CHOL	CARB	FIBER	SOD
Nantucket Nectars								
100% Juice	8 oz	120	0	0	0	28	–	0
NutraShake								
Fourtified	1 pkg (4 oz)	50	0	0	0	12	4	0
Ocean Spray								
100% Juice	8 oz	120	0	0	0	31	0	35
Shasta Plus								
Orange Drink	1 can (11.5 oz)	160	0	0	0	40	0	45
Snapple								
Orangeade	8 fl oz	120	0	0	0	29	–	10
Tang								
Orange Drink as prep	1 serv (8 oz)	90	0	0	0	23	0	0
Sugar Free Orange as prep	1 serv (8 oz)	5	0	0	0	0	0	0
Tropicana								
Double Vitamin C	8 fl oz	110	2	0	0	26	–	0
Juice	8 oz	110	2	0	0	26	–	0
Ruby Red	8 oz	110	2	0	0	26	–	0
Season's Best	8 oz	110	1	0	0	27	–	15
Season's Best Homestyle	8 fl oz	110	1	0	0	27	–	15
Tropical	8 oz	110	2	0	0	25	–	0
With Calcium	8 fl oz	110	2	0	0	26	–	0
Turkey Hill								
Orangeade	1 cup	120	–	0	0	30	–	–
Veryfine								
100% Juice	1 bottle (10 oz)	150	0	0	0	37	2	45
Chillers Artric Orange	8 fl oz	130	0	0	0	33	0	10
Juice Blend	1 can (11.5 oz)	160	0	0	0	39	0	10
Orange Drink	1 bottle (10 oz)	160	0	0	0	41	0	90
OREGANO								
ground	1 tsp	5	tr	tr	0	1	–	tr

ORGAN MEATS (*see* BRAINS, GIBLETS, GIZZARDS, HEART, KIDNEY, LIVER, SWEETBREADS)

ORIENTAL FOOD (*see* ASIAN FOOD, EGG ROLLS, DINNER, NOODLES, RICE, SUSHI)

OSTRICH								
cooked	3 oz	120	22	3	74	–	–	57

FOOD	PORTION	CAL	PROT	FAT	CHOL	CARB	FIBER	SOD
OYSTERS								
canned eastern	1 cup	170	18	6	136	10	–	277
canned eastern	3 oz	58	6	2	46	3	–	95
eastern cooked	6 med	58	6	2	46	3	–	94
eastern cooked	3 oz	117	12	4	93	7	–	190
eastern raw	6 med	58	6	2	46	3	–	94
eastern raw	1 cup	170	18	6	136	10	–	277
pacific raw	1 med	41	5	1	–	2	–	53
pacific raw	3 oz	69	8	2	–	4	–	90
steamed	1 med	41	5	1	–	2	–	53
steamed	3 oz	138	16	4	–	8	–	180
Bumble Bee								
Fancy Whole	2 oz	70	7	3	45	3	0	140
Smoked	½ can (1.9 oz)	120	10	7	35	6	0	210
TAKE-OUT								
breaded & fried	6 (4.9 oz)	368	13	18	109	40	–	677
oysters rockefeller	3 oysters	66	7	2	38	5	–	80
stew	1 cup	278	15	18	100	15	tr	928
PANCAKE/WAFFLE SYRUP								
low calorie	1 tbsp	12	0	0	0	3	0	–
maple	1 cup (11.1 oz)	824	tr	1	0	212	–	27
maple	1 tbsp (0.8 oz)	52	0	0	0	13	–	2
pancake syrup	1 tbsp (0.7 oz)	57	0	0	0	15	–	17
pancake syrup	1 cup (11 oz)	903	0	0	0	238	–	290
pancake syrup light	1 oz	46	0	0	0	13	–	57
pancake syrup w/ butter	1 tbsp (0.7 oz)	59	0	tr	1	15	–	20
pancake syrup w/ butter	1 cup (11 oz)	933	tr	5	14	234	–	307
Estee								
Maple	¼ cup	80	0	0	0	20	0	125
Mrs. Butter-worth's								
Original	¼ cup (2 oz)	230	0	0	0	56	–	95
Smucker's								
Breakfast Syrup Sugar Free	¼ cup (2 oz)	30	0	0	0	8	–	60
PANCAKES								
FROZEN								
buttermilk	1 (4 in diam)	83	2	1	3	16	–	183
plain	1 (4 in diam)	83	2	1	3	16	–	183

FOOD	PORTION	CAL	PROT	FAT	CHOL	CARB	FIBER	SOD
Eggo								
Buttermilk	3 (4.1 oz)	270	7	8	15	44	1	610
MIX								
buckwheat	1 (4 in diam)	62	2	2	20	9	–	160
buttermilk	1 (4 in diam)	74	2	1	–	14	tr	239
plain	1 (4 in diam)	74	2	1	–	14	tr	239
sugar free low sodium	1 (3 in diam)	44	1	tr	0	9	–	58
whole wheat	1 (4 in diam)	92	4	3	27	13	–	252
Betty Crocker								
Buttermilk as prep	3	200	5	3	10	20	1	540
Original as prep	3	200	6	3	10	39	2	540
Bisquick								
Shake 'N Pour Blueberry as prep	3	210	6	4	0	40	1	640
Bruce								
Sweet Potato Pancakes	2	210	6	3	0	39	2	670
Estee								
Pancake Mix as prep	4 (4 in diam)	180	4	0	0	40	1	255
Hodgson Mill								
Buckwheat	⅓ cup (1.8 oz)	160	5	1	0	36	5	590
Hungry Jack								
Potato as prep	3 (3 in diam)	90	3	2	50	16	1	380
Robin Hood								
Buttermilk as prep	3	230	8	6	60	35	1	560
TAKE-OUT								
blueberry	1 (4 in diam)	84	2	4	21	11	–	157
buckwheat	1 (4 in diam)	55	2	2	20	6	–	125
potato	1 (4 in diam)	78	2	6	60	4	tr	238
w/ butter & syrup	2 (8.1 oz)	520	8	14	58	91	–	1104
PAPAYA								
fresh	1	117	2	tr	0	30	–	8
fresh cubed	1 cup	54	1	tr	0	14	–	4
Sonoma								
Dried Pieces	2 pieces (2 oz)	200	0	4	0	41	6	60
Sunfresh								
In Extra Light Syrup	½ cup (4.5 oz)	70	1	0	0	17	1	5

FOOD	PORTION	CAL	PROT	FAT	CHOL	CARB	FIBER	SOD
PAPAYA JUICE								
nectar	1 cup	142	tr	tr	0	36	–	14
Everfresh								
Premium Drink	1 can (8 oz)	140	0	0	0	35	0	0
Nantucket Nectars								
Cocktail	8 oz	120	0	0	0	30	–	0
PAPRIKA								
paprika	1 tsp	6	tr	tr	0	1	–	1
PARSLEY								
dry	1 tsp	1	tr	tr	0	tr	–	1
dry	1 tbsp	1	tr	tr	0	tr	–	2
fresh chopped	½ cup	11	1	tr	0	2	–	17
PARSNIPS								
fresh cooked	1 (5.6 oz)	130	2	tr	0	31	–	17
fresh sliced cooked	½ cup	63	1	tr	0	15	–	8
raw sliced	½ cup	50	1	tr	0	12	–	7
PASSION FRUIT								
purple fresh	1	18	tr	tr	0	4	–	5
PASSION FRUIT JUICE								
purple	1 cup	126	1	tr	0	34	–	–
yellow	1 cup	149	2	tr	0	36	–	15
PASTA *(see also* NOODLES, PASTA DINNERS, PASTA SALAD*)*								
DRY								
corn cooked	1 cup (4.9 oz)	176	4	1	0	39	7	0
corn spaghetti	2 oz	180	4	2	0	35	3	5
elbows	1 cup	389	13	2	0	78	–	8
elbows cooked	1 cup (4.9 oz)	197	7	1	0	40	2	1
shells small cooked	1 cup (4 oz)	162	5	1	0	33	2	1
shells small protein fortified cooked	1 cup (4 oz)	189	9	tr	0	36	–	6
spaghetti cooked	1 cup (4.9 oz)	197	7	1	0	40	2	1
spaghetti protein fortified cooked	1 cup (4.9 oz)	230	11	tr	0	44	2	7
spinach spaghetti cooked	1 cup (4.9 oz)	182	6	1	0	37	–	20
spirals cooked	1 cup (4.7 oz)	189	6	tr	0	38	2	1

FOOD	PORTION	CAL	PROT	FAT	CHOL	CARB	FIBER	SOD
vegetable cooked	1 cup (4.7 oz)	172	6	tr	0	36	6	8
whole wheat cooked	1 cup (4.9 oz)	174	7	tr	0	37	4	4
whole wheat spaghetti cooked	1 cup (4.9 oz)	174	7	1	0	37	6	4
Annie Chun's								
Soba Noodles	2 oz	200	8	1	0	39	3	390
Barilla								
Conchiglie Rigate	1 cup (2 oz)	200	6	1	0	40	2	0
Gemelli as prep	1 cup (2 oz)	200	7	1	0	42	2	0
Pennette Rigate	1⅓ cups (2 oz)	200	7	1	0	42	2	0
Creamette								
Linguini Egg	2 oz	221	—	3	70	—	—	—
Rotelle	2 oz	210	—	1	0	—	—	—
Rotini Rainbow	2 oz	210	—	1	0	—	—	—
Spaghetti Egg	2 oz	221	—	3	70	—	—	—
Spaghetti Thin	2 oz	210	—	1	0	—	—	—
Ziti	2 oz	210	—	1	0	—	—	—
Cuore								
Capellini cooked	1⅓ cup (2 oz)	190	7	1	0	39	3	0
Fusilli cooked	1⅓ cup (2 oz)	190	7	1	0	39	3	0
Tortiglioni cooked	1⅓ cup (2 oz)	190	7	1	0	39	3	0
De Bole's								
Whole Wheat Organic Elbows	2 oz	210	7	2	0	40	5	0
DeCecco								
Whole Wheat Linguine cooked	2 oz	180	8	2	<5	33	7	0
Duc Amici								
Pasta Lite Low Carb Fusilli	2 oz	160	28	1	0	10	7	50
Eden								
Organic Extra Fine	2 oz	210	9	2	0	40	3	0
Organic Gemelli	2 oz	210	8	2	0	40	5	0
Organic Pesto Gemelli	2 oz	210	8	1	0	41	4	0
Organic Ribbons Saffron	2 oz	210	9	2	0	40	3	0

FOOD	PORTION	CAL	PROT	FAT	CHOL	CARB	FIBER	SOD
Organic Spaghetti Semolina	2 oz	200	8	1	0	40	2	0
Organic Spaghetti 50% Whole Grain	2 oz	210	8	1	0	41	4	0
Organic Spirals Kamut Vegetable	2 oz	210	8	2	0	40	6	45
Organic Spirals Sesame Rice	2 oz	200	8	2	0	37	4	0
Organic Spirals Mixed Grain	2 oz	210	8	2	0	41	7	15
Organic Spirals Spinach	2 oz	210	8	1	0	41	4	30
Organic Vegetable Alphabets	2 oz	200	8	1	0	40	2	15
Spirals Rye	2 oz	200	6	0	0	44	8	10
Goya								
Coditos not prep	½ cup	230	8	1	0	47	3	0
Hodgson Mill								
Four Color Veggie Bows	2 oz	200	8	1	0	41	1	15
Four Color Veggie Rotini Spirals	2 oz	200	8	1	0	41	1	15
Four Color Veggie Wagon Wheels	2 oz	200	8	1	0	41	1	15
Pastamania! Durum Wheat Fettuccine	2 oz	200	8	2	30	38	1	20
Pastamania! Fettuccine Garlic & Parsley	2 oz	200	8	2	30	38	1	20
Pastamania! Fettuccine w/ Jerusalem Artichoke	2 oz	210	8	2	0	41	2	10
Pastamania! Fettucinne w/ Mushroom	2 oz	210	8	2	35	41	2	15
Pastamania! Fusilli Tre Colore w/ Tomato & Spinach	2 oz	200	7	1	0	40	2	20

FOOD	PORTION	CAL	PROT	FAT	CHOL	CARB	FIBER	SOD
Pastamania! Pesto Fettuccine	2 oz	200	8	2	30	38	1	20
Pastamania! Sea Shell Mix	2 oz	200	8	1	0	40	1	10
Pastamania! Spinach Fettuccine	2 oz	200	8	2	40	37	2	35
Pastamania! Thin Linguine	2 oz	200	8	2	30	38	1	20
Pastamania! Tomato Spinach & Durum Wheat	2 oz	210	8	2	35	40	2	29
Spaghetti Whole Wheat	2 oz	190	9	1	0	34	6	10
Lundberg								
Spaghetti Organic Brown Rice	2 oz	210	4	2	0	44	3	5
Ronzoni								
Lasagne	2 ½ pieces (2 oz)	210	7	1	0	42	2	0
San Giorgio								
Mostaccioli Rigati	2 oz	210	–	1	0	–	–	–
FRESH								
cooked	2 oz	75	3	1	33	14	–	3
spinach cooked	2 oz	74	3	1	19	14	–	3
Di Giorno								
Angel's Hair	1 cup	160	6	2	0	31	2	115
Beef & Roasted Garlic Tortellini	1 cup	340	14	11	50	46	1	390
Fettuccine	1 cup	200	8	2	0	38	2	140
Four Cheese Raviolo	1 cup	350	14	15	70	40	2	390
Herb Linguine	1 cup	200	8	2	0	38	2	140
Italian Sausage Ravioli In Green Bell Pepper Pasta	1¼ cup	350	14	12	55	45	3	570
Lemon Chicken Tortellini In Cracked Black Pepper Pasta	1 cup	270	13	5	40	42	1	290
Light Cheese Ravioli	1 cup	280	15	7	40	40	2	400

FOOD	PORTION	CAL	PROT	FAT	CHOL	CARB	FIBER	SOD
Linguine	1 cup	200	8	2	0	38	2	140
Mozzarella Garlic Tortelloni	1 cup	300	15	8	45	42	1	400
Pesto Tortelloni	1 cup	320	16	8	45	46	3	430
Portabello Mushroom Tortelloni	1 cup	310	13	7	40	48	3	490
Red Bell Pepper Fettuccine	1 cup	200	8	2	0	38	2	140
Spinach Fettuccine	1 cup	190	8	2	0	38	2	160
Sun-Dried Tomato Ravioli	1⅓ cup	380	17	14	55	48	3	600
Three Cheese Tortellini	¾ cup	250	11	7	35	37	2	300

PASTA DINNERS *(see also PASTA SALAD)*
CANNED
Chef Boyardee

FOOD	PORTION	CAL	PROT	FAT	CHOL	CARB	FIBER	SOD
99% Fat Free Beef Ravioli	1 cup (8.6 oz)	210	9	1	15	41	3	1150
99% Fat Free Cheese Ravioli	1 cup (8.8 oz)	210	7	1	<5	44	4	860
Beef Ravioli	1 cup (8.6 oz)	230	9	5	20	37	4	1150
Beefaroni	1 cup (8.7 oz)	260	10	7	25	37	5	870
Macaroni & Cheese	½ can (7.5 oz)	180	8	2	20	35	2	1090
Mini Ravioli	1 cup (8.8 oz)	252	8	6	20	37	3	1180
Spaghetti & Meat Balls	1 cup (8.4 oz)	240	9	10	25	32	3	950
Tortellini Cheese	½ can (7 oz)	230	9	1	15	48	5	770
Tortellini Meat	½ can (7 oz)	260	10	4	30	48	4	810
Franco-American								
Beef Raviolios	1 can (7.7 oz)	250	9	5	12	39	4	911
Beefy Mac	1 can (7.5 oz)	228	9	8	10	30	3	1144
Elbow Macaroni & Cheese	1 can (7.5 oz)	187	6	6	7	25	2	875
Spaghetti 'N Beef	1 can (7.5 oz)	226	10	8	14	30	3	1063
Spaghetti w/ Meatballs	1 can (7.2 oz)	249	10	9	14	33	4	917

FOOD	PORTION	CAL	PROT	FAT	CHOL	CARB	FIBER	SOD
Kid's Kitchen								
Microwave Meals Cheezy Mac & Beef	1 cup (7.5 oz)	260	15	7	30	33	1	910
Microwave Meals Noodle Rings & Chicken	1 cup (7.5 oz)	150	10	4	30	17	1	1110
Microwave Meals Spaghetti Rings & Franks	1 cup (7.5 oz)	240	9	9	30	32	1	810
Progresso								
Beef Ravioli	1 cup (9.1 oz)	260	9	5	5	45	4	940
Cheese Ravioli	1 cup (9.1 oz)	220	7	2	<5	43	4	930
FROZEN								
Amy's Organic								
Macaroni & Cheese	1 pkg (9 oz)	390	17	14	40	50	4	550
Macaroni & Soy Cheese	1 pkg (9 oz)	360	16	14	0	42	4	500
Pasta Primavera	1 pkg (9.5 oz)	320	15	12	65	39	3	680
Ravioli w/ Sauce	1 pkg (9.5 oz)	340	15	12	20	44	6	580
Tofu Vegetable Lasagna	1 pkg (9.5 oz)	300	18	10	0	41	4	630
Vegetable Lasagna	1 pkg (9.5 oz)	300	15	10	15	39	5	680
Whole Meals Cannelloni	1 pkg (9 oz)	260	11	11	20	32	5	560
Banquet								
Chicken Pasta Primavera	1 meal (9.5 oz)	320	11	12	25	40	6	840
Family Size Egg Noodles w/ Beef & Brown Gravy	1 serv	150	11	5	35	16	2	1120
Family Size Lasagna w/ Meat Sauce	1 cup	270	14	10	45	33	2	900
Family Size Macaroni & Cheese	1 cup	230	8	7	10	32	3	1290
Fettuccine Alfredo	1 meal (9.5 oz)	350	11	16	25	40	4	850
Homestyle Noodles & Chicken	1 meal (12 oz)	390	12	19	50	44	7	1080

FOOD	PORTION	CAL	PROT	FAT	CHOL	CARB	FIBER	SOD
Lasagna w/ Meat Sauce	1 meal (9.5 oz)	260	10	8	15	38	3	820
Macaroni & Cheese	1 meal (12 oz)	420	15	14	20	57	5	1330
Birds Eye								
Pasta Secrets Italian Pesto	2⅓ cups (6.4 oz)	240	9	9	5	32	2	700
Pasta Secrets Primavera	2⅓ cups (6.6 oz)	230	9	10	10	26	3	430
Pasta Secrets Ranch	2⅓ cups (6.6 oz)	300	7	15	25	29	2	460
Pasta Secrets Three Cheese	2 cups (6.1 oz)	230	9	8	5	31	2	590
Pasta Secrets White Cheddar	2 cups (6.3 oz)	240	7	10	10	30	2	560
Pasta Secrets Zesty Garlic	2 cups (5.9 oz)	240	7	10	5	31	2	310
Green Giant								
Create A Meal Creamy Alfredo as prep	1¼ cups (10 oz)	380	34	12	75	33	4	990
Create A Meal Creamy Cheddar as prep	1½ cups (10 oz)	290	20	10	45	29	4	1470
Create A Meal Creamy Chicken Noodle as prep	1½ cups (10 oz)	350	28	11	65	34	3	970
Pasta Accents Alfredo	2 cups (5.6 oz)	210	9	5	15	25	4	480
Pasta Accents Creamy Cheddar	2⅓ cups (6.7 oz)	250	9	8	15	36	5	700
Pasta Accents Florentine	2 cups (7.3 oz)	310	13	9	20	44	5	910
Pasta Accents Garden Herb Seasoning	2 cups (6.8 oz)	230	9	7	15	32	7	750
Pasta Accents Garlic Seasoning	2 cups (6.6 oz)	260	7	10	15	36	5	640
Pasta Accents Primavera	2¼ cups (7 oz)	320	13	12	20	40	7	500

FOOD	PORTION	CAL	PROT	FAT	CHOL	CARB	FIBER	SOD
Pasta Accents White Cheddar Sauce	1¾ cups (5.6 oz)	300	10	12	20	38	4	570
Healthy Choice								
Beef Macaroni	1 meal (8.5 oz)	220	12	4	20	34	5	450
Bowls Cheese & Chicken Tortellini	1 meal (8.7 oz)	250	11	5	20	40	6	600
Breaded Chicken Breast Stips w/ Macaroni & Cheese	1 meal (8 oz)	270	22	5	40	34	1	600
Cheese Ravioli Parmigiana	1 meal (9 oz)	260	11	5	20	44	6	290
Chicken Fettuccine Alfredo	1 meal (8.5 oz)	280	21	7	35	30	4	600
Fettuccine Alfredo	1 meal (8 oz)	240	11	5	20	37	2	560
Lasagna Roma	1 meal (13.5 oz)	420	26	9	35	59	6	580
Macaroni & Cheese	1 meal (9 oz)	240	12	5	20	36	3	600
Manicotti w/Three Cheeses	1 meal (11 oz)	300	15	9	35	40	5	550
Spaghetti & Sauce w/ Seasoned Beef	1 meal (10 oz)	260	14	8	30	43	5	470
Stuffed Pasta Shells	1 meal (10.35 oz)	370	18	6	20	60	5	570
Kid Cuisine								
Magical Macaroni & Cheese	1 meal (10.6 oz)	440	10	13	15	72	4	670
Lean Cuisine								
Cafe Classics Bow Tie Pasta & Chicken	1 pkg (9.5 oz)	220	15	4	40	32	5	690
Cafe Classics Cheese Lasagna w/ Chicken Scaloppini	1 pkg (10 oz)	270	22	8	35	27	4	690
Cafe Classics Shrimp & Angel Hair Pasta	1 pkg (10 oz)	240	15	5	45	35	2	670
Everyday Favorites	1 pkg (10 oz)	270	13	6	10	40	5	590
Everyday Favorites Alfredo Pasta Primavera	1 pkg (10 oz)	290	11	7	10	46	3	570

FOOD	PORTION	CAL	PROT	FAT	CHOL	CARB	FIBER	SOD
Everyday Favorites Angel Hair Pasta	1 pkg (10 oz)	240	9	4	5	43	4	500
Everyday Favorites Cheese Cannelloni	1 pkg (9.1 oz)	230	21	4	15	28	4	590
Everyday Favorites Cheese Ravioli	1 pkg (8.5 oz)	260	12	7	35	38	4	590
Everyday Favorites Chicken Lasagna	1 pkg (10 oz)	280	20	7	40	34	2	590
Everyday Favorites Classic Cheese Lasagna	1 pkg (11.5 oz)	290	20	6	25	38	4	590
Everyday Favorites Fettucini Alfredo	1 pkg (9.25 oz)	280	13	7	15	42	3	540
Everyday Favorites Fettucini Primavera	1 pkg (10 oz)	270	13	7	15	38	4	580
Everyday Favorites Lasagna w/ Meat Sauce	1 pkg (10.5 oz)	300	23	8	30	35	4	570
Everyday Favorites Macaroni & Cheese	1 pkg (10 oz)	290	15	7	20	42	2	630
Everyday Favorites Macaroni & Beef	1 pkg (10 oz)	270	15	4	25	43	4	590
Everyday Favorites Penne Pasta	1 pkg (10 oz)	260	9	4	0	47	5	390
Everyday Favorites Spaghetti w/ Meat Sauce	1 pkg (11.5 oz)	290	11	5	20	50	7	570
Everyday Favorites Spaghetti w/ Meatballs	1 pkg (9.5 oz)	270	16	6	20	37	4	590
Everyday Favorites	1 pkg (9.25 oz)	270	21	6	40	33	3	620
Family Style Favorites Five Cheese Lasagna	1 serv (8 oz)	210	14	5	20	27	3	690
Skillet Sensations Chicken Alfredo	1 serv	280	20	6	30	36	3	590

FOOD	PORTION	CAL	PROT	FAT	CHOL	CARB	FIBER	SOD
Marie Callender's								
Cheese Ravioli In Marinara Sauce w/ Spirals & Garlic Bread	1 meal (16 oz)	750	25	29	30	96	11	1070
Extra Cheese Lasagna	1 meal (15 oz)	590	27	27	50	61	7	1230
Fettuccine Alfredo & Garlic Bread	1 meal (14 oz)	920	23	55	90	62	3	1270
Fettuccine Alfredo Supreme	1 meal (13 oz)	450	15	27	80	35	4	680
Fettuccine Primavera w/ Tortellini	1 meal (14 oz)	750	19	49	65	57	6	1130
Fettuccine w/ Broccoli & Chicken	1 meal (13 oz)	710	26	43	85	53	6	910
Lasagna w/ Meat Sauce	1 meal (15 oz)	630	29	31	75	59	3	1230
Macaroni & Cheese	1 meal (12 oz)	540	25	24	50	55	5	1930
Skillet Meal Chicken Alfredo	½ pkg	490	28	29	75	32	7	1220
Skillet Meal Penne Pasta & Meatballs	½ pkg	600	26	31	45	53	4	1360
Skillet Meal Rigatoni Vegetables In Cheese Sauce	1 cup	290	12	12	30	32	4	640
Spaghetti w/ Meat Sauce & Garlic Bread	1 meal (17 oz)	670	27	25	35	65	9	1100
Stuffed Pasta Trio	1 meal (10.5 oz)	380	15	16	50	40	5	950
Morton								
Macaroni & Cheese	1 serv (8 oz)	240	9	8	20	34	3	1190
Spaghetti w/ Meat Sauce	1 meal (8.5 oz)	200	5	6	5	30	4	750
Quorn								
Fettuccine Alfredo	1 pkg (10.5 oz)	360	17	16	45	40	4	920
Lasagna	1 pkg (10.5 oz)	360	23	12	15	43	4	910
Stouffer's								
Cheddar Pasta w/ Beef & Tomatoes	1 pkg (11 oz)	450	25	19	51	45	3	1130

FOOD	PORTION	CAL	PROT	FAT	CHOL	CARB	FIBER	SOD
Cheese Manicotti	1 pkg (9 oz)	380	18	17	45	38	4	880
Cheese Ravioli	1 pkg (10.6 oz)	380	15	13	100	51	6	700
Chicken Lasagna	1 serv (7.8 oz)	320	13	17	30	29	4	750
Fettucini Alfredo	1 pkg (10 oz)	520	16	28	100	17	4	1060
Fettucini Primavera	1 pkg (10 oz)	430	13	20	50	49	5	1100
Five Cheese Lasagna	1 pkg (10.75 oz)	360	21	13	35	40	6	960
Grilled Chicken & Angel HairPasta	1 pkg (10.9 oz)	380	25	13	40	40	5	750
Homestyle Chicken Fettucini	1 pkg (10.5 oz)	390	31	15	65	32	3	1250
Homestyle Chicken Parmigiana w/ Spaghetti	1 pkg (12 oz)	460	24	16	45	54	5	1060
Homestyle Veal Parmigiana w/ Spaghetti	1 pkg (11.9 oz)	430	21	17	80	49	6	1120
Lasagna Bake	1 pkg (10.25 oz)	370	18	12	30	47	6	900
Lasagna w/ Meat Sauce	1 pkg (10.5 oz)	370	23	14	45	39	4	1050
Macaroni & Cheese	1 cup (6 oz)	320	13	16	30	31	3	990
Macaroni & Cheese w/ Broccoli	1 pkg (10.5 oz)	360	15	17	25	37	5	1050
Macaroni & Beef	1 pkg (11.5 oz)	420	20	20	50	40	5	1530
Noodles Romanoff	1 pkg (12 oz)	490	18	25	60	48	4	1400
Pasta Shells w/ American Cheese	1 cup (6 oz)	260	11	10	20	31	2	1190
Salisbury Steak w/ Macaroni & Cheese	1 serv (11.3 oz)	410	26	19	70	34	2	1230
Spaghetti w/ Meat Sauce	1 pkg (10 oz)	350	15	12	35	46	5	570
Spaghetti w/ Meatballs	1 pkg (12.6 oz)	440	19	15	50	56	5	830
Tuna Noodle Casserole	1 pkg (10 oz)	320	20	10	40	37	0	1130
Turkey Tettrazini	1 pkg (10 oz)	360	19	17	55	33	1	1060
Vegetable Lasagna	1 pkg (10.5 oz)	440	21	20	35	43	5	1110
Weight Watchers								
Garden Lasagna	1 pkg (11 oz)	270	14	7	30	36	5	610

FOOD	PORTION	CAL	PROT	FAT	CHOL	CARB	FIBER	SOD
Homestyle Macaroni & Cheese	1 pkg (9 oz)	290	12	7	10	45	2	630
Smart Ones Angel Hair Pasta	1 pkg (9 oz)	180	9	2	0	32	4	600
Smart Ones Bowtie Pasta & Mushrooms Marsala	1 pkg (9.65 oz)	270	11	7	40	40	4	520
Smart Ones Chicken Fettucini	1 pkg (10 oz)	300	21	7	70	39	4	590
Smart Ones Creamy Rigatoni w/ Broccoli & Chicken	1 pkg (9 oz)	230	14	2	20	40	4	670
Smart Ones Fettucini Alfredo w/ Broccoli	1 pkg (8.5 oz)	230	13	6	20	32	3	540
Smart Ones Lasagna Florentine	1 pkg (10 oz)	200	11	2	10	33	5	640
Smart Ones Lasagna Alfredo	1 pkg (9 oz)	300	14	7	25	46	3	680
Smart Ones Lasagna w/ Meat Sauce	1 pkg (10.25 oz)	270	18	6	55	36	6	570
Smart Ones Lasagna w/ Meat Sauce	1 pkg (9 oz)	240	13	2	10	43	4	520
Smart Ones Macaroni & Cheese	1 pkg (9 oz)	220	9	2	5	42	4	640
Smart Ones Pasta & Spinach Romano	1 pkg (10.4 oz)	260	12	8	15	35	4	510
Smart Ones Pasta w/ Tomato Basil Sauce	1 pkg (9.6 oz)	260	10	7	10	40	3	360
Smart Ones Penne Pasta w/ Sun-Dried Tomatoes	1 pkg (10 oz)	280	11	8	15	40	3	560
Smart Ones Penne Pollo	1 pkg (10 oz)	290	22	6	55	38	3	590
Smart Ones Ravioli Florentine	1 pkg (8.5 oz)	220	9	2	5	43	4	490

FOOD	PORTION	CAL	PROT	FAT	CHOL	CARB	FIBER	SOD
Smart Ones Spaghetti Marinara	1 pkg (9 oz)	280	9	7	5	46	4	690
Smart Ones Spaghetti w/ Meat Sauce	1 pkg (10 oz)	280	15	6	15	41	4	560
Smart Ones Spicy Penne & Ricotta	1 pkg (10.2 oz)	280	11	6	5	45	4	400
Smart Ones Tuna Noodle Casserole	1 pkg (9.5 oz)	270	13	7	45	38	4	670
Smart Ones Zita Mozzarella	1 pkg (9 oz)	290	11	7	5	47	5	600
Yves								
Veggie Lasagna	1 pkg (10.5 oz)	300	17	3	0	51	4	650
Veggie Macaroni	1 pkg (10.5 oz)	230	14	2	0	38	3	580
Veggie Penne	1 pkg (10.5 oz)	220	12	2	0	36	4	730
MIX								
Hamburger Helper								
Ravioli as prep	1 cup	280	20	10	50	30	1	840
Ravioli w/ White Cheese Topping as prep	1 cup	310	20	10	50	34	1	960
Hodgson Mill								
Macaroni & Cheese Whole Wheat	1 serv	250	11	2	<5	45	6	570
Kraft								
Light Deluxe Macaroni & Cheese as prep	1 cup (6.5 oz)	290	14	5	15	48	1	810
Macaroni & Cheese All Shapes as prep	1 cup (6.9 oz)	410	12	18	10	49	1	750
Macaroni & Cheese Original as prep	1 cup (6.9 oz)	410	12	18	10	49	1	750
Spaghetti Classics Mild Italian as prep	1 cup (9.1 oz)	240	11	3	<5	46	3	850
Spaghetti Classics Tangy Italian as prep	1 cup (8.9 oz)	240	11	2	0	46	3	830
Spaghetti Classics Zesty Cheese as prep	1 cup (8.6 oz)	240	11	2	5	46	3	800

FOOD	PORTION	CAL	PROT	FAT	CHOL	CARB	FIBER	SOD
Spaghetti Classics w/ Meat Sauce as prep	1 cup (8.2 oz)	330	11	10	15	47	3	810
Lipton								
Pasta & Sauce Angel Hair Chicken Broccoli as prep	1 cup	260	8	8	0	43	2	810
Pasta & Sauce Angel Hair Parmesan as prep	1 cup	280	8	11	10	41	2	960
Pasta & Sauce Bow Tie Chicken Primavera as prep	1 cup	290	9	10	10	43	2	820
Pasta & Sauce Bow Tie Italian Cheese as prep	1 cup	300	10	12	15	41	tr	900
Pasta & Sauce Butter & Herbs as prep	1 cup	270	7	10	5	40	2	830
Pasta & Sauce Cheddar Broccoli as prep	1 cup	340	11	11	15	49	1	970
Pasta & Sauce Chicken Herb Parmesan as prep	1 cup	80	8	9	5	43	2	910
Pasta & Sauce Chicken Stir-Fry as prep	1 cup	270	8	8	0	43	2	900
Pasta & Sauce Creamy Garlic as prep	1 cup	350	10	13	15	50	1	980
Pasta & Sauce Creamy Mushroom as prep	1 cup	320	10	11	15	46	0	870
Pasta & Sauce Garlic & Butter Linguine as prep	1 cup	260	7	9	5	40	2	850

FOOD	PORTION	CAL	PROT	FAT	CHOL	CARB	FIBER	SOD
Pasta & Sauce Mild Cheddar Cheese as prep	1 cup	290	10	10	10	41	tr	930
Pasta & Sauce Roasted Garlic Chicken as prep	1 cup	290	9	10	10	43	tr	880
Pasta & Sauce Rotini Primavera as prep	1 cup	320	10	12	15	45	2	980
Pasta & Sauce Savory Herb w/ Garlic as prep	1 cup	280	8	9	5	52	2	890
Pasta & Sauce Three Cheese Rotini as prep	1 cup	320	11	12	15	44	tr	970
Melting Pot								
Terrazza Black Beans & Penne	1 cup	180	8	1	0	36	2	480
Terrazza Florentine Red Beans & Fusilli	1 cup	220	10	1	<5	43	2	350
Terrazza Red Lentils & Bow Ties	1 cup	240	13	2	40	42	5	390
Terrazza Tuscan White Beans & Gemell	1 cup	220	10	1	<5	44	3	450
Velveeta								
Rotini & Cheese w/ Broccoli as prep	1 cup (7.2 oz)	400	18	16	50	47	2	1230
Shells & Cheese Bacon as prep	1 cup (6.8 oz)	360	17	14	40	43	1	1140
Shells & Cheese Original as prep	1 cup (6.6 oz)	360	16	13	40	44	1	1030
Shells & Cheese Salsa as prep	1 cup (7.5 oz)	380	17	14	40	47	2	1180
READY-TO-EAT								
Tyson								
Rosemary Penne	1 pkg (12.5 oz)	330	25	5	45	45	5	860

FOOD	PORTION	CAL	PROT	FAT	CHOL	CARB	FIBER	SOD
SHELF-STABLE								
Hormel								
Microcup Meals Lasagna	1 cup (7.5 oz)	250	8	14	25	24	1	950
Microcup Meals Macaroni & Cheese	1 cup (7.5 oz)	260	11	11	35	30	1	690
Microcup Meals Ravioli w/ Tomato Sauce	1 cup (7.5 oz)	220	8	6	15	34	2	840
Microcup Meals Spaghetti & Meatballs	1 cup (7.5 oz)	220	11	7	25	28	1	930
Kid's Kitchen								
Microwave Meals Beefy Macaroni	1 cup (7.5 oz)	190	11	6	30	23	2	790
Microwave Meals Macaroni & Cheese	1 cup (7.5 oz)	260	11	11	35	30	1	690
Microwave Meals Mini Ravioli	1 cup (7.5 oz)	240	10	7	20	34	1	950
Microwave Meals Spaghetti & Meatballs	1 cup (7.5 oz)	220	11	7	25	28	1	950
Microwave Meals Spaghetti Ring & Meatballs	1 cup (7.5 oz)	250	11	7	20	35	3	1200
Lunch Bucket								
Beef Ravioli In Tomato Sauce	1 pkg (7.5 oz)	180	5	4	5	32	3	740
Italian Pasta w/ Chicken	1 pkg (7.5 oz)	130	5	2	10	24	2	610
Lasagna 'n Meatsauce	1 pkg (7.5 oz)	160	5	3	5	29	2	850
Macaroni 'n Beef in Meatsauce	1 pkg (7.5 oz)	180	0	5	10	10	8	820
Macaroni'n Cheese	1 pkg (7.5 oz)	190	7	7	20	24	2	930
Pasta'n Chicken	1 pkg (7.5 oz)	150	5	5	20	22	2	810
Spaghetti'n Meatsauce	1 pkg (7.5 oz)	160	5	3	5	29	2	850

FOOD	PORTION	CAL	PROT	FAT	CHOL	CARB	FIBER	SOD
TAKE-OUT								
lasagna	1 piece (2.5 in x 2.5 in)	374	22	21	107	25	2	668
macaroni & cheese	1 cup	230	9	10	24	26	–	730
manicotti	¾ cup (6.4 oz)	273	14	12	77	28	2	414
rigatoni w/ sausage sauce	¾ cup	260	10	12	59	28	3	106
spaghetti w/ meatballs & cheese	1 cup	407	21	19	104	38	–	696

PASTA SALAD

MIX
Kraft

FOOD	PORTION	CAL	PROT	FAT	CHOL	CARB	FIBER	SOD
Herb & Garlic as prep	¾ cup (4.9 oz)	280	6	14	0	34	2	670
Pasta Salad Classic Ranch w/ Bacon as prep	¾ cup (4.7 oz)	350	7	22	10	32	2	480
Pasta Salad Creamy Ceasar as prep	¾ cup (4.8 oz)	340	7	21	15	31	2	630
Pasta Salad Garden Primavera as prep	¾ cup (5 oz)	240	8	8	<5	35	2	710
Pasta Salad Italian 97% Fat Free as prep	¾ cup (4.9 oz)	190	8	2	<5	34	2	740
Pasta Salad Parmesan Peppercorn as prep	¾ cup (4.9 oz)	360	7	23	15	29	2	570

Suddenly Salad

FOOD	PORTION	CAL	PROT	FAT	CHOL	CARB	FIBER	SOD
Classic Pasta	¾ cup	250	7	8	0	38	2	910
Classic Pasta Reduced Fat Recipe	¾ cup	210	7	4	0	38	2	910
Garden Italian 98% Fat Free	¾ cup	140	5	1	0	28	2	520

TAKE-OUT

FOOD	PORTION	CAL	PROT	FAT	CHOL	CARB	FIBER	SOD
elbow macaroni salad	3.5 oz	160	3	5	0	26	–	590
italian style pasta salad	3.5 oz	140	3	7	0	15	–	480
mustard macaroni salad	3.5 oz	190	4	10	0	23	–	560

FOOD	PORTION	CAL	PROT	FAT	CHOL	CARB	FIBER	SOD
pasta salad w/ vegetables	3.5 oz	140	4	4	0	21	–	210

PATE

FOOD	PORTION	CAL	PROT	FAT	CHOL	CARB	FIBER	SOD
antipasto pate	1 can (2.25 oz)	110	3	9	5	3	1	530
chicken liver canned	1 oz	238	4	4	–	2	–	–
chicken liver canned	1 tbsp (13 g)	109	2	2	–	1	–	–
duck pate	1 oz	96	4	8	–	1	–	–
fish pate	1 oz	76	3	7	–	1	–	286
goose liver smoked canned	1 tbsp (13 g)	60	1	6	20	1	–	–
goose liver smoked canned	1 oz	131	3	12	43	1	–	–
liver canned	1 oz	90	4	8	–	tr	–	198
liver canned	1 tbsp (13 g)	41	5	4	–	tr	–	91
mushroom anchovy pate	1 can (2.25 oz)	130	2	11	5	7	1	400
pate foie gras	1 oz	127	3	13	109	1	–	211
pork pate	1 oz	107	3	10	51	1	0	189
pork pate en croute	1 oz	91	3	7	32	3	tr	214
rabbit pate	1 oz	66	5	5	21	1	–	97
salmon pate	1 can (2.25 oz)	140	6	10	10	6	0	420
shrimp	1 can (2.25 oz)	140	6	10	25	7	0	450
smoked turkey	1 can (2.25 oz)	170	6	13	15	7	0	480

PEACH

CANNED

FOOD	PORTION	CAL	PROT	FAT	CHOL	CARB	FIBER	SOD
halves in heavy syrup	1 half	60	tr	tr	0	16	–	5
halves in light syrup	1 half	44	tr	tr	0	12	–	4
halves juice pack	1 half	34	tr	tr	0	9	–	3
halves water pack	1 half	18	tr	tr	0	5	–	3
spiced in heavy syrup	1 cup	180	1	tr	0	49	–	9
spiced in heavy syrup	1 fruit	66	tr	tr	0	18	–	3

Del Monte

FOOD	PORTION	CAL	PROT	FAT	CHOL	CARB	FIBER	SOD
Fruit Cup Diced Extra Light Syrup	1 pkg (4 oz)	50	0	0	0	13	1	10
Fruit Cup Diced In Heavy Syrup	1 serv (4 oz)	80	0	0	0	20	1	10
Fruit Cup Fruit Naturals Diced	1 pkg (4 oz)	50	0	0	0	13	1	10

FOOD	PORTION	CAL	PROT	FAT	CHOL	CARB	FIBER	SOD
Fruit Pleasures Raspberry Flavor	½ cup (4.5 oz)	80	1	0	0	20	1	10
Fruit To Go Banana Berry Peaches	1 pkg (4 oz)	70	1	0	0	17	1	10
Fruitrageous Peachy Pie	1 pkg (4 oz)	80	1	0	0	21	1	10
Fruitrageous Wild Raspberry Flavor	1 pkg (4 oz)	80	1	0	0	20	1	10
Halves Ginger Flavor	½ cup (4.5 oz)	90	0	0	0	22	1	10
Halves In Extra Light Syrup	½ cup (4.4 oz)	60	0	0	0	15	1	10
Halves In Heavy Syrup	½ cup (4.5 oz)	100	0	0	0	24	1	10
Halves Melba In Heavy Syrup	½ cup (4.5 oz)	100	0	0	0	24	1	10
Slice Fruit Natural	½ cup (4.4 oz)	60	0	0	0	15	1	10
Sliced In Extra Light Syrup	½ cup (4.4 oz)	60	0	0	0	14	1	10
Sliced In Heavy Syrup	½ cup (4.5 oz)	100	0	0	0	24	1	10
Sliced Natural Raspberry Flavor	½ cup (4.4 oz)	80	0	0	0	20	1	10
Sliced Natural Harvest Spice Flavor	½ cup (4.5 oz)	80	1	0	0	21	1	10
Whole Spiced In Heavy Syrup	½ cup (4.2 oz)	100	0	0	0	24	1	10
DRIED								
halves	1 cup	383	6	1	0	98	13	12
halves	10	311	5	1	0	80	11	9
halves cooked w/ sugar	½ cup	139	1	tr	0	36	–	3
halves cooked w/o sugar	½ cup	99	1	tr	0	25	–	3
Sonoma								
Pieces	3–5 pieces (1.4 oz)	120	1	0	0	31	1	0

FOOD	PORTION	CAL	PROT	FAT	CHOL	CARB	FIBER	SOD
FRESH								
peach	1	37	1	tr	0	10	1	0
sliced	1 cup	73	1	tr	0	19	–	1
Chiquita								
Peach	1 med (3.4 oz)	40	14	0	0	10	2	0
FROZEN								
slices sweetened	1 cup	235	2	tr	0	60	–	16
PEACH JUICE								
nectar	1 cup	134	1	tr	0	35	–	17
Nantucket Nectars								
The Original	8 oz	120	0	0	0	30	–	15
PEANUT BUTTER								
chunky	2 tbsp	188	8	16	0	7	2	156
chunky	1 cup	1520	62	129	0	56	17	1255
chunky w/o salt	1 cup	1520	62	129	0	56	17	44
chunky w/o salt	2 tbsp	188	8	16	0	7	2	5
smooth	2 tbsp	188	8	16	0	7	2	153
smooth	1 cup	1517	63	128	0	53	15	1234
smooth w/o salt	2 tbsp	188	8	16	0	7	2	5
smooth w/o salt	1 cup	1517	63	129	0	53	15	44
Estee								
Creamy Low Sodium	2 tbsp (1 oz)	190	7	15	0	7	2	0
Jif								
Apple Cinnamon	2 tbsp (1.3 oz)	200	6	16	0	11	2	115
Berry Blend	2 tbsp (1.2 oz)	200	6	17	0	10	1	115
Chocolate Silk	2 tbsp (1.3 oz)	190	5	15	0	14	1	115
Creamy	2 tbsp (1.1 oz)	190	8	16	0	7	2	150
Extra Crunchy	2 tbsp (1.1 oz)	190	8	16	0	7	2	130
Reduced Fat Creamy	2 tbsp (1.3 oz)	190	8	12	0	15	2	250
Reduced Fat Crunchy	2 tbsp (1.3 oz)	190	8	12	0	15	2	220
Simply	2 tbsp (1.1 oz)	190	8	16	0	6	2	1
Peanut Wonder								
Low Sodium	2 tbsp	100	4	3	0	13	0	95
Regular	2 tbsp	100	4	3	0	13	0	220
Reese's								
Peanut Butter Chips	1 tbsp (0.5 oz)	80	3	4	0	7	–	35

FOOD	PORTION	CAL	PROT	FAT	CHOL	CARB	FIBER	SOD
PEANUTS								
chocolate coated	10 (1.4 oz)	208	5	13	4	20	–	16
chocolate coated	1 cup (5.2 oz)	773	19	50	13	74	–	61
cooked	½ cup	102	4	7	0	7	–	240
dry roasted	1 cup	855	35	73	0	31	12	1187
dry roasted w/ salt	30 nuts (1 oz)	170	7	14	0	6	2	230
oil roasted	1 oz	163	7	14	0	5	2	121
oil roasted	1 cup	837	38	71	0	27	13	624
oil roasted w/o salt	1 cup	837	38	71	0	27	13	9
oil roasted w/o salt	1 oz	163	7	14	0	5	2	2
spanish oil roasted	1 oz	162	8	14	0	5	2	121
spanish oil roasted w/o salt	1 oz	162	8	14	0	5	2	2
unroasted	1 oz	159	7	14	0	5	–	5
valencia oil roasted	1 cup	848	39	74	0	23	9	1111
valencia oil roasted	1 oz	165	8	14	0	5	2	216
valencia oil roasted w/o salt	1 oz	165	8	14	0	5	2	2
valencia oil roasted w/o salt	1 cup	848	40	74	0	23	9	9
virginia oil roasted	1 oz	161	8	14	0	5	–	121
virginia oil roasted	1 cup	826	37	70	0	28	–	619
Estee								
Candy Coated	¼ cup	200	5	9	<5	23	1	45
Frito Lay								
Honey Roasted	1 serv (1.5 oz)	270	10	21	0	10	3	80
Hot	1 serv (1.1 oz)	190	7	16	0	6	2	250
Salted	1 oz	200	7	16	0	5	2	180
Lance								
Honey Toasted	1 pkg (1⅜ oz)	220	9	15	0	13	3	170
Roasted	1 pkg (1¾ oz)	190	9	14	0	6	4	0
Salted	1 pkg (1⅛ oz)	200	9	15	0	6	4	150
Salted Long Tube	¼ cup (1 oz)	180	8	14	0	5	3	135
Little Debbie								
Salted	¼ cup (1 oz)	160	7	14	0	5	2	130
Pennant								
Oil Roasted	1 oz	170	7	14	0	6	3	115
Planters								
Cocktail Lightly Salted Oil Roasted	1 oz	170	7	15	0	5	2	55

FOOD	PORTION	CAL	PROT	FAT	CHOL	CARB	FIBER	SOD
Cocktail Oil Roasted	1 oz	170	7	14	0	6	3	115
Cocktail Unsalted Oil Roasted	1 oz	170	7	14	0	6	2	0
Dry Roasted	1 oz	160	7	13	0	6	3	250
Fun Size! Oil Roasted	2 pkg (1 oz)	170	7	15	0	6	2	140
Heat Hot Spicy Oil Roasted	1 pkg (1.7 oz)	290	12	25	0	9	4	370
Heat Hot Spicy Oil Roasted	1 oz	160	7	14	0	5	2	190
Heat Hot Spicy Oil Roasted	1 pkg (2 oz)	330	14	29	0	10	5	390
Heat Mild Spicy Oil Roasted	1 oz	160	7	14	0	5	2	130
Honey Roasted	1 oz	160	6	13	0	8	2	90
Honey Roasted Dry Roasted	1 pkg (1.7 oz)	260	10	19	0	17	3	260
Lightly Salted Dry Roasted	1 oz	160	8	14	0	5	3	110
Lightly Salted Dry Roasted	1 pkg (1.75 oz)	290	13	25	0	9	4	190
Lightly Salted Oil Roasted	1 pkg (1.8 oz)	300	13	27	0	8	4	95
Reduced Fat Honey Roasted	⅓ cup (1 oz)	130	6	7	0	12	2	150
Salted Oil Roasted	1 pkg (1 oz)	170	7	15	0	5	2	110
Spanish Oil Roasted	1 oz	170	7	14	0	5	2	105
Spanish Raw	1 oz	150	7	13	0	6	3	5
Sweet N Crunchy	1 oz	140	4	7	0	16	2	20
Unsalted Dry Roasted	1 oz	160	8	14	0	6	3	0
Tom's								
Double Coated	1 pkg (1.35 oz)	220	8	15	0	15	1	60
Toasted	1 pkg (1.4 oz)	240	11	19	0	7	2	160
Weight Watchers								
Honey Roasted	1 pkg (0.7 oz)	100	7	5	0	7	2	100

PEAR
CANNED
halves in heavy syrup	1 cup	188	1	tr	0	49	–	13
halves in heavy syrup	1 half	68	tr	tr	0	15	–	4
halves in light syrup	1 half	45	tr	tr	0	12	–	4

FOOD	PORTION	CAL	PROT	FAT	CHOL	CARB	FIBER	SOD
halves juice pack	1 cup	123	1	tr	0	32	–	10
halves water pack	1 half	22	tr	tr	0	6	–	41
Del Monte								
Fruit Cup Diced In Heavy Syrup	1 pkg (4 oz)	80	0	0	0	20	1	10
Fruit Cup Diced Extra Light Syrup	1 pkg (4 oz)	50	0	0	0	13	1	10
Fruit To Go Peachy Peaches	1 pkg (4 oz)	70	1	0	0	17	1	10
Halves Fruit Naturals	½ cup (4.4 oz)	60	0	0	0	15	1	10
Halves In Extra Light Syrup	½ cup (4.4 oz)	60	0	0	0	15	1	10
Halves In Heavy Syrup	½ cup (4.5 oz)	100	0	0	0	24	1	10
Orchard Select Sliced Bartlett	½ cup (4.4 oz)	80	1	0	0	20	2	10
Sliced In Extra Light Syrup	½ cup (4.5 oz)	60	0	0	0	15	1	10
DRIED								
halves	10	459	3	1	0	122	–	10
halves	1 cup	472	3	1	0	125	–	10
halves cooked w/ sugar	½ cup	196	1	tr	0	52	–	4
halves cooked w/o sugar	½ cup	163	tr	tr	0	43	–	4
Sonoma								
Pieces	3–4 pieces (1.4 oz)	120	1	0	0	33	3	0
FRESH								
asian	1 (4.3 oz)	51	1	tr	0	13	–	0
pear	1	98	1	1	0	25	4	1
sliced w/ skin	1 cup	97	1	1	0	25	4	1
Chiquita								
Pear	1 med (5.8 oz)	100	18	1	0	25	4	0
PEAR JUICE								
nectar	1 cup	149	tr	tr	0	39	–	9
PEAS								
CANNED								
green	½ cup	59	4	tr	0	11	–	186
green low sodium	½ cup	59	4	tr	0	11	–	2

FOOD	PORTION	CAL	PROT	FAT	CHOL	CARB	FIBER	SOD
Del Monte								
Sweet	½ cup (4.4 oz)	60	3	0	0	13	4	390
Sweet No Salt Added	½ cup (4.4 oz)	60	3	0	0	11	4	10
Sweet Very Young Small	½ cup (4.4 oz)	60	3	0	0	10	4	360
Green Giant								
Sweet	½ cup (4.3 oz)	60	4	0	0	11	4	390
Sweet 50% Less Sodium	½ cup (4.3 oz)	60	4	0	0	11	3	195
LeSueur								
Early Peas	½ cup (4.2 oz)	60	4	0	0	12	3	380
Early Peas 50% Less Sodium	½ cup (4.2 oz)	60	4	0	0	11	4	190
Sweet	½ cup (4.2 oz)	60	4	0	0	12	3	380
Sweet 50% Less Sodium	½ cup (4.2 oz)	60	4	0	0	11	4	190
Owatonna								
Early June or Sweet	½ cup	70	–	0	0	–	–	–
S&W								
Petite	½ cup (4.4 oz)	70	4	0	0	12	4	330
Small	½ cup (4.4 oz)	70	4	0	0	12	4	330
DRIED								
split cooked	1 cup	231	16	1	0	41	–	4
Bascom's								
Yellow Split as prep	½ cup	110	8	0	0	20	–	0
Hurst								
HamBeens Green Split Peas w/ Ham	1 serv	120	8	1	0	21	4	63
FRESH								
green cooked	½ cup	67	4	tr	0	13	–	2
green raw	½ cup	58	4	tr	0	11	–	3
snap peas cooked	½ cup	34	3	tr	0	6	2	3
snap peas raw	½ cup	30	2	tr	0	5	2	3
FROZEN								
green cooked	½ cup	63	4	tr	0	11	–	70
snap peas cooked	½ cup	42	3	tr	0	7	–	4
snap peas cooked	1 pkg (10 oz)	132	9	1	0	23	–	12
Birds Eye								
Butter Peas	½ cup (2.7 oz)	110	7	1	0	20	4	10

FOOD	PORTION	CAL	PROT	FAT	CHOL	CARB	FIBER	SOD
Crowder	½ cup (3 oz)	120	8	1	0	22	4	10
Field Peas w/ Snaps	⅔ cup (3.4 oz)	130	9	1	0	24	4	15
Green	½ cup	70	–	0	0	–	5	125
Purple Hull Peas	½ cup (2.8 oz)	110	7	1	0	21	4	10
Sugar Snap	½ cup	40	–	0	0	–	2	10
Tiny Tender	¾ cup	40	–	0	0	–	2	40
Green Giant								
Butter Sauce	¾ cup (4 oz)	100	4	2	<5	16	5	400
Butter Sauce LeSueur Baby	¾ cup (4 oz)	100	5	2	<5	16	4	370
Harvest Fresh LeSueur Baby	⅔ cup (3.2 oz)	70	4	0	0	13	4	220
Harvest Fresh Sugar Snap	⅔ cup (3.2 oz)	50	3	0	0	10	3	95
Harvest Fresh Sweet	⅔ cup (3.3 oz)	60	4	0	0	12	4	200
LaSueur Baby Sweet	⅔ cup (2.8 oz)	60	5	0	0	11	5	150
LaSueur Early June	⅔ cup (2.8 oz)	80	5	0	0	11	5	150
LaSueur Early June w/ Mushrooms	¾ cup (3 oz)	60	4	0	0	10	4	105
Select Sugar Snap	¾ cup (2.8 oz)	35	2	0	0	7	3	0
Sweet	⅔ cup (3.1 oz)	70	4	0	0	13	4	135
La Choy								
Snow Pea Pods	½ pkg (3 oz)	35	2	2	0	4	2	0
Tree Of Life								
Peas	⅔ cup (3.1 oz)	70	5	0	0	12	4	100
TAKE-OUT								
pea & potato curry	1 serv (7 oz)	284	5	22	–	19	6	–
pea curry	1 serv (4.4 oz)	438	5	42	–	11	4	–
PECANS								
dry roasted	1 oz	187	2	18	0	6	–	0
dry roasted salted	1 oz	187	2	18	0	6	–	260
halves dry roasted w/ salt	20 (1 oz)	200	3	21	0	4	3	110
halves dried	1 cup	721	8	73	0	20	7	1
oil roasted	1 oz	195	2	20	0	5	–	0
oil roasted salted	1 oz	195	2	20	0	5	–	252

FOOD	PORTION	CAL	PROT	FAT	CHOL	CARB	FIBER	SOD
Planters								
Chips	1 pkg (2 oz)	390	5	40	0	9	7	5
Gold Measure Halves	1 pkg (2 oz)	390	5	40	0	9	3	5
Halves	1 oz	190	3	20	0	4	2	0
Honey Roasted	1 oz	180	2	16	0	9	2	75
Pieces	1 oz	190	3	20	0	4	2	0
Pieces	1 pkg (2 oz)	390	5	40	0	9	3	5
PECTIN								
powder	1 pkg (1.75 oz)	163	tr	tr	0	45	–	100
powder	¼ pkg (0.4 oz)	39	0	0	0	11	–	24
Slim Set								
Packet	1 pkg	208	0	0	0	44	14	42
Powder	1 tbsp	3	0	0	0	1	tr	1
Sure Jell								
For Lower Sugar Recipes	1 tsp (2.8 g)	20	0	0	0	4	0	40
Fruit Pectin	1 tsp (3.6 g)	20	0	0	0	4	0	0
PEPEAO								
dried	½ cup	36	1	tr	0	10	–	8
raw sliced	1 cup	25	tr	tr	0	7	–	9
PEPPER								
black	1 tsp	5	tr	tr	0	1	–	1
cayenne	1 tsp	6	tr	tr	0	1	–	1
red	1 tsp	6	tr	tr	0	1	–	1
white	1 tsp	7	tr	tr	0	2	–	tr
PEPPERS								
CANNED								
chili green	1 cup (5.5 oz)	29	1	tr	0	6	2	552
chili green hot chopped	½ cup	17	1	tr	0	4	–	–
chili red hot	1 (2.6 oz)	18	1	tr	0	4	–	–
chili red hot chopped	½ cup	17	1	tr	0	4	–	–
green halves	½ cup	13	1	tr	0	3	–	958
jalapeno chopped	½ cup	17	1	tr	0	3	–	995
red halves	½ cup	13	1	tr	0	3	–	958
Chi-Chi's								
Chilies Diced Green	2 tbsp (1.2 oz)	10	0	0	0	1	0	20
Chilies Green Whole	¾ pepper (1 oz)	10	0	0	0	1	0	15

FOOD	PORTION	CAL	PROT	FAT	CHOL	CARB	FIBER	SOD
Old El Paso								
Green Chilies Chopped	2 tbsp (1 oz)	5	0	0	0	1	1	110
Green Chilies Whole	1 (1.2 oz)	10	0	0	0	2	1	230
Jalapenos Peeled	3 (1 oz)	10	0	0	0	1	1	200
Jalapenos Pickled	2 (0.9 oz)	5	0	0	0	1	0	380
Jalapenos Slices	2 tbsp (1.1 oz)	15	0	0	0	3	1	400
Progresso								
Cherry Sliced & So Hot	2 tbsp (1 oz)	25	0	2	0	2	1	30
Hot Cherry	1 (1 oz)	10	0	0	0	2	tr	150
Pepper Salad (drained)	2 tbsp (1 oz)	15	0	1	0	1	tr	160
Roasted	1 piece (1 oz)	10	0	0	0	3	0	55
Sweet Fried w/ Onions	2 tbsp (0.9 oz)	20	0	2	0	2	1	130
Tuscan	3 (1 oz)	10	0	0	0	2	1	450
Rosarita								
Chilies Diced Green	2 tbsp (1 oz)	6	tr	tr	0	1	1	85
Chilies Green Strips	¼ cup (1.2 oz)	5	tr	tr	0	1	1	74
Chilies Whole Green	2 tbsp (1.2 oz)	5	tr	tr	0	1	1	74
Jalapeno Whole w/ Escabeche	¼ cup (1.2 oz)	8	1	tr	0	1	1	430
Jalapenos Diced	2 tbsp (1 oz)	5	tr	tr	0	1	1	121
Jalapenos Nacho Sliced	2 tbsp (1 oz)	2	tr	tr	0	1	tr	224
Vlasic								
Hot Sliced Cherry	1 oz	5	0	0	0	1	—	480
Jalapeno Sliced	1 oz	10	0	0	0	2	—	480
Mild Cherry	1 oz	5	0	0	0	1	—	480
Pepper Rings Hot	1 oz	5	0	0	0	1	—	480
Pepper Rings Mild	1 oz	5	0	0	0	1	—	480
DRIED								
ancho	1 (0.6 oz)	48	2	1	0	9	4	7
green	1 tbsp	1	tr	tr	0	tr	—	1
pasilla	1 (7 g)	24	1	1	0	4	2	6
red	1 tbsp	1	tr	tr	0	tr	—	1
FRESH								
banana fresh	1 (4 in) (1.2 oz)	9	1	tr	0	2	1	4
banana fresh	1 cup (4.4 oz)	33	2	1	0	7	4	16

FOOD	PORTION	CAL	PROT	FAT	CHOL	CARB	FIBER	SOD
chili green hot fresh	1	18	1	tr	0	4	—	3
chili green hot fresh chopped	½ cup	30	2	tr	0	7	—	5
chili red fresh chopped	½ cup	30	2	tr	0	7	—	5
chili red hot fresh	1 (1.6 oz)	18	1	tr	0	4	—	3
green chopped cooked	½ cup	19	1	tr	0	5	—	1
green cooked	1 (2.6 oz)	20	1	tr	0	5	—	1
green fresh	1 (2.6 oz)	20	1	tr	0	5	1	1
green fresh chopped	½ cup	13	tr	tr	0	3	1	1
habanero chile	1 tsp	9	1	tr	0	2	1	2
hungarian fresh	1 (0.9 oz)	8	tr	tr	0	2	0	tr
jalapeno fresh	1 (0.5 oz)	4	tr	tr	0	1	tr	tr
jalapeno fresh sliced	1 cup (3.2 oz)	27	1	1	0	5	3	1
red chopped cooked	½ cup	19	1	tr	0	5	—	1
red cooked	1 (2.6 oz)	20	1	tr	0	5	—	1
red fresh	1 (2.6 oz)	20	1	tr	0	5	1	1
red fresh chopped	½ cup	13	tr	tr	0	3	1	1
serrano fresh	1 (6 g)	2	tr	tr	0	tr	tr	1
serrano fresh chopped	1 cup (3.7 oz)	34	2	tr	0	7	4	11
yellow fresh	10 strips	14	1	tr	0	3	—	1
yellow fresh	1 (6.5 oz)	50	2	tr	0	12	—	3
Chiquita								
Pepper	1 med (5.2 oz)	30	1	0	0	7	2	0
FROZEN								
green chopped not prep	1 oz	6	tr	tr	0	1	—	1
red chopped	1 oz	6	tr	tr	0	1	—	1
Birds Eye								
Diced Green	¾ cup (2.9 oz)	20	1	0	0	4	2	10

PERCH

FRESH

FOOD	PORTION	CAL	PROT	FAT	CHOL	CARB	FIBER	SOD
cooked	3 oz	99	21	1	98	0	—	67
cooked	1 fillet (1.6 oz)	54	11	1	53	0	—	36
ocean perch atlantic cooked	3 oz	103	20	2	46	0	—	82

FOOD	PORTION	CAL	PROT	FAT	CHOL	CARB	FIBER	SOD
ocean perch atlantic cooked	1 fillet (1.8 oz)	60	12	1	27	0	–	48
ocean perch atlantic raw	3 oz	80	16	1	36	0	–	64
raw	3 oz	77	16	1	76	0	–	52
red raw	3.5 oz	114	18	4	–	0	–	80
FROZEN								
Van De Kamp's								
Battered Fillets	2 (4 oz)	300	12	20	25	19	0	480
PERSIMMONS								
dried japanese	1	93	tr	tr	0	25	–	1
fresh	1	32	tr	tr	0	8	–	0
fresh japanese	1	118	1	tr	0	31	–	3
Sonoma								
Dried	6–8 pieces (1.4 oz)	140	1	0	0	35	3	10
PHEASANT								
breast w/o skin raw	½ breast (6.4 oz)	243	44	6	–	0	–	60
leg w/o skin raw	1 (3.6 oz)	143	24	5	–	0	–	48
roasted	3.5 oz	215	33	9	120	0	0	100
w/ skin raw	½ pheasant (14 oz)	723	91	37	–	0	–	161
w/o skin raw	½ pheasant (12.4 oz)	470	83	13	–	0	–	131
PHYLLO DOUGH								
phyllo dough	1 oz	85	2	2	0	15	–	137
sheet	1	57	1	1	0	10	–	92
PICANTE (see SALSA)								
PICKLES								
dill	1 (2.3 oz)	12	tr	tr	0	3	–	833
dill low sodium	1 (2.3 oz)	12	tr	tr	0	3	1	12
dill low sodium sliced	1 slice	1	tr	tr	0	tr	tr	1
dill sliced	1 slice	1	tr	tr	0	tr	tr	77
gerkins	1 oz	6	tr	tr	0	1	–	274
kosher dill	1 (2.3 oz)	12	tr	tr	0	3	1	833
polish dill	1 (2.3 oz)	12	tr	tr	0	3	1	833

FOOD	PORTION	CAL	PROT	FAT	CHOL	CARB	FIBER	SOD
quick sour	1 (1.2 oz)	4	tr	tr	0	1	–	423
quick sour low sodium	1 (1.2 oz)	4	tr	tr	0	1	–	6
quick sour sliced	1 slice	1	tr	tr	0	tr	–	85
sweet	1 (1.2 oz)	41	tr	tr	0	11	tr	328
sweet gherkin	1 sm (½ oz)	20	tr	tr	0	5	–	107
sweet low sodium	1 (1.2 oz)	41	tr	tr	0	11	tr	6
sweet sliced	1 slice	7	tr	tr	0	2	tr	56
Claussen								
Bread 'N Butter Chips	4 slices (1 oz)	20	0	0	0	4	0	170
Deli Style Hearty Garlic Whole	½ (1 oz)	5	0	0	0	1	0	260
Kosher Dills Halves	1 half (1 oz)	5	0	0	0	1	0	330
Kosher Dills Mini	1 (0.8 oz)	5	0	0	0	1	0	300
Kosher Dills Spears	1 spear (1.2 oz)	5	0	0	0	1	0	320
Kosher Dills Whole	½ (1 oz)	5	0	0	0	1	0	330
New York Deli Style Half Sours Whole	½ (1 oz)	5	0	0	0	1	0	260
Sandwich Slices Bread 'N Butter	2 (1.2 oz)	25	0	0	0	5	0	210
Sandwich Slices Deli Style Hearty Garlic	2 (1.2 oz)	5	0	0	0	1	0	320
Sandwich Slices Kosher Dills	2 (1.2 oz)	5	0	0	0	1	0	440
Super Slices For Burgers	1 (0.8 oz)	5	0	0	0	1	0	320
Vlasic								
Hamburger Dill Chips	1 oz	5	0	0	0	1	–	400
Kosher Cross Cuts	1 oz	5	0	0	0	1	–	220
Kosher Spears	1 oz	5	0	0	0	1	–	220
Kosher Whole	1 oz	5	0	0	0	1	–	220
Sweet Butter Chips	1 oz	30	0	0	0	7	–	190
Sweet Gerkins	1 oz	35	0	0	0	9	–	260
Whole Dills	1 oz	5	0	0	0	1	–	390

PIE (see also PIE CRUST)
FROZEN
Amy's Organic

FOOD	PORTION	CAL	PROT	FAT	CHOL	CARB	FIBER	SOD
Apple	1 serv (8 oz)	280	4	12	–	42	–	180

FOOD	PORTION	CAL	PROT	FAT	CHOL	CARB	FIBER	SOD
Mrs. Smith's								
Apple	1 slice (4.3 oz)	350	3	19	0	41	3	430
Blueberry	1 slice (4.6 oz)	330	3	17	0	43	3	500
Cappuccino	1 slice (4.2 oz)	300	4	13	0	45	2	260
Cherry	1 slice (4.3 oz)	320	3	17	0	41	2	490
Cherry Crumb	1 slice (4.2 oz)	320	3	12	0	52	1	250
Chocolate Cream	1 slice (4.6 oz)	340	3	18	15	43	2	380
Chocolate Mint Cream	1 slice (4.3 oz)	360	3	15	0	53	2	240
Coconut Custard	1 slice (4.4 oz)	260	6	14	70	28	tr	310
Cookies 'N Cream	1 slice (4.3 oz)	360	4	16	0	52	2	290
Dutch Apple	1 slice (4.4 oz)	330	3	13	0	50	2	300
French Silk	1 slice (4.4 oz)	560	4	40	55	48	1	280
Key West Lime	1 slice (4.3 oz)	430	5	18	15	62	1	290
Lemon Cream	1 slice (5 oz)	440	3	26	0	49	tr	180
Lemonade	1 slice (4.3 oz)	340	3	15	0	51	1	280
Mince	1 slice (4.6 oz)	380	3	17	0	53	2	520
Mixed Berry	1 slice (4.2 oz)	300	2	13	0	44	2	360
Peach	1 slice (4.6 oz)	320	3	17	0	40	2	450
Peach Lattice	1 slice (4.2 oz)	290	2	13	0	42	2	280
Peanut Butter Silk	1 slice (4.6 oz)	600	8	41	55	51	2	330
Pecan	1 slice (4.8 oz)	560	6	27	65	75	2	450
Pumpkin Custard	1 slice (4.6 oz)	270	5	13	40	35	2	330
Raspberry	1 slice (4.6 oz)	330	3	17	0	44	1	510
S'Mores Cream	1 slice (4.3 oz)	360	3	16	0	53	2	300
Strawberry Banana	1 slice (4.3 oz)	330	3	15	0	48	1	270
Sweet Potato Custard	1 slice (4.6 oz)	340	4	17	40	44	2	240
Sara Lee								
Apple 45% Reduced Fat	⅙ pie (4.5 oz)	290	4	8	<5	51	2	400
Chocolate Silk	⅕ pie (4.8 oz)	500	4	32	<5	49	<2	440
Coconut Cream	⅕ pie (4.8 oz)	480	4	31	0	47	2	430
Homestyle Apple	⅛ pie (4.6 oz)	340	3	16	0	46	1	310
Homestyle Blueberry	⅛ pie (4.6 oz)	360	3	15	0	54	2	340
Homestyle Cherry	⅛ pie (4.6 oz)	320	3	16	0	42	2	290
Homestyle Dutch Apple	⅛ pie (4.6 oz)	350	3	15	0	53	2	320
Homestyle Mince	⅛ pie (4.6 oz)	390	3	17	0	56	3	450
Homestyle Peach	⅛ pie (4.6 oz)	320	3	14	0	46	2	250

FOOD	PORTION	CAL	PROT	FAT	CHOL	CARB	FIBER	SOD
Homestyle Pecan	⅛ pie (4.2 oz)	520	5	24	45	70	3	480
Homestyle Pumpkin	⅛ pie (4.6 oz)	260	4	11	30	37	2	460
Homestyle Raspberry	⅛ pie (4.6 oz)	380	3	19	<5	48	2	330
Lemon Meringue	⅙ pie (5 oz)	350	2	11	0	59	5	460
Weight Watchers								
Mississippi Mud	1 piece (2.45 oz)	160	4	5	5	26	1	120
MIX								
Jell-O								
No Bake Chocolate Silk as prep	⅙ pie (4.4 oz)	320	5	16	5	37	tr	490
SNACK								
Dolly Madison								
Apple	1 (4.5 oz)	480	3	22	15	67	2	390
Blueberry	1 (4.5 oz)	480	3	21	20	70	2	460
Cherry	1 (4.5 oz)	470	3	22	20	65	1	470
Chocolate Pudding	1 (4.5 oz)	530	4	25	30	71	1	410
Lemon	1 (4.5 oz)	500	3	24	20	66	0	430
Peach	1 (4.5 oz)	480	3	21	25	66	1	460
Pecan	1 (3 oz)	360	3	19	70	44	1	320
Pecan Fried	1 (4.5 oz)	530	4	21	10	80	1	430
Pineapple	1 (4.5 oz)	460	4	21	15	62	1	340
Hostess								
Apple	1 (4.5 oz)	480	3	22	15	67	2	390
Blackberry	1 (4.5 oz)	520	3	21	15	79	2	400
Blueberry	1 (4.5 oz)	480	3	21	20	70	2	460
Cherry	1 (4.5 oz)	470	3	22	20	65	1	470
French Apple	1 (4.5 oz)	480	3	22	15	67	2	390
Lemon	1 (4.5 oz)	500	3	24	20	66	0	430
Peach	1 (4.5 oz)	480	3	21	25	68	1	460
Pineapple	1 (4.5 oz)	460	4	21	15	62	1	430
Strawberry	1 (4.5 oz)	510	3	23	15	71	2	360
Lance								
Pecan	1 (3 oz)	350	4	17	25	46	3	200
Tastykake								
Apple	1 (4 oz)	270	3	11	0	41	1	300
Blueberry	1 (4 oz)	300	3	11	0	49	1	300
Cherry	1 (4 oz)	290	3	11	0	46	tr	300
Coconut Creme	1 (4 oz)	370	5	21	55	42	1	420

FOOD	PORTION	CAL	PROT	FAT	CHOL	CARB	FIBER	SOD
French Apple	1 (4.2 oz)	310	3	11	0	52	1	290
Lemon	1 (4 oz)	300	3	13	40	44	tr	320
Peach	1 (4 oz)	280	3	11	0	43	1	300
Pineapple	1 (4 oz)	290	3	12	20	45	1	310
Pineapple Cheese	1 (4 oz)	320	5	12	20	50	1	410
Pumpkin	1 (4 oz)	340	4	14	35	47	1	530
Strawberry	1 (3.5 oz)	320	3	12	0	51	1	300
Tastyklair	1 (4 oz)	400	5	20	90	50	0	290
Tom's								
Apple	1 pkg (3 oz)	330	2	17	5	42	1	250
Banana Marshmallow	1 pkg (2.75 oz)	320	3	11	0	54	0	190
Cherry	1 pkg (3 oz)	320	2	18	5	37	1	240
Chocolate Marshmallow	1 pkg (2.75 oz)	320	3	11	0	53	tr	190
TAKE-OUT								
apple	⅛ of 9 in pie (5.4 oz)	411	4	19	0	58	3	327
banana cream	⅛ of 9 in pie (5.2 oz)	398	7	20	75	49	–	355
blueberry	⅛ of 9 in pie (5.2 oz)	360	4	18	0	49	–	272
butterscotch	⅛ of 9 in pie (4.5 oz)	355	6	18	78	42	–	335
cherry	⅛ of 9 in pie (6.3 oz)	486	5	22	0	69	–	343
coconut creme	⅛ of 9 in pie (4.7 oz)	396	6	21	77	46	–	356
coconut custard	⅙ of 8 in pie (3.6 oz)	271	6	14	36	32	–	348
custard	⅛ of 9 in pie (4.5 oz)	262	7	11	87	34	2	256
lemon meringue	⅛ of 9 in pie (4.5 oz)	362	5	16	68	50	2	307
mince	⅛ of 9 in pie (5.8 oz)	477	18	18	0	79	–	419
pecan	⅙ of 8 in pie (4 oz)	452	5	21	36	65	4	480
pumpkin	⅙ of 8 in pie (3.8 oz)	229	4	10	22	30	3	308
vanilla cream	⅛ of 9 in pie (4.4 oz)	350	6	18	78	41	–	327

PIE CRUST

FOOD	PORTION	CAL	PROT	FAT	CHOL	CARB	FIBER	SOD
FROZEN								
baked	⅛ of 9 in pie (0.6 oz)	82	1	5	–	8	–	104
baked	9 in shell (4.4 oz)	647	6	41	–	63	–	815
puff pastry baked	1 shell (1.4 oz)	223	3	15	0	18	–	101
Pepperidge Farm								
Puff Pastry Sheets	⅙ sheet (1.4 oz)	170	3	11	0	14	0	200
Puff Pastry Shell	1 (1.6 oz)	190	4	13	0	16	0	230
Puff Pastry Squares	1 sq (2 oz)	240	4	16	0	19	0	250

FOOD	PORTION	CAL	PROT	FAT	CHOL	CARB	FIBER	SOD
Pet-Ritz								
Deep Dish	⅛ pie (0.7 oz)	90	1	5	<5	11	0	75
Regular	⅛ pie (0.6 oz)	80	tr	5	<5	9	0	60
Tart Shells	1 (1 oz)	130	1	8	0	13	0	170
MIX								
as prep	9 in crust (5.6 oz)	801	11	49	0	81	—	1167
as prep	⅛ of 9 in pie (0.7 oz)	100	1	6	0	10	—	146
Betty Crocker								
Pie Crust as prep	⅛ crust	110	1	8	0	9	—	135
READY-TO-EAT								
chocolate cookie crumb baked	⅛ of 9 in pie (1 oz)	139	1	9	0	15	—	185
chocolate cookie crumb baked	9 in crust (7.7 oz)	1130	12	69	3	122	—	1502
chocolate cookie crumb chilled	9 in crust (7.8 oz)	1127	12	69	3	121	—	1499
chocolate cookie crumb chilled	⅛ of 9 in pie (1 oz)	142	1	9	0	15	—	188
graham cracker baked	⅛ of 9 in pie (1 oz)	148	1	8	0	20	—	171
graham cracker baked	9 in crust (8.4 oz)	1181	10	60	0	156	—	1365
graham cracker chilled	⅛ of 9 in pie (1 oz)	150	1	8	0	20	—	173
graham cracker chilled	9 in crust (8.6 oz)	1182	10	60	0	155	—	1365
vanilla wafer cracker crumbs baked	9 in crust (6.1 oz)	937	7	64	69	89	—	909
vanilla wafer cracker crumbs baked	⅛ of 9 in pie (0.8 oz)	119	1	8	9	11	—	116
vanilla wafer cracker crumbs chilled	⅛ of 9 in pie (0.8 oz)	117	1	8	9	11	—	113
vanilla wafer cracker crumbs chilled	9 in crust (6.2 oz)	934	7	64	69	88	—	906

FOOD	PORTION	CAL	PROT	FAT	CHOL	CARB	FIBER	SOD
Keebler								
GrahamSingle Serve	1 (0.8 oz)	120	1	6	0	15	tr	150
Reduced Fat Graham	⅛ pie (0.7 oz)	90	1	4	0	14	0	85
REFRIGERATED								
All Ready								
Crust	⅛ pie (0.9 oz)	120	tr	7	5	13	0	100
PIE FILLING								
apple	⅛ can (2.6 oz)	74	tr	tr	0	19	1	32
apple	1 can (21 oz)	599	1	1	0	156	6	259
cherry	⅛ can (2.6 oz)	85	tr	tr	0	22	–	7
cherry	1 can (21 oz)	683	3	1	0	175	–	54
pumpkin pie mix	1 cup	282	3	tr	0	71	–	561
Comstock								
MoreFruit Light Cherry	⅓ cup (2.9 oz)	60	0	0	0	13	0	30
Red Ruby Cherry	⅓ cup (3.1 oz)	90	0	0	0	23	1	25
Libby								
Pumpkin Pie Mix	⅓ cup	90	tr	1	0	20	2	115
Smucker's								
Pie Glaze Strawberry	2 oz	80	0	0	0	21	–	0
PIEROGI								
pierogi	¾ cup (4.4 oz)	307	11	19	49	24	–	369
Health Is Wealth								
Potato & Cheddar	2 (2.8 oz)	140	5	2	0	27	3	360
Potato & Onion	2 (2.8 oz)	140	4	2	0	27	3	300
Mrs. T's								
Jalapeno & Cheddar	3 (4.2 oz)	190	7	3	10	35	2	490
Potato & Cheddar	3 (4.2 oz)	180	7	3	10	34	2	430
Potato & Onion	3 (4.2 oz)	180	6	2	<5	34	2	340
Sweet Potato	3 (4.2 oz)	300	5	0	<5	35	3	250
PIG'S EARS AND FEET								
ear simmered	1	184	18	12	100	tr	0	185
feet pickled	1 oz	58	4	5	26	tr	0	262
feet pickled	1 lb	921	61	73	417	tr	0	4187
feet simmered	3 oz	165	16	11	85	0	0	26
Hormel								
Pickled Feet	2 oz	80	7	6	45	0	0	530
Pickled Hocks	2 oz	110	9	8	45	0	0	530

FOOD	PORTION	CAL	PROT	FAT	CHOL	CARB	FIBER	SOD
PIGEON								
w/ skin & bone	3.5 oz	169	21	10	110	0	–	90
PIGEON PEAS								
dried cooked	½ cup	102	6	tr	0	20	–	5
dried cooked	1 cup	204	11	1	0	39	–	9
PIGNOLIA (see PINE NUTS)								
PIKE								
northern cooked	½ fillet (5.4 oz)	176	38	1	78	0	–	76
northern cooked	3 oz	96	21	1	43	0	–	42
northern raw	3 oz	75	16	1	33	0	–	33
roe raw	1 oz	37	7	tr	103	tr	–	–
walleye baked	3 oz	101	21	1	94	0	–	56
walleye fillet baked	4.4 oz	147	30	2	137	0	–	81
PILLNUTS								
canarytree dried	1 oz	204	3	23	0	1	–	1
PIMIENTOS								
canned	1 tbsp	3	tr	tr	0	1	–	2
canned	1 slice	0	tr	0	0	tr	–	0
Dromedary								
Peeled	½ tsp (4 g)	0	0	0	0	0	0	0
Unpeeled	½ tsp (4 g)	0	0	0	0	0	0	0
PINE NUTS								
pignolia dried	1 tbsp	51	2	5	0	1	–	0
pignolia dried	1 oz	146	7	14	0	4	–	1
pinyon dried	1 oz	161	3	17	0	5	–	20
Progresso								
Pignoli	1 jar (1 oz)	170	10	13	0	2	0	0
PINEAPPLE								
CANNED								
chunks in heavy syrup	1 cup	199	1	tr	0	52	–	3
chunks juice pack	1 cup	150	1	tr	0	39	–	4
crushed in heavy syrup	1 cup	199	1	tr	0	52	–	3
slices in heavy syrup	1 slice	45	tr	tr	0	12	–	1
slices in light syrup	1 slice	30	tr	tr	0	8	–	1
slices juice pack	1 slice	35	tr	tr	0	9	–	1

FOOD	PORTION	CAL	PROT	FAT	CHOL	CARB	FIBER	SOD
slices water pack	1 slice	19	tr	tr	0	5	—	1
tidbits in heavy syrup	1 cup	199	1	tr	0	52	—	3
tidbits in juice	1 cup	150	1	tr	0	19	—	4
tidbits in water	1 cup	79	1	tr	0	20	—	3
Del Monte								
Chunks In Heavy Syrup	½ cup (4.3 oz)	90	0	0	0	24	1	10
Chunks In Its Own Juice	½ cup (4.3 oz)	70	0	0	0	17	1	10
Crushed In Heavy Syrup	½ cup (4.3 oz)	90	0	0	0	24	1	10
Crushed In Its Own Juice	½ cup (4.3 oz)	70	0	0	0	17	1	10
Fruit Cup Tidbits	1 pkg (4 oz)	50	1	0	0	15	1	10
Sliced In Heavy Syrup	2 slices (4.1 oz)	90	0	0	0	23	1	10
Sliced In Its Own Juice	½ cup (4 oz)	60	0	0	0	16	1	10
Spears In Its Own Juice	½ cup (4.3 oz)	70	0	0	0	17	1	10
Tidbits In Its Own Juice	½ cup (4.3 oz)	70	0	0	0	17	1	10
Wedges In Its Own Juice	½ cup (4.3 oz)	70	0	0	0	17	1	10
Dole								
Chunks Juice Pack	½ cup	60	0	0	0	15	1	10
Sunfresh								
In Extra Light Syrup	½ cup (4.6 oz)	80	0	0	0	17	0	65
DRIED								
Sonoma								
Pieces	2 pieces (1.4 oz)	140	0	2	0	30	2	30
FRESH								
diced	1 cup	77	1	tr	0	19	2	1
slice	1 slice	42	tr	tr	0	10	1	1
Bonita Hill								
Golden Extra Sweet	2 slices (3.9 oz)	60	1	0	0	16	1	10
FROZEN								
chunks sweetened	½ cup	104	tr	tr	0	27	—	2

FOOD	PORTION	CAL	PROT	FAT	CHOL	CARB	FIBER	SOD
PINEAPPLE JUICE								
canned	1 cup	139	1	tr	0	34	—	2
frzn as prep	1 cup	129	1	tr	0	32	—	3
frzn not prep	6 oz	387	3	tr	0	96	—	6
After The Fall								
Mandarin Pineapple	1 can (12 oz)	150	1	0	0	37	0	25
Del Monte								
Juice From	6 fl oz	80	1	0	0	20	0	5
Dole								
Chilled	8 oz	130	0	0	0	30	—	10
PINK BEANS								
dried cooked	1 cup	252	15	1	0	47	—	3
PINTO BEANS								
CANNED								
pinto	1 cup	186	11	1	0	35	—	998
Chi-Chi's								
Pinto Beans	½ cup (4.3 oz)	100	6	1	0	18	3	540
Eden								
Organic Spicy	½ cup (4.6 oz)	125	6	0	0	24	2	195
Green Giant								
Pinto Beans	½ cup (4.4 oz)	110	6	1	0	20	5	280
Old El Paso								
Pinto Beans	½ cup (4.6 oz)	110	6	1	0	19	7	420
Progresso								
Pinto Beans	½ cup (4.6 oz)	110	7	1	0	18	7	250
DRIED								
cooked	1 cup	235	14	1	0	44	—	3
Hurst								
HamBeens w/ Ham	3 tbsp (1.2 oz)	120	7	1	0	20	6	63
FROZEN								
cooked	3 oz	152	9	tr	0	29	—	—
PISTACHIOS								
dried	1 cup	739	26	62	0	32	14	7
dry roasted	1 oz	172	4	15	0	8	—	2
dry roasted salted	1 cup	776	19	68	0	35	—	1040
dry roasted salted	1 oz	172	4	15	0	8	—	260
dry roasted w/ salt	47 nuts (1 oz)	160	6	13	0	8	3	120

FOOD	PORTION	CAL	PROT	FAT	CHOL	CARB	FIBER	SOD
Lance								
Pistachios	1 pkg (1.1 oz)	90	4	7	0	4	2	105
Planters								
Munch'N Go Singles Shelled Dry Roasted	1 pkg (2 oz)	330	11	29	0	14	6	450
Red Salted Dry Roasted	1 pkg	160	5	14	0	7	3	250
Uncolored Dry Roasted	½ cup	160	5	14	0	7	3	180
Sonoma								
Salted Shelled	¼ cup (1 oz)	190	6	14	0	9	3	220
PITANGA								
fresh	1	2	tr	tr	0	1	–	0
fresh	1 cup	57	1	1	0	13	–	5
PIZZA (see also PIZZA DOUGH, PIZZA SAUCE)								
Amy's Organic								
Cheese	1 (13 oz)	310	13	11	15	39	2	490
Pocket Sandwich Cheese Pizza	1 (4.5 oz)	290	14	9	20	38	3	390
Pocket Sandwich Veggie Pepperoni Pizza	1 (4.5 oz)	220	12	7	15	28	3	490
Roasted Vegetable	1 (12 oz)	270	6	8	0	43	3	470
Spinach	1 (14 oz)	320	13	11	15	40	2	490
Appian Way								
Pizza Mix Thick Crust	⅓ pie (4.2 oz)	290	10	5	10	51	2	830
Pizza Mix Thin Crust	⅓ pie (4.1 oz)	250	7	3	0	48	2	740
Banquet								
Pepperoni	1 pie (6.75 oz)	490	11	23	35	56	5	790
Pizza Snack Cheese	6 pieces (7.5 oz)	200	9	8	20	24	2	360
Pizza Snack Pepperoni	6 pieces (7.5 oz)	230	8	11	20	23	2	430
Pizza Snack Pepperoni & Sausage	6 pieces (7.5 oz)	210	8	9	20	24	2	440
Croissant Pocket								
Stuffed Sandwich Pepperoni Pizza	1 piece (4.5 oz)	350	16	15	30	39	3	870

FOOD	PORTION	CAL	PROT	FAT	CHOL	CARB	FIBER	SOD
Di Giorno								
Rising Crust 12 inch Four Cheese	⅙ pie (4.9 oz)	320	16	11	25	39	3	870
Rising Crust 12 inch Italian Sausage	⅙ pie (5.3 oz)	360	18	14	35	40	3	1000
Rising Crust 12 inch Pepperoni	⅙ pie (5.2 oz)	370	18	16	35	40	3	1080
Rising Crust 12 inch Supreme	⅙ pie (5.8 oz)	380	18	17	40	40	3	1100
Rising Crust 12 inch Three Meat	⅙ pie (5.4 oz)	380	19	16	40	40	3	1100
Rising Crust 12 inch Vegetable	⅙ pie (5.6 oz)	310	15	10	20	41	3	830
Rising Crust 8 inch Chicken Supreme	⅓ pie (4.8 oz)	270	16	9	30	33	2	740
Rising Crust 8 inch Four Cheese	⅓ pie (4 oz)	260	14	9	20	33	2	720
Rising Crust 8 inch Italian Sausage	⅓ pie (4.4 oz)	300	15	12	25	33	2	830
Rising Crust 8 inch Pepperoni	⅓ pie (4.2 oz)	300	15	13	30	33	2	880
Rising Crust 8 inch Spinach	⅓ pie (4.3 oz)	250	15	8	15	33	3	670
Rising Crust 8 inch Supreme	⅓ pie (4.7 oz)	310	15	14	30	34	2	900
Rising Crust 8 inch Three Meat	⅓ pie (4.4 oz)	310	15	13	30	34	2	900
Rising Crust 8 inch Vegetable	⅓ pie (4.6 oz)	250	13	8	15	33	2	680
Health Is Wealth								
Pizza Munchees	6 (3 oz)	190	2	5	0	9	1	560
Healthy Choice								
French Bread Cheese	1 piece (6 oz)	340	22	5	15	51	5	480
French Bread Pepperoni	1 piece (6 oz)	340	24	5	20	49	6	580
French Bread Sausage	1 piece (6 oz)	320	21	5	25	48	5	580
French Bread Supreme	1 piece (6.35 oz)	330	21	5	20	51	6	580

FOOD	PORTION	CAL	PROT	FAT	CHOL	CARB	FIBER	SOD
French Bread Vegetable	1 piece (6 oz)	280	17	4	10	44	5	480
Hot Pocket								
Stuffed Sandwich Pepperoni & Sausage Pizza	1 (4.5 oz)	340	12	16	30	38	3	630
Stuffed Sandwich Pepperoni Pizza	1 (4.5 oz)	350	13	17	30	38	2	780
Jack's								
Great Combinations 12 inch Double Cheese	¼ pie (4.9 oz)	380	21	19	50	32	2	670
Great Combinations 12 inch Pepperoni	¼ pie (5.2 oz)	410	19	19	40	42	3	830
Great Combinations 12 inch Sausage	¼ pie (5.4 oz)	390	18	18	40	40	3	700
Great Combinations 12 inch Supreme	¼ pie (5.2 oz)	350	17	18	40	30	5	750
Great Combinations 9 inch Double Cheese	½ pie (5.5 oz)	430	23	21	55	38	3	740
Naturally Rising 12 inch Bacon Cheeseburger	⅙ pie (5 oz)	350	18	15	40	35	2	680
Naturally Rising 12 inch Canadian Bacon	⅙ pie (4.9 oz)	280	16	9	30	34	2	590
Naturally Rising 12 inch Cheese	⅙ pie (4.5 oz)	290	15	10	25	35	2	500
Naturally Rising 12 inch Pepperoni	⅙ pie (4.9 oz)	350	17	16	40	35	2	710
Naturally Rising 12 inch Pepperoni Supreme	⅙ pie (5.1 oz)	340	16	16	35	34	2	670
Naturally Rising 12 inch Sausage	⅙ pie (5.1 oz)	340	17	15	35	34	2	600

FOOD	PORTION	CAL	PROT	FAT	CHOL	CARB	FIBER	SOD
Naturally Rising 12 inch Spicy Italian Sausage	⅙ pie (5.1 oz)	330	17	14	40	34	2	680
Naturally Rising 12 inch The Works	⅙ pie (5.3 oz)	330	16	14	35	34	2	580
Naturally Rising 9 inch Cheese	⅓ pie (4.7 oz)	300	15	10	25	38	2	500
Naturally Rising 9 inch Pepperoni	⅓ pie (5.2 oz)	360	17	16	40	38	2	720
Naturally Rising 9 inch Sausage	⅓ pie (5.4 oz)	360	17	16	35	38	2	620
Naturally Rising 9 inch The Works	¼ pie (4.5 oz)	280	13	12	30	29	2	480
Original 12 inch Canadian Bacon	¼ pie (4.4 oz)	280	16	10	30	31	2	620
Original 12 inch Cheese	⅓ pie (5 oz)	360	19	13	30	41	3	650
Original 12 inch Hamburger	¼ pie (4.4 oz)	300	16	14	35	28	2	580
Original 12 inch Pepperoni	¼ pie (4.3 oz)	330	16	15	35	31	2	720
Original 12 inch Sausage	¼ pie (4.3 oz)	300	15	14	30	28	2	580
Original 12 inch Spicy Italian Sausage	¼ pie (4.3 oz)	290	15	13	35	29	2	650
Original 9 inch Pepperoni	½ pie (5 oz)	380	18	18	40	37	3	820
Original 9 inch Sausage	½ pie (5.1 oz)	360	17	16	35	36	3	660
Pizza Bursts Combination Sausage & Pepperoni	6 pieces (3 oz)	250	8	12	20	26	2	500
Pizza Bursts Pepperoni	6 pieces (3 oz)	260	9	14	20	25	2	560
Pizza Bursts Sausage	6 pieces (3 oz)	250	8	12	20	25	2	490

FOOD	PORTION	CAL	PROT	FAT	CHOL	CARB	FIBER	SOD
Pizza Bursts Supercheese	6 pieces (3 oz)	250	9	12	20	25	2	460
Pizza Bursts Supreme	6 pieces (3 oz)	250	8	13	20	26	2	520
Kid Cuisine								
Backpacking Pizza Snack	6 pieces	230	8	11	20	23	1	480
Big League Hamburger	1 meal (8.3 oz)	400	14	11	35	61	5	550
Fire Chief Cheese	1 pie (5.2 oz)	340	19	10	20	44	2	760
Pirate Pizza w/ Cheese	1 meal (8 oz)	430	12	11	30	71	5	480
Poolside Pepperoni	1 (5.2 oz)	380	18	14	35	44	2	990
Lean Cuisine								
Everyday Favorites French Bread Cheese	1 pkg (6 oz)	320	15	7	15	48	4	580
Everyday Favorites French Bread Deluxe	1 pkg (6.1 oz)	290	16	6	25	43	3	550
Everyday Favorites French Bread Pepperoni	1 pkg (5.25 oz)	300	15	8	25	43	3	590
Everyday Favorites French Bread Sun Dried Tomatoes	1 serv (6 oz)	340	19	8	20	48	3	580
Lean Pockets								
Stuffed Sandwich Pizza Deluxe	1 (4.5 oz)	270	12	8	25	37	2	680
Marie Callender's								
French Bread Cheese	1 (7.2 oz)	530	28	24	60	50	4	980
French Bread Pepperoni	1 (7.5 oz)	570	29	28	65	50	4	1160
French Bread Supreme	1 (7.5 oz)	510	26	23	50	50	4	1200
Old El Paso								
Pizza Burrito Cheese	1 (3.5 oz)	320	13	9	20	27	0	430
Pizza Burrito Pepperoni	1 (3.5 oz)	260	12	10	20	31	0	510

FOOD	PORTION	CAL	PROT	FAT	CHOL	CARB	FIBER	SOD
Pizza Burrito Sausage	1 (3.5 oz)	260	11	9	15	32	0	420
Pepperidge Farm								
Gourmet Crust Cheese	1 (4.4 oz)	390	12	20	90	39	6	770
Gourmet Crust Pepperoni	1 (4.5 oz)	420	15	23	90	39	5	810
Stouffer's								
French Bread Bacon Cheddar	1 piece (5.7 oz)	430	15	21	25	46	4	880
French Bread Cheese	1 piece (5.2 oz)	370	14	16	15	43	3	880
French Bread Cheeseburger	1 piece (6 oz)	420	17	20	30	44	3	800
French Bread Deluxe	1 piece (6.2 oz)	430	17	21	20	49	3	990
French Bread Double Cheese	1 piece (5.9 oz)	400	16	16	25	49	4	950
French Bread Pepperoni	1 piece (5.6 oz)	430	16	20	15	46	3	990
French Bread Pepperoni & Mushroom	1 piece (6.1 oz)	440	15	20	30	49	5	910
French Bread Sausage	1 piece (6 oz)	420	17	18	20	48	3	1260
French Bread Sausage & Pepperoni	1 piece (6.25 oz)	470	18	23	25	47	3	1340
French Bread Three Meat	1 piece (6.25 oz)	460	20	21	35	48	5	1200
French Bread Vegetable Deluxe	1 piece (6.4 oz)	380	14	16	20	46	4	780
French Bread White Pizza	1 piece (5.1 oz)	460	18	23	20	45	5	700
Tombstone								
Double Top Pepperoni	⅙ pie (4.5 oz)	340	18	19	45	24	2	810
Double Top Sausage	⅙ pie (4.6 oz)	320	18	17	40	25	2	760
Double Top Sausage & Pepperoni	⅙ pie (4.6 oz)	340	19	19	45	25	2	820
Double Top Supreme	⅙ pie (4.7 oz)	330	18	18	40	25	2	780
Double Top Two Cheese	⅙ pie (5.2 oz)	380	22	19	50	29	2	760

FOOD	PORTION	CAL	PROT	FAT	CHOL	CARB	FIBER	SOD
For One ½ Less Fat Cheese	1 pie (6.5 oz)	460	23	10	20	43	3	940
For One ½ Less Fat Vegetable	1 pie (7.2 oz)	360	21	9	10	48	5	860
For One Extra Cheese	1 pie (6.9 oz)	520	26	28	50	47	3	940
For One Pepperoni	1 pie (6.9 oz)	550	25	32	55	41	3	1160
For One Supreme	1 pie (7.5 oz)	550	24	32	55	42	3	1090
Light Supreme	⅕ pie (4.8 oz)	270	17	9	20	30	3	720
Light Vegetable	⅕ pie (4.6 oz)	240	14	7	10	31	3	500
Original 12 inch Canadian Bacon	¼ pie (5.5 oz)	350	20	14	35	36	3	890
Original 12 inch Deluxe	⅕ pie (4.8 oz)	310	15	14	30	29	3	690
Original 12 inch Extra Cheese	¼ pie (5.1 oz)	350	18	15	30	35	3	680
Original 12 inch Hamburger	⅕ pie (4.4 oz)	310	15	15	30	29	2	670
Original 12 inch Pepperoni	¼ pie (5.3 oz)	400	19	21	40	35	3	930
Original 12 inch Sausage	⅕ pie (4.4 oz)	300	15	14	30	29	2	680
Original 12 inch Sausage & Mushroom	⅕ pie (4.6 oz)	300	15	14	30	29	3	680
Original 12 inch Sausage & Pepperoni	⅕ pie (4.4 oz)	320	15	16	30	29	2	740
Original 12 inch Supreme	⅕ pie (5.1 oz)	320	15	16	30	29	2	730
Original 9 inch Deluxe	⅓ pie (4.4 oz)	280	14	13	25	27	2	630
Original 9 inch Extra Cheese	½ pie (5.6 oz)	380	19	19	30	40	3	740
Original 9 inch Hamburger	⅓ pie (4 oz)	280	14	13	25	27	2	600
Original 9 inch Pepperoni	⅓ pie (4 oz)	300	14	15	30	27	2	680
Original 9 inch Pepperoni & Sausage	⅓ pie (4.1 oz)	300	14	15	30	27	2	710

FOOD	PORTION	CAL	PROT	FAT	CHOL	CARB	FIBER	SOD
Original 9 inch Sausage	⅓ pie (4 oz)	280	14	13	25	27	2	610
Original 9 inch Supreme	⅓ pie (4.4 oz)	310	15	16	30	27	2	720
Oven Rising Italian Sausage	⅙ pie (5.1 oz)	320	16	13	30	35	2	700
Oven Rising Pepperoni	⅙ pie (4.9 oz)	340	17	15	35	34	2	750
Oven Rising Supreme	⅙ pie (5.1 oz)	320	16	14	30	34	2	720
Oven Rising Three Cheese	⅙ pie (4.8 oz)	320	16	13	35	34	2	580
Oven Rising Three Meat	⅙ pie (5.1 oz)	340	17	15	35	34	2	750
Thin Crust Four Meat Combo	¼ pie (5 oz)	380	19	23	45	26	2	890
Thin Crust Italian Sausage	¼ pie (5 oz)	370	18	22	45	26	2	840
Thin Crust Pepperoni	¼ pie (4.8 oz)	400	18	25	50	25	2	920
Thin Crust Supreme	¼ pie (5 oz)	380	18	22	45	26	2	840
Thin Crust Supreme Taco	¼ pie (5.1 oz)	370	16	23	50	27	2	740
Thin Crust Three Cheese	¼ pie (4.7 oz)	360	19	21	45	25	2	690
Weight Watchers								
Smart Ones Deluxe Combo	1 (6.57 oz)	380	23	11	40	47	6	550
Smart Ones Pepperoni	1 (5.56 oz)	390	23	12	45	46	4	650
TAKE-OUT								
cheese	12 in pie	1121	61	26	74	164	—	2680
cheese	⅛ of 12 in pie	140	8	3	9	21	—	336
cheese deep dish individual	1 (5.5 oz)	460	15	24	20	47	2	750
cheese meat & vegetables	12 in pie	1472	104	43	165	170	—	3054
cheese meat & vegetables	⅛ of 12 in pie	184	13	5	21	21	—	382
pepperoni	12 in pie	1445	81	56	115	157	—	2133
pepperoni	⅛ of 12 in pie	181	10	7	14	20	—	267

FOOD	PORTION	CAL	PROT	FAT	CHOL	CARB	FIBER	SOD
PIZZA DOUGH								
crust	1 slice (1.7 oz)	130	4	2	0	25	1	230
Betty Crocker								
Italian Herb Crust Mix	¼ crust (1.6 oz)	180	4	2	0	32	1	350
Boboli								
Thin Crust	⅕ crust (2 oz)	160	6	4	0	24	1	300
Pillsbury								
Crust	⅕ crust (2 oz)	150	5	2	0	27	tr	380
Robin Hood								
Crust	¼ crust	160	4	2	0	33	1	340
PIZZA SAUCE								
Hunt's								
Fully Prepared	¼ cup (2.2 oz)	21	1	1	0	4	2	251
Pizza Sauce	¼ cup (2.2 oz)	27	1	1	0	5	2	190
Prima Choice Supper Heavy	¼ cup (2.2 oz)	28	2	1	0	6	3	36
Muir Glen								
Organic	¼ cup (2.2 oz)	40	1	0	0	6	2	230
Progresso								
Pizza Sauce	¼ cup (2.1 oz)	20	tr	0	0	4	1	170
PLANTAINS								
fresh uncooked	1 (6.3 oz)	218	2	1	0	57	–	7
sliced cooked	½ cup	89	1	tr	0	24	–	4
Chifles								
Plantain Chips	1 pkg (2 oz)	170	tr	11	0	17	2	14
TAKE-OUT								
ripe fried	2.8 oz	214	1	7	–	38	4	–
PLUMS								
CANNED								
purple in heavy syrup	3	119	tr	tr	0	31	–	26
purple in heavy syrup	1 cup	320	1	tr	0	60	–	50
purple in light syrup	3	83	tr	tr	0	22	–	26
purple in light syrup	1 cup	158	1	tr	0	41	–	50
purple juice pack	3	55	tr	tr	0	14	–	1
purple juice pack	1 cup	146	1	tr	0	38	–	3
purple water pack	1 cup	102	1	tr	0	27	–	2
purple water pack	3	39	tr	tr	0	10	–	1

FOOD	PORTION	CAL	PROT	FAT	CHOL	CARB	FIBER	SOD
Eden								
Umeboshi Paste	1 tsp	5	0	0	0	1	0	600
Umeboshi Plums	1	5	0	0	0	1	0	710
FRESH								
plum	1	36	1	tr	0	9	–	0
sliced	1 cup	91	1	1	0	21	–	1
Chiquita								
Purple	2 med (4.6 oz)	80	1	1	0	19	2	0
POI								
poi	½ cup	134	tr	tr	0	33	–	14
POKEBERRY SHOOTS								
cooked	½ cup	16	2	tr	0	3	–	–
raw	½ cup	18	2	tr	0	3	–	–
POLENTA								
Frieda's								
Dried Tomato	4 oz	80	2	0	0	17	2	250
Italian Herb	4 oz	80	2	0	0	17	2	45
Mexicana	4 oz	80	2	0	0	17	2	200
Original	4 oz	80	2	0	0	16	2	198
Wild Mushroom	4 oz	80	2	0	0	17	2	200
Melissa's								
Original	4 oz	80	2	0	0	16	2	198
POLLACK								
altantic fillet baked	5.3 oz	178	38	2	137	0	–	166
atlantic baked	3 oz	100	21	1	77	0	–	94
POMEGRANATE								
fresh	1	104	1	tr	0	26	–	5
Cortas								
Concentrated Juice	1 tbsp (0.6 oz)	40	0	0	0	9	0	0
POMPANO								
florida cooked	3 oz	179	20	10	54	0	–	65
florida raw	3 oz	140	16	8	43	0	–	55
POPCORN (see also POPCORN CAKES)								
air-popped	1 cup (0.3 oz)	31	1	tr	0	6	2	0
air-popped	1 oz	108	3	1	0	22	4	1
caramel coated	1 oz	122	1	4	–	22	1	58

FOOD	PORTION	CAL	PROT	FAT	CHOL	CARB	FIBER	SOD
caramel coated	1 cup (1.2 oz)	152	1	5	–	28	2	72
carmel coated w/ peanuts	⅔ cup (1 oz)	114	2	2	0	23	1	84
cheese	1 oz	149	3	9	3	15	3	252
cheese	1 cup (0.4 oz)	58	1	4	1	6	1	98
oil popped	1 oz	142	3	8	0	16	3	251
oil popped	1 cup (0.4 oz)	55	1	3	0	6	1	97
Chester's								
Butter	3 cups	160	2	12	0	15	2	330
Caramel Craze	¾ cup	130	1	2	0	27	1	220
Cheddar Cheese	3 cups	190	3	13	<5	17	3	300
Microwave Butter	5 cups	200	3	12	0	22	4	300
Cracker Jack								
Fat Free Butter Toffee	¾ cup	110	1	0	0	26	1	85
Fat Free Caramel	¾ cup	110	tr	0	0	26	1	70
Original	½ cup (1 oz)	120	2	2	0	23	1	70
Estee								
Caramel	1 cup	120	tr	2	0	26	1	90
Herr's								
Regular	3 cups (1 oz)	140	2	11	0	11	3	250
Jolly Time								
America's Best 94% Fat Free	1 cup	20	tr	0	0	5	1	10
Blast O Butter	1 cup	45	1	3	0	5	1	85
Blast O Butter Light	1 cup	30	tr	2	0	4	1	75
Butter Licious	1 cup	35	tr	2	0	4	1	40
Butter Licious Light	1 cup	30	tr	2	0	4	tr	25
Crispy & White	1 cup	40	tr	3	0	4	1	40
Crispy & White Light	1 cup	25	tr	1	0	4	1	25
Healthy Pop 94% Fat Free	1 cup	20	tr	0	0	5	1	10
White Air Popped	5 cups	100	4	1	0	24	6	0
Yellow Air Popped	5 cups	100	4	1	0	24	6	0
Lance								
Cheese	1 pkg (0.6 oz)	90	2	5	0	9	2	210
Plain	1 pkg (0.5 oz)	70	1	3	0	10	1	135
White Cheddar	1 pkg (0.6 oz)	100	1	8	0	7	1	170
White Cheddar	1 pkg (0.9 oz)	150	2	11	0	10	1	240

FOOD	PORTION	CAL	PROT	FAT	CHOL	CARB	FIBER	SOD
Newman's Own								
Microwave Butter Flavor	3½ cups	170	2	11	0	16	3	180
Microwave Light Butter	3½ cups	110	2	3	0	20	3	90
Microwave Light Natural	3½ cups	110	2	3	0	20	3	90
Microwave Natural	3½ cups	170	2	11	0	16	3	180
Popcorn unpopped	3 tbsp	110	4	2	0	27	7	0
Orville Redenbacher's								
Gourmet Original	3 cups	92	3	1	0	22	5	2
Hot Air	3 cups	92	3	1	0	22	5	2
Microwave Butter	3 cups	168	2	13	0	15	4	388
Microwave Butter No Salt Added	3 cups	176	3	12	0	19	4	2
Microwave Butter Light	3 cups	122	3	6	0	20	5	357
Microwave Caramel	1 serv	179	1	10	0	23	3	47
Microwave Golden Cheddar	1 serv	169	2	13	0	15	3	373
Microwave Natural	3 cups	164	2	11	0	18	4	512
Microwave Natural No Salt Added	3 cups	174	3	12	0	19	5	2
Microwave Natural Light	3 cups	118	3	5	0	19	5	382
Microwave Smartpop	1 serv	96	3	3	0	20	5	445
Microwave Smartpop Butter Snack Size	1 bag	155	5	4	0	34	0	477
Microwave Snack Size Butter	1 bag	287	3	22	0	25	6	647
Microwave Snack Size Butter Light	1 bag	183	4	8	0	30	7	539
Microwave White Cheddar	1 serv	169	2	13	0	15	3	373
Redenbudders Microwave Herb & Garlic	1 serv	176	2	13	0	16	4	499
Redenbudders Microwave Zesty Butter	1 serv	177	2	13	0	16	4	429

FOOD	PORTION	CAL	PROT	FAT	CHOL	CARB	FIBER	SOD
Redenbudders Movie Theater Butter Light	1 serv	113	3	5	0	20	5	321
Redenbudders Movie Theater Microwave Butter	1 serv	176	2	13	0	16	4	499
Smart Pop Movie Theater Butter	1 serv	92	3	2	0	20	5	307
White	3 cups	92	3	1	0	22	5	2
Planters								
Fiddle Faddle Caramel Fat Free	1 cup (1 oz)	110	tr	0	0	28	1	210
Pop Secret								
94% Fat Free Butter	1 cup (5 g)	20	tr	0	0	4	tr	40
94% Fat Free Natural	1 cup (5 g)	20	tr	0	0	4	tr	40
Butter	1 cup (7 g)	35	tr	3	0	4	tr	50
Cheddar Cheese	1 cup (6 g)	30	tr	2	0	3	tr	45
Jumbo Pop Butter	1 cup (7 g)	40	tr	3	0	4	tr	55
Jumbo Pop Movie Theater Butter	1 cup (7 g)	40	tr	3	0	4	tr	55
Light Butter	1 cup (5 g)	20	tr	1	0	4	tr	45
Light Movie Theater Butter	1 cup (5 g)	25	tr	1	0	4	tr	45
Light Natural	1 cup (5 g)	25	tr	1	0	4	tr	45
Movie Theater Butter	1 cup (7 g)	40	tr	3	0	3	tr	55
Nacho Cheese	1 cup (6 g)	30	tr	2	0	3	tr	50
Natural	1 cup (7 g)	35	tr	3	0	4	tr	65
Real Butter	1 cup (7 g)	35	tr	3	0	4	tr	60
Smartfood								
Butter	3 cups	150	2	9	5	15	1	240
Low Fat Toffee Crunch	¾ cup	110	1	1	0	25	1	220
Reduced Fat Golden Butter	3⅓ cups	130	3	4	0	21	4	410
Reduced Fat White Cheddar	3 cups	140	4	6	<5	19	3	280
White Cheddar	2 cups	190	3	12	5	17	2	310
Snyder's Of Hanover								
Butter	⅝ oz	110	1	10	0	6	0	150

FOOD	PORTION	CAL	PROT	FAT	CHOL	CARB	FIBER	SOD
Tom's								
Caramel Corn	1 pkg (1.6 oz)	180	1	3	0	39	2	110
Utz								
Au Natural	3 cups (1 oz)	120	3	1	0	25	5	0
Butter	2 cups (1 oz)	170	2	12	0	13	3	210
Cheese	2 cups (1 oz)	150	2	10	5	14	3	250
Hulless Puff'N Corn	2 cups (1 oz)	180	1	15	0	11	0	150
Hulless Puff'N Corn Hot Cheese	1 pkg (1.75 oz)	290	3	22	0	21	0	680
Hulless Pull'N Corn Cheese	2 cups (1 oz)	170	2	12	<5	13	0	210
White Cheddar	2 cups (1 oz)	150	3	9	<5	15	3	270
Weight Watchers								
Butter	1 pkg (0.66 oz)	90	2	3	0	14	3	100
Butter Toffee	1 pkg (0.9 oz)	110	1	3	0	21	1	90
Caramel	1 pkg (0.9 oz)	100	1	1	0	22	1	45
Microwave	1 pkg (1 oz)	100	3	1	0	20	7	0
White Cheddar Cheese	1 pkg (0.66 oz)	90	2	4	0	12	2	125

POPCORN CAKES

FOOD	PORTION	CAL	PROT	FAT	CHOL	CARB	FIBER	SOD
Orville Redenbacher's								
BBQ Mini	8 (0.5 oz)	55	0	1	0	12	1	124
Butter	2 (0.6 oz)	134	2	1	tr	13	2	79
Butter Mini	8 (0.5 oz)	56	2	1	1	11	1	71
Caramel	1 (0.4 oz)	34	1	tr	0	8	1	16
Caramel Mini	7 (0.5 oz)	50	1	tr	tr	12	1	24
Nacho Cheese Mini	8 (0.5 oz)	56	2	1	1	11	1	85
Peanut Crunch Mini	7 (0.5 oz)	55	2	1	tr	11	1	39
White Cheddar	2 (0.6 oz)	63	0	1	tr	13	2	83
White Cheddar Mini	8 (0.5 oz)	56	2	1	tr	12	1	67
Quaker								
Blueberry Crunch	1 (0.5 oz)	50	1	0	0	11	–	0
Butter Mini	6 (0.5 oz)	50	2	1	0	11	2	140
Butter Popped	1 (0.3 oz)	35	1	0	0	7	–	45
Caramel	1 (0.5 oz)	50	1	0	0	12	–	30
Caramel Mini	5 (0.5 oz)	50	1	1	0	12	1	70
Cheddar Cheese Mini	6 (0.5 oz)	50	2	1	0	11	1	200
Lightly Salted Mini	7 (0.5 oz)	50	2	1	0	12	2	120
Monterey Jack	1 (0.4 oz)	40	1	0	0	8	–	80

FOOD	PORTION	CAL	PROT	FAT	CHOL	CARB	FIBER	SOD
Strawberry Crunch	1 (0.5 oz)	50	1	0	0	11	–	0
White Cheddar	1 (0.4 oz)	40	1	0	0	8	–	90

POPOVER

FOOD	PORTION	CAL	PROT	FAT	CHOL	CARB	FIBER	SOD
home recipe as prep w/ 2% milk	1 (1.4 oz)	87	4	3	46	11	–	82
home recipe as prep w/ whole milk	1 (1.4 oz)	90	4	3	47	11	–	82
mix as prep	1 (1.2 oz)	67	3	2	–	10	–	143

POPPY SEEDS

FOOD	PORTION	CAL	PROT	FAT	CHOL	CARB	FIBER	SOD
poppy seeds	1 tsp	15	1	1	0	1	–	1

PORGY

FOOD	PORTION	CAL	PROT	FAT	CHOL	CARB	FIBER	SOD
fresh	3 oz	77	18	tr	–	0	0	52

PORK *(see also BACON, CANADIAN BACON, DELI MEATS/COLD CUTS, HAM, PORK DISHES, SAUSAGE)*

CANNED

Hormel

FOOD	PORTION	CAL	PROT	FAT	CHOL	CARB	FIBER	SOD
Pickled Tidbits	2 oz	100	8	8	45	0	0	530

FRESH

FOOD	PORTION	CAL	PROT	FAT	CHOL	CARB	FIBER	SOD
boston blade roast lean & fat cooked	3 oz	229	20	16	73	0	0	57
boston blade steak lean & fat cooked	3 oz	220	22	14	81	0	0	59
center loin roast lean bone in cooked	3 oz	169	23	8	67	0	0	56
center loin chop lean bone in cooked	3 oz	172	25	7	72	0	0	53
center rib chop lean & fat bone in cooked	3 oz	213	23	13	62	0	0	34
center rib roast lean & fat bone in cooked	3 oz	217	23	13	62	0	0	39
fresh ham rump lean roasted	3 oz	175	26	7	82	0	0	55

FOOD	PORTION	CAL	PROT	FAT	CHOL	CARB	FIBER	SOD
fresh ham rump lean & fat roasted	3 oz	214	25	12	82	0	0	53
fresh ham shank lean roasted	3 oz	183	24	9	78	0	0	54
fresh ham shank lean & fat roasted	3 oz	246	22	17	78	0	0	50
fresh ham whole lean roasted	3 oz	179	25	8	80	0	0	54
fresh ham whole lean roasted diced	1 cup	285	40	13	127	0	0	86
fresh ham whole lean & fat roasted	3 oz	232	23	15	80	0	0	51
fresh ham whole lean & fat roasted diced	1 cup	369	36	24	127	0	0	81
ground cooked	3 oz	252	22	18	80	0	0	62
leg loin & shoulder lean only roasted	3 oz	198	–	11	79	–	–	–
loin chop lean bone in braised	3 oz	191	21	11	71	0	0	53
loin chop lean bone in broiled	3 oz	199	22	12	71	0	0	68
loin roast lean bone in roasted	3 oz	210	23	13	79	0	0	25
loin whole lean & fat braised	3 oz	203	23	12	68	0	0	41
loin whole lean & fat broiled	3 oz	206	23	12	68	0	0	53
loin whole lean & fat roasted	3 oz	211	23	12	70	0	0	50
lungs braised	3 oz	84	14	3	329	0	0	69
pancreas cooked	3 oz	186	24	9	268	0	0	36
ribs country style lean & fat braised	3 oz	252	20	18	74	0	0	50
shoulder arm picnic lean & fat roasted	3 oz	269	20	20	80	0	0	60

FOOD	PORTION	CAL	PROT	FAT	CHOL	CARB	FIBER	SOD
shoulder whole lean & fat roasted	3 oz	248	20	18	77	0	0	58
shoulder whole lean & fat roasted diced	1 cup	394	31	29	122	0	0	92
shoulder whole lean roasted	3 oz	196	22	12	77	0	0	64
shoulder whole lean roasted diced	1 cup	311	34	18	122	0	0	101
sirloin chop lean & fat bone in braised	3 oz	208	22	13	70	0	0	43
sirloin roast lean & fat bone in cooked	3 oz	222	23	14	74	0	0	51
spareribs braised	3 oz	338	25	26	103	0	0	79
spleen braised	3 oz	127	24	3	428	0	0	91
tail simmered	3 oz	336	15	30	110	0	0	21
tenderloin lean roasted	3 oz	139	24	4	67	0	0	48
top loin chop boneless lean & fat cooked	3 oz	198	24	11	64	0	0	36
top loin roast bonless lean & fat cooked	3 oz	192	24	10	66	0	0	37
Freirich								
Porkette	4 oz	220	16	18	70	1	0	660
Oscar Mayer								
Sweet Morsel Smoked Boneless Pork Shoulder Butt	3 oz	180	11	15	50	0	0	990
READY-TO-EAT								
Tyson								
Pork Pattie	1 (3.8 oz)	200	15	11	40	9	3	270
TAKE-OUT								
chicharrones pork cracklings fried	1 cup	844	27	72	–	22	tr	128

FOOD	PORTION	CAL	PROT	FAT	CHOL	CARB	FIBER	SOD

PORK DISHES
Thomas E. Wilson

FOOD	PORTION	CAL	PROT	FAT	CHOL	CARB	FIBER	SOD
Lemon Pepper Pork Roast	1 serv (3 oz)	110	19	3	30	2	0	680

TAKE-OUT

FOOD	PORTION	CAL	PROT	FAT	CHOL	CARB	FIBER	SOD
pork roast	2 oz	70	10	3	40	0	–	390
tourtiere	1 piece (4.9 oz)	451	15	34	–	21	–	–

POT PIE
Amy's Organic

FOOD	PORTION	CAL	PROT	FAT	CHOL	CARB	FIBER	SOD
Broccoli	1 (7.5 oz)	430	11	22	45	46	4	630
Country Vegetable	1 (7.5 oz)	370	12	16	40	47	4	580
Shepard's	1 (8 oz)	160	5	4	0	27	5	490
Vegetable	1 (7.5 oz)	360	7	18	45	44	4	540
Vegetable Non-Dairy	1 (7.5 oz)	320	9	9	0	50	4	590

Banquet

FOOD	PORTION	CAL	PROT	FAT	CHOL	CARB	FIBER	SOD
Beef	1 (7 oz)	400	9	23	30	38	1	1000
Cheesy Potato & Broccoli w/ Ham	1 (7 oz)	410	9	23	25	40	2	1220
Chicken	1 (7 oz)	380	10	22	40	36	1	950
Chicken & Broccoli	1 (7 oz)	350	10	20	35	32	2	830
Family Size Hearty Chicken	1 cup	460	11	29	35	39	2	1010
Macaroni & Cheese	1 pkg (6.5 oz)	210	7	5	10	34	1	750
Turkey	1 (7 oz)	370	10	20	45	38	3	850
Vegetable Cheese	1 (7 oz)	340	6	17	10	39	1	920

Healthy Choice

FOOD	PORTION	CAL	PROT	FAT	CHOL	CARB	FIBER	SOD
Colonial Chicken	1 (9.5 oz)	310	22	7	45	40	5	570

Lean Cuisine

FOOD	PORTION	CAL	PROT	FAT	CHOL	CARB	FIBER	SOD
Everyday Favorites Chicken Pie	1 pkg (9.5 oz)	300	19	8	30	38	–	580
Everyday Favorites Vegetable Eggroll	1 pkg (9 oz)	300	7	5	0	57	4	610

Marie Callender's

FOOD	PORTION	CAL	PROT	FAT	CHOL	CARB	FIBER	SOD
Beef	1 (9.5 oz)	680	16	42	20	53	1	1430
Chicken	1 (9.5 oz)	680	14	48	20	53	3	1100
Chicken & Broccoli	1 (9.5 oz)	670	16	43	25	54	4	1000
Chicken Au Gratin	1 (9.5 oz)	690	19	46	30	50	4	1300
Turkey	1 (9.5 oz)	680	13	46	15	56	5	1100

FOOD	PORTION	CAL	PROT	FAT	CHOL	CARB	FIBER	SOD
Morton								
Macaroni & Cheese	1 (6.5 oz)	210	7	5	10	34	1	750
Vegetable w/ Beef	1 (7 oz)	340	5	21	20	33	2	1380
Vegetable w/ Chicken	1 (7 oz)	320	8	18	25	32	2	1040
Vegetable w/ Turkey	1 (7 oz)	310	8	18	25	29	2	1060
Mrs. Paterson's								
Aussie Pie Chicken	1 (5.5 oz)	460	12	25	90	45	2	770
Aussie Pie Chicken Low Fat	1 (5.5 oz)	380	13	17	35	44	1	930
Aussie Pie Philly Steak	1 (5.5 oz)	420	11	24	40	39	2	860
Stouffer's								
Beef Pie	1 pkg (10 oz)	450	19	26	65	36	3	1140
Chicken Pie	1 pkg (10 oz)	540	23	33	25	38	4	1080
Turkey	1 pkg (10 oz)	530	21	33	65	36	3	1040
Swanson								
Beef	1 (7 oz)	376	12	19	22	39	5	739
Chicken	1 (7 oz)	416	9	22	19	45	2	814
Turkey	1 (7 oz)	440	12	24	18	44	2	748
TAKE-OUT								
beef	⅓ of 9 in pie (7.4 oz)	515	21	30	42	39	–	596
chicken	⅓ of 9 in pie (7.4 oz)	545	23	31	56	42	–	594

POTATO (see also CHIPS, KNISH, PANCAKES)

FOOD	PORTION	CAL	PROT	FAT	CHOL	CARB	FIBER	SOD
CANNED								
potatoes	½ cup	54	1	tr	0	12	–	–
Del Monte								
New Sliced	⅔ cup (5.4 oz)	60	1	0	0	13	2	360
New Whole	2 med (5.5 oz)	60	1	0	0	13	2	360
Hormel								
Au Gratin & Bacon	1 can (7.5 oz)	250	8	14	25	23	2	840
S&W								
Whole Small	2 (5.5 oz)	60	1	0	0	13	2	360
FRESH								
baked skin only	1 skin (2 oz)	115	2	tr	0	27	2	12
baked w/ skin	1 (6.5 oz)	220	5	tr	0	51	–	16
baked w/o skin	1 (5 oz)	145	3	tr	0	34	2	8
baked w/o skin	½ cup	57	1	tr	0	13	1	3
boiled	½ cup	68	1	tr	0	16	1	3
microwaved	1 (7 oz)	212	5	tr	0	49	–	16

FOOD	PORTION	CAL	PROT	FAT	CHOL	CARB	FIBER	SOD
microwaved w/o skin	½ cup	78	2	tr	0	18	–	5
raw w/o skin	1 (3.9 oz)	88	2	tr	0	20	–	7
PurelyIdaho								
Oven Roasts	1 serv (3 oz)	70	2	0	0	17	2	0
Yukon Gold								
Fresh	1 (5.3 oz)	110	–	0	0	–	–	–
FROZEN								
french fries	10 strips	111	2	4	0	17	2	15
french fries thick cut	10 strips	109	2	4	0	17	–	23
hashed brown	½ cup	170	2	9	–	22	–	27
potato puffs	½ cup	138	2	7	0	19	–	462
potato puffs as prep	1	16	tr	1	0	2	–	52
Birds Eye								
Baby Gourmet	7 (4 oz)	100	2	0	0	21	1	15
Whole	3 (2.6 oz)	50	1	0	0	13	1	25
Healthy Choice								
Cheddar Broccoli Potatoes	1 meal (10.5 oz)	330	13	7	25	53	6	550
Lean Cuisine								
Everyday Favorites Deluxe Cheddar Potato	1 pkg (10.4 oz)	250	13	6	20	37	5	590
Everyday Favorites Roasted Potatoes w/ Broccoli	1 pkg (10.25 oz)	260	12	6	15	39	7	590
MicroMagic								
French Fries Low Fat	1 pkg (3 oz)	130	3	3	0	23	3	35
Oh Boy!								
Stuffed w/ Cheddar Cheese	1 (5 oz)	130	3	4	<5	22	2	270
Stouffer's								
Au Gratin	½ cup (5.75 oz)	130	4	6	15	15	1	590
Scalloped	½ cup (5.75 oz)	140	4	6	<5	17	2	450
Tree Of Life								
Organic French Fries	20 pieces (3 oz)	110	2	3	0	19	1	75
Weight Watchers								
Smart Ones Baked Broccoli & Cheese	1 pkg (10 oz)	250	11	6	20	39	6	570

FOOD	PORTION	CAL	PROT	FAT	CHOL	CARB	FIBER	SOD
MIX								
au gratin as prep	4½ oz	127	3	6	–	18	–	601
instant mashed flakes as prep w/ whole milk & butter	½ cup	118	2	6	15	16	–	349
instant mashed flakes not prep	½ cup	78	2	tr	0	18	–	24
instant mashed granules as prep w/ whole milk & butter	½ cup	114	2	5	15	15	–	270
instant mashed granules not prep	½ cup	372	8	1	0	86	–	67
scalloped as prep	4½ oz	127	3	6	–	18	–	467
Betty Crocker								
Au Gratin Low Fat Recipe	½ cup	110	3	1	<5	22	1	560
Au Gratin as prep	½ cup	150	3	6	5	22	1	600
Cheddar & Bacon	½ cup	150	3	6	<5	21	1	650
Cheddar & Bacon Low Fat Recipe	½ cup	120	3	3	0	21	1	620
Cheddar & Sour Cream	½ cup	130	3	3	5	25	1	580
Chicken & Vegetable	⅔ cup	140	4	4	<5	23	2	520
Chicken & Vegetable Low Fat Recipe	⅔ cup	120	4	3	<5	23	2	510
Hash Browns	½ cup	190	3	8	0	30	3	620
Homestyle Broccoli Au Gratin	½ cup	140	3	6	<5	21	2	530
Homestyle Broccoli Au Gratin Low Fat Recipe	½ cup	110	3	3	0	21	2	530
Homestyle Cheddar Cheese	½ cup	120	3	3	<5	21	1	600
Homestyle Cheddar Cheese Stove Top Recipe	½ cup	140	3	5	5	21	1	680

FOOD	PORTION	CAL	PROT	FAT	CHOL	CARB	FIBER	SOD
Homestyle Cheesy Scalloped	½ cup	140	3	6	<5	21	2	540
Homestyle Cheesy Scalloped Low Fat Recipe	½ cup	110	3	3	<5	21	3	540
Julienne	½ cup	150	3	6	<5	21	1	630
Mashed Butter & Herb	½ cup	160	3	8	5	20	1	470
Mashed Butter & Herb Reduced Fat Recipe	½ cup	130	3	5	<5	20	1	450
Mashed Chicken & Herb	½ cup	150	3	7	<5	21	1	520
Mashed Chicken & Herb Reduced Fat Recipe	½ cup	120	3	4	0	21	1	490
Mashed Four Cheese	½ cup	150	3	7	<5	20	2	570
Mashed Four Cheese Reduced Fat Recipe	½ cup	120	3	4	0	20	2	540
Mashed Potato Buds	⅔ cup	160	3	8	<5	19	1	460
Mashed Potato Buds Reduced Fat Recipe	⅔ cup	120	3	4	0	19	1	420
Mashed Roasted Garlic	½ cup	150	3	8	<5	19	2	400
Mashed Roasted Garlic Reduced Fat Recipe	½ cup	130	3	5	0	19	2	380
Mashed Sour Cream & Chives	½ cup	150	3	7	5	21	1	440
Potato Shakers Original	⅔ cup	140	3	4	<5	23	2	580
Potato Shakers Original Low Fat Recipe	⅔ cup	120	3	2	<5	23	2	560
Ranch	½ cup	160	3	6	<5	25	2	610
Scalloped	½ cup	150	3	6	<5	23	1	620
Scalloped Low Fat Recipe	⅔ cup	110	3	1	0	23	1	580

FOOD	PORTION	CAL	PROT	FAT	CHOL	CARB	FIBER	SOD
Sour Cream'n Chive	½ cup	160	3	7	5	22	2	600
Three Cheese	½ cup	150	3	6	<5	23	1	600
Twice Baked Cheddar & Bacon Low Fat Recipe	⅔ cup	130	6	3	<5	22	1	530
Twice Baked Cheddar & Bacon as prep	⅔ cup	210	6	11	85	22	1	580
Hungry Jack								
Au Gratin as prep	½ cup	150	3	5	10	24	1	620
Cheddar & Bacon as prep	½ cup	150	4	5	10	24	2	540
Cheesy Scalloped as prep	½ cup	150	3	5	10	24	1	570
Creamy Scalloped as prep	½ cup	150	3	5	10	24	2	460
Mashed Butter Flavored as prep	½ cup	150	3	7	<5	19	1	350
Mashed Flakes as prep	½ cup	160	3	7	<5	20	1	240
Mashed Garlic Flavored as prep	½ cup	150	3	7	<5	19	1	360
Mashed Parsley Butter as prep	½ cup	150	3	7	<5	19	1	380
Mashed Sour Cream 'n Chives as prep	½ cup	150	3	7	<5	19	1	380
Sour Cream & Chives as prep	½ cup	160	3	6	15	23	1	510
Idaho								
Mashed Potato Flakes as prep	½ cup	150	3	6	<5	20	1	240
Mashed Potato Granules as prep	½ cup	160	3	7	<5	22	2	300
Shake 'N Bake								
Perfect Potatoes Crispy Cheddar	⅛ pkg (7 g)	30	2	2	5	2	0	380
Perfect Potatoes Herb & Garlic	⅛ pkg (7 g)	20	0	0	0	5	0	380
Perfect Potatoes Home Fries	⅛ pkg (7 g)	20	0	0	0	5	0	410

FOOD	PORTION	CAL	PROT	FAT	CHOL	CARB	FIBER	SOD
Perfect Potatoes Parmesan Peppercorn	⅙ pkg (7 g)	25	1	1	<5	3	0	300
Perfect Potatoes Savory Onion	⅙ pkg (7 g)	20	0	0	0	5	0	280
SHELF-STABLE								
Lunch Bucket								
Scalloped w/ Ham Chunks	1 pkg (7.5 oz)	170	2	7	10	24	3	660
Micro Cup Meals								
Microcup Meals Scalloped Potatoes w/ Ham	1 cup (7.5 oz)	240	7	14	35	20	2	920
TAKE-OUT								
au gratin w/ cheese	½ cup	178	7	10	18	17	–	548
baked topped w/ cheese sauce	1	475	15	29	19	47	–	381
baked topped w/ cheese sauce & bacon	1	451	18	26	30	44	–	973
baked topped w/ cheese sauce & broccoli	1	402	14	14	20	47	–	484
baked topped w/ cheese sauce & chili	1	481	23	22	31	56	–	701
baked topped w/ sour cream & chives	1	394	7	22	23	50	–	182
curry	1 serv (6 oz)	292	4	16	–	36	4	–
french fries	1 reg	235	3	12	0	29	–	124
french fries	1 lg	355	5	19	0	44	–	187
hash brown	½ cup (2.5 oz)	151	2	9	9	16	–	290
indian yogurt potatoes	1 serv	315	7	9	18	52	0	216
mashed	½ cup	111	2	4	2	18	–	309
mustard potato salad	3.5 oz	120	1	6	0	16	–	393
o'brien	1 cup	157	5	3	7	30	–	421
potato dumpling	3.5 oz	334	7	1	–	74	3	1

FOOD	PORTION	CAL	PROT	FAT	CHOL	CARB	FIBER	SOD
potato pancakes	1 (1.3 oz)	101	2	7	35	11	–	188
potato salad	½ cup	179	3	10	86	14	–	661
potato salad w/ vegetables	3.5 oz	120	2	3	0	20	–	390
scalloped	½ cup	127	4	5	7	18	–	435

POTATO STARCH

FOOD	PORTION	CAL	PROT	FAT	CHOL	CARB	FIBER	SOD
potato starch	1 oz	96	tr	tr	0	24	–	1

POUT

FOOD	PORTION	CAL	PROT	FAT	CHOL	CARB	FIBER	SOD
ocean baked	3 oz	86	18	1	57	0	–	66
ocean fillet baked	4.8 oz	139	29	2	91	0	–	107

PRETZELS

FOOD	PORTION	CAL	PROT	FAT	CHOL	CARB	FIBER	SOD
chocolate covered	1 (0.4 oz)	50	1	2	–	8	–	–
dutch twist	4 (2.1 oz)	229	6	2	0	48	2	1029
rods	4 (2 oz)	229	6	2	0	48	2	1029
sticks	10	10	tr	tr	tr	2	–	48
twists	10 (2.1 oz)	229	6	2	0	48	2	1029
whole wheat	2 sm (1 oz)	103	3	1	0	23	–	58
Bachman								
Thin'n Right	12 (1 oz)	120	3	1	0	23	1	650
Estee								
Chocolate Covered	7	130	2	6	0	19	tr	270
Dutch	2 (1.1 oz)	130	3	1	0	26	1	40
Unsalted	23 (1 oz)	120	3	1	0	25	1	30
Gardetto's								
Mustard	1 pkg (0.5 oz)	50	1	1	0	10	tr	110
Herr's								
Hard Sourdough	1 (1 oz)	100	3	0	0	23	2	450
Lance								
Pretzels	1 pkg (1.25 oz)	140	4	1	0	28	tr	470
Little Debbie								
Mini Twists	1 pkg (1.2 oz)	140	4	1	0	28	1	470
Nabisco								
Air Crisps Fat Free	23 pieces (1 oz)	110	2	0	0	23	tr	550
Nestle								
Flipz Milk Chocolate Covered	9 pieces (1 oz)	130	2	5	<5	19	tr	135
Flipz White Fudge Covered	9 pieces (1 oz)	130	2	6	0	19	0	130

FOOD	PORTION	CAL	PROT	FAT	CHOL	CARB	FIBER	SOD
Newman's Own								
Salted Rounds Organic	1 pkg (1.4 oz)	150	3	2	0	31	1	530
Planters								
Twists	1 pkg (1.5 oz)	160	4	1	0	35	1	640
Twists	1 oz	100	3	1	0	23	1	420
Rold Gold								
Crispy's Thins	4 (1 oz)	110	3	2	0	22	1	670
Fat Free Cheddar Cheese	17 (1 oz)	110	3	0	0	23	1	440
Fat Free Honey Mustard	17 (1 oz)	110	3	0	0	23	1	380
Fat Free Sticks	48 (1 oz)	110	3	0	0	23	1	530
Fat Free Thins	12 pieces (1 oz)	110	2	0	0	24	1	520
Fat Free Tiny Twists	18 pieces (1 oz)	110	3	0	0	23	1	420
Honey Mustard	16 (1 oz)	110	3	1	0	22	1	370
Rods	3 (1 oz)	110	3	1	0	22	1	610
Sour Dough Nuggets	11 (1 oz)	110	2	0	0	24	1	330
Snyder's Of Hanover								
Dips White Fudge	1 oz	130	2	6	0	19	0	80
Hard Sourdough	1 oz	100	3	0	0	22	1	240
Hard Sourdough Unsalted	1 oz	100	3	0	0	22	1	90
Logs	1 oz	110	3	1	0	21	tr	360
Mini	1 oz	120	3	0	0	25	tr	250
Mini Unsalted	1 oz	110	3	0	0	25	tr	75
Nibblers	1 oz	120	3	0	0	25	tr	200
Nibblers Honey Mustard & Onions	1 oz	130	3	3	0	23	tr	95
Nibblers Oat Bran	1 oz	130	3	3	0	23	3	170
Nibblers Unsalted	1 oz	120	3	0	0	25	tr	50
Oat Bran	1 oz	100	3	3	0	22	2	260
Old Fashioned Dipping Stix	1 oz	100	3	0	0	22	1	330
Old Tyme Unsalted	1 oz	120	3	1	0	24	1	75
Olde Tyme	1 oz	120	3	1	0	24	1	120
Olde Tyme Stix	1 oz	120	3	1	0	23	1	150
Pieces Buttermilk Ranch	1 oz	130	3	5	0	19	tr	250

FOOD	PORTION	CAL	PROT	FAT	CHOL	CARB	FIBER	SOD
Pieces Cheddar Cheese	1 oz	190	2	6	0	18	tr	260
Pieces Honey Mustard & Onions	1 oz	140	2	7	0	18	tr	240
Pieces Peppered Pizza	1 oz	150	2	8	0	16	tr	340
Rods	1 oz	120	4	2	0	24	tr	400
Snaps	24 (1 oz)	120	3	1	0	25	tr	390
Thin	1 oz	130	3	0	0	23	tr	430
Whole Wheat Honey	1 oz	120	3	1	0	24	2	20
Utz								
Country Store Stix	5 (1 oz)	110	3	1	0	22	1	470
Fat Free Hard	1 (0.8 oz)	90	2	0	0	18	tr	470
Fat Free Hard No Salt Added	1 (0.8 oz)	90	2	0	0	19	tr	50
Fat Free Sour Dough Nuggets	10 (1 oz)	100	2	0	0	22	1	470
Fat Free Stix	14 (1 oz)	100	3	0	0	23	1	280
Fat Free Thin	10 (1 oz)	100	2	0	0	22	1	480
Honey Mustard & Onion	⅓ cup (1 oz)	130	2	6	0	18	tr	270
Rods	3 (1 oz)	120	3	1	0	24	1	400
Specials	5 (1 oz)	110	3	1	0	21	1	470
Specials Extra Dark	5 (1 oz)	110	3	1	0	21	1	470
Specials Unsalted	5 (1 oz)	110	3	1	0	21	1	80
Wheels	20 (1 oz)	100	2	0	0	22	1	480
Weight Watchers								
Oat Bran Nuggets	1 pkg (1.5 oz)	170	4	3	0	33	3	250

PRUNE JUICE

canned	1 cup	181	2	tr	0	45	3	11

PRUNES

canned in heavy syrup	5	90	1	tr	0	24	–	2
canned in heavy syrup	1 cup	245	2	tr	0	65	–	6
dried	10	201	2	tr	0	53	6	3
dried	1 cup	385	4	1	0	101	12	6

FOOD	PORTION	CAL	PROT	FAT	CHOL	CARB	FIBER	SOD
dried cooked w/ sugar	½ cup	147	1	tr	0	39	7	2
dried cooked w/o sugar	½ cup	113	1	tr	0	30	6	2
Sonoma								
Pitted	¼ cup (1.4 oz)	120	1	0	0	29	3	5

PUDDING (see also CUSTARD, PUDDING POPS)
MIX
Betty Crocker

FOOD	PORTION	CAL	PROT	FAT	CHOL	CARB	FIBER	SOD
Rice as prep	1 serv	200	1	3	9	33	–	70
Jell-O								
Americana Rice as prep w/ skim milk	½ cup (5.2 oz)	140	5	0	<5	29	0	160
Americana Tapioca as prep w/ skim milk	½ cup (5.1 oz)	130	4	0	<5	28	0	180
Banana Cream as prep w/ 2% milk	½ cup (5.1 oz)	140	4	3	10	26	0	240
Butterscotch as prep w/ 2% milk	½ cup (5.2 oz)	160	4	3	10	30	0	190
Chocolate as prep w/ 2% milk	½ cup (5.2 oz)	150	5	3	10	28	tr	170
Chocolate Fudge as prep w/ 2% milk	½ cup (5.2 oz)	150	5	3	10	28	1	170
Coconut Cream as prep w/ 2% milk	½ cup (5.1 oz)	150	4	5	10	24	tr	210
Fat Free Chocolate as prep w/ skim milk	½ cup (5.2 oz)	130	5	0	<5	29	0	170
Fat Free Vanilla as prep w/ skim milk	½ cup (5.1 oz)	130	4	0	<5	28	0	200
Instant Banana Cream as prep w/ 2% milk	½ cup (5.2 oz)	150	4	3	10	29	0	410
Instant Butterscotch as prep w/ 2% milk	½ cup (5.2 oz)	150	4	3	10	29	0	450

FOOD	PORTION	CAL	PROT	FAT	CHOL	CARB	FIBER	SOD
Instant Chocolate as prep w/ 2% milk	½ cup (5.2 oz)	160	4	3	10	31	tr	470
Instant Chocolate Fudge as prep w/ 2% milk	½ cup (4.2 oz)	160	5	3	10	31	tr	440
Instant Coconut Cream as prep w/ 2% milk	½ cup (4.2 oz)	160	4	5	10	27	tr	320
Instant French Vanilla as prep w/ 2% milk	½ cup (4.2 oz)	150	4	3	10	29	0	410
Instant Lemon as prep w/ 2% milk	½ cup (4.2 oz)	150	4	3	10	29	0	370
Instant Pistachio as prep w/ 2% milk	½ cup (4.2 oz)	160	4	3	10	29	0	410
Instant Vanilla as prep w/ 2% milk	½ cup (4.2 oz)	150	4	3	10	29	0	410
Instant Fat Free Chocolate as prep w/ skim milk	½ cup (5.3 oz)	140	5	0	<5	31	tr	410
Instant Fat Free Devil's Food as prep w/ skim milk	½ cup (5.3 oz)	140	5	0	<5	31	tr	420
Instant Fat Free Sugar Free Banana as prep w/ skim milk	½ cup (4.6 oz)	70	4	0	<5	12	0	410
Instant Fat Free Sugar Free Vanilla as prep w/ skim milk	½ cup (4.6 oz)	70	4	0	<5	12	0	400
Instant Fat Free Vanilla as prep w/ skim milk	½ cup (5.2 oz)	140	4	0	<5	29	0	410

FOOD	PORTION	CAL	PROT	FAT	CHOL	CARB	FIBER	SOD
Instant Fat Free White Chocolate as prep w/ skim milk	½ cup (5.2 oz)	140	4	0	<5	29	0	410
Lemon as prep	½ cup (4.4 oz)	140	tr	2	75	29	0	75
Milk Chocolate as prep w/ 2% milk	½ cup (5.2 oz)	150	4	3	10	28	tr	170
Sugar Free Chocolate as prep w/ 2% milk	½ cup (4.6 oz)	90	5	3	10	13	tr	170
Sugar Free Vanilla as prep w/ 2% milk	½ cup (4.5 oz)	80	4	3	10	11	0	170
Vanilla as prep w/ 2% milk	½ cup (5.1 oz)	150	0	3	9	30	0	408
Louisiana Purchase								
Bread	1 serv (1.3 oz)	150	3	3	0	28	2	220
Lundberg								
Elegant Rice Cinnamon Raisin	½ cup (3.9 oz)	70	0	0	0	16	1	0
Elegant Rice Coconut	½ cup (3.9 oz)	70	0	2	0	13	1	0
Elegant Rice Honey Almond	½ cup (3.9 oz)	70	2	1	0	15	1	0
Uncle Ben's								
Rice Pudding Cinnamon & Raisins as prep	½ cup (1.5 oz)	160	2	1	0	37	1	150
READY-TO-EAT								
Handi-Snacks								
Banana	1 serv (3.5 oz)	120	1	4	0	22	0	150
Butterscotch	1 serv (3.5 oz)	120	1	4	0	22	0	150
Chocolate	1 serv (3.5 oz)	130	2	4	0	23	tr	125
Chocolate Fudge	1 serv (3.5 oz)	130	2	4	0	23	tr	130
Fat Free Chocolate	1 serv (3.5 oz)	90	2	0	0	21	0	170
Fat Free Vanilla	1 serv (3.5 oz)	90	1	0	0	21	0	180
Tapioca	1 serv (3.5 oz)	120	2	4	0	21	0	120
Vanilla	1 serv (3.5 oz)	120	1	4	0	21	0	150

FOOD	PORTION	CAL	PROT	FAT	CHOL	CARB	FIBER	SOD
Healthy Choice								
Low Fat Chocolate Raspberry	½ cup (3.5 oz)	102	3	2	0	19	0	111
Low Fat Chocolate Almond	½ cup (3.5 oz)	109	3	2	0	21	0	109
Low Fat Double Chocolate Fudge	½ cup (3.5 oz)	101	3	1	0	20	0	116
Low Fat French Vanilla	½ cup (3.5 oz)	98	2	1	0	20	0	122
Low Fat Tapioca	½ cup (3.5 oz)	101	2	1	1	21	0	115
Hunt's								
Snack Pack Banana	1 serv (3.5 oz)	119	2	4	2	18	0	155
Snack Pack Butterscotch	1 serv (3.5 oz)	130	2	4	2	21	0	164
Snack Pack Chocolate	1 serv (3.5 oz)	143	2	5	1	22	0	139
Snack Pack Chocolate Fudge	1 serv (3.5 oz)	147	2	5	1	23	0	153
Snack Pack Chocolate Marshmallow	1 serv (3.5 oz)	134	2	5	1	21	0	212
Snack Pack Fat Free Chocolate	1 serv (3.5 oz)	86	2	tr	1	19	0	134
Snack Pack Fat Free Tapioca	1 serv (3.5 oz)	82	2	tr	0	18	0	141
Snack Pack Fat Free Vanilla	1 serv (3.5 oz)	81	2	tr	0	18	0	146
Snack Pack Lemon	1 serv (3.5 oz)	124	tr	3	0	24	0	47
Snack Pack Milk Chocolate Variety	1 serv (3.5 oz)	143	2	5	2	22	0	136
Snack Pack Swirl Chocolate Caramel	1 serv (3.5 oz)	143	2	5	1	23	0	143
Snack Pack Swirl Chocolate Peanut Butter	1 serv (3.5 oz)	146	3	6	2	21	0	156
Snack Pack Swirl Smores	1 serv (3.5 oz)	136	2	5	1	21	0	94
Snack Pack Tapioca	1 serv (3.5 oz)	125	1	4	1	21	0	144
Snack Pack Toppers Chocolate w/ Fun Chips	1 serv (4 ox)	176	2	6	1	28	tr	153

FOOD	PORTION	CAL	PROT	FAT	CHOL	CARB	FIBER	SOD
Snack Pack Vanilla	1 serv (3.5 oz)	135	2	5	1	21	0	147
Imagine								
Banana	1 pkg (4 oz)	150	1	3	0	30	0	40
Butterscotch	1 pkg (4 oz)	150	1	3	0	31	0	45
Chocolate	1 pkg (4 oz)	170	1	3	0	38	1	65
Lemon	1 pkg (4 oz)	150	1	3	0	33	1	50
Jell-O								
Chocolate	1 serv (4 oz)	160	3	5	0	28	0	190
Chocolate Marshmallow	1 serv (4 oz)	160	3	5	0	27	0	180
Chocolate Vanilla Swirls	1 serv (4 oz)	160	3	5	0	27	0	180
Free Chocolate	1 serv (4 oz)	100	3	0	0	23	tr	190
Free Chocolate Vanilla Swirl	1 serv (4 oz)	100	3	0	0	23	tr	210
Free Devil's Food	1 serv (4 oz)	100	3	0	0	23	tr	210
Free Rocky Road	1 serv (4 oz)	100	3	0	0	23	tr	210
Free Vanilla	1 serv (4 oz)	100	2	0	0	23	0	240
Tapioca	1 serv (4 oz)	140	2	4	0	26	0	160
Tapioca	1 serv (4 oz)	100	2	0	0	23	0	240
Vanilla	1 serv (4 oz)	160	2	5	0	25	0	170
Kozy Shack								
Banana	1 pkg (4 oz)	130	3	3	10	22	1	150
Chocolate	1 pkg (4 oz)	140	3	4	5	24	1	150
Light Chocolate	1 pkg (4 oz)	110	4	1	5	22	1	150
Light Vanilla	1 pkg (4 oz)	110	4	1	10	22	0	160
Rice	1 pkg (4 oz)	130	4	3	17	23	1	140
Tapioca	1 pkg (4 oz)	140	3	3	5	25	0	160
Vanilla	1 pkg (4 oz)	130	3	3	10	22	1	150
NutraBalance								
Low Lactose All Flavors	1 serv (4 oz)	225	7	8	0	31	—	220
Swiss Miss								
Butterscotch	1 pkg (4 oz)	156	2	6	1	24	0	182
Chocolate	1 pkg (4 oz)	166	3	6	1	26	0	177
Chocolate Fudge	1 pkg (4 oz)	175	3	6	1	28	0	207
Fat Free Chocolate	1 pkg (4 oz)	98	2	tr	0	22	0	141
Fat Free Chocolate Fudge	1 pkg (4 oz)	101	2	tr	0	23	0	147

FOOD	PORTION	CAL	PROT	FAT	CHOL	CARB	FIBER	SOD
Fat Free Tapioca	1 pkg (4 oz)	98	2	tr	0	22	0	184
Fat Free Vanilla	1 pkg (4 oz)	93	2	tr	0	21	0	168
Fat Free Parfait Vanilla Chocolate	1 pkg (4 oz)	96	2	tr	0	21	0	143
Milk Chocolate	1 pkg (4 oz)	166	2	6	1	26	0	165
Parfait Vanilla Chocolate	1 pkg (4 oz)	164	3	6	1	25	0	196
Swirl Chocolate Caramel	1 pkg (4 oz)	169	2	6	1	26	1	178
Swirl Chocolate Vanilla	1 pkg (4 oz)	169	2	6	1	26	0	159
Swirl Chocolate Vanilla Chocolate	1 pkg (4 oz)	169	3	6	1	26	0	159
Tapioca	1 pkg (4 oz)	138	2	4	1	24	0	180
Vanilla	1 pkg (4 oz)	156	2	6	1	24	0	181
TAKE-OUT								
blancmange	1 serv (4.7 oz)	154	4	5	—	25	tr	—
bread pudding	1 serv (6.7 oz)	564	11	18	—	94	6	—
bread pudding	½ cup (4.4 oz)	212	7	7	83	31	—	291
bread w/ raisins	½ cup	180	5	5	77	31	—	185
chocolate	½ cup (5.5 oz)	206	5	4	9	41	—	157
queen of puddings	1 serv (4.4 oz)	266	6	10	—	41	tr	—
rice pudding	1 serv (3 oz)	110	4	—	3	17	tr	—
rice w/ raisins	½ cup	246	7	6	136	42	4	270
tapioca	½ cup (5.3 oz)	189	7	7	124	26	—	288
vanilla	½ cup (4.3 oz)	130	4	4	17	20	—	113
yorkshire	1 serv (3 oz)	177	6	8	57	22	tr	168
PUDDING POPS								
chocolate	1 (1.6 oz)	72	2	2	1	12	—	77
vanilla	1 (1.6 oz)	75	2	2	1	13	—	50
PUFFERFISH								
raw	3 oz	72	17	0	—	0	0	120
PUMMELO								
fresh	1	228	5	tr	0	59	—	7
sections	1 cup	71	1	tr	0	18	—	2

FOOD	PORTION	CAL	PROT	FAT	CHOL	CARB	FIBER	SOD
PUMPKIN								
CANNED								
Libby								
Solid Pack	½ cup	40	2	1	0	9	5	5
Owatonna								
Pumpkin	½ cup	40	–	1	0	–	–	–
FRESH								
cooked mashed	½ cup	24	1	tr	0	6	–	2
flowers cooked	½ cup	10	1	tr	0	2	–	4
leaves cooked	½ cup	7	1	tr	0	1	–	3
SEEDS								
dried	1 oz	154	7	13	0	5	–	5
roasted	1 oz	148	9	12	0	4	–	5
salted & roasted	1 oz	148	9	12	0	4	–	144
PURSLANE								
cooked	1 cup	21	2	tr	0	4	–	51
raw	1 cup	7	1	tr	0	1	–	20
QUAIL								
breast w/o skin raw	1 (2 oz)	69	13	2	–	0	–	31
w/ skin raw	1 quail (3.8 oz)	210	21	13	–	0	–	58
w/o skin raw	1 quail (3.2 oz)	123	20	4	–	0	–	47
QUICHE								
TAKE-OUT								
cheese	1 slice (3 oz)	283	11	20	–	16	1	–
lorraine	⅛ of 8 in pie	600	13	48	285	29	–	653
mushroom	1 slice (3 oz)	256	9	18	–	17	1	–
QUINCE								
fresh	1	53	tr	tr	0	14	–	4
QUINOA								
quinoa not prep	1 cup (6 oz)	636	22	10	0	117	10	36
RABBIT								
domestic w/o bone roasted	3 oz	167	25	7	70	0	–	40
wild w/o bone stewed	3 oz	147	28	3	104	0	–	38
RACCOON								
roasted	3 oz	217	25	12	–	0	–	–

FOOD	PORTION	CAL	PROT	FAT	CHOL	CARB	FIBER	SOD
RADICCHIO								
raw shredded	½ cup	5	tr	tr	0	1	—	4
RADISHES								
chinese dried	½ cup	157	5	tr	0	37	—	161
chinese raw	1 (12 oz)	62	2	tr	0	14	—	71
chinese raw sliced	½ cup	8	tr	tr	0	2	—	9
chinese sliced cooked	½ cup	13	tr	tr	0	3	—	10
daikon dried	½ cup	157	5	tr	0	37	—	161
daikon raw	1 (12 oz)	62	2	tr	0	14	—	71
daikon raw sliced	½ cup	8	tr	tr	0	2	—	9
daikon sliced cooked	½ cup	13	tr	tr	0	3	—	10
red raw	10	7	tr	tr	0	2	—	11
red sliced	½ cup	10	tr	tr	0	2	—	14
white icicle raw	1 (½ oz)	2	tr	tr	0	tr	—	3
white icicle raw sliced	½ cup	7	1	tr	0	1	—	8
Eden								
Daikon Dried Shredded	2 tbsp	45	1	0	0	9	3	20
Daikon Pickled	2 slices	5	0	0	0	1	0	250
TAKE-OUT								
korean kimchee	½ cup	31	2	1	—	6	—	—
moo namul saengche korean salad	1 serv (3.7 oz)	34	1	tr	0	8	2	547
RAISINS								
chocolate coated	10 (0.4 oz)	39	tr	2	0	7	—	4
chocolate coated	1 cup (6.7 oz)	741	8	28	5	130	—	68
golden seedless	1 cup	437	5	1	0	115	8	17
seedless	1 cup	434	5	1	0	115	8	17
seedless	1 tbsp	27	tr	tr	0	7	—	—
sultanas	1 oz	88	1	0	—	23	2	—
Cinderella								
Seedless	½ cup	250	—	0	0	—	—	—
Dole								
CinnaRaisins	1 pkg (1 oz)	95	1	0	0	22	2	5
Estee								
Chocolate Covered	¼ cup	180	3	6	<5	27	1	45

FOOD	PORTION	CAL	PROT	FAT	CHOL	CARB	FIBER	SOD
Mariana								
Fruitn Yogurt Milk Chocolate Covered Raisins	32 pieces (1 oz)	130	1	5	0	20	2	40
Nestle								
Chocolate Covered	1⅓ tbsp	70	tr	3	0	11	tr	0
Sonoma								
Monukka Thompson	¼ cup (1.4 oz)	130	1	0	0	31	2	10
Tree Of Life								
Organic	¼ cup (1.4 oz)	130	1	0	0	31	2	10
RASPBERRIES								
canned in heavy syrup	½ cup	117	1	tr	0	30	–	4
fresh	1 cup	61	1	1	0	14	–	0
fresh	1 pint	154	3	2	0	36	–	0
frozen sweetened	1 cup	256	2	tr	0	65	–	1
frozen sweetened	1 pkg (10 oz)	291	2	tr	0	74	–	1
Birds Eye								
Red	5 oz	90	1	0	0	22	5	5
Tree Of Life								
Organic	⅔ cup (5 oz)	50	1	0	0	12	2	0
RASPBERRY JUICE								
Crystal Light								
Raspberry Ice Drink	1 serv (8 oz)	5	0	0	0	0	0	20
Raspberry Ice Drink Mix as prep	1 serv (8 oz)	5	0	0	0	0	0	0
Dole								
Country Raspberry	8 fl oz	140	0	0	0	35	–	35
Fresh Samantha								
Raspberry Dream	1 cup (8 oz)	120	2	1	–	10	8	0
Kool-Aid								
Drink Mix as prep	1 serv (8 oz)	60	0	0	0	17	0	0
Raspberry Drink as prep w/ sugar	1 serv (8 oz)	100	0	0	0	25	0	30
Splash Blue Raspberry Drink	1 serv (8 oz)	120	0	0	0	30	0	35

FOOD	PORTION	CAL	PROT	FAT	CHOL	CARB	FIBER	SOD
RED BEANS								
CANNED								
Green Giant								
Red Beans	½ cup (4.5 oz)	100	6	1	0	19	6	350
Hunt's								
Small	½ cup (4.5 oz)	89	6	1	0	19	6	713
Van Camp								
Red Beans	½ cup (4.6 oz)	90	6	0	0	20	5	560
DRIED								
Hurst								
HamBeens w/ Ham	1 serv	120	8	1	0	20	10	63
MIX								
Bean Cuisine								
Pasta & Beans Barcelona Red w/ Radiatore	1 serv	210	7	1	0	29	4	15
RELISH								
cranberry orange	½ cup	246	tr	tr	0	64	–	44
hamburger	1 tbsp	19	tr	tr	0	5	–	164
hamburger	½ cup	158	1	1	0	42	–	1338
hot dog	1 tbsp	14	tr	tr	0	4	–	164
hot dog	½ cup	111	2	1	0	28	–	1332
piccalilli	1.4 oz	13	tr	tr	–	2	1	–
sweet	1 tbsp	19	tr	tr	0	5	–	122
sweet	½ cup	159	tr	1	0	43	–	990
Claussen								
Sweet Pickle	1 tbsp (0.5 oz)	15	0	0	0	3	0	85
Green Giant								
Corn	1 tbsp (0.6 oz)	20	0	0	0	5	0	40
Old El Paso								
Jalapeno	1 tbsp (0.5 oz)	5	0	0	0	1	0	110
Vlasic								
Fancy Sweet	1 tbsp	15	0	0	0	4	–	140
RENNIN								
tablet	1 (0.9 g)	1	0	0	–	tr	–	234
RHUBARB								
fresh	½ cup	13	1	tr	0	3	–	2
frozen	½ cup	60	tr	tr	0	3	–	1
frzn as prep w/ sugar	½ cup	139	tr	tr	0	37	–	2

FOOD	PORTION	CAL	PROT	FAT	CHOL	CARB	FIBER	SOD
RICE *(see also* FLOUR, RICE CAKES, WILD RICE*)*								
brown long grain cooked	1 cup (6.8 oz)	216	2	0	5	45	4	10
brown medium grain cooked	1 cup (6.8 oz)	218	5	2	0	46	4	2
glutinous cooked	1 cup (6.1 oz)	169	4	tr	0	37	2	9
starch	1 oz	98	tr	0	0	24	–	17
white long grain cooked	1 cup (5.5 oz)	205	4	tr	0	45	1	2
white long grain instant cooked	1 cup (5.8 oz)	162	3	tr	0	35	1	5
white medium grain cooked	1 cup (6.5 oz)	242	4	tr	0	53	1	0
white short grain cooked	1 cup (6.5 oz)	242	4	tr	0	53	–	0
Birds Eye								
Rice & Broccoli In Cheese Sauce	1 pkg	290	8	9	15	15	2	1110
White & Wild w/ Green Beans	1 cup (6.6 oz)	180	4	4	10	31	2	480
Carolina								
Red Beans & Rice as prep	¼ pkg	190	6	1	0	40	6	790
Chun King								
Fried Rice Mix	½ cup (1.4 oz)	126	4	tr	0	29	1	691
Goya								
Arroz Amarillo	¼ cup (1.6 oz)	170	4	0	0	37	1	546
Green Giant								
Rice & Broccoli	1 pkg (10 oz)	320	8	12	15	44	2	1000
Rice Medley	1 pkg (10 oz)	240	6	3	5	46	2	880
Rice Pilaf	1 pkg (10 oz)	230	6	3	5	44	3	1020
White & Wild	1 pkg (10 oz)	250	6	5	0	45	3	1000
Kitchen Del Sol								
Mediterranean Paella Costa Brave as prep	½ cup (1.2 oz)	130	3	2	0	23	1	312
Mediterranean Sunny Lemon Pilaf as prep	½ cup (1.2 oz)	110	3	1	0	22	1	210

FOOD	PORTION	CAL	PROT	FAT	CHOL	CARB	FIBER	SOD
Mediterranean Tomato & Basil w/ Pine Nuts	½ cup (1 oz)	110	2	4	0	18	1	270
La Choy								
Fried Rice	1 cup (4.9 oz)	236	5	1	0	53	2	1024
Lipton								
Golden Saute Onion Mushroom	½ cup (2.1 oz)	240	6	4	0	45	2	850
Oriental Stir Fry as prep	1 cup	270	5	8	0	47	1	860
Rice & Sauce Alfredo Broccoli as prep	1 cup	320	9	12	15	46	1	990
Rice & Sauce Beef as prep	1 cup	270	6	8	0	47	1	1010
Rice & Sauce Cajun Style as prep	1 cup	270	7	7	0	46	1	910
Rice & Sauce Cajun Style w/ Beans as prep	1 cup	310	10	8	0	52	7	530
Rice & Sauce Cheddar Broccoli as prep	1 cup	280	7	9	5	46	1	1010
Rice & Sauce Chicken & Parmesan Risotto as prep	1 cup	270	6	9	0	43	tr	830
Rice & Sauce Chicken Broccoli as prep	1 cup	280	7	9	0	46	2	910
Rice & Sauce Chicken Flavor as prep	1 cup	280	7	9	5	45	1	960
Rice & Sauce Creamy Chicken as prep	1 cup	290	6	11	0	45	1	830
Rice & Sauce Herb & Butter as prep	1 cup	280	6	11	10	43	tr	880
Rice & Sauce Medley as prep	1 cup	270	7	9	5	44	2	870

FOOD	PORTION	CAL	PROT	FAT	CHOL	CARB	FIBER	SOD
Rice & Sauce Mushroom as prep	1 cup	270	6	8	0	45	1	960
Rice & Sauce Mushroom & Herb as prep	1 cup	290	6	8	0	49	1	620
Rice & Sauce Oriental as prep	1 cup	280	7	8	0	48	2	940
Rice & Sauce Pilaf as prep	1 cup	260	6	11	0	44	1	930
Rice & Sauce Scampi Style as prep	1 cup	270	6	9	5	44	1	900
Rice & Sauce Spanish as prep	1 cup	270	6	8	0	47	2	900
Rice & Sauce Teriyaki as prep	1 cup	270	5	8	0	45	1	910
Roasted Chicken as prep	1 cup	260	4	8	0	46	1	880
Salsa Style as prep	1 cup	220	4	7	0	37	2	540
Southwestern Chicken Flavor as prep	1 cup	260	5	11	0	47	1	840
Lundberg								
One-Step Curry	1 cup (7.4 oz)	160	5	1	0	38	5	400
Quick Brown Rice Savory Vegetarian Chicken	1 cup (2.5 oz)	260	6	3	—	53	5	910
Risotto Tomato Basil	1 serv	140	4	1	0	30	1	630
Melting Pot								
Risotto Melanese w/ Saffron	1 cup	210	4	0	0	48	0	70
Risotto Primavera	1 cup	200	5	1	0	44	1	85
Risotto Sun-Dried Tomatoes & Peas	1 cup	200	5	1	0	45	1	75
Risotto Three Cheese	1 cup	200	5	2	5	44	0	410
Risotto Wild Mushroom	1 cup	200	5	1	0	44	2	50

FOOD	PORTION	CAL	PROT	FAT	CHOL	CARB	FIBER	SOD
Minute								
Boil-In-Bag White as prep	1 cup (5.7 oz)	190	4	0	0	42	tr	10
Instant Brown as prep	⅔ cup	170	4	2	0	34	2	10
Instant White as prep	1 cup (5.7 oz)	160	3	0	0	36	tr	5
Long Grain & Wild Seasoned w/ Herbs as prep	1 cup (7.8 oz)	230	6	1	0	50	1	950
Old El Paso								
Mexican	½ cup (4 oz)	410	8	2	0	90	3	1350
Spanish	1 cup (8.6 oz)	130	3	1	0	28	2	1340
Success								
Brown & Wild Mix as prep	½ cup	120	3	3	0	21	2	432
TastyBite								
Green Peas Pilaf	½ pkg (4.5 oz)	208	6	4	0	36	4	487
Van Camp								
Spanish	½ cup (4.5 oz)	90	2	2	0	19	2	645
Zatarain's								
Dirty Rice Mix as prep w/o meat and oil	½ cup	130	3	0	0	29	0	680
Red Beans & Rice as prep w/o oil	½ cup	100	4	0	0	21	4	490
TAKE-OUT								
congee	½ cup (4.1 oz)	44	1	–	–	10	–	–
nasi goreng indonesian rice & vegetables	1 cup (4.9 oz)	130	4	0	0	28	1	530
paella	1 serv (7 oz)	308	23	16	92	17	3	580
pilaf	½ cup	84	4	3	22	11	3	362
risotto	6.6 oz	426	6	18	–	65	3	–
spanish	¾ cup	363	11	27	35	19	–	1339

RICE CAKES *(see also POPCORN CAKES)*

FOOD	PORTION	CAL	PROT	FAT	CHOL	CARB	FIBER	SOD
Estee								
Banana Nut	5	60	1	1	0	14	0	30
Cinnamon Spice	5	60	1	0	0	14	0	5
Granny Smith Apple	5	60	1	0	0	13	0	5

FOOD	PORTION	CAL	PROT	FAT	CHOL	CARB	FIBER	SOD
Mixed Berry	5	60	1	0	0	14	0	0
Peanut Butter Crunch	5	60	1	0	0	13	tr	80
Lundberg								
Nutra Farmed Brown Rice	1 (0.7 oz)	70	1	0	0	15	—	55
Nutra Farmed Sesame Tamari	1 (0.7 oz)	70	2	1	0	16	2	120
Organic Koku Semsame	1 (0.7 oz)	80	2	0	0	17	2	35
Quaker								
Apple Cinnamon	1 (0.5 oz)	50	1	0	0	11	—	0
Banana Crunch	1 (0.5 oz)	50	1	0	0	11	—	45
Cinnamon Crunch	1 (0.5 oz)	50	1	0	0	11	—	25
Mini Apple Cinnamon	5 (0.5 oz)	50	1	0	0	12	—	0
Mini Banana Nut	5 (0.5 oz)	50	1	0	0	12	—	40
Mini Butter Popped Corn	6 (0.5 oz)	50	1	0	0	12	—	120
Mini Caramel Corn	5 (0.5 oz)	50	1	0	0	12	—	25
Mini Chocolate Crunch	5 (0.5 oz)	50	1	0	0	12	—	10
Mini Cinnamon Crunch	5 (0.5 oz)	50	1	0	0	12	—	25
Mini Honey Nut	5 (0.5 oz)	50	1	0	0	12	—	25
Mini Monterey Jack	6 (0.5 oz)	50	1	0	0	11	—	100
Mini White Cheddar	6 (0.5 oz)	50	1	0	0	11	—	120
Salt-Free	1 (0.3 oz)	35	1	0	0	7	—	0
Salted	1 (0.3 oz)	35	1	0	0	7	—	15
Weight Watchers								
Apple Cinnamon	1 oz	110	2	1	0	25	1	0
Butter	1 oz	110	2	2	0	21	1	280
Caramel	1 oz	110	2	1	0	24	1	30
White Cheddar	1 oz	100	3	1	0	22	1	280

ROCKFISH

FOOD	PORTION	CAL	PROT	FAT	CHOL	CARB	FIBER	SOD
pacific cooked	1 fillet (5.2 oz)	180	36	3	66	0	—	114
pacific cooked	3 oz	103	20	2	38	0	—	65
pacific raw	3 oz	80	16	1	29	0	—	51

ROE *(see also individual names)*

FOOD	PORTION	CAL	PROT	FAT	CHOL	CARB	FIBER	SOD
fish	1 oz	11	2	tr	30	tr	—	—

FOOD	PORTION	CAL	PROT	FAT	CHOL	CARB	FIBER	SOD
fresh baked	3 oz	173	24	7	408	2	–	–
fresh baked	1 oz	58	8	2	136	1	–	–

ROLL

FROZEN

New York

Garlic	1 (2 oz)	210	3	10	0	26	1	370

Sara Lee

Deluxe Cinnamon Rolls w/o Icing	1 (2.7 oz)	370	5	15	40	41	1	300

READY-TO-EAT

bialy	1 (2.2 oz)	138	14	0	0	32	1	167
brioche sweet roll	1 (3.5 oz)	410	10	23	190	41	3	495
brown & serve	1 (1 oz)	85	2	2	0	14	–	148
cheese	1 (2.3 oz)	238	5	12	–	29	–	236
cinnamon raisin	1 (2¾ in)	223	4	10	40	31	1	229
dinner	1 (1 oz)	85	2	2	0	14	–	148
egg	1 (2½ in)	107	3	2	–	18	1	191
french	1 (1.3 oz)	105	3	2	0	19	–	232
hamburger	1 (1½ oz)	123	4	2	–	22	–	241
hamburger multi-grain	1 (1½ oz)	113	4	2	0	19	2	197
hamburger reduced calorie	1 (1½ oz)	84	4	1	0	18	3	190
hard	1 (3½ in)	167	6	2	0	30	–	310
hot cross bun	1	202	5	4	–	38	1	–
hotdog	1 (1½ oz)	123	4	2	–	22	–	241
hotdog reduced calorie	1 (1½ oz)	84	4	1	0	18	3	190
hotdog whole wheat	1 (1.5 oz)	110	5	2	0	19	2	220
kaiser	1 (3½ in)	167	6	2	0	30	–	310
oat bran	1 (1.2 oz)	78	3	2	0	13	1	136
rye	1 (1 oz)	81	3	1	0	15	–	253
submarine	1 (4.7 oz)	155	5	2	tr	30	–	313
wheat	1 (1 oz)	77	2	2	0	13	–	96
whole wheat	1 (1 oz)	75	3	1	0	15	–	135

Bread Du Jour

Cracked Wheat	1 (1.2 oz)	100	3	1	0	17	1	200
Italian	1 (1.2 oz)	90	3	1	0	16	0	190
Sourdough	1 (1.2 oz)	90	3	1	0	17	0	190

FOOD	PORTION	CAL	PROT	FAT	CHOL	CARB	FIBER	SOD
Country Kitchen								
Frankfurt	1	120	–	2	0	–	–	–
Freihofer's								
Brown 'N Serve	1 (1 oz)	80	3	2	0	13	1	160
Pepperidge Farm								
Brown & Serve Club	1 (1.6 oz)	120	5	1	0	22	2	240
Dinner Rolls Finger Poppy	1 (0.9 oz)	80	3	2	<5	12	tr	125
Parker House	1 (0.9 oz)	80	2	2	<5	13	tr	120
Stroehmann								
Hamburger	1 (1.4 oz)	100	3	2	0	21	tr	210
Hamburger Potato	1 (1.9 oz)	140	4	2	0	28	tr	260
Hot Dog	1 (1.4 oz)	100	3	2	0	21	tr	210
Hot Dog Potato	1 (1.9 oz)	140	4	2	0	28	tr	260
Wonder								
Brown & Serve	1 (1 oz)	80	2	2	0	13	0	150
Brown & Serve Sourdough	1 (1 oz)	70	2	2	0	13	0	130
Brown & Serve Wheat	1 (1 oz)	80	2	2	0	13	0	140
Bun	1 (3 oz)	220	7	3	0	42	1	430
Club French	1 (1.6 oz)	120	4	2	0	23	0	230
Club Grain	1 (1.6 oz)	120	4	2	0	23	1	210
Club Sourdough	1 (1.6 oz)	120	4	2	0	23	0	230
Dinner	2 (1.6 oz)	130	4	1	0	25	1	240
Dinner Honey Rich	1 (1.3 oz)	100	3	2	0	17	0	160
Dinner Wheat	2 (1.6 oz)	140	3	3	0	24	1	240
Hamburger	1 (2.5 oz)	190	5	3	0	36	1	370
Hamburger	1 (2 oz)	150	4	2	0	28	1	290
Hamburger	1 (2.5 oz)	180	7	3	0	32	2	370
Hamburger	1 (1.5 oz)	110	3	2	0	21	0	220
Hamburger Wheat	1 (1.9 oz)	140	5	2	0	24	2	280
Hamburger Wheat	1 (1.5 oz)	120	4	2	0	21	1	210
Hoagie French	1 (3 oz)	220	7	3	0	41	1	410
Hoagie Grain	1 (3 oz)	220	7	3	0	41	2	370
Hoagie Sourdough	1 (3 oz)	220	8	3	0	41	1	410
Hot Dog	1 (2 oz)	160	4	3	0	29	0	300
Kaiser	1 (2.2 oz)	180	5	3	0	33	1	270
Kaiser Hoagie	1 (3 oz)	220	7	3	0	41	1	410
Multigrain	1 (1.8 oz)	140	4	2	0	25	1	210

FOOD	PORTION	CAL	PROT	FAT	CHOL	CARB	FIBER	SOD
Potato Bun	1 (1.5 oz)	110	4	1	0	22	1	220
Steak	1 (2.5 oz)	190	6	3	0	36	1	360
REFRIGERATED								
cinnamon w/ frosting	1	109	2	4	–	17	–	250
crescent	1 (1 oz)	98	2	4	0	14	–	341
Pillsbury								
Apple Cinnamon	1 (1.5 oz)	150	2	6	0	23	tr	320
Caramel	1 (1.7 oz)	170	2	7	0	24	tr	330
Cinnamon w/ Icing	1 (1.5 oz)	150	2	6	0	23	tr	340
Cinnamon w/ Icing Reduced Fat	1 (1.5 oz)	140	2	4	0	24	tr	340
Cinnamon Raisin w/ Icing	1 (1.7 oz)	170	2	6	0	26	tr	320
Cornbread Twists	1 (1.4 oz)	140	3	6	0	18	0	330
Crecents Reduced Fat	1 (1 oz)	100	2	5	0	12	0	230
Crescent	1 (1 oz)	110	2	6	0	11	0	220
Dinner	1 (1.4 oz)	110	4	2	0	18	1	270
Dinner Wheat	1 (1.4 oz)	110	4	2	0	18	1	270
Orange Sweet Roll w/ Icing	1 (1.7 oz)	150	2	7	0	25	tr	340
ROSE APPLE								
fresh	3.5 oz	32	1	tr	0	7	–	–
ROSE HIP								
fresh	1 oz	26	1	0	0	5	–	42
ROSELLE								
fresh	1 cup	28	1	tr	0	6	–	3
ROSEMARY								
dried	1 tsp	4	tr	tr	0	1	–	1
ROUGHY								
orange baked	3 oz	75	16	1	22	0	–	69
RUTABAGA								
cooked mashed	½ cup	41	1	tr	0	9	–	22
raw cubed	½ cup	25	1	tr	0	6	–	14
SABLEFISH								
baked	3 oz	213	15	17	53	0	–	61
fillet baked	5.3 oz	378	26	30	95	0	–	108

FOOD	PORTION	CAL	PROT	FAT	CHOL	CARB	FIBER	SOD
smoked	1 oz	72	5	6	18	0	–	206
smoked	3 oz	218	15	17	55	0	–	626

SAFFLOWER

seeds dried	1 oz	147	5	11	0	10	–	–

SAFFRON

saffron	1 tsp	2	tr	tr	0	tr	–	1

SAGE

ground	1 tsp	2	tr	tr	0	tr	–	tr

SALAD (see also LETTUCE, PASTA SALAD)

MIX

Dole

All American Toss	2 cups (3.5 oz)	50	4	1	<5	7	2	160
American Blend	1½ cups (3 oz)	15	1	0	0	3	1	10
Classic	1½ cups (3 oz)	15	1	0	0	4	1	15
Classic Romaine Blend	1½ cups (3 oz)	15	1	0	0	3	1	10
Coleslaw	1½ cups (3 oz)	25	1	0	0	5	2	25
European Special Blend	2 cups (3 oz)	15	1	0	0	3	1	15
Garlic Caesar Complete w/ Dressing	1½ cups (3.5 oz)	180	3	15	5	8	1	420
Greek Marinade	1½ cups (3.5 oz)	100	2	8	<5	5	1	340
Greener Selection	1½ cups (3 oz)	15	1	0	0	3	1	10
Light Caesar Complete w/ Dressing	1½ cups (3.5 oz)	60	3	1	0	10	2	390
Light Herb Ranch Complete w/ Dressing	1½ cups (3.5 oz)	50	2	1	5	10	2	280
Light Roasted Garlic Caesar Complete w/ Dressing	1½ cups (3.5 oz)	60	3	1	0	11	1	400
Light Zesty Italian Complete w/ Dressing	1½ cups (3.5 oz)	50	2	1	0	11	1	290

FOOD	PORTION	CAL	PROT	FAT	CHOL	CARB	FIBER	SOD
Mediterranean Marinade	2 cups (3.5 oz)	90	1	8	0	5	1	180
Oriental Complete w/ Dressing	1½ cups (3.5 oz)	120	2	6	0	13	2	240
Romano Complete w/ Dressing	1½ cups (3.5 oz)	150	3	12	0	9	2	570
Sunflower Ranch Complete w/ Dressing	1½ cups (3.5 oz)	160	2	16	5	5	2	220
Tomato & Mozzarella Medley	2 cups (3.5 oz)	60	4	2	5	7	2	80
Triple Cheese Toss	2 cups (3.5 oz)	80	5	5	15	4	1	120
Earthbound Farm								
Baby Caesar Mix	1 pkg (5 oz)	25	2	0	0	3	2	10
Caesar w/ Garlic Croutons	1 serv (3.5 oz)	170	3	15	10	7	1	230
Italian Salad Organic	1⅔ cups (2.9 oz)	15	1	0	0	3	1	10
Mixed Baby Greens Organic	1 pkg (4 oz)	30	3	0	0	4	2	100
Organic Baby Greens w/ Vinaigrette & Garlic Croutons	1 serv (3.5 oz)	230	3	20	0	11	1	290
Organic Italian Salad w/ Blue Cheese Dressing & Walnuts	1 serv (3.5 oz)	190	4	17	15	4	1	210
Romaine Blend Organic	1⅔ cups (2.9 oz)	15	1	0	0	3	1	10
Fresh Express								
Fancy Field Greens	1½ cups (3 oz)	15	1	0	0	3	2	15
Original Iceberg Garden w/ Zip	1½ cups (3 oz)	15	1	0	0	3	1	10
Veggie Lover's	1½ cups (3 oz)	20	1	0	0	4	1	15
Suddenly Salad								
Caesar	¾ cup	220	5	9	0	30	1	580
Caesar Low Fat Recipe	¾ cup	170	5	3	0	30	1	580
Italian Pepperoni	1 cup	190	6	4	0	35	2	680
Italian Pepperoni Low Fat Recipe	1 cup	180	6	2	0	35	2	680

FOOD	PORTION	CAL	PROT	FAT	CHOL	CARB	FIBER	SOD
Ranch & Bacon	¾ cup	330	7	20	15	30	1	480
Ranch & Bacon Low Fat Recipe	¾ cup	180	7	2	<5	30	1	530
Weight Watchers								
Caesar Salad	1 serv (3.5 oz)	60	2	0	0	11	1	600
Caesar Salad w/ Cookies	1 pkg (4.3 oz)	160	4	3	0	29	3	670
European Salad	1 serv (3.5 oz)	60	0	0	2	13	2	530
European Salad w/ Cookies	1 pkg (4.3 oz)	160	3	3	0	31	2	620
Garden Salad	1 serv (3.5 oz)	60	0	0	2	12	1	270
Garden Salad w/ Cookies	1 pkg (4 oz)	120	3	2	0	24	2	340
TAKE-OUT								
caesar	2 cups (5 oz)	235	5	20	10	11	1	440
chef w/o dressing	1½ cups	386	24	28	244	9	–	279
tossed w/o dressing	¾ cup	16	1	0	0	3	–	27
tossed w/o dressing	1½ cups	32	3	tr	0	7	–	53
tossed w/o dressing w/ cheese & egg	1½ cups	102	9	6	98	5	–	119
tossed w/o dressing w/ chicken	1½ cups	105	17	2	72	4	–	209
tossed w/o dressing w/ pasta & seafood	1½ cups (14.6 oz)	380	16	21	50	32	–	1572
tossed w/o dressing w/ shrimp	1½ cups	107	15	2	180	7	–	487
waldorf	½ cup	79	1	6	8	6	1	49

SALAD DRESSING
MIX
Et Tu

FOOD	PORTION	CAL	PROT	FAT	CHOL	CARB	FIBER	SOD
Caesar Salad Kit	1 serv	140	2	12	5	6	0	115
Good Seasons								
Cheese Garlic as prep	2 tbsp (1 oz)	140	0	16	0	1	0	330
Fat Free Honey Mustard as prep	2 tbsp (1.2 oz)	20	0	0	0	5	0	280
Fat Free Italian as prep	2 tbsp (1.1 oz)	10	0	0	0	2	0	290

FOOD	PORTION	CAL	PROT	FAT	CHOL	CARB	FIBER	SOD
Fat Free Ranch as prep	2 tbsp (1.2 oz)	20	0	0	0	5	0	250
Fat Free Zesty Herb as prep	2 tbsp (1.1 oz)	10	0	0	0	2	0	260
Garlic & Herbs as prep	2 tbsp (1 oz)	140	0	15	0	1	0	340
Gourmet Caesar as prep	2 tbsp (1.1 oz)	150	0	16	0	3	0	300
Gourmet Parmesan Italian as prep	2 tbsp (1.1 oz)	150	0	16	0	2	0	330
Honey French as prep	2 tbsp (1.2 oz)	160	0	15	0	5	0	250
Honey Mustard as prep	2 tbsp (1.1 oz)	150	0	15	0	3	0	240
Italian as prep	2 tbsp (1 oz)	140	0	15	0	1	0	320
Mexican Spice as prep	2 tbsp (1.1 oz)	140	0	15	0	2	0	310
Mild Italian as prep	2 tbsp (1.1 oz)	150	0	15	0	2	0	370
Oriental Sesame as prep	2 tbsp (1.1 oz)	150	0	16	0	3	0	360
Reduced Calorie Italian as prep	2 tbsp (1 oz)	50	0	5	0	2	0	280
Reduced Calorie Zesty Italian as prep	2 tbsp (1 oz)	50	0	5	0	2	0	260
Roasted Garlic as prep	2 tbsp (1.1 oz)	150	0	15	0	2	0	340
Zesty Italian as prep	2 tbsp (1 oz)	140	0	15	0	1	0	220
McCormick								
Mediterrenean Potato Salad	1 tbsp	25	tr	0	–	4	1	460
Pasta Salad Vinagarette	1 tsp (5 g)	15	0	0	–	2	–	590
READY-TO-EAT								
blue cheese	1 tbsp	77	1	8	–	1	–	–
french	1 tbsp	67	tr	6	–	3	–	214
french reduced calorie	1 tbsp	22	0	1	1	4	–	128
italian	1 tbsp	69	tr	7	–	2	–	116

FOOD	PORTION	CAL	PROT	FAT	CHOL	CARB	FIBER	SOD
italian reduced calorie	1 tbsp	16	tr	2	1	1	–	118
russian	1 tbsp	76	tr	8	–	2	–	133
russian reduced calorie	1 tbsp	23	tr	1	1	5	–	141
sesame seed	1 tbsp	68	1	7	0	1	–	153
thousand island	1 tbsp	59	tr	6	–	2	–	109
thousand island reduced calorie	1 tbsp	24	tr	2	2	3	–	153
Benecol								
Creamy Italian	2 tbsp	100	0	10	0	10	0	170
French	2 tbsp (0.8 oz)	130	0	11	0	6	0	170
Ranch	2 tbsp	130	0	13	0	3	0	250
Thousand Island	2 tbsp	130	0	12	0	5	0	210
Estee								
Creamy French	2 tbsp (1 oz)	10	0	0	0	2	–	80
Italian	2 tbsp	5	0	0	0	1	0	80
Hellmann's								
Citrus Splash Ruby Red Ginger	2 tbsp (1 oz)	90	0	7	–	8	–	400
Kraft								
⅓ Less Fat Catalina	2 tbsp (1.2 oz)	80	0	5	0	9	0	400
⅓ Less Fat Cucumber Ranch	2 tbsp (1.1 oz)	60	0	5	0	2	0	480
⅓ Less Fat Italian	2 tbsp (1.1 oz)	70	0	7	0	3	0	240
⅓ Less Fat Ranch	2 tbsp (1.1)	110	0	11	10	1	0	310
⅓ Less Fat Thousand Island	2 tbsp (1.2 oz)	70	0	5	10	7	0	340
Bacon & Tomato	2 tbsp (1.1 oz)	140	tr	14	<5	2	0	280
Buttermilk Ranch	2 tbsp (1.1 oz)	150	0	16	<5	1	0	240
Caesar Italian	2 tbsp (1.1 oz)	100	tr	10	0	2	0	480
Caesar Ranch	2 tbsp (1.1 oz)	110	1	11	10	1	0	290
Catalina	2 tbsp (1.1 oz)	120	0	10	0	7	0	390
Catalina w/ Honey	2 tbsp (1.1 oz)	130	0	11	0	7	0	320
Classic Caesar	2 tbsp (1.1 oz)	110	1	11	10	1	0	290
Coleslaw	2 tbsp (1.1 oz)	130	0	11	15	7	0	410
Creamy French	2 tbsp (1.1 oz)	160	0	15	0	5	0	270
Creamy Garlic	2 tbsp (1.1 oz)	110	0	11	0	2	0	360
Creamy Italian	2 tbsp (1.1 oz)	110	0	11	0	2	0	250

FOOD	PORTION	CAL	PROT	FAT	CHOL	CARB	FIBER	SOD
Cucumber Ranch	2 tbsp (1.1 oz)	140	0	15	0	2	0	220
Free Blue Cheese	2 tbsp (1.2 oz)	45	0	0	0	11	1	360
Free Caesar Italian	2 tbsp (1.2 oz)	25	tr	0	0	4	0	480
Free Catalina	2 tbsp (1.2 oz)	35	0	0	0	8	tr	320
Free Classic Caesar	2 tbsp (1.2 oz)	45	tr	0	0	11	tr	360
Free Creamy Italian	2 tbsp (1.2 oz)	50	0	0	0	12	tr	330
Free French	2 tbsp (1.2 oz)	45	0	0	0	11	tr	300
Free Garlic Ranch	2 tbsp (1.2 oz)	45	0	0	0	11	1	320
Free Honey Dijon	2 tbsp (1.2 oz)	45	0	0	0	10	1	330
Free Italian	2 tbsp (1.2 oz)	20	0	0	0	4	0	430
Free Peppercorn Ranch	2 tbsp (1.2 oz)	45	0	0	0	11	tr	330
Free Ranch	1 tbsp (1.2 oz)	50	0	0	0	11	1	350
Free Red Wine Vinegar	2 tbsp (1.1 oz)	15	0	0	0	3	0	410
Free Thousand Island	2 tbsp (1.2 oz)	40	0	0	0	9	1	280
Garlic Ranch	2 tbsp (1.1 oz)	180	0	19	10	1	0	270
Herb Vinaigrette	2 tbsp (1.1 oz)	140	0	15	0	tr	0	250
Honey Dijon	2 tbsp (1.1 oz)	110	0	10	0	6	0	210
Honey Mustard	2 tbsp (1.1 oz)	110	0	10	0	6	0	210
House Italian w/ Olive Oil Blend	2 tbsp (1.1 oz)	120	0	12	<5	2	0	240
Peppercorn Ranch	2 tbsp (1 oz)	170	tr	18	10	1	0	270
Pesto Italian	2 tbsp (1.1 oz)	90	0	9	0	2	0	310
Ranch	2 tbsp (1 oz)	170	0	18	10	1	0	280
Roka Blue Cheese	2 tbsp (1.1 oz)	130	tr	13	<5	2	tr	310
Russian	2 tbsp (1.2 oz)	130	0	10	0	10	0	310
Sour Cream & Onion Ranch	2 tbsp (1 oz)	170	0	18	10	1	0	250
Thousand Island	2 tbsp (1.1 oz)	110	0	10	10	5	0	310
Thousand Island w/ Bacon	2 tbsp (1.1 oz)	130	0	12	0	5	0	200
Tomato & Herb Italian	2 tbsp (1.1 oz)	100	0	9	0	3	0	340
Zesty Italian	2 tbsp (1.1 oz)	110	0	11	0	2	0	540
LaMartinique								
Blue Cheese Vinaigrette	2 tbsp	160	2	17	5	0	0	450

FOOD	PORTION	CAL	PROT	FAT	CHOL	CARB	FIBER	SOD
Poppy Seed	2 tbsp	170	0	15	0	8	0	330
Nasoya								
Creamy Dill	2 tbsp	70	0	7	0	2	0	135
Creamy Italian	2 tbsp	60	0	6	0	2	0	180
Garden Herb	2 tbsp	70	0	7	0	2	0	140
Sesame Garlic	2 tbsp	60	0	6	0	2	0	130
Thousand Island	2 tbsp	70	0	6	0	3	0	115
Newman's Own								
Balsamic Vinaigrette	2 tbsp (1.1 oz)	90	0	9	0	3	0	350
Caesar	2 tbsp (1.1 oz)	150	1	16	<5	1	0	450
Light Italian	2 tbsp (1.1 oz)	20	0	1	0	3	0	380
Olive Oil & Vinegar	2 tbsp (1 oz)	150	0	16	0	1	0	150
Ranch	2 tbsp (1 oz)	180	1	19	<5	2	0	170
Old Dutch								
Sweet & Sour	2 tbsp	50	0	0	0	13	0	480
Seven Seas								
⅓ Less Fat Creamy Italian	2 tbsp (1.1 oz)	60	0	5	0	2	0	500
⅓ Less Fat Italian w/ Olive Oil Blend	2 tbsp (1.1 oz)	45	0	4	0	2	0	460
⅓ Less Fat Ranch	2 tbsp (1.1 oz)	100	0	9	0	5	0	320
⅓ Less Fat Red Wine Vinegar & Oil	2 tbsp (1.1 oz)	45	0	4	0	3	0	320
⅓ Less Fat Viva Italian	2 tbsp (1.1 oz)	45	0	4	0	2	0	320
2 Cheese Italian	2 tbsp (1.1 oz)	70	0	7	0	3	0	240
Chunky Blue Cheese	2 tbsp (1.1 oz)	130	tr	13	<5	2	tr	310
Classic Caesar	2 tbsp (1.1 oz)	100	tr	10	0	2	0	480
Creamy Italian	2 tbsp (1.1 oz)	120	0	12	0	1	0	510
Free Ranch	2 tbsp (1.2 oz)	45	0	0	0	11	1	330
Free Red Wine Vinegar	2 tbsp (1.1 oz)	15	0	0	0	3	0	410
Free Sour Cream & Onion Ranch	2 tbsp (1.2 oz)	50	0	0	0	11	1	300
Free Viva Italian	2 tbsp (1.1 oz)	10	0	0	0	2	1	480
Green Goddess	2 tbsp (1.1 oz)	130	0	13	0	1	0	260
Herbs & Spices	2 tbsp (1.1 oz)	90	0	9	0	1	0	290
Ranch	2 tbsp (1.1 oz)	160	0	17	<5	2	0	260
Red Wine Vinegar & Oil	2 tbsp (1.1 oz)	90	0	9	0	2	0	500

FOOD	PORTION	CAL	PROT	FAT	CHOL	CARB	FIBER	SOD
Viva Italian	2 tbsp (1.1 oz)	90	0	9	0	2	0	370
Viva Russian	2 tbsp (1.1 oz)	150	0	16	0	3	0	210
Weight Watchers								
Fat Free Caesar	1 pkg (0.75 oz)	5	0	0	0	1	0	290
Fat Free Caesar	2 tbsp	10	0	0	0	1	0	390
Fat Free Creamy Italian	2 tbsp	30	0	0	0	7	0	360
Fat Free French Style	2 tbsp	40	0	0	0	9	0	200
Fat Free Honey Dijon	2 tbsp	45	0	0	0	11	0	150
Fat Free Italian	2 tbsp	10	0	0	0	2	0	360
Fat Free Ranch	1 pkg (0.75 oz)	25	0	0	0	6	0	200
Fat Free Ranch	2 tbsp	35	0	0	0	7	0	270
Wishbone								
Caesar	2 tbsp (1 oz)	90	1	10	5	2	0	300
Chunky Blue Cheese	2 tbsp (1 oz)	150	1	17	0	3	0	290
Classic House Italian	2 tbsp (1 oz)	140	0	14	5	2	0	360
Classic Olive Oil Italian	2 tbsp (1 oz)	60	0	5	0	4	0	350
Creamy Caesar	2 tbsp (1 oz)	180	1	18	10	1	0	290
Creamy Italian	2 tbsp (1 oz)	110	1	10	0	4	0	240
Creamy Roasted Garlic	2 tbsp (1 oz)	110	1	10	0	3	0	240
Deluxe French	2 tbsp (1 oz)	120	0	11	0	5	0	170
Fat Free Chunky Blue Cheese	2 tbsp (1 oz)	35	0	0	0	7	tr	290
Fat Free Creamy Italian	2 tbsp (1 oz)	35	0	0	0	9	tr	250
Fat Free Creamy Roasted Garlic	2 tbsp (1 oz)	40	0	0	0	9	0	280
Fat Free Deluxe French	2 tbsp (1 oz)	30	0	0	0	7	tr	230
Fat Free Honey Dijon	2 tbsp (1 oz)	45	1	0	0	10	0	270
Fat Free Italian	2 tbsp (1 oz)	10	0	0	0	2	0	280
Fat Free Parmesan & Onion	2 tbsp (1 oz)	45	1	0	0	9	tr	320
Fat Free Ranch	2 tbsp (1 oz)	40	0	0	0	9	tr	280
Fat Free Red Wine Vinaigrette	2 tbsp (1 oz)	35	0	0	0	7	0	230
Fat Free Sweet N' Spicy French	2 tbsp (1 oz)	30	0	0	0	7	0	220

FOOD	PORTION	CAL	PROT	FAT	CHOL	CARB	FIBER	SOD
Fat Free Thousand Island	2 tbsp (1 oz)	35	0	0	0	9	tr	290
Italian	2 tbsp (1 oz)	80	0	8	0	3	0	490
Lite French	2 tbsp (1 oz)	50	0	2	5	8	0	240
Lite Italian	2 tbsp (1 oz)	15	0	1	0	2	0	500
Lite Ranch	2 tbsp (1 oz)	100	0	8	5	5	0	300
Olive Oil Vinaigrette	2 tbsp (1 oz)	60	0	5	0	4	0	250
Oriental	2 tbsp (1 oz)	70	0	5	0	5	0	440
Parmesan & Onion	2 tbsp (1 oz)	110	1	10	5	5	0	260
Ranch	2 tbsp (1 oz)	160	0	17	10	1	0	200
Red Wine Vinaigrette	2 tbsp (1 oz)	80	0	5	0	9	0	230
Robusto Italian	2 tbsp (1 oz)	90	0	8	0	4	0	550
Russian	2 tbsp (1 oz)	110	0	6	0	15	0	350
Sweet N' Spicy French	2 tbsp (1 oz)	140	0	12	0	6	0	330
Thousand Island	2 tbsp (1 oz)	140	0	12	10	7	0	340

SALMON
CANNED

FOOD	PORTION	CAL	PROT	FAT	CHOL	CARB	FIBER	SOD
chum w/ bone	1 can (13.9 oz)	521	79	20	144	0	–	1797
chum w/ bone	3 oz	120	18	5	33	0	–	414
pink w/ bone	3 oz	118	17	5	–	0	–	471
pink w/ bone	1 can (15.9 oz)	631	90	27	–	0	–	2514
sockeye w/ bone	1 can (12.9 oz)	566	76	27	161	0	–	1987
sockeye w/ bone	3 oz	130	17	6	37	0	–	458

Bumble Bee

FOOD	PORTION	CAL	PROT	FAT	CHOL	CARB	FIBER	SOD
Keta	½ cup (3.5 oz)	160	20	8	–	0	–	490
Red	½ cup (3.5 oz)	180	20	10	–	0	–	490

Libby

FOOD	PORTION	CAL	PROT	FAT	CHOL	CARB	FIBER	SOD
Keta	½ can (3.8 oz)	140	–	6	–	–	–	–
Pink	½ can (3.8 oz)	150	–	7	–	–	–	–

FRESH

FOOD	PORTION	CAL	PROT	FAT	CHOL	CARB	FIBER	SOD
atlantic baked	3 oz	155	22	7	60	0	–	48
chinook baked	3 oz	196	22	11	72	0	–	51
chum baked	3 oz	131	22	4	81	0	–	54
coho cooked	½ fillet (5.4 oz)	286	42	12	76	0	–	91
coho cooked	3 oz	157	23	6	42	0	–	50
coho raw	3 oz	124	18	5	33	0	–	39
pink baked	3 oz	127	22	4	57	0	–	73
roe raw	1 oz	59	7	3	–	tr	–	–

FOOD	PORTION	CAL	PROT	FAT	CHOL	CARB	FIBER	SOD
sockeye cooked	3 oz	183	23	9	74	0	–	102
sockeye cooked	½ fillet (5.4 oz)	334	42	17	135	0	–	102
sockeye raw	3 oz	143	18	7	53	0	–	40
SMOKED								
chinook	3 oz	99	16	4	20	0	–	666
chinook	1 oz	33	5	1	7	0	–	220
Lascco								
Nova Sliced	2 oz	60	10	1	20	3	0	960
Nathan's								
Nova	2 oz	80	13	3	30	1	0	1150
TAKE-OUT								
roulette w/ spinach stuffing	1 serv (4 oz)	160	13	6	45	10	tr	400
salmon cake	1 (3 oz)	241	18	15	104	6	–	602
SALSA								
black bean & corn	2 tbsp (1 oz)	15	1	0	0	3	tr	45
cirtus	2 tbsp (1 oz)	10	0	0	0	2	0	7
Chi-Chi's								
Con Queso	2 tbsp (1.1 oz)	90	3	7	15	4	0	480
Hot	2 tbsp (1 oz)	10	0	0	0	2	0	160
Medium	2 tbsp (1 oz)	10	0	0	0	2	0	140
Mild	2 tbsp (1 oz)	10	0	0	0	1	0	140
Picante Hot	2 tbsp (1 oz)	10	0	0	0	2	0	270
Picante Medium	2 tbsp (1 oz)	10	0	0	0	2	0	200
Picante Mild	2 tbsp (1 oz)	10	0	0	0	2	0	210
Verde Medium	2 tbsp (1.2 oz)	15	0	0	0	3	0	180
Verde Mild	2 tbsp (1.2 oz)	15	0	0	0	3	0	180
Guiltless Gourmet								
Roasted Red Pepper	2 tbsp (1 oz)	10	0	0	0	2	0	120
Southwestern Grill	2 tbsp (1 oz)	10	0	0	0	2	0	150
Hunt's								
Alfresco All Varieties	2 tbsp (1.1 oz)	10	tr	tr	0	2	tr	161
Hot	2 tbsp (1.1 oz)	27	1	tr	0	6	1	236
Medium	2 tbsp (1.1 oz)	27	1	tr	0	6	1	236
Mild	2 tbsp (1.1 oz)	27	1	tr	0	6	1	236
Picante All Varieties	2 tbsp (1.1 oz)	11	1	tr	0	2	tr	256
Squeeze Mild & Medium	2 tbsp (1.1 oz)	27	1	tr	0	6	1	236

FOOD	PORTION	CAL	PROT	FAT	CHOL	CARB	FIBER	SOD
Muir Glen								
Black Bean & Corn Medium	2 tbsp (1.1 oz)	15	1	0	0	3	tr	125
Chipotle Medium	2 tbsp (1.1 oz)	10	0	0	0	2	0	125
Fire Roasted Tomato Medium	2 tbsp (1.1 oz)	10	0	0	0	2	0	125
Garlic Cilantro Medium	2 tbsp (1.1 oz)	10	0	0	0	2	0	125
Habanero Hot	2 tbsp (1.1 oz)	10	0	0	0	2	0	125
Organic Medium	2 tbsp (1.1 oz)	10	0	0	0	2	0	125
Organic Mild	2 tbsp (1.1 oz)	10	0	0	0	2	0	125
Roasted Garlic Medium	2 tbsp (1.1 oz)	10	0	0	0	2	0	125
Newman's Own								
Bandito Hot	2 tbsp (1.1 oz)	10	0	0	0	2	tr	150
Bandito Medium	2 tbsp (1.1 oz)	10	0	0	0	2	tr	105
Bandito Mild	2 tbsp (1.1 oz)	10	0	0	0	2	tr	105
Peach	2 tbsp (1.1 oz)	25	0	0	0	6	1	90
Pineapple	2 tbsp (1.1 oz)	15	0	0	0	3	1	90
Roasted Garlic	2 tbsp (1.1 oz)	10	1	0	0	2	1	150
Old El Paso								
Green Chili Medium	2 tbsp (1 oz)	10	0	0	0	2	tr	110
Homestyle	2 tbsp (1 oz)	5	0	0	0	1	0	110
Homestyle Mild	2 tbsp (1 oz)	5	0	0	0	1	0	110
Picante Hot	2 tbsp (1 oz)	10	0	0	0	2	0	230
Picante Medium	2 tbsp (1 oz)	10	0	0	0	2	0	230
Picante Mild	2 tbsp (1 oz)	10	0	0	0	2	0	230
Picante Thick'n Chunky Hot	2 tbsp (1 oz)	10	0	0	0	2	0	160
Picante Thick'n Chunky Medium	2 tbsp (1 oz)	10	0	0	0	2	0	140
Picante Thick'n Chunky Mild	2 tbsp (1 oz)	10	0	0	0	2	0	130
Pico De Gallo Hot	2 tbsp (1 oz)	5	0	0	0	2	tr	260
Pico De Gallo Medium	1 tbsp (1 oz)	5	0	0	0	2	tr	260
Salsa Verde	2 tbsp (1 oz)	10	0	0	0	2	0	95
Thick'n Chunky Hot	2 tbsp (1 oz)	10	0	0	0	2	0	130

FOOD	PORTION	CAL	PROT	FAT	CHOL	CARB	FIBER	SOD
Thick'n Chunky Medium	2 tbsp (1 oz)	10	0	0	0	2	0	140
Thick'n Chunky Mild	2 tbsp (1 oz)	10	0	0	0	2	0	140
Pace								
Picante Mild or Medium	2 tbsp	10	0	0	0	2	0	220
Thick & Chunky Mild or Medium	2 tbsp	10	0	0	0	2	0	220
Rosarita								
Extra Chunky Medium	2 tbsp (1 oz)	7	tr	tr	0	1	tr	229
Green Tomatillo Medium	2 tbsp (1 oz)	8	tr	tr	0	2	1	188
Picante Zesty Jalapeno Hot	2 tbsp (1 oz)	8	tr	tr	0	2	1	246
Picante Zesty Jalapeno Medium	2 tbsp (1 oz)	9	tr	tr	0	2	1	254
Picante Zesty Jalapeno Mild	2 tbsp (1 oz)	8	tr	tr	0	2	tr	239
Roasted Mild	2 tbsp (1 oz)	10	tr	tr	0	2	1	233
Traditional Medium	2 tbsp (1 oz)	7	tr	tr	0	2	1	234
Traditional Mild	2 tbsp (1 oz)	7	1	tr	0	1	1	247
Snyder's Of Hanover								
Mild	2 tbsp	10	0	0	0	2	0	220
Taco Bell								
Smooth 'N Zesty Picante Medium	2 tbsp (1.1 oz)	15	0	0	0	3	tr	190
Smooth 'N Zesty Picante Mild	2 tbsp (1.1 oz)	15	0	0	0	3	tr	190
Thick 'N Chunky Salsa Hot	2 tbsp (1.1 oz)	15	0	0	0	2	tr	240
Thick 'N Chunky Salsa Medium	2 tbsp (1.1 oz)	15	0	0	0	2	tr	240
Thick 'N Chunky Salsa Mild	2 tbsp (1.1 oz)	15	tr	0	0	3	tr	240
Tostitos								
Con Queso	2.3 oz	80	2	5	<10	10	<2	560

FOOD	PORTION	CAL	PROT	FAT	CHOL	CARB	FIBER	SOD
Hot	2.3 oz	30	2	0	0	6	2	520
Low Fat Con Queso	2.5 oz	80	2	3	<10	8	tr	560
Medium	2.3 oz	30	2	0	0	6	2	520
Mild	2.3 oz	30	2	0	0	6	2	520
Restaurant Style	2.2 oz	30	<2	0	0	6	<2	420
Ultimate Garden	2.4 oz	30	2	0	0	6	2	460
Tree Of Life								
Medium	2 tbsp (1 oz)	10	0	0	0	2	–	30
Mild	2 tbsp (1 oz)	10	0	0	0	2	–	30
Utz								
Chunky	2 tbsp (1 fl oz)	60	2	0	0	14	4	190
SALSIFY								
fresh sliced cooked	½ cup	46	2	tr	0	10	–	11
raw sliced	½ cup	55	2	tr	0	12	–	13
SALT/SEASONED SALT								
salt	1 tbsp (18 g)	0	0	0	0	0	–	6976
salt	1 tsp (6 g)	0	0	0	0	0	–	2325
Eden								
Atlantic Sea Salt	¼ tsp	0	0	0	0	0	0	467
Brittany Sea Salt	¼ tsp	0	0	0	0	0	0	552
Morton								
Garlic	1 tsp	3	–	tr	0	–	–	–
Iodized	1 tsp	tr	–	0	0	–	–	–
Kosher	1 tsp	0	–	0	0	–	–	–
Lite	¼ tsp (1.4 g)	tr	0	0	0	tr	–	280
Nature's Season Seasoning Blend	1 tsp	3	–	tr	0	–	–	–
Non-Iodized	1 tsp	0	–	0	0	–	–	–
Seasoned	1 tsp	4	–	tr	0	–	–	–
SALT SUBSTITUTES								
Cardia								
Salt Alternative	1 pkg (0.6 g)	0	0	0	0	0	–	135
Eden								
Shiso Leaf Powder	1 tsp	0	0	0	0	0	2	200
Estee								
Salt-It	¼ tsp	0	0	0	0	0	0	560
Halsosalt								
All Flavors	¼ tsp (7 g)	1	0	0	0	0	–	0

FOOD	PORTION	CAL	PROT	FAT	CHOL	CARB	FIBER	SOD
Morton								
Salt Substitute	¼ tsp (1.2 g)	tr	0	0	0	tr	–	tr
Mrs. Dash								
Onion & Herb	⅛ tsp (0.02 oz)	2	tr	0	0	tr	–	1
NoSalt								
Salt Alternative	1 pkg (0.75 g)	0	2	0	0	0	–	0
Papa Dash								
Lite Salt	½ tsp (1 g)	0	0	0	0	1	–	170
SANDWICHES								
Croissant Pocket								
Stuffed Sandwich Chicken Broccoli & Cheddar	1 piece (4.5 oz)	300	14	11	35	37	5	640
Stuffed Sandwich Ham & Cheddar	1 piece (4.5 oz)	360	13	17	45	39	5	710
Healthy Choice								
Bread Stuffs Chicken & Broccoli	1 (6.1 oz)	310	17	4	25	50	2	600
Bread Stuffs Ham & Cheese w/ Broccoli	1 (6.1 oz)	320	21	5	20	46	1	590
Bread Stuffs Italian Style Meatball	1 (6.1 oz)	330	16	5	20	52	4	600
Bread Stuffs Philly Beef Steak	1 (6.1 oz)	310	17	5	20	50	3	600
Hot Pocket								
Stuffed Sandwich Barbecue	1 (4.5 oz)	340	13	12	25	45	1	850
Stuffed Sandwich Beef & Cheddar	1 (4.5 oz)	360	14	18	50	36	tr	830
Stuffed Sandwich Beef Fajita	1 (4.5 oz)	360	14	17	40	39	5	780
Stuffed Sandwich Chicken & Cheddar w/ Broccoli	1 (4.5 oz)	300	12	12	30	37	tr	620
Stuffed Sandwich Ham & Cheese	1 (4.5 ox)	340	14	15	45	37	4	840
Stuffed Sandwich Turkey & Ham w/ Cheese	1 (4.5 oz)	320	14	13	35	38	1	680

FOOD	PORTION	CAL	PROT	FAT	CHOL	CARB	FIBER	SOD
Lean Pockets								
Stuffed Sandwich Beef & Broccoli	1 (4.5 oz)	250	9	7	50	37	7	710
Stuffed Sandwich Chicken Fajita	1 (4.5 oz)	260	12	8	40	36	3	770
Stuffed Sandwich Chicken Parmesan	1 (4.5 oz)	260	12	8	25	34	1	630
Stuffed Sandwich Glazed Chicken Supreme	1 (4.5 oz)	240	10	7	30	34	1	600
Stuffed Sandwich Turkey & Ham w/ Cheddar	1 (4.5 oz)	260	15	7	35	35	4	810
Stuffed Sandwich Turkey Broccoli & Cheese	1 (4.5 oz)	260	12	8	35	35	4	710
Smucker's								
Uncrustables Grape	1 (2 oz)	200	7	8	0	27	2	260
TAKE-OUT								
chicken fillet plain	1	515	24	29	60	39	—	957
croque monsieur	1 (12.4 oz)	765	41	46	152	43	2	1018
fish fillet w/ tartar sauce	1	431	17	55	—	41	—	615
fish fillet w/ tartar sauce & cheese	1	524	21	29	68	48	—	939
fried egg w/ cheese	1	340	16	19	291	26	—	804
fried egg w/ cheese & ham	1	348	19	16	245	31	—	1005
ham w/ cheese	1	353	21	15	58	33	—	772
roast beef w/ cheese	1	402	32	18	77	27	—	1634
roast beef plain	1	346	22	14	52	33	—	792
steak w/ tomato lettuce salt & mayonnaise	1	459	30	14	73	52	—	798
submarine w/ salami ham cheese lettuce tomato onion & oil	1	456	22	19	35	51	—	1650
tuna salad submarine sandwich w/ lettuce & oil	1	584	30	28	47	55	—	1294

FOOD	PORTION	CAL	PROT	FAT	CHOL	CARB	FIBER	SOD
SAPODILLA								
fresh	1	140	1	2	0	34	—	20
fresh cut up	1 cup	199	1	3	0	48	—	29
SAPOTES								
fresh	1	301	5	1	0	76	—	21
SARDINES								
CANNED								
atlantic in oil w/ bone	2	50	6	3	34	0	—	121
atlantic in oil w/ bone	1 can (3.2 oz)	192	23	11	131	0	—	465
pacific in tomato sauce w/ bone	1 can (13 oz)	658	61	44	225	0	—	1532
pacific in tomato sauce w/ bone	1	68	6	5	23	0	—	157
Bumble Bee								
In Hot Sauce	½ can (2 oz)	109	9	8	30	tr	0	230
In Mustard	½ can (2 oz)	88	10	5	35	1	0	260
In Oil	½ can (2 oz)	125	15	7	39	0	0	240
In Water	½ can (2 oz)	83	15	3	60	0	0	190
FRESH								
raw	3.5 oz	135	19	5	—	0	—	100
SAUCE *(see also* BARBECUE SAUCE, GRAVY, PIZZA SAUCE, SALSA, SPAGHETTI SAUCE, TOMATO*)*								
JARRED								
fish sauce chinese	1 tbsp	9	2	0	—	tr	0	1224
fish sauce vietnamese nuoc mam	1 tbsp	6	1	0	0	1	0	1390
hoisin	1 tbsp	35	1	1	0	7	tr	258
oyster	1 tbsp	8	tr	0	0	2	0	437
teriyaki	1 tbsp	15	1	0	0	3	—	690
Armour								
Chili Hot Dog	¼ cup (2.2 oz)	120	4	9	20	5	0	310
Meatless Sloppy Joe Sauce	¼ cup (2.2 oz)	30	0	0	0	7	0	430
Boar's Head								
Ham Glaze Brown Sugar & Spice	2 tbsp (1.4 oz)	120	0	0	0	30	0	95
Cheez Whiz								
Cheese	2 tbsp (1.2 oz)	90	4	7	20	3	0	540

FOOD	PORTION	CAL	PROT	FAT	CHOL	CARB	FIBER	SOD
Cheese Jalapeno Pepper	2 tbsp (1.2 oz)	90	4	7	25	3	0	510
Cheese Mild Salsa	2 tbsp (1.2 oz)	100	4	7	25	3	0	530
Chi-Chi's								
Enchilada	¼ cup (2.1 oz)	30	0	2	0	3	0	210
Taco	1 tbsp (0.5 oz)	10	0	0	0	1	0	75
Chun King								
Sweet And Sour	2 tbsp (1.2 oz)	58	tr	tr	0	14	0	104
Teriyaki	1 tbsp (0.6 oz)	17	1	tr	0	3	0	917
Teriyaki Hot	1 tbsp (0.6 oz)	17	2	tr	0	3	0	995
Del Monte								
Seafood Cocktail	¼ cup (2.7 oz)	100	1	0	0	24	0	910
Sloppy Joe Hickory Flavor	¼ cup (2.4 oz)	70	1	0	0	18	0	700
Sloppy Joe Original	¼ cup (2.4 oz)	70	1	0	0	16	0	680
Fritos								
Texas-Style Chili Hearty Topping	2.3 oz	50	2	2	10	8	1	330
Utimate Taco Hearty Topping	2.3 oz	50	2	2	10	8	1	330
Gebhardt								
Enchilada Sauce	¼ cup (2.2 oz)	35	1	2	0	4	1	218
Hot Dog Chili Sauce	¼ cup (2.2 oz)	60	3	3	1	6	2	274
Hot Sauce	1 tsp (5 g)	1	tr	tr	0	tr	0	89
Green Giant								
Sloppy Joe	¼ cup (2.6 oz)	50	2	0	0	11	2	420
Sloppy Joe as prep w/ meat	1 serv (4.4 oz)	200	14	11	45	11	2	470
Hormel								
Not-So-Sloppy-Joe Sauce	¼ cup (2.2 oz)	70	1	0	0	15	1	720
House Of Tsang								
Bangkok Padang	1 tbsp (0.6 oz)	45	1	3	0	4	0	240
Hoisin	1 tsp (6 g)	15	0	0	0	4	0	120
Mandarin Marinade	1 tbsp (0.6 oz)	25	0	0	0	6	0	680
Saigon Sizzle	1 tbsp (0.6 oz)	40	1	0	0	8	0	350
Spicy Brown Bean	1 tsp (6 g)	15	0	0	0	3	0	130
Stir Fry Classic	1 tbsp (0.6 oz)	25	0	1	0	4	0	570

FOOD	PORTION	CAL	PROT	FAT	CHOL	CARB	FIBER	SOD
Stir Fry Sweet & Sour	1 tbsp (0.6 oz)	30	0	0	0	7	0	45
Stir Fry Szechuan Spicy	1 tbsp (0.6 oz)	20	0	1	0	4	0	490
Sweet & Sour Concentrate	1 tsp (6 g)	10	0	0	0	3	0	15
Teriyaki Korean	1 tbsp (0.6 oz)	30	0	1	0	6	0	430
Hunt's								
Light w/ Mushrooms	½ cup (4.4 oz)	42	2	tr	0	8	2	438
Steak	1 tbsp (0.6 oz)	10	tr	tr	0	2	tr	256
Just Rite								
Hot Dog	¼ cup (2.2 oz)	50	2	3	2	5	2	265
Kraft								
Cocktail	¼ cup (2.3 oz)	60	1	1	0	13	1	800
Fat Free Tartar Sauce	2 tbsp (1.1 oz)	25	0	0	0	5	0	200
Lemon & Herb Tartar Sauce	2 tbsp (1 oz)	150	0	16	15	tr	0	170
Reduced Fat Sandwich Spread	1 tbsp (0.5 oz)	35	0	3	0	3	0	130
Sandwich Spread	1 tbsp (0.5 oz)	50	0	4	<5	3	0	105
Sweet'n Sour	2 tbsp (1.2 oz)	60	0	0	0	14	0	125
Tartar	2 tbsp (1.1 oz)	90	0	9	10	4	2	170
La Choy								
Duck Sauce Sweet & Sour	2 tbsp (1.3 oz)	61	tr	tr	0	15	0	128
Sweet & Sour	2 tbsp (1.2 oz)	58	tr	tr	0	14	0	104
Teriyaki	1 tbsp (0.6 oz)	17	1	tr	0	3	0	917
Lea & Perrins								
Worcestershire	1 tsp	5	0	0	0	1	–	65
Manwich								
BBQ Sloppy Joe	¼ cup (2.2 oz)	57	1	tr	0	14	1	887
Bold	¼ cup (2.2 oz)	62	1	1	0	13	1	802
Mexican	¼ cup (2.2 oz)	27	1	tr	0	5	1	552
Original	¼ cup (2.2 oz)	32	1	tr	0	6	1	365
Taco Season	¼ cup (2.2 oz)	27	1	tr	0	6	1	552
Thick & Chunky	¼ cup (2.3 oz)	44	1	tr	0	9	1	737
McCormick								
Flavor Medleys Garlic & Herb	2 tbsp	50	0	5	–	5	–	390
Flavor Medleys Italian Herb	2 tbsp	50	0	4	–	4	–	370

FOOD	PORTION	CAL	PROT	FAT	CHOL	CARB	FIBER	SOD
Flavor Medleys Lemon Pepper	2 tbsp	50	0	4	–	4	–	450
Flavor Medleys Tomato & Basil	2 tbsp	50	0	3	–	4	–	400
Mrs. Dash								
Steak	1 tbsp (0.4 oz)	17	tr	tr	0	4	–	10
Newman's Own								
Spicy Simmer Sauce Diavolo	½ cup (4.4 oz)	70	0	3	0	10	3	510
Old El Paso								
Enchilada Hot	¼ cup (2 oz)	30	0	2	0	4	0	190
Enchilada Mild	¼ cup (2 oz)	25	0	1	0	4	0	160
Green Chili Enchilada Sauce	¼ cup (2.1 oz)	30	tr	2	0	3	0	330
Taco Hot	1 tbsp (0.5 oz)	5	0	0	0	1	0	90
Taco Medium	1 tbsp (0.5 oz)	5	0	0	0	1	0	70
Taco Mild	1 tbsp (0.5 oz)	5	0	0	0	1	0	85
Taco Sauce	1 tbsp (0.5 oz)	5	0	0	0	1	0	85
Taco Sauce Extra Chunky Medium	1 tbsp (0.5 oz)	5	0	0	0	1	0	80
Taco Sauce Extra Chunky Mild	1 tbsp (0.5 oz)	5	0	0	0	1	0	80
Open Range								
Hot Dog Chili	¼ cup (2.2 oz)	61	3	3	3	6	2	255
Ortega								
Taco Western Style	1 oz	8	–	0	0	–	–	–
Pace								
Enchilada Sauce	¼ cup	36	0	0	0	6	0	290
Taco Sauce	¼ cup	32	0	2	0	4	0	150
Progresso								
Alfredo	½ cup (4.4 oz)	200	8	15	50	7	1	850
Sauce Arturo								
Original	¼ cup (2.2 fl oz)	50	1	1	0	8	0	680
Tabasco								
Caribbean Steak Sauce	1 tbsp (0.6 oz)	15	0	0	0	4	0	160
Garlic Basting Sauce	1 tbsp (0.6 oz)	20	0	0	0	4	0	250
Habanero Sauce	1 tsp (0.2 oz)	5	0	0	0	1	0	140
Hot Sauce w/ Garlic	1 tsp (0.2 oz)	0	0	0	0	0	0	95

FOOD	PORTION	CAL	PROT	FAT	CHOL	CARB	FIBER	SOD
Jalepeno Pepper Sauce	1 tbsp	15	tr	0	0	3	tr	3200
New Orleans Steak Sauce	1 tbsp (0.6 oz)	15	0	0	0	4	0	270
Pepper Sauce	1 tsp (0.2 oz)	0	0	0	0	0	0	30
Taco Bell								
Taco Sauce Medium	2 tbsp (1.1 oz)	15	0	0	0	3	tr	160
Taco Sauce Mild	2 tbsp (1.1 oz)	15	0	0	0	3	tr	160
The Restaurant Hot Sauce	1 tsp (5 g)	0	0	0	0	0	0	50
Tostitos								
Beef Fiesta Nacho	2.4 oz	120	4	8	10	6	tr	500
Chicken Quesadilla Topping	2.5 oz	90	4	6	10	6	tr	600
MIX								
Durkee								
A La King as prep	1 cup	60	1	4	0	8	0	800
Cheese as prep	¼ cup	25	1	2	2	4	0	260
Hollandaise as prep	2 tbsp	10	0	0	0	2	0	70
White as prep	¼ cup	20	0	1	0	5	0	330
French's								
Cheese as prep	¼ cup	25	1	1	0	4	0	250
Hollandaise as prep	2 tbsp	10	0	0	0	2	0	75
Manwich								
Mix	¼ oz	22	tr	tr	0	5	tr	355
McCormick								
Bernaise Blend	1 tsp (3 g)	10	0	0	—	1	—	130
Chicken Dijon Blend	1⅔ tbsp (10 g)	40	tr	2	<5	5	—	420
Green Peppercorn Blend as prep	¼ cup	20	tr	0	—	3	—	360
Grill Mates Mesquite Marinade as prep	1 tbsp	15	0	0	—	2	—	610
Grill Mates Southwest Marinade	2 tsp (5 g)	15	0	0	—	2	tr	440
Hollandaise Blend	2 tsp (4 g)	15	0	0	15	1	—	110
Hunter Blend as prep	¼ cup	25	tr	0	—	4	—	270
Meat Marinade	1 tsp (4 g)	15	0	0	—	2	—	240

FOOD	PORTION	CAL	PROT	FAT	CHOL	CARB	FIBER	SOD
Pepper Medley Blend as prep	¼ cup	30	1	2	–	3	–	310
White Blend	2 tsp (6 g)	20	tr	1	–	3	–	300
SHELF-STABLE								
Cheez Whiz								
Cheese Sqeezable	2 tbsp (1.2 oz)	100	2	8	15	4	0	470
TAKE-OUT								
bearnaise	1 oz	177	1	19	21	1	tr	257

SAUERKRAUT

FOOD	PORTION	CAL	PROT	FAT	CHOL	CARB	FIBER	SOD
canned	½ cup	22	1	tr	0	5	–	780
B&G								
Sauerkraut	2 tbsp (1 oz)	6	0	0	0	1	1	180
Boar's Head								
Sauerkraut	2 tbsp (1 oz)	5	0	0	0	1	tr	180
Claussen								
Sauerkraut	¼ cup (1.1 oz)	5	0	0	0	1	1	210
Del Monte								
Bavarian Style	2 tbsp (1 oz)	15	0	0	0	4	0	180
Sauerkraut	2 tbsp (1 oz)	0	0	0	0	1	1	180
Eden								
Organic	½ cup	25	2	0	0	4	3	580
S&W								
Canned	2 tbsp (1 oz)	5	0	0	0	1	0	220
Red Cabbage	2 tbsp (1 oz)	15	0	0	0	3	0	160

SAUSAGE

FOOD	PORTION	CAL	PROT	FAT	CHOL	CARB	FIBER	SOD
bierschinken	3.5 oz	174	18	11	–	tr	–	753
bierwurst	3.5 oz	258	16	21	–	0	–	–
blutwurst uncooked	3.5 oz	424	13	39	–	0	–	680
bockwurst	3.5 oz	276	12	25	–	0	–	700
bratwurst pork cooked	1 link (3 oz)	256	12	22	51	2	–	473
brotwurst pork & beef	1 link (2.5 oz)	226	10	19	44	2	–	778
chipolata	3.5 oz	342	14	32	66	1	0	747
chorizo	3.5 oz	499	20	45	70	4	tr	2300
fleischwurst	3.5 oz	305	12	29	–	0	–	829
gelbwurst uncooked	3.5 oz	363	12	33	–	0	–	640
italian pork cooked	1 (3 oz)	268	17	21	65	1	–	765
jagdwurst	3.5 oz	211	16	16	–	0	–	818

FOOD	PORTION	CAL	PROT	FAT	CHOL	CARB	FIBER	SOD
kielbasa pork	1 oz	88	8	8	19	1	–	305
knockwurst pork & beef	1 (2.4 oz)	209	8	19	39	1	–	687
mettwurst uncooked	3.5 oz	483	13	45	–	0	–	1090
plockwurst uncooked	3.5 oz	312	19	45	–	0	–	–
regensburger uncooked	3.5 oz	354	13	31	–	0	–	–
vienna canned	1 (½ oz)	45	2	4	8	tr	–	152
weisswurst uncooked	3.5 oz	305	11	27	–	0	–	620
zungenwurst (tongue)	3.5 oz	285	17	24	–	0	–	–
Armour								
Vienna Sausage 25% Less Fat	3 (1.9 oz)	130	6	11	50	1	0	420
Vienna Sausage 50% Less Fat	3 (1.9 oz)	90	5	7	40	1	0	420
Vienna Sausage Chicken & Beef	3 (1.9 oz)	120	6	10	65	1	0	620
Vienna Sausage Hot'n Spicy	3 (2.1 oz)	150	5	13	50	2	0	660
Vienna Sausage In BBQ Sauce	3 (2.1 oz)	150	5	13	50	3	0	580
Vienna Sausage In Beef Stock	3 (1.9 oz)	150	5	14	50	0	0	430
Vienna Sausage Jalapeno In Beef Stock	3 (1.9 oz)	170	5	16	50	1	0	420
Banner								
Sausage Stomachs	2 oz	90	0	5	95	0	0	430
Sausage Tripe	2 oz	90	9	5	85	2	0	430
Bilinski's								
Chicken & Vegetable	1 (3 oz)	80	14	2	40	2	tr	530
Boar's Head								
Bratwurst	1 (4 oz)	300	19	25	75	0	0	650
Hot Smoked	1 (3.2 oz)	280	12	25	55	1	0	740
Kielbasa	2 oz	120	9	10	50	0	0	440
Knockwurst	1 (4 oz)	310	15	27	50	1	0	950

FOOD	PORTION	CAL	PROT	FAT	CHOL	CARB	FIBER	SOD
Brown'N Serve								
Turkey	3 (2.1 oz)	120	10	8	35	2	0	370
Healthy Choice								
Low Fat Smoked	2 oz	70	8	2	25	4	1	590
Low Fat Smoked Polska Kielbasa	2 oz	70	8	2	25	4	1	590
Hormel								
Kielbasa	2 oz	150	8	13	40	–	–	530
Light & Lean 97 Dinner Smoked	2 oz	60	8	2	20	2	0	640
Pickled Hot	6 (2 oz)	140	8	11	40	1	0	380
Pickled Smoked	6 (2 oz)	140	8	11	40	1	0	380
Smoked Summer	2 oz	200	8	18	55	2	0	970
Vienna	2 oz	140	5	14	45	0	0	420
Vienna Chicken	2 oz	110	6	9	55	1	0	400
Little Sizzlers								
Brown & Serve	3 links (2.1 oz)	190	8	22	45	1	0	670
Brown & Serve	2 patties (1.8 oz)	190	7	18	40	1	0	560
Cooked	2 patties (1.8 oz)	230	8	22	45	0	0	610
Cooked	3 links (1.8 oz)	230	8	22	45	0	0	610
Heat & Serve Pork cooked	3 links (1.8 oz)	230	8	22	45	0	0	610
Louis Rich								
Polska Kielbasa	2 oz	90	8	5	35	2	0	490
Turkey Hot	2.5 oz	120	12	8	55	1	0	430
Turkey Original	2.5 oz	120	12	8	55	1	0	430
Turkey Smoked	2 oz	90	8	5	30	2	0	490
Old Smokehouse								
Summer Sausage	2 oz	200	8	18	55	2	0	970
Oscar Mayer								
Pork cooked	2 links (1.7 oz)	170	9	15	40	1	0	410
Smokies Beef	1 (1.5 oz)	120	5	11	30	1	0	420
Smokies Cheese	1 (1.5 oz)	130	6	12	30	1	0	450
Smokies Link	1 (1.5 oz)	130	5	12	25	1	0	430
Smokies Little	6 (2 oz)	170	7	15	35	1	0	570
Smokies Little Cheese	6 (2 oz)	180	7	16	40	1	0	590
Perdue								
Hot Italian Turkey Cooked	1 link (2.4 oz)	150	16	9	60	1	–	470

FOOD	PORTION	CAL	PROT	FAT	CHOL	CARB	FIBER	SOD
Sweet Italian Turkey Cooked	1 link (2.4 oz)	150	16	9	60	1	—	490
Shady Brook								
Turkey Breakfast	2 oz	80	10	4	35	—	—	480
Turkey Hot Italian	2 oz	100	12	5	40	—	—	460
Turkey Old World Style	4 oz	190	20	11	65	—	—	850
Turkey Sweet Italian	2 oz	100	12	5	40	—	—	420
Turkey Store								
Breakfast	2 links (2 oz)	140	8	11	45	1	—	360
Wampler								
Breakfast Turkey	2 (2.4 oz)	110	13	6	45	1	—	440
Italian Turkey	1 (2.7 oz)	120	14	6	50	1	—	480
TAKE-OUT								
pork	1 link (0.5 oz)	48	3	4	11	tr	—	168
pork	1 patty (1 oz)	100	5	8	22	tr	—	349

SAUSAGE DISHES
TAKE-OUT

FOOD	PORTION	CAL	PROT	FAT	CHOL	CARB	FIBER	SOD
italian sausage w/ peppers & onions	1 cup	210	17	11	70	14	—	1120
sausage roll	1 (2.3 oz)	311	5	24	—	22	1	—

SAUSAGE SUBSTITUTES

FOOD	PORTION	CAL	PROT	FAT	CHOL	CARB	FIBER	SOD
nonmeat sausage	1 patty (38 g)	97	7	7	0	4	—	137
nonmeat sausage	1 link (25 g)	64	5	5	0	2	—	222
Boca Burgers								
Breakfast Patties	1 (1.3 oz)	70	9	3	0	4	2	300
GardenSausage								
Patty	1 (2.5 oz)	140	7	3	5	20	5	460
Lightlife								
Gimme Lean	2 oz	70	9	0	0	8	1	290
Lean Links Breakfast	1 (1.2 oz)	60	4	3	0	4	0	130
Lean Links Italian	1 (1.4 oz)	60	5	2	0	5	0	160
Light	2 patties (2.3 oz)	80	11	0	0	10	1	340
Loma Linda								
Linketts	1 (1.2 oz)	70	7	5	0	1	1	160
Little Links	2 (1.6 oz)	90	8	6	0	2	2	230
Morningstar Farms								
Breakfast Links	2 (1.6 oz)	60	8	2	0	2	2	340

FOOD	PORTION	CAL	PROT	FAT	CHOL	CARB	FIBER	SOD
Breakfast Patties	1 (1.3 oz)	80	10	3	0	3	2	270
Grillers	1 patty (2.2 oz)	140	14	7	0	5	3	260
Sausage Style Recipe Crumbles	⅔ cup (1.9 oz)	90	11	3	0	5	2	370
Natural Touch								
Vegan Sausage Crumbles	½ cup (1.9 oz)	60	10	0	0	4	2	300
Worthington								
Leanies	1 link (1.4 oz)	100	7	7	0	2	1	430
Prosage Links	2 (1.6 oz)	60	8	3	0	2	2	340
Saucettes	1 link (1.3 oz)	90	6	6	0	1	1	200
Super Links	1 (1.7 oz)	110	7	8	0	2	1	350
Veja Links	1 (1.1 oz)	50	5	3	0	1	0	190
Yves								
Veggie Breakfast Links	1 (1.6 oz)	60	11	0	0	3	2	390
Veggie Breakfast Patties	1 (2 oz)	70	11	2	0	4	2	350
SAVORY								
ground	1 tsp	4	tr	tr	0	1	–	tr
SCALLOP								
raw	3 oz	75	14	1	28	2	–	137
TAKE-OUT								
breaded & fried	2 lg	67	6	3	19	3	–	144
SCONE								
apricot scone	1	232	5	7	34	39	–	201
Finnegan's								
Cranberry	1 (2.7 oz)	90	2	2	0	20	1	176
Health Valley								
Apple Kiwi	1	180	4	0	0	43	5	190
Cinnamon Raisin	1	180	4	0	0	43	5	190
Cranberry Orange	1	180	4	0	0	43	5	190
Mountain Blueberry	1	180	4	0	0	43	5	190
Pineapple Banana	1	180	4	0	0	43	5	190
TAKE-OUT								
cheese	1 (1.75 oz)	182	5	9	–	22	1	–
fruit	1 (1.75 oz)	158	4	5	–	27	2	–
orange poppy	1 (3 oz)	260	6	6	30	47	2	400

FOOD	PORTION	CAL	PROT	FAT	CHOL	CARB	FIBER	SOD
plain	1 (1.75 oz)	181	4	7	–	27	1	–
raisin	1 (3 oz)	270	6	6	25	50	2	400
SCUP								
fresh baked	3 oz	115	21	3	–	0	–	46
SEA BASS (see BASS)								
SEA CUCUMBER								
dried	1 oz	74	14	1	17	1	0	1411
fresh	1 oz	20	5	tr	14	tr	0	143
SEA TROUT (see TROUT)								
SEA URCHIN								
canned	1 oz	39	4	1	–	3	0	–
fresh	1 oz	36	4	1	–	3	tr	32
roe paste	1 tbsp	19	2	tr	–	3	0	658
SEAWEED								
agar dried	1 oz	87	2	tr	0	23	–	29
agar fresh	1 oz	tr	tr	tr	0	2	–	3
hijiki dried	1 tbsp	9	1	0	0	2	1	–
irishmoss fresh	1 oz	14	tr	tr	0	4	–	19
kelp fresh	1 oz	12	tr	tr	0	3	–	66
kombu fresh	1 oz	12	tr	tr	0	3	–	66
laver fresh	1 oz	10	2	tr	0	1	–	14
nori fresh	1 oz	10	2	tr	0	1	–	14
nori sheet dried	1 (8 x 8 in)	5	1	0	0	1	1	18
seahair dried	1 tbsp	13	1	0	0	3	tr	–
spirulina dried	1 oz	83	16	2	0	7	–	309
spirulina fresh	1 oz	7	2	tr	0	1	–	28
tangle fresh	1 oz	12	tr	tr	0	3	–	66
wakame fresh	1 oz	13	1	tr	0	3	–	249
SEITAN (see WHEAT)								
SEMOLINA								
dry	1 cup (5.9 oz)	601	21	2	0	122	7	2
SESAME								
seeds dried	1 tbsp	52	2	5	0	2	–	1
sesame butter	1 tbsp	95	3	8	0	4	1	2

FOOD	PORTION	CAL	PROT	FAT	CHOL	CARB	FIBER	SOD
sesame crunch candy	20 pieces (1.2 oz)	181	4	12	0	18	–	–
tahini from roasted & toasted kernels	1 tbsp	89	3	8	0	3	–	17
Eden								
Organic Seaweed Gomasio	1 serv (1.5 oz)	10	0	1	0	0	0	35
Organic Gomasio	½ tsp	10	0	1	0	0	tr	40
Organic Gomasio Garlic	½ tsp	10	0	1	0	0	tr	35
Planters								
Nut Mix	1 oz	150	5	12	0	9	2	240
SESBANIA								
flower	1	1	tr	0	0	tr	–	0
flowers	1 cup	5	tr	tr	0	1	–	3
flowers cooked	1 cup	23	1	tr	0	5	–	11
SHAD								
american baked	3 oz	214	18	15	–	0	–	56
roe baked w/ butter & lemon	1 oz	36	6	1	–	tr	–	21
roe raw	1 oz	37	7	tr	103	tr	–	–
SHARK								
batter-dipped & fried	3 oz	194	16	12	50	5	–	103
fin dried	1 oz	32	7	tr	–	–	–	5
raw	3 oz	111	18	4	43	0	–	67
SHEEPSHEAD FISH								
cooked	3 oz	107	22	1	–	0	–	62
cooked	1 fillet (6.5 oz)	234	48	3	–	0	–	136
raw	3 oz	92	17	2	–	0	–	61
SHELLFISH *(see individual names,* SHELLFISH SUBSTITUTES*)*								
SHELLFISH SUBSTITUTES								
crab imitation	3 oz	87	10	1	17	1	–	715
scallop imitation	3 oz	84	11	tr	18	9	–	676
shrimp imitation	3 oz	86	11	1	31	8	–	599
surimi	3 oz	84	13	1	25	6	–	122
surimi	1 oz	28	4	tr	8	2	–	40

FOOD	PORTION	CAL	PROT	FAT	CHOL	CARB	FIBER	SOD
Louis Kemp								
Crab Delights	½ cup (3 oz)	90	10	0	10	12	2	410
Lobster Delights	½ cup (3 oz)	80	8	0	10	12	0	420
Scallop Delights	13 pieces (3 oz)	80	9	0	10	12	0	550
SHELLIE BEANS								
canned	½ cup	37	2	tr	0	8	—	408
SHERBET (*see also* ICES AND ICE POPS)								
orange	½ cup (4 fl oz)	132	1	2	5	29	—	44
orange	½ gal	2158	17	31	113	469	—	706
orange	1 bar (2.75 fl oz)	91	1	1	3	20	—	30
orange home recipe	½ cup	120	2	2	9	24	—	30
Breyers								
Fat Free Orange	½ cup (3 oz)	110	2	0	0	27	0	25
Fat Free Rainbow	½ cup (3 oz)	110	1	0	0	28	0	25
Fat Free Raspberry	½ cup (3 oz)	120	2	0	0	28	0	20
Fat Free Tropical	½ cup (3 oz)	110	1	0	0	27	0	25
Orange	½ cup (3 oz)	120	1	1	5	26	0	25
Rainbow	½ cup (3 oz)	120	1	2	5	27	0	15
Raspberry	½ cup (3 oz)	120	1	2	5	28	0	15
Tropical	½ cup (3 oz)	120	1	1	5	27	0	15
Turkey Hill								
Fruit Rainbow	½ cup	120	—	1	5	26	—	20
Orange Grove	½ cup	120	—	1	5	26	—	20
SHRIMP								
canned	3 oz	102	20	2	147	1	—	143
canned	1 cup	154	30	3	222	1	—	216
chinese shrimp paste	1 tbsp	15	3	tr	45	1	—	2000
cooked	3 oz	84	18	1	166	0	—	190
cooked	4 large	22	5	tr	43	0	—	49
raw	4 large	30	6	tr	43	tr	—	42
raw	3 oz	90	17	1	130	1	—	126
Bumble Bee								
Medium	⅓ can (2 oz)	45	10	tr	115	0	0	650
Orleans Tiny Cocktail	½ can (3 oz)	44	—	0	114	0	0	650
Gorton's								
Popcorn Garlic & Herb	22 pieces (3.6 oz)	270	11	14	90	24	—	600

FOOD	PORTION	CAL	PROT	FAT	CHOL	CARB	FIBER	SOD
Popcorn Original	20 pieces (3.2 oz)	240	9	13	65	22	–	780
Van De Kamp's								
Breaded Butterfly	7 (4 oz)	280	12	14	55	28	2	580
Breaded Popcorn	20 (4 oz)	270	11	13	35	28	1	610
Breaded Whole	7 (4 oz)	240	13	10	50	26	2	520
TAKE-OUT								
breaded & fried	3 oz	206	18	10	150	10	–	292
jambalaya	¾ cup	188	11	5	50	26	8	83
SMELT								
rainbow cooked	3 oz	106	19	3	76	0	–	65
rainbow raw	3 oz	83	15	2	60	0	–	51

SMOOTHIE (see FRUIT DRINKS)

SNACKS
Baken-ets

FOOD	PORTION	CAL	PROT	FAT	CHOL	CARB	FIBER	SOD
BBQ	9 (0.5 oz)	70	7	5	10	tr	tr	400
Hot N'Spicy	7 (0.5 oz)	70	8	5	20	tr	tr	440
Hot N'Spicy Cracklins	8 (0.5 oz)	80	7	5	20	tr	tr	320
Regular	9 (0.5 oz)	80	8	5	20	tr	tr	330
Regular Cracklins	8 (0.5 oz)	40	7	6	15	tr	tr	550
Barbara's Bakery								
Cheese Puffs Bakes	1½ cups (1 oz)	160	2	11	0	13	0	190
Cheese Puffs Jalapeno	¾ cup (1 oz)	150	2	10	0	16	0	130
Cheese Puffs Original	¾ cup (1 oz)	150	2	10	0	16	0	130
Big Dipper								
Bagel Chips Lowfat Barbeque	12 (1 oz)	110	4	2	0	21	1	190
Bagel Chips Lowfat Garlic	12 (1 oz)	120	4	2	0	21	1	295
Bagel Chips Lowfat Original	12 (1 oz)	110	4	2	0	21	1	150
Bugles								
Baked Cheddar Cheese	1½ cups (1 oz)	130	2	4	0	23	0	430
Baked Original	1½ cups (1 oz)	130	2	4	0	23	0	350
Baked Original	1 pkg (1.4 oz)	170	2	5	0	30	tr	460
Nacho	1⅓ cups (1 oz)	160	1	9	0	18	0	320

FOOD	PORTION	CAL	PROT	FAT	CHOL	CARB	FIBER	SOD
Nacho	1 pkg (0.9 oz)	130	1	7	0	15	0	280
Original	1 pkg (1.5 oz)	230	2	13	0	25	tr	440
Original	1⅓ cups (1 oz)	160	1	9	0	18	tr	310
Ranch	1⅓ cups (1 oz)	160	2	9	0	18	tr	310
Smokin BBQ	1⅓ cups (1 oz)	150	1	8	0	19	0	330
Sour Cream & Onion	1⅓ cups (1 oz)	160	1	9	0	18	0	290
Cheetos								
Crunchy	21 pieces (1 oz)	160	2	10	0	15	tr	290
Curls	15 pieces (1 oz)	150	2	10	0	15	1	290
Flamin' Hot	21 pieces (1 oz)	160	2	10	0	15	tr	280
Nacho Cheese	23 pieces (1 oz)	160	2	10	0	15	tr	260
Puffed Balls	38 pieces (1 oz)	150	2	10	0	15	tr	300
Puffs	29 pieces (1 oz)	160	2	10	0	15	tr	370
Zig Zags	17 pieces (1 oz)	170	2	11	<5	17	tr	370
Chex Mix								
Bold'n Zesty	1 pkg (1.7 oz)	230	4	9	0	33	3	610
Cheddar Cheese	1 pkg (1.7 oz)	220	5	9	0	33	2	550
Hot'n Spicy	⅔ cup (1 oz)	130	3	5	0	21	2	410
Hot'n Spicy	1 pkg (1.7 oz)	210	4	7	0	35	3	90
Traditional	1 pkg (1.7 oz)	210	4	7	0	35	2	680
Combos								
Cheddar Cheese Cracker	1 pkg (1.7 oz)	250	5	13	5	28	1	520
Cheddar Cheese Cracker	1 oz	140	3	8	5	16	0	300
Cheddar Cheese Pretzel	1 oz	130	3	5	0	18	0	310
Cheddar Cheese Pretzel	1 pkg (1.8 oz)	240	5	9	5	33	1	560
Chili Cheese w/ Corn Shell	1 oz	140	2	6	0	17	1	420
Chili Cheese w/ Corn Shell	1 pkg (1.7 oz)	230	4	11	5	29	2	710
Mustard Pretzel	1 pkg (1.8 oz)	230	4	8	0	35	1	500
Mustard Pretzel	1 oz	130	2	4	0	19	1	270
Nacho Cheese Pretzel	1 pkg (1.7 oz)	230	5	8	0	34	1	580
Nacho Cheese Pretzel	1 oz	130	3	5	0	19	1	320
Nacho Cheese w/ Tortilla Shell	1 oz	140	2	6	0	17	1	380

FOOD	PORTION	CAL	PROT	FAT	CHOL	CARB	FIBER	SOD
Nacho Cheese w/ Tortilla Shell	1 pkg (1.7 oz)	230	4	11	0	30	1	640
Peanut Butter Cracker	1 oz	140	4	8	0	15	1	260
Pepperoni & Cheese Pizza	1 oz	140	2	7	5	17	0	280
Pepperoni & Cheese Pizza	1 pkg (1.7 oz)	240	4	11	5	30	1	480
Pizzeria Pretzel	1 pkg (1.8 oz)	230	5	8	0	35	1	520
Pizzeria Pretzel	1 oz	130	3	5	0	19	1	290
Tortilla Ranch	1 bag (1.7 oz)	240	4	12	5	29	1	610
Tortilla Ranch	1 oz	140	2	7	5	17	1	350
Dakota Gourmet								
Amazing Corn Classic	1 pkg (1 oz)	360	10	7	0	78	5	813
Amazing Corn Cool Ranch	1 pkg (1 oz)	367	10	9	2	74	5	1073
Amazing Corn Mesquite BBQ	1 pkg (1 oz)	369	11	8	0	76	5	725
Heart Smart Toasted Corn	⅓ cup (1 oz)	110	3	2	0	22	3	280
Toasted Corn Heart Smart	1 pkg (1.75 oz)	177	5	3	0	39	2	470
Trail Mix Heart Smart	1 pkg (1.75 oz)	172	4	0	0	39	3	156
Eden								
Rice Puffs Five Flavor Arare	1 oz	110	3	0	0	24	2	160
Frito Lay								
Funyuns	13 (1 oz)	140	2	7	0	18	tr	270
Munchos	16 (1 oz)	160	1	10	0	16	1	230
Munchos BBQ	14 (1 oz)	160	1	10	0	15	1	250
Hapi								
Chili Bits	½ cup (1 oz)	110	3	0	0	25	1	180
Health Valley								
Cheddar Lites Green Onion	1¾ cups	120	3	3	5	21	1	170
Cheddar Lites Original	1¾ cups	120	3	3	5	21	1	170

FOOD	PORTION	CAL	PROT	FAT	CHOL	CARB	FIBER	SOD
Corn Puffs Caramel	2 cups	120	2	2	0	25	1	80
Low Fat Potato Puffs Cheddar Cheese	1½ cups	110	2	3	5	21	1	260
Low Fat Potato Puffs Garlic w/ Cheese	1½ cups	260	2	3	0	21	1	260
Low Fat Potato Puffs Zesty Ranch	1½ cups	110	2	3	0	21	1	260
Innovative Foods								
Roasted Sweet Corn	1 pkg (0.8 oz)	76	3	0	0	17	2	5
Lance								
Cheese Balls	1 pkg (1 oz)	150	2	8	0	16	0	300
Crunchy Cheese Twists	1 pkg (1.25 oz)	190	2	4	0	15	0	280
Gold-N-Chees	1 pkg (1 oz)	130	3	5	0	18	1	290
Onion Rings	1 pkg (0.9 oz)	100	1	8	0	7	1	170
Pork Skins	1 pkg (0.4 oz)	65	6	4	10	1	0	230
Pork Skins BBQ	1 pkg (0.4 oz)	60	6	4	10	1	0	330
Mr. Peanut								
Peanut Butter Crisps Graham	12 pieces (1.1 oz)	150	4	8	0	18	2	100
Old Dutch Foods								
Baked Cheese Curls	2 cups (1.1 oz)	180	2	12	0	15	tr	340
Cheese Puffcorn Curls	2 cups (1.1 oz)	170	2	12	0	15	0	310
Pita Puffs								
Barbeque	35 (1 oz)	120	4	3	0	20	1	150
Lowfat Garlic	35 (1 oz)	110	3	1	0	22	1	125
Lowfat Original	35 (1 oz)	110	3	1	0	22	1	170
Lowfat Salsa	35 (1 oz)	110	3	1	0	21	1	290
Pizza	35 (1 oz)	120	4	2	0	21	1	230
Ranch	35 (1 oz)	120	4	2	0	21	1	195
Planters								
Cheez Balls	1 oz	150	2	10	2	15	1	300
Cheez Balls	1 pkg (1 oz)	150	2	10	2	15	1	330
Cheez Curls	1 pkg (1.2 oz)	190	2	12	2	19	1	380
Cheez Mania Original	42 pieces (1 oz)	150	2	10	<5	15	1	300
Heat Snack Mix	1 oz	140	5	8	0	13	2	230

FOOD	PORTION	CAL	PROT	FAT	CHOL	CARB	FIBER	SOD
Robert's American Gourmet								
Pirate's Booty Puffed Rice & Corn w/ Cheddar	1 oz	120	3	3	0	22	4	137
Rold Gold								
Snack Mix Colossal Cheddar	1 pkg (1 oz)	140	3	7	0	17	1	230
Snyder's Of Hanover								
Cheese Twists	1 oz	230	1	14	0	10	0	280
Fried Pork Skins	1 oz	80	8	4	30	1	0	115
Fried Pork Skins Barbecue	1 oz	80	8	4	20	1	0	106
Kruncheez	1.25 oz	200	2	10	0	19	tr	210
Onion Toasters	1 oz	188	2	10	0	21	tr	350
Utz								
Caramel Corn Clusters	1⅛ cups (1 oz)	120	tr	2	0	24	tr	140
Cheese Balls	50 (1 oz)	150	2	9	0	16	tr	260
Cheese Curls	18 (1 oz)	150	2	9	0	16	tr	260
Cheese Curls Crunchy	30 (1 oz)	160	2	10	0	16	0	200
Cheese Curls Reduced Fat	32 (1 oz)	140	3	6	<5	18	2	300
Onion Rings	41 (1 oz)	140	1	7	0	18	0	340
Party Mix	¾ cup (1 oz)	140	2	6	0	19	1	250
Pork Cracklins	0.5 oz	90	6	7	15	0	—	300
Pork Cracklins Hot & Spicy	0.5 oz	80	8	5	15	0	—	340
Pork Rinds	0.5 oz	80	8	5	15	0	—	230
Pork Rinds BBQ	0.5 oz	80	8	5	15	0	—	280
Weight Watchers								
Cheese Curls	1 pkg (0.5 oz)	70	1	3	0	10	0	85
SNAIL								
cooked	3 oz	233	41	1	110	13	—	350
raw	3 oz	117	20	tr	55	7	—	175
TAKE-OUT								
escargot cooked	5	25	4	0	15	1	0	25
SNAKE								
fresh	3 oz	78	17	tr	—	3	0	57

FOOD	PORTION	CAL	PROT	FAT	CHOL	CARB	FIBER	SOD
SNAPPER								
cooked	3 oz	109	22	1	40	0	–	48
cooked	1 fillet (6 oz)	217	45	3	80	0	–	96
raw	3 oz	85	17	1	31	0	–	54
SODA (see also DRINK MIXERS, ENERGY DRINKS, WATER)								
club	12 oz	0	0	0	0	0	–	75
cola	12 oz	151	tr	tr	0	39	–	14
cream	12 oz	191	0	0	0	49	–	43
diet cola	12 oz	2	tr	0	0	tr	–	21
diet cola w/ equal	12 oz	2	tr	0	0	tr	–	21
diet cola w/ saccharin	12 oz	2	tr	0	0	tr	–	57
ginger ale	12 oz can	124	tr	0	0	32	–	25
grape	12 oz	161	0	0	0	42	–	57
lemon lime	12 oz	149	0	0	0	38	–	41
orange	12 oz	177	0	0	0	46	–	49
pepper type	12 oz	151	0	tr	0	38	–	38
quinine	12 oz	125	0	0	0	32	–	15
root beer	12 oz	152	tr	0	0	39	–	49
tonic water	12 oz	125	0	0	0	32	–	15
7 Up								
Diet	1 oz	tr	–	0	0	–	–	–
Gold	1 oz	13	–	0	0	–	–	–
Original	1 can	140	0	0	0	39	–	75
A & W								
Root Beer	1 can	180	0	0	0	46	–	45
After The Fall								
Raspberry Ginger Ale	1 can (12 oz)	150	1	0	0	36	0	25
Barritts								
Ginger Beer	1 bottle (12 oz)	200	0	0	0	49	–	40
Best Health								
Root Beer	1 bottle (12 oz)	165	0	0	0	42	–	35
Vanilla Cream	1 bottle (12 oz)	170	0	0	0	43	–	30
Canada Dry								
Ginger Ale	1 can	120	0	0	0	33	0	40
Tonic Water	8 fl oz	90	0	0	0	24	0	15
Crush								
Tropical Fruit Punch	1 can (11.5 fl oz)	200	–	0	0	–	–	–

FOOD	PORTION	CAL	PROT	FAT	CHOL	CARB	FIBER	SOD
Dr Pepper								
Diet	1 oz	tr	–	0	0	–	–	–
Original	1 can	150	0	0	0	40	–	55
Health Valley								
Ginger Ale	1 bottle	160	0	0	0	40	0	0
Rootbeer Old Fashioned	1 bottle	160	0	0	0	40	0	0
Sarsaparilla Rootbeer	1 bottle	160	0	0	0	40	0	0
IBC								
Root Beer	1 can	160	0	0	0	43	–	55
Like								
Cola	1 oz	13	–	0	0	–	–	–
Cola Sugar Free	1 oz	tr	–	0	0	–	–	–
Lucozade								
Soda	7 oz	136	0	0	0	36	0	–
Saranac								
Diet Root Beer	1 bottle (12 oz)	35	0	0	0	9	–	55
Ginger Beer	1 bottle (12 oz)	160	0	0	0	42	–	55
Root Beer	1 bottle (12 oz)	180	04	0	0	46	–	55
Shasta								
Black Cherry	1 can (12 oz)	170	0	0	0	41	0	54
Caffeine Free Cola	1 can (12 oz)	160	0	0	0	41	–	45
Cherry Cola	1 can (12 oz)	160	0	0	0	39	–	45
Club Soda	1 can (12 oz)	0	0	0	0	0	–	90
Cola	1 can (12 oz)	170	0	0	0	42	0	45
Creme	1 can (12 oz)	190	0	0	0	47	0	45
Diet Black Cherry	1 can (12 oz)	0	0	0	0	0	0	55
Diet Caffeine Free Cola	1 can (12 oz)	0	0	0	0	0	0	55
Diet Cherry Cola	1 can (12 oz)	0	0	0	0	0	0	55
Diet Cola	1 can (12 oz)	0	0	0	0	0	0	45
Diet Creme	1 can (12 oz)	0	0	0	0	0	0	55
Diet Doc Shasta	1 can (12 oz)	0	0	0	0	0	0	45
Diet Ginger Ale	1 can (12 oz)	0	0	0	0	0	0	55
Diet Grape	1 can (12 oz)	0	0	0	0	0	0	55
Diet Grapefruit	1 can (12 oz)	0	0	0	0	0	0	55
Diet Kiwi-Strawberry	1 can (12 oz)	0	0	0	0	0	0	45

FOOD	PORTION	CAL	PROT	FAT	CHOL	CARB	FIBER	SOD
Diet Lemon-Lime Twist	1 can (12 oz)	0	0	0	0	0	0	55
Diet Orange	1 can (12 oz)	0	0	0	0	0	0	55
Diet Pineapple-Orange	1 can (12 oz)	0	0	0	0	0	0	55
Diet Raspberry Creme	1 can (12 oz)	0	0	0	0	0	0	45
Diet Red Pop	1 can (12 oz)	0	0	0	0	0	0	55
Diet Root Beer	1 can (12 oz)	0	0	0	0	0	0	55
Diet Strawberry	1 can (12 oz)	0	0	0	0	0	0	55
Diet Strawberry-Peach	1 can (12 oz)	0	0	0	0	0	0	55
Doc Shasta	1 can (12 oz)	160	0	0	0	39	0	45
Fruit Punch	1 can (12 oz)	200	0	0	0	50	0	45
Ginger Ale	1 can (12 oz)	130	0	0	0	32	0	45
Grape	1 can (12 oz)	190	0	0	0	48	0	45
Kiwi-Strawberry	1 can (12 oz)	170	0	0	0	43	0	45
Lemon-Lime Twist	1 can (12 oz)	150	0	0	0	38	0	45
Moon Mist	1 can (12 oz)	180	0	0	0	46	0	45
Orange	1 can (12 oz)	200	0	0	0	49	0	45
Peach	1 can (12 oz)	170	0	0	0	43	0	45
Pineapple	1 can (12 oz)	200	0	0	0	51	0	45
Pineapple-Orange	1 can (12 oz)	180	0	0	0	46	0	45
Quinine/Tonic	1 can (12 oz)	130	0	0	0	32	0	45
Raspberry Creme	1 can (12 oz)	170	0	0	0	44	0	45
Red Pop	1 can (12 oz)	170	0	0	0	43	0	45
Root Beer	1 can (12 oz)	170	0	0	0	42	0	45
Strawberry	1 can (12 oz)	190	0	0	0	46	0	45
Strawberry-Peach	1 can (12 oz)	170	0	0	0	42	0	45
Sunkist								
Orange	1 can	190	0	0	0	52	0	45
Welch's								
Sparkling Apple	12 oz	180	—	0	0	—	—	—
Sparkling Grape	12 oz	180	—	0	0	—	—	—
Sparkling Orange	12 oz	180	—	0	0	—	—	—
Sparkling Strawberry	12 oz	180	—	0	0	—	—	—
SOLE								
cooked	3 oz	99	21	1	58	0	—	89
cooked	1 fillet (4.5 oz)	148	31	2	86	0	—	133

FOOD	PORTION	CAL	PROT	FAT	CHOL	CARB	FIBER	SOD
lemon raw	3.5 oz	85	17	1	–	0	–	80
raw	3.5 oz	90	18	1	50	0	–	100
Van De Kamp's								
Lightly Breaded Fillets	1 (4 oz)	220	14	11	40	17	0	410
Natural Fillets	1 (4 oz)	110	23	2	50	0	0	125
TAKE-OUT								
battered & fried	3.2 oz	211	13	11	31	15	–	484
breaded & fried	3.2 oz	211	13	11	31	15	–	484

SORBET (see ICES AND ICE POPS)

SORGHUM

sorghum	1 cup (6.7 oz)	651	22	6	0	143	–	12

SOUFFLE

lemon chilled	1 cup	176	9	tr	2	34	–	108
raspberry chilled	1 cup	173	10	tr	3	34	–	108
spinach	1 cup	218	11	18	184	3	–	763

SOUP
CANNED
Boston Market

Chicken Broth Reduced Sodium	1 cup	15	1	1	0	1	0	760
Butterball								
Chicken Broth Reduced Sodium 99% Fat Free	1 cup	10	1	0	0	2	0	620
Campbell								
98% Fat Free Cream Of Chicken as prep	1 cup	80	3	3	10	10	0	830
Bean w/ Bacon as prep	1 cup	168	8	4	3	26	8	891
Beef Barley as prep	1 cup	81	6	2	10	11	2	915
Beef Noodle as prep	1 cup	73	5	2	12	8	1	908
Cheddar Cheese	1 cup	130	3	8	15	11	1	950
Cheddar Cheese as prep	1 cup	134	4	8	19	11	1	1083
Chicken Vegetable as prep	1 cup	74	3	3	9	9	1	985

FOOD	PORTION	CAL	PROT	FAT	CHOL	CARB	FIBER	SOD
Chicken & Pasta w/ Garden Vegetables	1 cup (8.4 oz)	90	6	1	5	14	1	850
Chicken Gumbo as prep	1 cup	55	2	1	5	9	1	985
Chunky Savory Chicken w/ White & Wild Rice	1 cup	140	9	3	25	18	2	840
Chunky Classic Chicken Noodle	1 cup (8.4 oz)	130	8	4	20	15	1	880
Clam Chowder New England as prep	1 cup	89	4	3	3	13	1	979
Classic Chicken Noodle	1 cup	70	3	2	15	10	1	890
Classic Chicken Rice	1 cup (8.4 oz)	80	2	2	5	14	1	850
Consomme as prep	1 cup	24	5	tr	tr	1	tr	817
Cream Of Asparagus as prep	1 cup	72	2	4	2	9	1	749
Cream Of Mushroom as prep	1 cup	108	2	7	2	9	2	872
Cream Of Celery as prep	1 cup	107	2	7	2	9	1	903
Cream Of Chicken as prep	1 cup	120	3	8	10	10	1	880
Cream Of Potato as prep	1 cup	102	2	4	7	15	1	951
Fiesta Tomato as prep	1 cup	72	1	tr	1	16	1	856
Garden Vegetable as prep	1 cup	69	3	2	3	11	1	857
Green Pea as prep	1 cup	173	9	3	1	29	4	888
Healthy Request Chicken Noodle as prep	1 cup	60	2	2	10	8	tr	450
Healthy Request Chicken Rice as prep	1 cup	60	2	2	10	8	tr	420
Healthy Request Cream Of Mushroom as prep	1 cup	66	2	2	4	10	1	475

FOOD	PORTION	CAL	PROT	FAT	CHOL	CARB	FIBER	SOD
Healthy Request Cream Of Chicken & Broccoli as prep	1 cup	78	3	3	6	10	1	460
Healthy Request Cream Of Chicken as prep	1 cup	70	2	3	10	12	tr	430
Healthy Request Hearty Pasta w/ Vegetables	1 cup	87	3	1	1	17	2	474
Healthy Request Tomato as prep	1 cup	91	2	2	1	18	2	456
Healthy Request Vegetable as prep	1 cup	84	3	1	1	17	2	473
Home Cookin' Chicken Vegetable	1 cup (8.4 oz)	130	6	4	10	20	3	820
Home Cookin' Chicken Rice	1 cup	110	6	1	10	20	2	920
Home Cookin' Chicken w/ Egg Noodles	1 cup (8.4 oz)	90	6	2	15	13	1	940
Home Cookin' Oriental Noodles w/ Vegetables	1 cup (8.4 oz)	100	4	1	10	18	3	890
Italian Tomato as prep	1 cup	105	2	tr	1	23	4	820
Low Sodium Chicken Broth	1 can (10.75 oz)	27	4	1	2	2	tr	75
Low Sodium Chicken w/ Noodles	1 can (10.75 oz)	162	14	5	40	16	2	85
Low Sodium Chunky Vegetable Beef	1 can (10.75 oz)	159	13	4	39	17	3	64
Low Sodium Cream of Mushroom	1 can (10.75 oz)	200	3	13	12	18	2	48
Low Sodium Green Pea	1 can (10.75 oz)	235	12	4	4	38	6	27
Low Sodium Tomato w/ Pieces	1 can (10.75 oz)	170	4	5	6	28	3	36
Minestrone as prep	1 cup	81	3	2	1	12	2	971
Plus! Hearty Minestrone	2 cup (8.4 oz)	130	5	1	0	25	4	670

FOOD	PORTION	CAL	PROT	FAT	CHOL	CARB	FIBER	SOD
Ready To Serve Bean w/ Bacon 'N Ham	1 can (10.5 oz)	274	14	7	13	41	11	1299
Ready To Serve Chicken Noodle	1 can (10.5 oz)	134	7	4	23	18	2	1323
Ready To Serve Chicken w/ Rice	1 can (10.5 oz)	122	5	2	11	20	2	1132
Ready-To-Serve Vegetable Beef	1 can (10.5 oz)	143	9	1	10	26	5	1243
Savory Tomato & Dill as prep	1 cup	99	2	2	tr	20	2	811
Select Chicken & Pasta w/ Roasted Garlic	1 cup (8.4 oz)	110	6	2	10	17	1	800
Select Chicken Rice	1 cup	110	7	1	10	18	2	890
Select Fiesta Vegetable	1 cup (8.4 oz)	120	4	1	0	24	3	810
Select Mushroom w/ White & Wild Rice	1 cup	90	6	1	0	16	2	820
Select Roasted Chicken w/ Rotini & Penne Pasta	1 cup	110	6	2	10	17	1	800
Select Split Pea w/ Ham	1 cup (8.4 oz)	170	10	2	10	30	6	860
Select Tuscany-Style Minestrone	1 cup (8.4 oz)	190	5	9	5	21	5	870
Simply Home Chicken Noodle	1 cup (8.4 oz)	80	5	1	10	12	1	810
Simply Home Chicken w/ Rice	1 cup (8.4 oz)	100	5	1	5	19	1	810
Tomato as prep	1 cup	80	2	0	0	18	2	730
Vegetable Beef as prep	1 cup	68	5	2	8	9	2	897
Vegetarian Vegetable as prep	1 cup	79	2	2	0	14	2	844
Gold's								
Russian Borscht	8 oz	70	1	0	0	17	2	750
Health Valley								
5 Bean Vegetable	1 cup	250	10	0	0	32	10	250

FOOD	PORTION	CAL	PROT	FAT	CHOL	CARB	FIBER	SOD
Beef Broth Fat Free	1 cup	20	5	0	0	0	0	160
Beef Broth Fat Free No Salt	1 cup	20	5	0	0	0	0	160
Black Bean & Vegetable	1 cup	110	11	0	0	24	9	280
Chicken Broth	1 cup	45	7	2	25	0	0	250
Chicken Broth Fat Free	1 cup	30	7	0	0	0	0	170
Chicken Broth No Salt	1 cup	45	7	2	25	0	0	25
Country Corn & Vegetable	1 cup	70	5	0	0	17	7	135
Garden Vegetable	1 cup	80	6	0	0	17	4	250
Italian Plus Carotene	1 cup	80	7	0	0	19	6	240
Lentil & Carrot	1 cup	100	10	0	0	25	10	220
Organic Black Bean	1 cup	110	8	0	0	28	10	45
Organic Lentil No Salt	1 cup	90	9	0	0	20	9	40
Organic Minestrone	1 cup	100	8	0	0	23	8	190
Organic Mushroom Barley No Salt	1 cup	60	5	0	0	15	5	95
Organic Potato Leek	1 cup	70	4	0	0	15	3	230
Organic Potato Leek No Salt	1 cup	70	4	0	0	15	3	35
Organic Split Pea	1 cup	110	10	0	0	23	8	160
Organic Split Pea No Salt	1 cup	110	10	0	0	23	8	115
Organic Tomato	1 cup	90	4	0	0	22	4	250
Organic Vegetable No Salt	1 cup	80	5	0	0	18	6	80
Pasta Bolognese	1 cup	100	4	0	0	20	4	290
Pasta Cacciatore	1 cup	100	4	0	0	20	4	290
Pasta Romano	1 cup	100	4	0	0	20	4	290
Real Italian Minestrone	1 cup	90	8	0	0	21	8	210
Rotini & Vegetable	1 cup	100	4	0	0	20	4	290
Split Pea & Carrots	1 cup	110	8	0	0	17	4	230
Super Broccoli Carotene	1 cup	70	6	0	0	16	7	240
Tomato Vegetable	1 cup	80	6	0	0	17	5	240

FOOD	PORTION	CAL	PROT	FAT	CHOL	CARB	FIBER	SOD
Vegetable Barley	1 cup	90	6	0	0	19	4	210
Vegetable Power Carotene	1 cup	70	5	0	0	17	6	240
Healthy Choice								
Bean & Ham	1 cup (8.7 oz)	166	9	1	4	31	7	570
Beef & Potato	1 cup (8.5 oz)	116	11	1	5	16	tr	452
Broccoli Cheddar	1 cup (8.4 oz)	116	4	2	4	22	2	304
Chicken Corn Chowder	1 cup (8.8 oz)	176	8	3	8	30	2	466
Chicken Pasta	1 cup (8.6 oz)	119	7	3	6	18	1	493
Chicken Rice	1 cup (8.4 oz)	119	9	2	6	19	3	324
Chili Beef	1 cup (9.1 oz)	189	15	2	12	32	5	441
Clam Chowder	1 cup (8.8 oz)	123	6	1	12	23	2	481
Classic Italian Bean and Pasta	1 cup (8 oz)	100	6	2	0	17	3	480
Country Vegetable	1 cup (8.6 oz)	112	5	1	0	24	3	453
Cream Of Mushroom	1 cup (8.8 oz)	77	4	1	tr	14	1	450
Cream Of Celery as prep	1 cup	73	1	2	3	14	3	366
Cream Of Chicken Vegetable	1 cup (8.9 oz)	127	7	2	10	21	1	384
Cream Of Roasted Chicken as prep	1 cup	80	2	3	4	13	3	349
Cream Of Roasted Garlic as prep	1 cup	57	1	1	2	13	3	489
Garden Tomato Herbs as prep	1 cup	80	2	1	0	18	3	298
Garden Vegetable	1 cup (8.6 oz)	108	5	1	tr	22	6	454
Hearty Chicken	1 cup (8.7 oz)	136	9	3	21	20	3	482
Lentil	1 cup (8.7 oz)	135	10	1	tr	28	5	472
Minestrone	1 cup (8.6 oz)	107	5	1	1	24	5	370
Old Fashion Chicken Noodle	1 cup (8.8 oz)	137	9	3	9	19	1	402
Split Pea & Ham	1 cup (8.8 oz)	164	11	2	7	26	5	468
Tomato Garden	1 cup (8.6 oz)	101	4	1	1	19	5	468
Turkey Wild Rice	1 cup (8.4 oz)	72	10	1	3	9	3	407
Vegetable Beef	1 cup (8.8 oz)	96	11	1	2	14	2	433

FOOD	PORTION	CAL	PROT	FAT	CHOL	CARB	FIBER	SOD
Herb-Ox								
Beef Liquid	2 tsp (0.4 oz)	20	2	0	0	2	0	570
Chicken Liquid	2 tsp (0.4 oz)	15	1	0	0	1	0	620
Imagine								
Creamy Broccoli	1 serv (8 oz)	70	3	2	0	10	2	370
Creamy Butternut Squash	1 serv (8 oz)	120	2	2	0	23	2	370
Creamy Mushroom	1 serv (8 oz)	80	4	3	0	10	2	310
Creamy Potato Leek	1 serv (8 oz)	90	2	3	0	14	2	380
Creamy Sweet Corn	1 serv (8 oz)	100	4	3	0	15	1	540
Creamy Tomato	1 serv (8 oz)	90	8	2	0	17	2	520
Vegetable Broth	1 serv (8 oz)	45	0	1	0	7	1	500
Zesty Gazpacho	1 serv (8 oz)	80	tr	0	0	8	tr	720
Natural Choice								
Orangic Vegan Classic Tomato	1 cup	100	2	1	0	22	2	317
Organic Vegan Classic Mushroom	1 cup	50	2	2	0	9	2	435
Organic Vegan Country Corn	1 cup	100	3	1	0	24	3	377
Organic Vegan Kabocha Squash	1 cup	60	2	1	0	14	1	370
Organic Vegan Southern Greens	1 cup	80	2	3	0	13	2	399
Organic Vegan Split Pea	1 cup	120	7	1	0	21	7	420
Organic Vegan Vegetable Curry	1 cup	110	4	4	0	17	2	392
Old El Paso								
Black Bean w/ Bacon	1 cup (8.6 oz)	160	11	2	5	26	7	960
Chicken Vegetable	1 cup (8.4 oz)	110	9	3	15	13	0	620
Chicken w/ Rice	1 cup (8.4 oz)	90	8	3	15	10	0	680
Garden Vegetable	1 cup (8.4 oz)	110	5	3	<5	17	0	710
Hearty Beef	1 cup (8.4 oz)	120	10	3	25	14	0	690
Hearty Chicken Noodle	1 cup (8.4 oz)	110	9	3	25	10	0	720
Pacific								
Free Range Organic Chicken Broth	1 cup	5	1	0	0	1	–	570

FOOD	PORTION	CAL	PROT	FAT	CHOL	CARB	FIBER	SOD
Progresso								
99% Fat Free Beef Barley	1 cup (8.5 oz)	140	11	2	20	20	3	470
99% Fat Free Beef Vegetable	1 cup (8.5 oz)	160	11	2	10	24	3	870
99% Fat Free Chicken Noodle	1 cup (8.3 oz)	90	7	2	20	13	1	950
99% Fat Free Chicken Rice w/ Vegetables	1 cup (8.4 oz)	110	7	2	10	16	1	780
99% Fat Free Creamy Mushroom Chicken	1 cup (8.3 oz)	90	7	2	10	12	1	840
99% Fat Free Lentil	1 cup (8.5 oz)	130	8	2	0	20	6	440
99% Fat Free Minestrone	1 cup (8.5 oz)	130	7	2	0	23	4	710
99% Fat Free Roasted Chicken w/ Italian Style Vegetable	1 cup (8 oz)	90	7	2	10	12	1	660
99% Fat Free Split Pea	1 cup (8.9 oz)	170	10	2	0	29	5	620
99% Fat Free Tomato Garden Vegetable	1 cup (8.6 oz)	100	3	2	0	19	2	660
99% Fat Free Vegetable	1 cup (8.4 oz)	70	2	1	0	13	2	870
99% Fat Free White Cheddar Potato	1 cup (8.6 oz)	140	4	3	5	26	2	930
Basil Rotini Tomato	1 cup (8.9 oz)	120	5	2	<5	22	2	890
Bean & Ham	1 cup (8.4 oz)	160	10	2	10	25	8	870
Beef Barley	1 cup (8.5 oz)	130	10	4	25	13	3	780
Beef Minestrone	1 cup (8.5 oz)	140	10	3	10	18	3	970
Beef Noodle	1 cup (8.5 oz)	140	13	4	30	15	1	950
Beef Vegetable & Rotini	1 cup (8.4 oz)	130	13	3	25	14	4	780
Cheese & Herb Tortellini Tomato	1 cup (8.6 oz)	140	4	3	<5	23	2	700

FOOD	PORTION	CAL	PROT	FAT	CHOL	CARB	FIBER	SOD
Chickarina	1 cup (8.3 oz)	130	8	5	20	12	tr	1010
Chicken Minestrone	1 cup (8.4 oz)	110	9	2	15	15	2	890
Chicken Vegetable	1 cup (8.4 oz)	90	7	2	15	13	2	820
Chicken & Wild Rice	1 cup (8.4 oz)	100	7	2	15	15	1	850
Chicken Barley	1 cup (8.5 oz)	110	8	2	15	16	3	850
Chicken Broth	1 cup (8.2 oz)	20	1	2	0	1	0	920
Chicken Noodle	1 cup (8.4 oz)	90	9	2	25	9	tr	950
Chicken Rice w/ Vegetable	1 cup (8.4 oz)	90	6	2	10	13	1	890
Clam & Rotini Chowder	1 cup (8.8 oz)	190	7	9	10	21	0	800
Escarole In Chicken Broth	1 cup (8.1 oz)	25	1	1	<5	3	1	930
Green Split Pea	1 cup (8.6 oz)	170	10	3	5	25	5	870
Hearty Black Bean	1 cup (8.5 oz)	170	8	2	<5	30	10	730
Hearty Penne In Chicken Broth	1 cup (8.4 oz)	80	4	1	0	14	tr	1020
Hearty Tomato	1 cup (8.7 oz)	100	2	2	0	19	1	800
Herb Rotini Vegetable	1 cup (9.1 oz)	120	5	2	0	21	4	990
Homestyle Chicken w/ Vegetable	1 cup (8.4 oz)	90	7	2	15	11	tr	900
Italian Herb Shells Minestrone	1 cup (9.1 oz)	120	5	2	0	22	4	1050
Lentil	1 cup (8.5 oz)	140	9	2	0	22	7	750
Macaroni & Bean	1 cup (8.6 oz)	160	7	4	<5	23	6	800
Manhattan Clam Chowder	1 cup (8.4 oz)	110	12	2	10	11	3	710
Meatballs & Pasta Pearls	1 cup (8.3 oz)	140	7	7	15	13	0	700
Minestrone	1 cup (8.4 oz)	120	5	2	0	21	5	960
Minestrone Parmesan	1 cup (8.3 oz)	100	3	3	0	16	3	700
New England Clam Chowder	1 cup (8.4 oz)	190	6	10	15	20	1	920
Oregano Penne Italian Style Vegetable	1 cup (8.7 oz)	90	3	2	0	15	1	960
Peppercorn Penne Vegetable	1 cup (9.1 oz)	100	3	1	0	20	2	920

FOOD	PORTION	CAL	PROT	FAT	CHOL	CARB	FIBER	SOD
Potato Broccoli & Cheese	1 cup (8.8 oz)	160	5	6	<5	21	1	960
Potato Ham & Cheese	1 cup (8.6 oz)	170	6	7	10	21	1	860
Roasted Garlic Pasta Lentil	1 cup (9.3 oz)	120	7	2	0	20	5	960
Rotisserie Seasoned Chicken	1 cup (8.5 oz)	100	7	2	15	15	2	920
Spicy Chicken & Penne	1 cup (8.5 oz)	110	9	2	15	14	1	950
Split Pea w/ Ham	1 cup (8.4 oz)	150	9	4	15	20	5	830
Tomato	1 cup (8.5 oz)	100	2	2	0	19	1	790
Tomato Basil	1 cup (8.8 oz)	100	2	2	0	19	1	790
Tomato Vegetable	1 cup (8.5 oz)	90	3	2	0	15	4	990
Tortellini In Chicken Broth	1 cup (8.3 oz)	70	3	2	10	10	2	970
Turkey Noodle	1 cup (8.4 oz)	90	7	2	20	11	tr	1080
Turkey Rice w/ Vegetables	1 cup (8.5 oz)	110	7	1	15	18	1	1040
Vegetable	1 cup (8.4 oz)	90	3	2	<5	15	2	810
White Meat Roasted Chicken Rotini	1 cup (8.1 oz)	80	6	2	15	11	tr	970
Swanson								
Beef Broth	1 cup	19	3	1	tr	1	1	813
Beef Broth Onion Seasoned	1 cup (8.4 oz)	20	2	0	0	2	tr	890
Chicken Broth 99% Fat Free	1 cup	15	1	1	0	1	–	980
Chicken Broth Seasoned Italian Herbs	1 cup (8.4 oz)	20	1	1	<5	3	tr	950
Vegetble Broth	1 cup	19	1	1	1	3	0	996
Ultra Slim-Fast								
Chicken Alfredo Pasta	1 cup (8.3 oz)	132	12	2	10	17	2	333
Walnut Acres								
Organic Country Corn Chowder	1 cup (8.8 oz)	150	4	3	10	28	2	690
Weight Watchers								
Chicken & Rice	1 can (10.5 oz)	110	6	2	10	17	4	720

FOOD	PORTION	CAL	PROT	FAT	CHOL	CARB	FIBER	SOD
Chicken Noodle	1 can (10.5 oz)	150	9	2	30	25	4	740
Minestrone	1 can (10.5 oz)	130	5	2	5	23	6	760
Vegetable	1 can (10.5 oz)	130	4	1	0	27	6	680
FROZEN								
Nature's Entree								
Chowder	1 pkg (12 oz)	230	16	6	15	26	5	960
Tortellini Minestone	1 pkg (12 oz)	360	22	9	10	48	5	960
MIX								
Armour								
Bouillon Cubes Beef	1 (4 g)	5	0	0	0	1	0	920
Bouillon Cubes Chicken	1 (4 g)	5	0	0	0	1	0	910
Azumaya								
Thin Cut Noodle	1 cup	120	5	0	0	24	tr	820
Wide Cut Noodle	1 cup	120	5	0	0	24	tr	800
Bean Cuisine								
13 Bean Bouillabisse	1 cup	220	6	0	0	17	5	0
Island Black Bean	1 cup	210	6	0	0	17	7	0
Lots of Lentil	1 cup	230	6	0	0	17	5	5
Mesa Maize	1 cup	160	6	0	0	18	6	10
White Bean Provencal	1 cup	250	10	1	0	32	11	15
Cup-a-Soup								
Broccoli & Cheese as prep	1 serv (6 oz)	70	2	3	5	9	tr	550
Chicken Vegetable as prep	1 serv (6 oz)	50	1	1	10	10	0	520
Chicken Broth as prep	1 serv (6 oz)	20	1	0	0	3	0	440
Chicken Broth w/Pasta Fat Free as prep	1 serv (6 oz)	45	2	0	0	8	0	450
Chicken Noodle as prep	1 serv (6 oz)	50	2	1	10	8	0	540
Cream Of Chicken as prep	1 serv (6 oz)	70	1	2	0	12	tr	640
Creamy Chicken Vegetable as prep	1 serv (6 oz)	80	2	5	0	10	tr	590
Creamy Mushroom as prep	1 serv (6 oz)	60	1	2	0	10	0	610

FOOD	PORTION	CAL	PROT	FAT	CHOL	CARB	FIBER	SOD
Green Pea as prep	1 serv (6 oz)	80	4	1	0	12	3	520
Hearty Chicken Noodle as prep	1 serv (6 oz)	60	3	1	15	10	0	590
Ring Noodle as prep	1 serv (6 oz)	50	2	1	10	9	0	560
Spring Vegetable as prep	1 serv (6 oz)	45	2	1	10	21	tr	500
Tomato as prep	1 serv (6 oz)	100	2	1	5	20	tr	510
George Washington								
Broth & Brown Seasoning	1 serv	6	–	0	–	–	–	–
Broth & Golden Seasoning	1 serv	6	–	0	–	–	–	–
Broth & Onion Seasoning	1 serv	12	–	0	–	–	–	–
Broth & Vegetable Seasoning	1 serv	12	–	0	–	–	–	–
Health Valley								
Chicken Noodles w/ Vegetables	1 serv	110	3	0	0	24	3	190
Corn Chowder w/ Tomatoes	1 serv	100	4	0	0	21	3	190
Creamy Potatoe w/ Broccoli	1 serv	70	4	0	0	17	3	190
Garden Split Pea w/ Carrots	1 serv	130	8	0	0	22	2	190
Lentil w/ Couscous	1 serv	130	7	0	0	28	5	190
Pasta Italiano	1 serv	140	5	0	0	31	3	190
Pasta Marinara	1 serv	100	5	0	0	20	1	190
Pasta Parmesan	1 serv	100	5	0	0	20	1	190
Spicy Black Bean w/ Couscous	1 serv	130	6	0	0	29	5	190
Zesty Black Bean w/ Rice	1 serv	100	5	0	0	22	4	190
Herb-Ox								
Beef Bouillon	1 cube (3.5 g)	5	0	0	0	tr	0	900
Beef Instant Bouillon Powder	1 tsp (4 g)	5	0	0	0	tr	0	1020
Beef Instant Broth & Seasoning Pack	1 pkg (4.5 g)	5	0	0	0	tr	0	1020

FOOD	PORTION	CAL	PROT	FAT	CHOL	CARB	FIBER	SOD
Beef Instant Broth & Seasoning Pack Low Sodium	1 pkg (4 g)	10	0	0	0	2	0	5
Chicken Bouillon	1 cube (4 g)	5	0	0	0	tr	0	1100
Chicken Instant Bouillon Powder	1 tsp (4 g)	5	0	0	0	tr	0	1100
Chicken Instant Broth & Seasoning Pack	1 pkg (4 g)	5	0	0	0	tr	0	1100
Chicken Instant Broth & Seasoning Pack Low Sodium	1 pkg (4 g)	10	0	0	0	2	0	5
Vegetable Bouillon	1 cube (4 g)	5	0	0	0	tr	0	980
Hodgson Mill								
Choice Bean not prep	¼ cup (1.5 oz)	150	9	0	0	27	11	5
Hurst								
15 Bean Soup Beef	1 serv (6 oz)	120	8	1	0	20	9	310
15 Bean Soup Cajun	1 serv	120	8	1	0	20	9	100
15 Bean Soup Chicken	1 serv (6 oz)	120	8	1	0	20	9	250
15 Bean Soup Chili	1 serv (6 oz)	120	8	1	0	20	9	170
15 Bean Soup Ham	1 serv	120	8	1	0	20	9	70
HamBeens Great Northern Bean	1 serv	120	7	1	0	22	11	470
HamBeens Navy Bean	1 serv	120	8	1	0	21	11	470
Pasta Fagioli	1 serv	120	8	1	0	23	9	540
Spanish American Pinto Bean	1 serv	120	7	1	0	22	6	350
Spanish-American Black Bean	1 serv	120	7	1	0	22	8	280
Lipton								
Chicken Noodle w/ White Chicken Meat as prep	1 cup	80	3	2	15	11	0	690
Extra Noodle w/ Chicken Broth as prep	1 cup	90	3	2	25	15	tr	680
Giggle Noodle w/ Chicken Broth as prep	1 cup	70	2	2	20	11	0	750

FOOD	PORTION	CAL	PROT	FAT	CHOL	CARB	FIBER	SOD
Recipe Secrets Beefy Mushroom	1½ tbsp (0.4 oz)	35	1	0	0	7	0	640
Recipe Secrets Beefy Onion	1 tbsp (0.3 oz)	25	1	1	0	5	0	610
Recipe Secrets Fiesta Herb w/ Red Pepper as prep	1 cup	30	1	0	0	6	0	560
Recipe Secrets Golden Herb w/ Lemon as prep	1 cup	35	tr	1	0	7	0	510
Recipe Secrets Golden Onion	1⅔ tbsp (0.5 oz)	50	1	1	0	9	0	700
Recipe Secrets Italian Herb w/ Tomato as prep	1 cup	40	tr	1	0	9	0	510
Recipe Secrets Onion as prep	1 cup	20	0	0	0	4	tr	610
Recipe Secrets Onion Mushroom as prep	1 cup	30	1	1	0	5	0	640
Recipe Secrets Savory Herb w/ Garlic as prep	1 cup	30	1	0	0	6	0	480
Recipe Secrets Vegetable as prep	1 cup	30	tr	0	0	7	1	600
Ring-O-Noodle w/ Chicken Broth as prep	1 cup	70	2	2	15	10	0	720
Soup Secrets Chicken 'N Onion as prep	1 cup	120	4	2	5	24	1	740
Soup Secrets Chicken w/ Pasta & Beans as prep	1 cup	110	5	2	5	19	3	700
Soup Secrets Country Chicken w/ Pasta & Herbs as prep	1 cup	100	4	2	5	18	1	740
Soup Secrets Homestyle Lentil w/ Bow Tie Pasta as prep	1 cup	130	7	1	0	22	5	750

FOOD	PORTION	CAL	PROT	FAT	CHOL	CARB	FIBER	SOD
Soup Secrets Minestrone as prep	1 cup	110	4	1	0	21	4	750
Spiral Pasta w/ Chicken Broth as prep	1 cup	60	2	1	0	11	0	660
Morga								
Vegetable Bouillon No Salt Added	½ cube (5 g)	25	tr	2	0	1	0	115
Vegetable Broth Fat Free	1 tsp (4 g)	10	tr	0	0	2	0	710
Ramen Noodle								
Beef Low Fat as prep	1 pkg (2.2 oz)	216	6	1	1	45	2	1361
Beef as prep	1 pkg (2.2 oz)	280	6	11	tr	40	3	1236
Chicken Low Fat as prep	1 pkg (2.2 oz)	216	7	1	tr	44	2	1335
Chicken as prep	1 pkg (2.2 oz)	279	6	11	1	40	6	1360
Oriental Low Fat as prep	1 pkg (2.2 oz)	217	7	1	0	45	2	1359
Shrimp Low Fat as prep	1 pkg (2.2 oz)	218	7	1	5	45	3	1111
Shrimp as prep	1 pkg (2.2 oz)	294	6	13	1	39	3	972
Tomato as prep	1 pkg (2.2 oz)	295	6	13	tr	39	2	822
Steero								
Beef Bouillon Cube	1 (3.5 g)	5	0	0	–	1	–	900
Beef Bouillon Cube Reduced Sodium	1 cube (3.5 oz)	5	0	0	–	1	–	600
Beef Bouillon Instant	1 tsp (3.5 oz)	5	0	0	–	1	–	900
Beef Bouillon Instant Reduced Sodium	1 tsp (3.5 oz)	5	0	0	–	1	–	600
Chicken Bouillon Cube	1 (3.5 g)	5	0	0	–	1	–	900
Chicken Bouillon Cube Reduced Sodium	1 (3.5 g)	5	0	0	–	1	–	600
Chicken Bouillon Cube Reduced Sodium	1 (3.5 g)	5	0	0	–	1	–	600
Chicken Bouillon Instant	1 tsp (3.5 g)	5	0	0	–	1	–	900

FOOD	PORTION	CAL	PROT	FAT	CHOL	CARB	FIBER	SOD
Chicken Bouillon Instant Reduced Sodium	1 tsp (3.5 g)	5	0	0	–	1	–	600
Thai Kitchen								
Rice Noodle Bowl Roasted Garlic	1 bowl	170	3	2	0	35	0	390
Rice Noodle Bowl Spring Onion	1 bowl	170	3	2	0	35	0	400
Weight Watchers								
Instant Beef Broth	1 pkg (0.16 oz)	10	0	0	0	2	0	800
Instant Chicken Broth	1 pkg (0.16 oz)	10	0	0	0	2	0	830
Wyler's								
Beef Bouillon Cube	1 (3.5 g)	5	0	0	–	1	–	900
Beef Bouillon Cube Reduced Sodium	1 (3.5 g)	5	0	0	–	1	–	600
Beef Bouillon Instant	1 tsp (3.5 g)	5	0	0	–	1	–	900
Beef Bouillon Instant Reduced Sodium	1 tsp (3.5 g)	5	0	0	–	1	–	600
Chicken Bouillon Cube	1 (3.5 g)	5	0	0	–	1	–	900
Chicken Bouillon Cube Reduced Sodium	1 (3.5 g)	5	0	0	–	1	–	900
Chicken Bouillon Instant	1 tsp (3.5)	5	0	0	–	1	–	900
Chicken Bouillon Instant Reduced Sodium	1 tsp (3.5 g)	5	0	0	–	1	–	600
SHELF-STABLE								
Hormel								
Micro Cup Bean & Ham	1 cup (7.5 oz)	190	9	4	15	29	7	680
Micro Cup Beef Vegetable	1 cup (7.5 oz)	90	6	1	10	15	1	790
Micro Cup Broccoli Cheese w/ Ham	1 cup (7.5 oz)	170	4	13	40	10	1	710
Micro Cup Chicken & Rice	1 cup (7.5 oz)	110	5	3	15	17	1	950
Micro Cup Chicken Noodle	1 cup (7.5 oz)	110	8	3	35	13	0	790

FOOD	PORTION	CAL	PROT	FAT	CHOL	CARB	FIBER	SOD
Micro Cup New England Clam Chowder	1 cup (7.5 oz)	130	5	5	25	17	1	820
Micro Cup Potato Cheese w/ Ham	1 cup (7.5 oz)	190	4	13	50	15	1	750
Lunch Bucket								
Chicken Noodle	1 pkg (7.25 oz)	80	2	2	10	13	0	830
Country Vegetable	1 pkg (7.25 oz)	60	1	1	0	14	3	750
TAKE-OUT								
beef stew soup	1 cup (8.8 oz)	221	23	5	60	20	—	461
black bean turtle soup	1 cup	241	15	1	0	45	—	6
brunswick stew soup	1 cup (8.5 oz)	232	27	6	71	17	—	438
corn & cheese chowder	¾ cup	215	9	12	66	21	3	386
gazpacho	1 cup	46	1	tr	0	5	—	63
greek	¾ cup	63	4	2	83	7	2	386
hot & sour	1 serv (14 oz)	173	15	8	87	8	1	475
onion soup gratinee	1 serv	492	25	27	77	38	4	1325
oxtail	5 oz	64	4	3	—	7	—	—
pasta e fagioli	1 cup (8.8 oz)	194	9	5	3	30	—	790
ratatouille	1 cup (7.5 oz)	266	2	25	0	12	—	329
vietnamese pho beef noodle	1 serv (7.8 oz)	480	15	12	46	78	1	43

SOUR CREAM

FOOD	PORTION	CAL	PROT	FAT	CHOL	CARB	FIBER	SOD
sour cream	1 tbsp (0.4 oz)	26	tr	3	5	1	—	6
sour cream	1 cup (8 oz)	493	7	48	102	10	—	123
Breakstone's								
Free	2 tbsp (1.1 oz)	35	2	0	<5	6	0	25
Reduced Fat	2 tbsp (1.1 oz)	45	1	4	15	2	0	20
Sour Cream	2 tbsp (1 oz)	60	tr	5	20	1	0	15
Knudsen								
Free	2 tbsp (1.1 oz)	35	2	0	<5	6	0	25
Hampshire	2 tbsp (1 oz)	60	tr	6	25	1	0	15
Light	2 tbsp (1.1 oz)	50	2	3	10	2	0	10
Land O Lakes								
Fat Free	2 tbsp (1.1 oz)	25	2	0	<5	4	0	40
Light	2 tbsp (1 oz)	40	1	3	10	3	0	35
Sour Cream	2 tbsp (1 oz)	60	tr	6	15	1	0	30

FOOD	PORTION	CAL	PROT	FAT	CHOL	CARB	FIBER	SOD
SOUR CREAM SUBSTITUTES								
nondairy	1 cup	479	6	45	0	15	–	235
nondairy	1 oz	59	1	6	0	2	–	29
SOURSOP								
fresh	1	416	6	2	0	105	–	87
fresh cut up	1 cup	150	2	1	0	38	–	31
SOY (see also CHEESE SUBSTITUTES, ICE CREAM AND FROZEN DESSERTS, MILK SUBSTITUTES, MISO, SOY SAUCE, SOYBEANS, TEMPEH, TOFU, YOGURT FROZEN)								
lecithin	1 tbsp	104	0	14	0	0	–	–
soy milk	1 cup	79	7	5	0	4	–	30
soya cheese	1.4 oz	128	7	11	–	tr	0	–
I.M. Healthy								
SoyNut Butter Chocolate	2 tbsp (1.1 oz)	190	5	14	0	12	4	50
SoyNut Butter Honey Creamy	2 tbsp (1.1 oz)	170	7	11	0	12	2	150
SoyNut Butter Original Creamy	2 tbsp (1.1 oz)	170	8	11	0	10	1	170
SoyNut Butter Unsweetened Chunky	2 tbsp (1.1 oz)	160	7	13	0	5	5	160
SoyNut Butter Unsweetened Creamy	2 tbsp (1.1 oz)	160	7	13	0	5	5	160
Loma Linda								
Soyagen All Purpose	¼ cup (1 oz)	130	6	6	0	12	3	150
Soyagen Carob	¼ cup (1 oz)	130	6	6	0	13	2	170
Soyagen No Sucrose	¼ cup (1 oz)	130	6	6	0	12	3	160
Natural Touch								
Roasted Soy Butter	2 tbsp (1.1 oz)	170	6	11	0	10	1	170
Revival								
Chocolate Soy Nuts!	12–14 pieces (0.5 oz)	70	2	4	2	7	tr	8
Soy Shake Plain as prep w/ water	1 pkg (1 oz)	110	20	2	0	2	0	360
Soy Shakes Chocolate Daydreams as prep w/ water	1 pkg (2.2 oz)	240	20	3	0	36	2	290
Soy Shakes Vanilla Pleasures as prep w/ water	1 pkg (2 oz)	220	20	2	0	31	0	290

FOOD	PORTION	CAL	PROT	FAT	CHOL	CARB	FIBER	SOD
Soy Wonder								
Creamy	2 tbsp	170	8	11	0	10	1	170
Crunchy	2 tbsp	170	8	11	0	10	1	170
SOY SAUCE								
shoyu	1 tbsp	9	1	tr	0	2	–	1029
soy sauce	1 tbsp	7	tr	tr	0	1	–	1024
tamari	1 tbsp	11	2	tr	0	1	–	1005
Chun King								
Lite	1 tbsp (0.5 oz)	15	2	tr	0	2	0	542
Soy Sauce	1 tbsp (0.6 oz)	11	2	tr	0	1	0	1227
Eden								
Organic Shoyu Reduced Sodium	1 tbsp	10	2	0	0	2	0	500
Organic Tamari	1 tbsp	15	2	0	0	2	0	860
Ponzu Sauce	1 tbsp	5	0	0	0	1	0	340
Shoyu	1 tbsp	15	2	0	0	2	0	1010
House Of Tsang								
Ginger Flavored	1 tbsp (0.6 oz)	20	1	0	0	4	0	730
Light	1 tbsp (0.6 oz)	5	1	0	0	0	0	900
Low Sodium	1 tbsp (0.6 oz)	5	0	0	0	0	0	280
Low Sodium Ginger	1 tbsp (0.6 oz)	10	0	0	0	2	0	280
Low Sodium Mushroom	1 tbsp (0.6 oz)	10	0	0	0	2	0	280
Just Rite								
Soy Sauce	1 tbsp (0.5 oz)	11	2	tr	0	1	0	1227
Kikkoman								
Lite	1 tbsp (0.5 oz)	10	1	0	0	1	–	575
Soy Sauce	1 tbsp (0.5 oz)	10	2	0	0	0	0	920
La Choy								
Lite	1 tbsp (0.5 oz)	15	2	tr	0	2	0	542
Soy Sauce	1 tbsp (0.6 oz)	11	2	tr	0	1	0	1227
Tree Of Life								
Shoyu	1 tbsp (0.5 oz)	15	2	0	0	1	–	960
Tamari Wheat Free	1 tbsp (0.5 oz)	15	2	0	0	1	–	940
SOYBEANS								
dried cooked	1 cup	298	29	15	0	17	–	1
dry roasted	½ cup	387	34	19	0	28	–	2
green cooked	½ cup	127	11	6	0	10	4	13

FOOD	PORTION	CAL	PROT	FAT	CHOL	CARB	FIBER	SOD
roasted	½ cup	405	30	22	0	29	–	140
sprouts steamed	½ cup	38	4	2	0	3	–	5
sprouts stir fried	1 cup	125	13	7	0	9	–	14
Dakota Gourmet								
Soy Nuts	1 oz	129	11	7	0	9	1	217
Eden								
Organic Black	½ cup (4.6 oz)	120	11	6	0	8	7	30
Seapoint Farms								
Edamame Organic	½ cup (2.6 oz)	100	8	3	0	9	4	30
Edamame In Pods frzn	½ cup (2.6 oz)	100	8	3	0	9	4	30
Edamame Rice Bowl Kung Pao Vegetable	1 pkg (12 oz)	420	15	6	0	72	6	960
Edamame Rice Bowl Szechwan Vegetables	1 pkg (12 oz)	420	13	4	0	80	6	510
Edamame Rice Bowl Teriyaki Vegetable	1 pkg (12 oz)	430	14	5	0	83	5	1130
Edamame Rice Bowl Vegetable Fried Rice	1 pkg (11 oz)	220	11	6	40	31	1	950
Edamane Shelled	½ cup (2.6 oz)	100	8	3	0	9	4	30

SPAGHETTI *(see* PASTA, PASTA DINNERS, PASTA SALAD, SPAGHETTI SAUCE*)*

SPAGHETTI SAUCE
JARRED
Colavita

FOOD	PORTION	CAL	PROT	FAT	CHOL	CARB	FIBER	SOD
Garden Style	½ cup (4.4 oz)	60	3	3	0	12	3	290
Del Monte								
Chunky Garlic & Herb	½ cup (4.4 oz)	60	2	2	0	11	1	490
Chunky Italian Herb	½ cup (4.4 oz)	60	2	1	0	12	1	520
Tomato & Basil	½ cup (4.4 oz)	70	2	1	0	16	3	600
Traditional	½ cup (4.4 oz)	60	2	1	0	15	3	590
With Garlic & Onion	½ cup (4.4 oz)	80	2	1	0	16	2	490
With Green Peppers & Mushrooms	½ cup (4.4 oz)	80	2	1	0	16	3	490
With Meat	½ cup (4.4 oz)	60	3	1	4	14	3	720
With Mushrooms	½ cup (4.4 oz)	60	2	1	0	14	2	630

FOOD	PORTION	CAL	PROT	FAT	CHOL	CARB	FIBER	SOD
Eden								
Organic Lightly Seasoned	½ cup (4.4 oz)	80	3	3	0	12	3	320
Francesco Rinaldi								
Alfredo	¼ cup (2.1 oz)	70	2	5	15	4	0	410
Chunky Garden Mushroom & Onion	½ cup (4.4 oz)	80	3	2	0	12	3	690
Chunky Garden Tomato Garlic & Onion	½ cup (4.4 oz)	80	3	2	0	12	3	690
Dolce Sweet & Tasty Tomato	½ cup (4.4 oz)	110	2	5	0	15	3	610
Dolce Three Cheese	½ cup (4.4 oz)	90	3	2	0	15	3	490
Dulce Super Mushroom	½ cup (4.4 oz)	110	3	5	0	15	3	490
Hearty Diavolo	½ cup (4.4 oz)	70	2	4	0	7	3	550
Hearty Mushroom Pepper & Onion	½ cup (4.4 oz)	80	3	3	0	10	3	690
Hearty Tomato & Basil	½ cup (4.4 oz)	80	2	3	0	11	4	730
Puttanesca	½ cup (4.3 oz)	70	2	4	0	8	tr	720
Tomato Alfredo	¼ cup (2.1 oz)	60	2	4	10	4	0	290
Traditional Meat Flavored	½ cup (4.4 oz)	90	2	4	4	11	3	700
Traditional Mushroom	1.2 cup (4.4 oz)	90	2	4	0	11	3	700
Traditional No Salt Added	½ cup (4.4 oz)	70	2	3	0	10	tr	25
Traditional Original	½ cup (4.4 oz)	90	2	4	0	11	3	700
Vodka Sauce	¼ cup (2.1 oz)	60	2	4	10	4	0	290
Healthy Choice								
Chunky Italian Vegetable	½ cup (4.4 oz)	40	2	tr	0	9	2	299
Chunky Mushroom	½ cup (4.4 oz)	42	2	tr	0	9	2	297
Garlic & Herbs	½ cup (4.4 oz)	49	2	tr	0	10	2	337
Garlic Lovers Garlic & Mushroom	½ cup (4.4 oz)	44	2	tr	0	10	2	362

FOOD	PORTION	CAL	PROT	FAT	CHOL	CARB	FIBER	SOD
Garlic Lovers Roasted Garlic	½ cup (4.4 oz)	52	2	tr	0	12	3	293
Garlic Lovers Roasted Garlic & Sun Dried Tomato	½ cup (4.4 oz)	52	2	tr	0	11	3	357
Super Chunky Mushroom & Sweet Peppers	½ cup (4.4 oz)	43	2	tr	0	9	2	308
Super Chunky Tomato Mushroom & Garlic	½ cup (4.4 oz)	45	2	tr	0	10	2	372
Super Chunky Vegetable Primavera	½ cup (4.4 oz)	43	2	tr	0	9	2	327
Traditional	½ cup (4.4 oz)	48	2	tr	0	11	2	378
With Mushrooms	½ cup (4.4 oz)	48	2	tr	0	11	2	378
Hunt's								
Angela Mia Marinara	¼ cup (2.2 oz)	24	1	1	0	4	2	252
Chunky	½ cup (4.4 oz)	38	1	1	0	8	2	467
Chunky Italian Sausage	½ cup (4.5 oz)	72	3	3	2	45	3	542
Chunky Italian Style Vegetable	½ cup (4.4 oz)	63	2	1	0	13	2	528
Chunky Marinara	½ cup (4.4 oz)	61	1	1	0	12	2	526
Chunky Tomato Garlic & Onion	½ cup (4.4 oz)	63	2	1	0	13	2	528
Classic Four Cheese	½ cup (4.4 oz)	50	3	1	0	9	3	600
Classic Garlic & Herb	½ cup (4.4 oz)	53	2	2	0	9	3	600
Classic Parmesan	½ cup (4.4 oz)	49	3	2	1	8	3	600
Classic Tomato & Basil	½ cup (4.4 oz)	48	2	1	0	9	2	563
Family Favorites Seasoned Diced Tomato Sauce	½ cup (4.3 oz)	50	2	1	0	11	2	810
Homestyle Meat Flavored	½ cup (4.4 oz)	51	2	2	0	9	3	600
Homestyle Mushrooms	½ cup (4.4 oz)	48	2	1	0	9	3	530

FOOD	PORTION	CAL	PROT	FAT	CHOL	CARB	FIBER	SOD
Homestyle Traditional	½ cup (4.4 oz)	49	2	1	0	9	3	598
Light Meat Flavored	½ cup (4.4 oz)	45	2	1	2	8	3	437
Light w/ Garlic & Herb	½ cup (4.5 oz)	40	2	1	0	7	3	380
Original Meat Flavored	½ cup (4.4 oz)	68	2	2	1	12	3	600
Original Traditional	½ cup (4.4 oz)	67	2	2	0	11	3	477
Original w/ Mushrooms	½ cup (4.4 oz)	62	2	2	0	11	3	605
Original w/ Italian Cheese & Garlic	½ cup (4.5 oz)	64	3	2	1	10	3	622
Tomato Bits	½ cup (4.5 oz)	49	2	tr	0	11	3	607
Traditional Light	½ cup (4.4 oz)	40	2	tr	0	7	1	400
Muir Glen								
Organic Balsamic Roasted Onion	½ cup (4.4 oz)	50	2	1	0	10	0	320
Organic Cabernet Marinara	½ cup (4.4 oz)	50	2	1	0	10	0	330
Organic Chunky Herb	½ cup (4.4 oz)	50	2	1	0	10	0	320
Organic Garden Vegetable	½ cup (4.4 oz)	50	2	1	0	10	0	120
Organic Garlic & Onion	½ cup (4.4 oz)	55	2	1	0	10	0	320
Organic Garlic Roasted Garlic	½ cup (4.4 oz)	50	2	1	0	10	0	320
Organic Green Olive	½ cup (4.4 oz)	60	2	2	0	10	0	350
Organic Italian Herb	½ cup (4.4 oz)	55	2	1	0	10	0	320
Organic Mushroom Marinara	½ cup (4.4 oz)	45	2	0	0	10	0	120
Organic Portabello Mushroom	½ cup (4.4 oz)	50	2	0	0	10	0	330
Organic Sun Dried Tomato	½ cup (4.4 oz)	55	2	1	0	10	1	170
Organic Tomato Basil	½ cup (4.4 oz)	50	2	1	0	12	0	370
Newman's Own								
Marinara Ventian	½ cup (4.4 oz)	60	2	2	0	9	3	590
Marinara Ventian w/ Mushrooms	½ cup (4.4 oz)	60	2	2	0	9	3	590

FOOD	PORTION	CAL	PROT	FAT	CHOL	CARB	FIBER	SOD
Pasta Sauce Bambolina	½ cup (4.5 oz)	100	1	5	0	15	5	590
Pasta Sauce Roasted Garlic & Red & Green Peppers	½ cup (4.7 oz)	70	2	3	0	11	4	460
Pasta Sauce Say Cheese	½ cup (4.4 oz)	90	3	3	<5	14	3	510
Sockarooni	½ cup (4.4 oz)	60	2	2	0	9	3	590
Prego								
Pasta Bake Sauce Tomato Garlic & Basil	1 serv (3.4 oz)	80	1	4	0	11	2	530
Traditional	½ cup (4.2 oz)	140	2	5	0	23	2	610
Progresso								
Marinara	½ cup (4.3 oz)	80	2	5	<5	8	2	480
Meat Flavored	½ cup (4.4 oz)	100	4	5	5	12	3	610
Sauce	½ cup (4.4 oz)	100	3	5	<5	12	2	620
Ragu								
Chunky Garden Style Tomato Garlic & Onion	½ cup (4.5 oz)	110	2	3	0	18	2	520
Sara Lee								
Chunky Garden Mushroom & Peppers	½ cup (4.4 oz)	80	3	2	0	12	3	690
Tree Of Life								
Pasta Sauce	½ cup (4 oz)	50	2	2	0	9	–	290
Pasta Sauce Fat Free Classic	½ cup (3.9 oz)	40	2	0	0	8	0	250
Pasta Sauce Fat Free Mushroom & Basil	½ cup (3.9 oz)	30	1	0	0	7	0	300
Pasta Sauce Fat Free Onion & Garlic	½ cup (3.9 oz)	30	1	0	0	7	0	240
Pasta Sauce Fat Free Sweet Pepper	½ cup (3.9 oz)	30	1	0	0	7	0	280
Pasta Sauce No Salt Added	½ cup (3.9 oz)	50	2	2	0	9	–	0

FOOD	PORTION	CAL	PROT	FAT	CHOL	CARB	FIBER	SOD
MIX								
Durkee								
Spaghetti Sauce as prep	½ cup	15	0	0	0	5	0	390
With Mushrooms as prep	½ cup	15	1	0	0	4	0	520
French's								
Italian as prep	½ cup	16	0	0	0	5	0	390
Mushroom as prep	½ cup	20	1	1	2	4	0	760
Thick as prep	½ cup	10	0	0	0	4	0	630
McCormick								
Alfredo Pasta Blend as prep	½ cup	60	–	2	10	4	0	680
Pasta Rosa Blend	1 tbsp (10 g)	40	1	2	<5	4	0	540
Pesto Pasta Sauce as prep	2 tsp (4 g)	10	tr	0	–	tr	–	480
Primavera Pasta Blend	1 tbsp (7 g)	30	0	1	–	4	–	490
Spaghetti Sauce	1 tbsp (8 g)	25	0	0	–	5	–	490
REFRIGERATED								
Di Giorno								
Alfredo	¼ cup (2.2 oz)	180	3	18	25	3	0	600
Basil Pesto	¼ cup (2.2 oz)	320	7	31	15	2	tr	530
Four Cheese	¼ cup (2.2 oz)	160	5	15	30	3	0	410
Garlic Pesto	¼ cup (2.1 oz)	340	7	33	15	3	tr	540
Light Alfredo Sauce	¼ cup (2.4 oz)	140	5	9	30	9	0	600
Marinara	½ cup (4.5 oz)	70	2	0	0	15	2	220
Plum Tomato Cream Sauce	½ cup (4.4 oz)	160	3	13	40	8	2	370
Plum Tomato & Mushroom	½ cup (4.4 oz)	60	2	0	0	13	2	260
Roasted Red Bell Pepper Cream Sauce	¼ cup (2.3 oz)	140	4	10	35	8	0	510
TAKE-OUT								
bolognese	5 oz	195	11	15	–	4	tr	–

FOOD	PORTION	CAL	PROT	FAT	CHOL	CARB	FIBER	SOD

SPANISH FOOD (see also BEANS, CHILI, CHIPS, DINNER, PEPPERS, SALSA, SAUCE, SNACKS, TORTILLA)

CANNED

Chi-Chi's

FOOD	PORTION	CAL	PROT	FAT	CHOL	CARB	FIBER	SOD
Pico De Gallo	2 tbsp (1.2 oz)	10	0	0	0	2	0	170
Derby								
Tamales	3 (6.5 oz)	253	7	17	23	21	4	1034
Gebhardt								
Enchiladas	2 (5.7 oz)	258	4	19	25	20	3	687
Tamales	2 (5.7 oz)	268	5	21	28	19	3	770
Tamales Jumbo	2 (6.9 oz)	332	6	25	34	24	3	930
Hormel								
Tamales Beef	3 (7.5 oz)	280	6	21	35	20	3	1010
Tamales Chicken	3 (7.5 oz)	210	6	11	50	22	2	1020
Tamales Hot Spicy Beef	3 (7.5 oz)	280	6	21	35	20	3	1010
Tamales Jumbo Beef	2 (6.9 oz)	270	5	20	35	18	3	940
Old El Paso								
Tamales	3 (7.2 oz)	330	7	19	30	31	5	590
Rosarita								
Enchilada Sauce Mild	¼ cup (2.1 oz)	23	1	1	0	3	0	409
Van Camp								
Tamales	2 (5 oz)	210	5	13	20	20	3	610
FROZEN								
Amy's Organic								
Black Bean Vegetable Enchilada	1 (4.75 oz)	130	4	4	0	20	2	390
Burritos Bean & Cheese	1 (6 oz)	280	10	8	10	43	6	460
Burritos Bean & Rice Non-Dairy	1 (6 oz)	250	9	5	0	44	6	450
Burritos Black Bean Vegetable	1 (6 oz)	320	9	8	0	54	4	480
Burritos Breakfast	1 (6 oz)	230	9	5	0	38	5	480
Cheese Enchilada	1 (4.7 oz)	210	11	9	20	16	2	390
Mexican Tamale Pie	1 (8 oz)	220	10	3	0	41	11	480
Pocket Sandwich Tamale	1 (4.5 oz)	250	8	7	10	39	3	580

FOOD	PORTION	CAL	PROT	FAT	CHOL	CARB	FIBER	SOD
Whole Meals Cheese Enchilada	1 pkg (9 oz)	330	15	14	30	38	6	680
Whole Meals Enchilada	1 pkg (10 oz)	250	7	8	0	41	5	680
Banquet								
Chimichanga Meal	1 meal (9.5 oz)	500	13	24	20	56	9	1180
Enchilada Beef	1 pkg (11 oz)	370	10	12	20	54	6	1330
Enchilada Cheese	1 pkg (11 oz)	360	12	10	20	56	6	1500
Enchilada Chicken	1 pkg (11 oz)	350	12	10	25	54	9	1580
Enchilada Beef & Tamale Combo	1 pkg (11 oz)	450	10	20	30	50	9	1530
Mexican Style Enchilada Combo	1 meal (11 oz)	360	10	11	20	55	9	1390
Chi-Chi's								
Burro Beef	1 pkg (15.9 oz)	590	27	19	55	76	11	2060
Burro Chicken	1 pkg (15.9 oz)	540	26	14	55	77	10	2110
Chimichanga Beef	1 pkg (15.9 oz)	630	28	24	55	75	10	2050
Chimichanga Chicken	1 pkg (15.9 oz)	580	25	19	50	78	10	2100
Enchilada Chicken Suprema	1 pkg (15.9 oz)	600	26	20	70	80	11	2310
Enchilida Baja	1 pkg (15.9 oz)	590	27	20	50	75	15	1920
Health Is Wealth								
Burrito Munchees	10 (5 oz)	310	11	7	5	53	6	610
Mexican Munchees	2 (1 oz)	49	2	1	0	8	1	110
Healthy Choice								
Chicken Enchilada Supreme	1 meal (11.3 oz)	300	13	7	40	46	4	560
Chicken Enchiladas Suiz	1 meal (10 oz)	280	14	6	40	43	5	440
Chicken Breast Con Queso Burrito	1 meal (10.55 oz)	350	14	6	35	60	6	590
Lean Cuisine								
Everyday Favorites Chicken Enchilada Suiza	1 pkg (9 oz)	280	11	5	25	48	3	520
Old El Paso								
Burrito Bean & Cheese	1 (4.9 oz)	290	12	9	15	44	3	840

FOOD	PORTION	CAL	PROT	FAT	CHOL	CARB	FIBER	SOD
Burrito Beef & Bean Hot	1 (5 oz)	320	12	10	15	45	3	850
Burrito Beef & Bean Medium	1 (5 oz)	320	12	10	15	46	3	800
Burrito Beef & Bean Mild	1 (5 oz)	330	12	9	15	48	4	690
Chimichanga Beef	1 (4.5 oz)	370	9	20	10	37	3	470
Chimichanga Chicken	1 (4.5 oz)	350	11	16	20	39	2	540
Patio								
Beef & Cheese Enchiladas Chili 'N Beans	1 meal (15.5 oz)	670	19	30	60	80	12	2400
Beef Enchiladas Chili 'N Beans	1 meal (15.5 oz)	540	12	27	50	73	12	2690
Burrito Bean & Cheese	1 (5 oz)	300	9	9	15	45	4	690
Burrito Beef & Bean Hot	1 (5 oz)	320	10	12	25	43	4	840
Burrito Beef & Bean Mild	1 (5 oz)	330	10	12	20	45	4	890
Burrito Chicken	1 (5 oz)	290	11	6	20	44	2	740
Burritos Beef & Bean Medium	1 (5 oz)	310	10	10	20	45	4	660
Burritos Beef & Bean Red Chili Pepper Red Hot	1 (5 oz)	320	10	12	20	42	4	850
Enchilada Beef	1 meal (12 oz)	320	12	12	25	52	9	1700
Enchilada Cheese	1 meal (12 oz)	370	11	12	25	54	7	1570
Enchilada Chicken	1 meal (12 oz)	400	13	12	35	60	8	1470
Fiesta	1 meal (12 oz)	350	11	11	25	53	7	1760
Mexican Style	1 meal (13.25 oz)	470	15	19	20	59	10	2210
Stouffer's								
Chicken Enchilada	1 serv (4.8 oz)	230	7	11	30	25	3	530
Tyson								
Beef Fajita	3½ pieces (12.5 oz)	550	28	16	20	75	6	1130
Chicken Fajita	3½ pieces (13.1 oz)	460	28	11	45	61	6	1220
Weight Watchers								
Smart Ones Chicken Enchiladas Suiza	1 pkg (9 oz)	270	15	9	50	33	2	660

FOOD	PORTION	CAL	PROT	FAT	CHOL	CARB	FIBER	SOD
Smart Ones Santa Fe Style Rice & Beans	1 pkg (10 oz)	290	12	8	20	43	6	590
MIX								
Gebhardt								
Menudo Mix	¼ tsp (0.4 g)	1	tr	tr	0	tr	tr	52
McCormick								
Burrito Seasoning	1 tbsp (8 g)	25	tr	1	—	5	tr	500
Fajitas Marinade Mix	2 tsp (4 g)	15	0	0	—	2	—	250
Taco Seasoning Hot	2 tsp (6 g)	20	tr	0	—	3	tr	430
Taco Seasoning Mild	2 tsp (7 g)	20	tr	0	—	4	tr	460
Old El Paso								
Burrito Seasoning Mix	2 tsp (6 g)	20	tr	0	0	3	1	290
Dinner Kit Burrito as prep	1	280	—	7	66	35	3	840
Dinner Kit Soft Taco as prep	2	380	—	10	63	45	3	1340
Dinner Kit Taco as prep	2	270	—	13	60	21	4	910
Enchilada Sauce Mix	2 tsp (4 g)	10	0	0	0	2	tr	540
Taco Mix 40% Less Sodium	2 tsp (6 g)	20	0	0	0	4	0	330
Taco Seasoning Mix	2 tsp (6 g)	20	0	0	0	5	0	550
Taco Bell								
Home Originals Chicken Fajita Dinner as prep	2 (6.9 oz)	340	21	9	40	45	3	1120
Home Originals Chicken Fajita Seasoning Mix	1 tbsp (8 g)	25	tr	0	0	5	2	540
Home Originals Soft Taco Dinner as prep	2 (6.3 oz)	410	21	18	60	41	2	1090
Home Originals Taco Dinner as prep	2 (4.4 oz)	280	16	15	50	19	2	580
Home Originals Taco Seasoning Mix	2 tsp (6 g)	20	tr	0	0	3	tr	450
Home Originals Ultimate Bean Burrito Dinner as prep	1 (4.4 oz)	200	6	5	0	34	3	710

FOOD	PORTION	CAL	PROT	FAT	CHOL	CARB	FIBER	SOD
Home Originals Ultimate Nachos as prep	12 pieces (4.6 oz)	240	6	11	0	31	4	680
READY-TO-EAT								
taco shell baked	1 med (0.5 oz)	61	1	3	0	8	tr	48
taco shell baked w/o salt	1 med (½ oz)	61	1	3	0	8	tr	2
Chi-Chi's								
Taco Shells White Corn	2 (1.2 oz)	170	3	8	0	22	2	0
Taco Shells Yellow Corn	2 shells (1.2 oz)	170	2	8	0	22	2	0
Gebhardt								
Taco Shells	3 (1.1 oz)	155	2	8	0	19	3	1
La Mexicana								
Flour Burritos	1 (1.6 oz)	160	4	5	0	26	2	580
Old El Paso								
Taco Shells Mini	7 (1.1 oz)	160	2	10	0	18	2	130
Taco Shells Regular	3 (1.1 oz)	170	2	10	0	18	2	130
Taco Shells Super	2 (1.3 oz)	190	3	12	0	21	2	150
Taco Shells White Corn	3 (1.1 oz)	170	2	10	0	18	2	30
Tostaco Shells	1 (0.8 oz)	130	2	7	0	14	1	10
Tostada Shells	3 (1.1 oz)	160	2	10	0	19	2	220
Rosarita								
Taco Shells	3 (1.1 oz)	155	2	8	0	19	3	1
Tostada Shells	2 (1 oz)	125	2	5	37	17	0	20
Taco Bell								
Home Originals Taco Shells	3 (1.1 oz)	150	2	6	0	21	2	5
TAKE-OUT								
burrito w/ apple	1 sm (2.6 oz)	231	3	10	3	35	—	211
burrito w/ apple	1 lg (5.4 oz)	484	5	20	7	73	—	443
burrito w/ beans	2 (7.6 oz)	448	14	14	5	71	—	986
burrito w/ beans & cheese	2 (6.5 oz)	377	15	12	27	55	—	1166
burrito w/ beans & chili peppers	2 (7.2 oz)	413	16	15	33	58	—	1043
burrito w/ beans & meat	2 (8.1 oz)	508	22	18	48	66	—	1335

FOOD	PORTION	CAL	PROT	FAT	CHOL	CARB	FIBER	SOD
burrito w/ beans cheese & beef	2 (7.1 oz)	331	15	13	125	40	—	990
burrito w/ beans cheese & chili peppers	2 (11.8 oz)	663	33	23	158	85	—	2060
burrito w/ beef	2 (7.7 oz)	523	27	21	65	59	—	1492
burrito w/ beef & chili peppers	2 (7.1 oz)	426	22	17	54	49	—	1116
burrito w/ beef cheese & chili peppers	2 (10.7 oz)	634	41	25	170	64	—	2091
burrito w/ cherry	1 sm (2.6 oz)	231	3	10	3	35	—	211
burrito w/ cherry	1 lg (5.4 oz)	484	5	20	7	73	—	443
chimichanga w/ beef	1 (6.1 oz)	425	20	20	9	43	—	910
chimichanga w/ beef & cheese	1 (6.4 oz)	443	20	23	51	39	—	956
chimichanga w/ beef & red chili peppers	1 (6.7 oz)	424	18	19	9	46	—	1169
chimichanga w/ beef cheese & red chili peppers	1 (6.3 oz)	364	15	18	50	38	—	895
enchilada eggplant	1	142	—	5	7	—	—	—
enchilada w/ cheese	1 (5.7 oz)	320	10	19	44	29	—	784
enchilada w/ cheese & beef	1 (6.7 oz)	324	12	18	40	30	—	1320
enchirito w/ cheese beef & beans	1 (6.8 oz)	344	18	16	49	34	—	1251
frijoles w/ cheese	1 cup (5.9 oz)	226	11	8	36	29	—	882
nachos w/ cheese	6 to 8 (4 oz)	345	9	19	18	36	—	816
nachos w/ cheese & jalapeno peppers	6 to 8 (7.2 oz)	607	17	34	83	60	—	1736
nachos w/ cheese beans ground beef & peppers	6 to 8 (8.9 oz)	568	20	31	21	56	—	1800
nachos w/ cinnamon & sugar	6 to 8 (3.8 oz)	592	7	36	39	63	—	439
taco	1 sm (6 oz)	370	21	21	57	27	—	802
taco salad	1½ cups	279	13	15	44	24	—	763

FOOD	PORTION	CAL	PROT	FAT	CHOL	CARB	FIBER	SOD
taco salad w/ chili con carne	1½ cups	288	17	13	4	27	—	886
tostada w/ beans & cheese	1 (5.1 oz)	223	10	10	30	27	—	543
tostada w/ beans beef & cheese	1 (7.9 oz)	334	16	17	75	30	—	870
tostada w/ beef & cheese	1 (5.7 oz)	315	19	16	41	23	—	896
tostada w/ guacamole	2 (9.2 oz)	360	12	23	39	32	—	789

SPICES (see individual names, HERBS/SPICES)

SPINACH
CANNED
spinach	½ cup	25	3	1	0	4	—	29
Del Monte								
Chopped	½ cup (4 oz)	30	2	0	0	4	2	360
No Salt Added	½ cup (4 oz)	30	2	0	0	4	2	85
Whole Leaf	½ cup (4 oz)	30	2	0	0	4	2	360
S&W								
Spinach	½ cup (4.5 oz)	30	3	0	0	4	2	440
FRESH								
cooked	½ cup	21	3	tr	0	3	2	63
malabar cooked	1 cup (1.5 oz)	10	1	tr	0	1	1	24
mustard chopped cooked	½ cup	14	2	tr	0	3	—	—
mustard raw chopped	½ cup	17	2	tr	0	3	—	—
new zealand chopped cooked	½ cup	11	1	tr	0	2	—	97
new zealand raw	½ cup	4	tr	tr	0	1	—	36
raw chopped	½ cup	6	1	tr	0	1	1	22
raw chopped	1 pkg (10 oz)	46	6	1	0	7	—	160
Dole								
Baby Spinach	3½ cups (3 oz)	35	2	0	0	9	4	135
FROZEN								
cooked	½ cup	27	3	tr	0	5	—	82
Amy's Organic								
Pocket Sandwich Spinach Feta	1 (4.5 oz)	200	9	7	15	27	2	420

FOOD	PORTION	CAL	PROT	FAT	CHOL	CARB	FIBER	SOD
Birds Eye								
Chopped	⅓ cup	20	0	0	–	–	2	80
Creamed	½ cup (4.3 oz)	100	3	7	35	7	1	660
Cut Leaf	1 cup (2.8 oz)	20	2	0	0	2	2	110
Green Giant								
Butter Sauce	½ cup (3.4 oz)	40	2	2	<5	5	2	280
Creamed	½ cup (3.8 oz)	80	4	3	0	10	2	520
Cut Leaf	¾ cup (2.6 oz)	25	3	0	0	3	3	65
Harvest Fresh	½ cup (3.5 oz)	25	3	0	0	3	2	240
Health Is Wealth								
Spinach Munchees	2 (1 oz)	60	2	3	0	9	1	105
Spinach Feta Munchees	2 (1 oz)	70	2	3	5	9	1	115
Stouffer's								
Creamed	1 serv (4.5 oz)	160	4	12	15	8	2	380
Souffle	1 serv (4 oz)	150	6	10	120	9	0	480
Tree Of Life								
Organic	1 cup (3 oz)	20	2	0	0	2	2	110
TAKE-OUT								
indian saag	1 serv	28	2	2	0	2	1	44
spanakopita spinach pie	1 cup (6 oz)	196	14	3	30	35	4	590

SPINACH JUICE

FOOD	PORTION	CAL	PROT	FAT	CHOL	CARB	FIBER	SOD
juice	7 oz	14	2	0	0	2	–	146

SPOT

FOOD	PORTION	CAL	PROT	FAT	CHOL	CARB	FIBER	SOD
baked	3 oz	134	20	5	–	0	–	32

SPORTS DRINKS (see ENERGY DRINKS)

SPROUTS

FOOD	PORTION	CAL	PROT	FAT	CHOL	CARB	FIBER	SOD
kidney bean	½ cup	27	4	tr	0	4	–	–
kidney bean cooked	1 lb	152	22	3	0	21	–	–
lentil sprouts	½ cup	40	3	tr	0	8	–	4
mung bean	½ cup	16	2	tr	0	3	–	3
mung bean canned	½ cup	8	1	tr	0	1	–	–
mung bean cooked	½ cup	13	1	tr	0	3	–	6
navy bean	½ cup	35	–	tr	0	–	–	–
navy bean cooked	3½ oz	78	–	1	0	–	–	–
pea	½ cup	77	5	tr	0	17	–	12
pinto bean	3½ oz	62	–	1	0	12	–	–

FOOD	PORTION	CAL	PROT	FAT	CHOL	CARB	FIBER	SOD
pinto bean cooked	3½ oz	22	–	tr	0	4	–	–
radish	½ cup	8	1	tr	0	1	–	1
Chun King								
Bean Sprouts	1 cup (3 oz)	11	1	tr	0	1	1	17
Fresh Alternatives								
BroccoSprouts	½ cup (1 oz)	10	1	0	0	1	1	0
Deli Blend	½ cup (1 oz)	10	1	0	0	1	tr	0
Salad Blend	½ cup (1 oz)	10	1	0	0	2	tr	0
Sandwich Blend	½ cup (1 oz)	5	1	0	0	1	tr	0
La Choy								
Bean Sprouts	1 cup (2.9 oz)	11	1	tr	0	1	1	17
TAKE-OUT								
mung bean stir fried	½ cup	31	3	tr	0	7	–	–

SQUAB

FOOD	PORTION	CAL	PROT	FAT	CHOL	CARB	FIBER	SOD
boneless baked	3.5 oz	175	37	3	75	0	0	100
breast w/o skin raw	1 (3.5 oz)	135	22	5	91	0	–	–
w/o skin raw	1 squab (5.9 oz)	239	29	13	–	0	–	–

SQUASH (see also ZUCCHINI)

FOOD	PORTION	CAL	PROT	FAT	CHOL	CARB	FIBER	SOD
seeds dried	1 oz	154	7	13	0	5	–	5
seeds whole roasted	1 oz	127	5	6	0	15	–	5
CANNED								
crookneck sliced	½ cup	14	1	tr	0	3	–	5
FRESH								
acorn cooked mashed	½ cup	41	1	tr	0	11	3	3
acorn cubed baked	½ cup	57	1	tr	0	15	2	4
butternut baked	½ cup	41	1	tr	0	11	2	4
crookneck raw sliced	½ cup	12	1	tr	0	3	1	1
crookneck sliced cooked	½ cup	18	1	tr	0	4	1	1
hubbard baked	½ cup	51	3	tr	0	11	3	8
hubbard cooked mashed	½ cup	35	2	tr	0	8	3	6
scallop raw sliced	½ cup	12	1	tr	0	3	1	1
scallop sliced cooked	½ cup	14	1	tr	0	3	1	1
spaghetti cooked	½ cup	23	1	tr	0	5	2	14
FROZEN								
butternut cooked mashed	½ cup	47	1	tr	0	12	3	2

FOOD	PORTION	CAL	PROT	FAT	CHOL	CARB	FIBER	SOD
crookneck sliced cooked	½ cup	24	1	tr	0	5	–	6
Birds Eye								
Cooked Squash	½ cup	50	–	0	0	–	4	0
Sliced Yellow	⅔ cup (2.7 oz)	15	tr	0	0	2	1	15
SEEDS								
dried	1 cup	747	34	63	0	25	–	24
roasted	1 cup	1184	75	96	0	31	–	40
salted & roasted	1 cup	1184	75	96	0	31	–	1294
SQUID								
fried	3 oz	149	15	6	221	7	–	260
raw	3 oz	78	13	1	198	3	–	37
SQUIRREL								
roasted	3 oz	147	26	4	103	0	–	102
STARFRUIT								
fresh	1	42	1	tr	0	10	–	2
Sonoma								
Dried	7–9 pieces (1.4 oz)	140	1	0	0	34	0	0
STRAWBERRIES								
CANNED								
in heavy syrup	½ cup	117	1	tr	0	30	–	5
FRESH								
strawberries	1 cup	45	1	1	0	10	4	2
strawberries	1 pint	97	2	1	0	22	–	4
FROZEN								
sweetened sliced	1 cup	245	1	tr	0	66	–	8
sweetened sliced	1 pkg (10 oz)	273	2	tr	0	74	–	9
unsweetened	1 cup	52	1	tr	0	14	–	3
whole sweetened	1 cup	200	1	tr	0	54	–	3
whole sweetened	1 pkg (10 oz)	223	1	tr	0	60	–	3
Birds Eye								
In Syrup	½ cup (4.7 oz)	120	1	0	0	31	1	0
Lite Syrup	1 pkg (10 oz)	120	1	0	0	31	1	0
Whole	½ cup (4.5 oz)	100	tr	0	0	25	1	0
Tree Of Life								
Organic	¾ cup (5 oz)	50	1	0	0	13	2	0

FOOD	PORTION	CAL	PROT	FAT	CHOL	CARB	FIBER	SOD

STRAWBERRY JUICE

Capri Sun

FOOD	PORTION	CAL	PROT	FAT	CHOL	CARB	FIBER	SOD
Strawberry Cooler Drink	1 pkg (7 oz)	90	0	0	0	25	0	20

Kool-Aid

FOOD	PORTION	CAL	PROT	FAT	CHOL	CARB	FIBER	SOD
Drink as prep w/ sugar	1 serv (8 oz)	100	0	0	0	25	0	30
Drink Mix as prep	1 serv (8 oz)	60	0	0	0	16	0	0

Veryfine

FOOD	PORTION	CAL	PROT	FAT	CHOL	CARB	FIBER	SOD
Juice-Ups	8 fl oz	140	0	0	0	36	0	15

STUFFING/DRESSING

FOOD	PORTION	CAL	PROT	FAT	CHOL	CARB	FIBER	SOD
bread as prep w/ water & fat	½ cup	251	5	15	tr	25	–	627
bread as prep w/ water egg & fat	½ cup	107	3	7	75	9	–	319
bread dry as prep	½ cup	178	3	9	–	22	3	543
cornbread as prep	½ cup	179	3	9	0	22	–	455

Kellogg's

FOOD	PORTION	CAL	PROT	FAT	CHOL	CARB	FIBER	SOD
Croutettes Mix	1 cup (1.2 oz)	120	5	0	0	25	0	460

Pepperidge Farm

FOOD	PORTION	CAL	PROT	FAT	CHOL	CARB	FIBER	SOD
Corn Bread	¾ cup (1.5 oz)	170	4	2	0	33	2	480
Herb Seasoned	¾ cup (1.5 oz)	170	5	2	0	33	3	600
Herb Seasoned Cubed	¾ cup (1.3 oz)	140	4	2	0	28	2	530
One Step Chicken	½ cup (1.2 oz)	140	4	4	<5	23	tr	440
One Step Southwestern Corn Bread	½ cup (1.2 oz)	150	4	5	0	23	tr	440
One Step Turkey	½ cup (1.2 oz)	150	4	5	<5	22	tr	500

Stove Top

FOOD	PORTION	CAL	PROT	FAT	CHOL	CARB	FIBER	SOD
Chicken as prep w/ margarine	½ cup (3.6 oz)	170	4	9	0	20	tr	510
Cornbread as prep w/ margarine	½ cup (3.6 oz)	170	3	8	0	21	1	580
Flexible Serve Chicken as prep w/ margarine	½ cup (3.3 oz)	170	3	8	0	19	tr	520

FOOD	PORTION	CAL	PROT	FAT	CHOL	CARB	FIBER	SOD
Flexible Serve Cornbread as prep w/ margarine	½ cup (3.3 oz)	160	3	8	0	19	1	560
Flexible Serve Homestyle Herb as prep w/ margarine	½ cup (3.3 oz)	170	3	8	0	19	1	500
For Beef as prep w/ margarine	½ cup (3.7 oz)	180	4	9	0	22	1	540
For Pork as prep w/ margarine	½ cup (3.6 oz)	170	4	9	0	20	1	530
For Turkey as prep w/ margarine	½ cup (3.6 oz)	170	4	9	0	20	tr	530
Long Grain & Wild Rice as prep w/ margarine	½ cup (3.7 oz)	180	4	9	0	22	tr	500
Lower Sodium Chicken as prep w/ margarine	½ cup (3.6 oz)	180	4	9	0	21	tr	340
Microwave Chicken as prep w/ margarine	½ cup (3.5 oz)	160	4	7	0	20	tr	480
Mushroom & Onion as prep w/ margarine	½ cup (3.6 oz)	180	4	9	0	20	tr	480
San Francisco Style as prep w/ margarine	½ cup (3.6 oz)	170	4	9	0	20	1	530
Savory Herb as prep w/ margarine	½ cup (3.6 oz)	170	4	9	0	20	1	530
Traditional Sage as prep w/ margarine	½ cup (3.6 oz)	180	4	9	0	21	1	530
TAKE-OUT								
bread	½ cup (3½ oz)	195	4	8	0	26	3	534
sausage	½ cup	292	8	11	12	40	1	258

FOOD	PORTION	CAL	PROT	FAT	CHOL	CARB	FIBER	SOD
STURGEON								
cooked	3 oz	115	18	4	–	0	–	–
raw	3 oz	90	14	3	–	0	–	–
roe raw	1 oz	59	7	3	–	tr	–	–
smoked	1 oz	48	9	1	–	0	–	–
smoked	3 oz	147	27	4	–	0	–	–
SUCKER								
white baked	3 oz	101	18	3	45	0	–	44
SUGAR								
brown packed	1 cup (7.7 oz)	828	0	0	0	214	–	86
brown unpacked	1 cup (5.1 oz)	546	0	0	0	141	–	57
maple	1 piece (1 oz)	100	0	tr	0	26	–	3
powdered	1 tbsp (0.3 oz)	31	0	0	0	8	–	0
powdered unsifted	1 cup (4.2 oz)	467	tr	tr	0	119	–	2
sugarcane stem	3 oz	54	1	0	0	14	3	–
white	1 cup (7 oz)	773	0	0	0	200	–	3
white	1 tbsp	45	0	0	0	12	–	tr
white	1 packet (6 g)	25	0	0	0	6	–	tr
white	1 tsp (4 g)	15	0	0	0	4	–	0
Domino								
Dark Brown	1 tsp	15	0	0	0	4	–	0
White	1 tsp	16	0	0	0	4	–	0
Maui Brand								
Raw Sugar	1 tsp	15	0	0	0	4	–	0
SUGAR SUBSTITUTES *(see also FRUCTOSE)*								
Mrs. Bateman's								
Sugarlike	1 tsp (4 g)	4	0	0	0	4	0	0
Weight Watchers								
Sweetener	1 serv (1 g)	5	0	0	0	1	0	30
SUGAR-APPLE								
fresh	1	146	3	tr	0	37	–	15
fresh cut up	1 cup	236	5	1	0	59	–	24
SUNCHOKE								
fresh raw sliced	½ cup	57	2	tr	0	13	–	–
SUNFISH								
pumpkinseed baked	3 oz	97	21	1	73	0	–	87

FOOD	PORTION	CAL	PROT	FAT	CHOL	CARB	FIBER	SOD
SUNFLOWER								
sunflower butter	1 tbsp	93	3	8	0	4	–	82
Dakota Gourmet								
Honey Roasted Kernels	1 pkg (1 oz)	158	6	12	0	8	1	56
Lightly Salted Kernels	1 pkg (1 oz)	168	6	14	0	5	2	85
Frito Lay								
Seeds	1 oz	180	7	15	0	5	2	25
Lance								
Seeds In Shell	⅔ cup (1.8 oz)	160	6	13	0	5	2	30
Seeds Roasted & Shelled	1 pkg (1⅛ oz)	190	7	16	0	6	2	100
Planters								
Kernels	1 pkg (2 oz)	340	13	29	0	11	8	310
Kernels	1 pkg (1.7 oz)	290	11	25	0	9	7	260
Kernels Barbecue	1 pkg (1.7 oz)	290	11	25	0	10	6	180
Kernels Honey Roasted	1 pkg (1.7 oz)	280	10	22	0	15	6	105
Kernels Salted	1 oz	170	7	14	0	4	4	140
Munch'N Go Singles Dry Roasted	1 pkg	120	4	11	0	4	1	70
Nuts Dry Roasted	¼ cup (1.1 oz)	190	7	17	0	6	4	230
Original w/ Shell Dry Roasted	¾ cup	160	6	15	0	5	2	35
SUSHI								
TAKE-OUT								
california roll	1 piece (0.8 oz)	28	1	1	1	4	–	37
sashimi	1 serv (6 oz)	198	24	7	63	4	–	718
tuna roll	1 piece (0.7 oz)	23	2	tr	3	3	–	33
vegetable roll	1 piece (1.2 oz)	27	1	1	0	5	–	47
vinegared ginger	⅓ cup (1.6 oz)	48	1	tr	0	12	–	6
wasabi	2 tsp (0.3 oz)	5	tr	tr	0	1	–	124
yellowtail roll	1 piece (0.6 oz)	25	1	1	0	3	–	32
SWAMP CABBAGE								
chopped cooked	½ cup	10	1	tr	0	2	–	60
raw chopped	1 cup	11	1	tr	0	2	–	63

FOOD	PORTION	CAL	PROT	FAT	CHOL	CARB	FIBER	SOD
SWEET POTATO *(see also YAM)*								
baked w/ skin	1 (3.5 oz)	118	2	tr	0	28	3	12
canned in syrup	½ cup	106	1	tr	0	25	–	38
canned pieces	1 cup	183	3	tr	0	42	–	107
fresh mashed	½ cup	172	3	tr	0	40	3	21
frzn cooked	½ cup	88	2	tr	0	21	–	7
leaves cooked	½ cup	11	1	tr	0	2	–	4
TAKE-OUT								
candied	3.5 oz	144	1	3	0	29	–	73
SWEETBREADS								
beef braised	3 oz	230	23	15	–	0	–	51
lamb braised	3 oz	199	19	13	340	0	–	44
veal braised	3 oz	218	25	12	–	0	–	–
SWISS CHARD								
cooked	½ cup	18	2	tr	0	4	–	158
raw chopped	½ cup	3	tr	tr	0	1	–	38
SWORDFISH								
cooked	3 oz	132	22	4	43	0	–	98
raw	3 oz	103	17	3	33	0	–	76
SYRUP								
corn	2 tbsp	122	0	0	0	32	–	19
date syrup	1 tbsp	63	tr	tr	–	15	0	–
malt	1 tbsp (0.8 oz)	76	2	0	0	17	–	8
maple	1 tbsp (0.8 oz)	52	0	0	0	13	–	2
raspberry	1 oz	76	tr	0	0	19	–	1
rose hip	1 oz	9	0	0	–	2	0	–
sorghum	1 tbsp (0.7 oz)	61	0	0	0	16	–	2
Eden								
Organic Barley Malt	1 tbsp	60	1	0	0	14	0	0
Estee								
Blueberry	¼ cup	80	0	0	0	20	0	70
Hershey								
Strawberry	2 tbsp (1.4 oz)	100	0	0	0	26	–	10
Karo								
Corn Syrup Light	2 tbsp (1 oz)	120	0	0	0	31	–	35
Quik								
Strawberry	2 tbsp (1.5 oz)	110	0	0	0	27	0	0

FOOD	PORTION	CAL	PROT	FAT	CHOL	CARB	FIBER	SOD
Smucker's								
Apricot	¼ cup	210	0	0	0	52	—	0
Blackberry	¼ cup	210	0	0	0	52	—	0
Plate Scapers Kiwi Lime	2 tbsp (1.3 oz)	100	0	0	0	25	—	10
Plate Scapers Mango Orange	2 tbsp	100	0	0	0	24	—	0
Plate Scapers Raspberry	2 tbsp (1.3 oz)	100	0	0	0	25	—	5

TACO (see SPANISH FOOD)

TAHINI (see SESAME)

TAMARIND

fresh	1	5	tr	tr	0	1	—	1
fresh cut up	1 cup	287	3	1	0	75	—	33

TANGERINE

CANNED								
in light syrup	½ cup	76	1	tr	0	20	—	8
juice pack	½ cup	46	1	tr	0	12	—	7
FRESH								
sections	1 cup	86	1	tr	0	22	—	3
tangerine	1	37	1	tr	0	9	—	1
Chiquita								
Tangerine	1 med (3.5 oz)	50	1	1	0	15	2	0

TANGERINE JUICE

canned sweetened	1 cup	125	1	1	0	30	—	2
fresh	1 cup	106	1	tr	0	25	—	2
frzn sweetened as prep	1 cup	110	1	tr	0	27	—	2
frzn sweetened not prep	6 oz	344	3	1	0	83	—	7
After The Fall								
Juice	1 can (12 oz)	170	2	0	0	40	0	35
Fresh Samantha								
Fresh Juice	1 cup (8 oz)	110	2	0	0	8	0	0

TAPIOCA

pearl dry	½ cup (2.7 oz)	272	tr	tr	0	67	1	1
starch	1 oz	98	17	tr	—	24	—	1

FOOD	PORTION	CAL	PROT	FAT	CHOL	CARB	FIBER	SOD
Minute								
Minute Tapioca	1½ tsp (6 g)	20	0	0	0	5	0	0
TARO								
chips	10 (0.8 oz)	115	1	6	0	16	–	79
chips	1 oz	141	1	7	0	19	–	97
leaves cooked	½ cup	18	2	tr	0	3	–	2
raw sliced	½ cup	56	1	tr	0	14	–	6
shoots sliced cooked	½ cup	10	1	tr	0	2	–	1
sliced cooked	½ cup (2.3 oz)	94	tr	tr	0	23	–	10
tahitian sliced cooked	½ cup	30	3	tr	0	5	–	37
TARPON								
fresh	3 oz	87	17	2	–	0	0	70
TARRAGON								
ground	1 tsp	5	tr	tr	0	1	–	1
TEA/HERBAL TEA *(see also* ICED TEA*)*								
HERBAL								
Celestial Seasonings								
Mandarin Orange Spice	1 tea bag	0	0	0	0	tr	–	0
Eden								
Organic Genmaicha Tea	1 cup	0	0	0	0	0	0	0
Organic Kukicha Tea	1 cup	0	0	0	0	0	0	0
Lipton								
Bedtime Story	1 tea bag	0	0	0	0	1	–	0
Cinnamon Apple	1 tea bag	0	0	0	0	1	–	0
Ginger Twist	1 tea bag	0	0	0	0	0	0	0
Lemon	1 tea bag	0	0	0	0	1	–	0
Orange	1 tea bag	0	0	0	0	1	–	0
Peppermint	1 tea bag	0	0	0	0	1	–	0
Quietly Chamomile	1 tea bag	0	0	0	0	1	–	0
REGULAR								
brewed tea	6 oz	2	0	0	0	tr	–	5
instant unsweetened as prep w/ water	8 oz	2	tr	0	0	tr	–	8

FOOD	PORTION	CAL	PROT	FAT	CHOL	CARB	FIBER	SOD
Activitea								
Green Tea	1 cup	36	0	0	0	3	—	3
General Foods								
International Instant Tea Island Orange Creme as prep	1 serv (8 oz)	70	0	2	0	13	0	65
Lipton								
Brisk Tea as prep	1 serv	0	0	0	0	0	0	0
Decaffeinated Brisk Tea as prep	1 serv	0	0	0	0	0	0	0
English Blend as prep	1 cup	0	0	0	0	0	0	0
Flavored Decaffeinated Orange & Spice	1 tea bag	0	0	0	0	0	—	0
Green Tea	1 tea bag	0	0	0	0	0	—	0
Loose Tea	1 tsp (2 g)	0	0	0	0	0	0	0
Paradise								
Tropical Tea	8 fl oz	1	0	0	0	tr	0	7
Tropical Tea Decafe	8 fl oz	1	0	0	0	tr	0	7
Tropical Tea Passion Fruit	8 fl oz	1	0	0	0	tr	0	7
Salada								
Green Tea	1 cup	0	0	0	0	0	0	0
Green Tea Decaffeinated	1 tea bag	0	0	0	0	0	—	0
Tetley								
British Blend Round Teabags	1 cup	0	0	0	0	0	0	0
Tea Bag as prep	1	0	0	0	0	0	0	0

TEMPEH

FOOD	PORTION	CAL	PROT	FAT	CHOL	CARB	FIBER	SOD
tempeh	½ cup	165	16	6	0	14	—	5
Lightlife								
Garden Vege	4 oz	200	21	8	0	12	6	399
Quinoa Sesame	4 oz	220	21	8	0	15	7	0
Smokey Strips	3 slices (2 oz)	80	8	3	0	6	1	230
Soy	4 oz	210	24	8	0	11	7	0

FOOD	PORTION	CAL	PROT	FAT	CHOL	CARB	FIBER	SOD
Three Grain	4 oz	200	20	7	0	13	6	0
Wild Rice	4 oz	190	19	7	0	13	6	0
Turtle Island								
Five Grain	3 oz	190	11	6	0	20	6	10
Low Fat Millet	3 oz	130	8	2	0	20	3	10
Soy	3 oz	160	13	4	0	20	7	15
Wild Rice Rhapsody	3 oz	160	13	4	0	20	7	15
THYME								
ground	1 tsp	4	tr	tr	0	1	–	1
TILEFISH								
cooked	½ fillet (5.3 oz)	220	37	7	–	0	–	88
cooked	3 oz	125	21	4	–	0	–	50
raw	3 oz	81	15	2	–	0	–	45
TOFU								
fresh fried	1 piece (0.5 oz)	35	2	3	0	1	tr	2
fuyu salted & fermented	1 block (⅓ oz)	13	1	1	0	1	tr	316
koyadofu dried frozen	1 piece (½ oz)	82	8	5	0	2	tr	1
okara	½ cup	47	2	1	0	8	1	6
Azumaya								
Baked Chili Picante	2 pieces	200	20	10	0	9	2	320
Baked Mesquite	2 pieces	100	20	10	0	6	2	480
Baked Spicy Thai Peanut	2 pieces	190	20	10	0	6	2	500
Baked Teriyaki	2 pieces	200	20	10	0	9	2	730
Extra Firm	1 serv (2.8 oz)	70	8	4	0	2	1	0
Firm	1 serv (2.8 oz)	70	7	4	0	2	0	0
Lite Extra Firm	1 serv (2.8 oz)	60	8	2	0	3	1	30
Lite Silken	1 serv (3.2 oz)	40	5	1	0	3	0	45
Silken	1 serv (3.2 oz)	40	4	2	0	1	–	0
Galaxy								
Slices Hickory Smoked	1 slice (1 oz)	50	2	2	0	5	0	340
Slices Italian Garlic Herb	1 slice (1 oz)	50	2	2	0	5	0	390
Slices Original	1 slice (1 oz)	50	2	2	0	5	0	340
Slices Savory	1 slice (1 oz)	50	2	2	0	5	0	390

FOOD	PORTION	CAL	PROT	FAT	CHOL	CARB	FIBER	SOD
Hinoichi								
Firm	1 inch slice (3 oz)	60	6	3	0	2	1	10
Long Life								
Tofu	3 oz	60	6	3	0	2	1	10
Nasoya								
5 Spice	1 serv (3 oz)	70	7	4	0	0	0	220
Baked Mesquite Smoke	2 pieces	220	21	9	0	17	3	560
Baked Teriyaki	2 pieces	230	20	9	0	21	3	700
Baked TexMex	2 pieces	230	21	9	0	21	4	360
Baked Thai Peanut	2 pieces	240	21	10	0	19	3	540
Extra Firm	1 serv (3 oz)	90	8	5	0	3	0	0
Firm	1 serv (3 oz)	70	7	4	0	2	tr	0
Frim Enriched	1 serv (3 oz)	45	7	1	0	0	0	30
Garlic & Onion	1 serv (3 oz)	70	7	4	0	1	0	250
Silken	1 serv (3.2 oz)	45	4	3	0	2	0	5
Soft	1 serv (3 oz)	60	7	4	0	1	0	0
TofuMate Breakfast Scramble	¼ pkg	15	1	0	0	3	–	330
TofuMate Eggless Salad	¼ pkg	15	0	0	0	4	–	310
TofuMate Mandarin Stirfry	¼ pkg	30	1	0	0	6	–	310
TofuMate Mediterranean Herb	¼ pkg	15	1	0	0	3	–	330
TofuMate Szechwan StirFry	¼ pkg	25	1	0	0	4	–	280
TofuMate Texas Taco	¼ pkg	15	1	0	0	3	0	360
Tree Of Life								
30% Reduced Fat Firm	⅓ block (3.2 oz)	90	10	4	0	4	2	5
Easymeal Pasta Primavera as prep	1 serv	460	20	16	10	54	3	790
Easymeal Southwest Medley as prep	1 serv	380	15	14	0	44	3	790
Easymeal Teriyaki Stir Fry as prep	1 serv	270	13	14	0	24	6	560
Easymeal Thai Stir Fry as prep	1 serv	270	14	14	0	21	6	230

FOOD	PORTION	CAL	PROT	FAT	CHOL	CARB	FIBER	SOD
Organic Baked	⅓ block (2.7 oz)	150	16	8	0	5	0	310
Organic Baked Island Spice	⅓ pkg (2.7 oz)	130	15	7	0	3	0	320
Organic Baked Oriental	⅓ pkg (2.7 oz)	130	15	7	0	5	0	330
Organic Baked Savory	⅓ block (2.7 oz)	140	15	7	0	4	0	310
Organic Firm	⅓ block (3.2 oz)	100	9	5	0	2	0	5
Raw Firm	⅓ block (3.2 oz)	100	9	5	0	2	0	5

TOMATILLO

FOOD	PORTION	CAL	PROT	FAT	CHOL	CARB	FIBER	SOD
fresh	1 (1.2 oz)	11	tr	tr	0	2	–	0
fresh chopped	½ cup	21	1	1	0	4	–	1

TOMATO (see also PIZZA SAUCE, SPAGHETTI SAUCE)
CANNED
Amore

FOOD	PORTION	CAL	PROT	FAT	CHOL	CARB	FIBER	SOD
Sun-Dried Tomato Paste	1 tsp (6 g)	15	0	1	0	tr	0	115
Big R								
Cajun Stewed	½ cup (4.2 oz)	25	1	0	0	4	1	150
Diced w/ Chilies	½ cup (4.2 oz)	25	1	0	0	4	1	340
Mexican Stewed	½ cups (4.2 oz)	25	1	0	0	5	1	190
Stewed	½ cup (4.2 oz)	25	1	0	0	5	1	190
Whole	½ cup (4.2 oz)	25	1	0	0	5	1	190
Claussen								
Halves	1 serv (1 oz)	5	0	0	0	1	tr	320
Contadina								
California Sliced	½ cup	40	–	tr	0	–	–	–
Paste	2 tbsp (1.2 oz)	30	2	0	0	6	1	20
Puree	¼ cup (2.2 oz)	20	tr	0	0	4	tr	15
Recipe Ready Diced Roasted Garlic	½ cup (4,3 oz)	45	1	0	0	10	tr	560
Del Monte								
Chunky Chili Style	½ cup (4.5 oz)	30	1	0	0	8	2	670
Chunky Pasta Style	½ cup (4.5 oz)	45	1	0	0	11	2	560
Crushed Italian Recipe	½ cup (4.4 oz)	45	2	0	0	9	1	390
Crushed Original Recipe	½ cup (4.4 oz)	45	2	0	0	9	1	390

FOOD	PORTION	CAL	PROT	FAT	CHOL	CARB	FIBER	SOD
Crushed w/ Garlic	½ cup (4.4 oz)	50	2	0	0	11	1	510
Diced	½ cup (4.4 oz)	25	1	0	0	6	2	160
Diced No Salt Added	½ cup (4.4 oz)	25	1	0	0	6	2	50
Diced w/ Basil Garlic & Oregano	½ cup (4.4 oz)	50	2	0	0	11	1	650
Diced w/ Garlic & Onion	½ cup (4.4 oz)	40	2	1	0	8	1	610
Diced w/ Green Pepper & Onion	½ cup (4.4 oz)	40	1	0	0	9	2	480
Paste	2 tbsp (1.2 oz)	30	1	0	0	7	2	25
Sauce	¼ cup (2.1 oz)	20	1	0	0	4	1	340
Sauce No Salt Added	¼ cup (2.1 oz)	20	0	0	0	4	1	20
Stewed Cajun Recipe	½ cup (4.4 oz)	35	1	0	0	9	2	460
Stewed Italian Recipe	½ cup (4.4 oz)	30	1	0	0	8	2	420
Stewed Mexican Recipe	½ cup (4.4 oz)	35	1	0	0	9	2	400
Stewed Original	½ cup (4.4 oz)	35	1	0	0	9	2	360
Stewed Original No Salt Added	½ cup (4.4 oz)	35	1	0	0	9	2	50
Wedges	½ cup (4.4 oz)	35	1	0	0	9	2	380
Zesty Diced w/ Mild Green Chilies	½ cup (4.4 oz)	30	1	0	0	6	1	550
Eden								
Organic Diced	½ cup	30	1	0	0	6	2	5
Organic Diced w/ Green Chilies	½ cup	30	2	0	0	5	2	35
Hunt's								
Angela Mia Puree	¼ cup (2.2 oz)	16	1	tr	0	3	tr	21
Choice Cut	½ cup (4.2 oz)	23	1	tr	0	5	1	325
Choice Cut Diced Tomatoes & Italian Herb	½ cup (4.2 oz)	24	1	0	0	5	1	600
Choice Cut Diced Tomatoes & Roasted Garlic	½ cup (4.2 oz)	24	1	0	0	5	1	505
Choice Cut Diced Tomatoes w/ Red Pepper & Basil	¼ cup (4.2 oz)	27	1	tr	0	6	1	396

FOOD	PORTION	CAL	PROT	FAT	CHOL	CARB	FIBER	SOD
Crushed Pear Tomatoes	½ cup (4.2 oz)	29	1	tr	0	7	2	286
Diced In Juice	½ cup (4.2 oz)	20	1	tr	0	4	1	477
Diced In Puree	½ cup (4.3 oz)	23	1	tr	0	5	1	304
Diced w/ Green Chilies	2 tbsp (0.4 oz)	1	tr	tr	0	tr	tr	24
Paste	2 tbsp (1.2 oz)	30	1	tr	0	6	2	88
Paste Italian	2 tbsp (1.2 oz)	27	1	tr	0	6	2	264
Paste No Salt Added	2 tbsp (1.2 oz)	30	1	tr	0	6	2	7
Paste w/ Garlic	2 tbsp (1.2 oz)	28	2	tr	0	6	2	281
Puree	¼ cup (2.2 oz)	24	1	tr	0	5	2	98
Ready Sauce Chunky Chili	¼ cup (2.2 oz)	22	1	tr	0	4	1	320
Ready Sauce Chunky Italian	¼ cup (2.2 oz)	30	1	1	0	4	1	179
Ready Sauce Chunky Mexican	¼ cup (2.2 oz)	21	1	tr	0	4	1	390
Ready Sauce Chunky Salsa	¼ cup (2.2 oz)	18	1	tr	0	3	1	357
Ready Sauce Chunky Tomato	¼ cup (2.2 oz)	15	1	tr	0	3	1	403
Ready Sauce Garlic & Herb	¼ cup (2.2 oz)	26	1	tr	0	5	1	202
Sauce	¼ cup (2.2 oz)	16	1	tr	0	3	1	366
Sauce Herb	¼ cup (2.2 oz)	32	1	1	0	5	1	271
Sauce Italian	¼ cup (2.2 oz)	32	1	1	0	5	1	210
Sauce Meatloaf Fixins	¼ cup (2.2 oz)	23	1	tr	0	4	1	600
Sauce No Salt Added	¼ cup (2.2 oz)	16	1	tr	0	3	1	12
Sauce Special	¼ cup (2.2 oz)	21	1	1	0	4	1	144
Stewed	½ cup (4.2 oz)	33	1	tr	0	7	2	357
Stewed No Salt Added	½ cup (4.2 oz)	33	1	tr	0	7	2	31
Whole Peeled	2 (5.2 oz)	24	2	tr	0	5	1	433
Whole Peeled No Salt Added	2 (4.8 oz)	21	2	tr	0	4	1	9
Muir Glen								
Diced Fire Roasted	¼ cup	30	1	0	0	6	1	290
Diced w/ Green Chilies	½ cup (4.5 oz)	25	1	0	0	4	1	290

FOOD	PORTION	CAL	PROT	FAT	CHOL	CARB	FIBER	SOD
Organic Chunky Sauce	¼ cup (2.3 oz)	20	tr	0	0	4	1	160
Organic Crushed Fire Roasted	¼ cup	20	1	0	0	5	1	160
Organic Diced	½ cup (4.5 oz)	25	1	0	0	4	1	290
Organic Diced No Salt Added	½ cup (4.5 oz)	25	1	0	0	4	1	45
Organic Diced w/ Basil & Garlic	½ cup (4.5 oz)	25	1	0	0	4	1	290
Organic Diced w/ Italian Herbs	½ cup (4.4 oz)	25	1	0	0	4	1	290
Organic Ground Peeled	¼ cup (2.3 oz)	10	tr	0	0	2	1	100
Organic Paste	2 tbsp (1.2 oz)	30	2	0	0	6	1	20
Organic Puree	¼ cup (2.2 oz)	20	1	0	0	5	1	20
Organic Sauce	¼ cup (2.2 oz)	20	tr	0	0	5	1	310
Organic Sauce No Salt Added	¼ cup (2.2 oz)	20	tr	0	0	5	1	30
Organic Stewed	½ cup (4.5 oz)	30	1	0	0	7	tr	290
Organic Whole Peeled	½ cup (4.6 oz)	30	1	0	0	5	1	260
Whole Peeled w/ Basil	½ cup (4.6 oz)	30	1	0	0	5	1	260
Old El Paso								
Tomatoes & Jalapenos	¼ cup (2 oz)	15	1	0	0	3	1	290
Tomatoes & Green Chilies	¼ cup (2 oz)	10	0	0	0	2	0	310
Progresso								
Crushed	¼ cup (2.1 oz)	20	1	0	0	4	1	95
Italian Style Peeled	½ cup (4.2 oz)	20	1	0	0	4	1	220
Paste	2 tbsp (1.2 oz)	30	2	0	0	6	1	20
Puree	¼ cup (2.2 oz)	25	1	0	0	5	1	15
Puree Thick Style	¼ cup (2.2 oz)	20	tr	0	0	5	1	15
Sauce	¼ cup (2.1 oz)	20	1	0	0	4	1	260
Whole Peeled	½ cup (4.2 oz)	25	1	0	0	5	1	220
Red Pack								
Puree	¼ cup (2.2 oz)	25	1	0	0	5	1	10

FOOD	PORTION	CAL	PROT	FAT	CHOL	CARB	FIBER	SOD
Ro-Tel								
Diced Tomatoes & Green Chilies	½ cup (4.4 oz)	20	tr	0	0	4	1	370
Sonoma								
Dried Spice Medley oil drained	1 tbsp (0.5 oz)	50	1	4	0	3	1	200
Pesto	¼ cup (2 oz)	110	3	9	2	6	1	125
Tapenade	1 tbsp (0.7 oz)	70	1	6	0	4	1	5
DRIED								
sun dried	1 cup	140	8	2	0	30	—	1131
sun dried	1 piece	5	tr	tr	0	1	—	42
sun dried in oil	1 cup (4 oz)	235	6	15	0	26	—	293
sun dried in oil	1 piece (3 g)	6	tr	tr	0	1	—	8
sun-dried	5 pieces (0.5 oz)	40	2	0	0	7	3	90
Sonoma								
Bits	2–3 tsp (5 g)	15	1	0	0	3	1	5
Dried	2–3 halves (5 g)	15	1	0	0	3	1	5
Julienne	7–9 pieces (5 g)	15	1	0	0	3	1	5
Pasta Toss	½ cup (0.7 oz)	70	4	0	0	13	3	75
Season It	2–3 tsp (5 g)	20	1	0	0	3	1	25
FRESH								
cooked	½ cup	32	1	1	0	7	—	13
green	1	30	1	tr	0	6	—	16
red	1 (4.5 oz)	26	1	tr	0	6	2	11
red chopped	1 cup	35	2	tr	0	8	2	16
Chiquita								
Tomato	1 med (5.2 oz)	35	1	1	0	7	1	5
Eurofresh								
Tomatoes On The Vine	1 med (5.2 oz)	35	1	1	0	—	1	5
TAKE-OUT								
stewed	1 cup	80	2	3	0	13	—	460
TOMATO JUICE								
beef broth & tomato	5½ oz	61	1	tr	—	14	—	220
clam & tomato	1 can (5½ oz)	77	1	tr	—	18	—	664
tomato juice	6 oz	32	1	tr	0	8	—	658
tomato juice	½ cup	21	1	tr	0	5	—	441

FOOD	PORTION	CAL	PROT	FAT	CHOL	CARB	FIBER	SOD
Campbell								
Juice	8 oz	51	2	1	–	10	2	683
Del Monte								
Juice	8 fl oz	50	2	0	0	10	1	760
Snap-E-Tom Chile Cocktail	6 fl oz	40	2	0	0	8	1	500
Dole								
Juice	1 bottle (12 oz)	85	4	0	0	17	2	1000
Hunt's								
Juice	1 can (6 oz)	22	1	tr	0	5	1	452
No Salt Added	8 fl oz	34	2	tr	0	8	2	12
Mott's								
Tomato Juice	8 fl oz	40	2	0	0	9	–	850
Muir Glen								
Organic	5.5 oz	40	1	0	0	8	4	420
TONGUE								
beef simmered	3 oz	241	19	18	91	tr	–	51
lamb braised	3 oz	234	18	17	161	0	–	57
pork braised	3 oz	230	20	16	124	0	0	93
TORTILLA								
corn	1 (6 in diam)	56	1	1	0	12	1	40
corn w/o salt	1–6 in diam (.9 oz)	56	1	1	0	12	1	3
flour w/o salt	1–8 in diam (1.2 oz)	114	3	3	0	20	1	167
La Mexicana								
Corn	1 (0.8 oz)	50	1	1	0	10	1	0
Flour	1 (0.8 oz)	80	2	3	0	13	1	260
Tortillas de Trigo	1 (1 oz)	140	2	7	0	18	1	75
Mariachi								
Tortilla	1	112	3	3	–	20	–	174
Old El Paso								
Flour	1 (1.4 oz)	130	3	4	0	21	0	290
Soft Taco Tortilla	2 (1.8 oz)	180	5	4	0	33	0	410
Tyson								
Flour	1 (1.7 oz)	150	3	4	0	24	1	310
Flour Heat Pressed	2 (2 oz)	170	4	4	0	30	2	410
White Corn	2 (1.8 oz)	100	2	1	0	21	3	70
Whole Wheat Heat Pressed	1 (1.4 oz)	120	4	3	0	20	3	240
Yellow Corn	3 (1.9 oz)	140	3	2	0	27	3	20

FOOD	PORTION	CAL	PROT	FAT	CHOL	CARB	FIBER	SOD
TORTILLA CHIPS (see CHIPS)								
TREE FERN								
chopped cooked	½ cup	28	tr	tr	0	8	–	3
TRITICALE								
dry	1 cup (6.7 oz)	645	25	4	0	138	–	10
triticale not prep	1 oz	94	4	tr	–	18	2	7.4
TROUT								
baked	3 oz	162	23	7	63	0	–	57
rainbow cooked	3 oz	129	22	4	62	0	–	29
seatrout baked	3 oz	113	18	4	90	0	–	63
TRUFFLES								
fresh	0.5 oz	4	2	tr	0	9	2	39
TUMERIC								
ground	1 tsp	8	tr	tr	0	1	–	1
TUNA								
CANNED								
light in oil	1 can (6 oz)	399	50	14	30	0	–	606
light in oil	3 oz	169	25	7	15	0	–	301
light in water	3 oz	99	22	1	25	0	–	287
light in water	1 can (5.8 oz)	192	42	1	49	0	–	558
white in oil	1 can (6.2 oz)	331	47	14	55	0	–	704
white in oil	3 oz	158	23	7	26	0	–	336
white in water	3 oz	116	23	2	35	0	–	333
white in water	1 can (6 oz)	234	46	4	72	0	–	673
Bumble Bee								
Albacore In Water	2 oz	60	12	1	–	0	–	310
Chunk Light In Water	2 oz	60	12	1	–	0	–	310
Chunk Light In Water Pouch	2 oz	60	13	1	30	0	0	250
Solid White In Water	2 oz	70	15	1	25	0	0	250
Progresso								
In Olive Oil drained	¼ cup (2 oz)	160	13	12	30	0	0	250
StarKist								
Chunk Light No Drain Package	¼ cup (2 oz)	60	13	1	30	0	0	250
Low Sodium Chunk White In Water	2 oz	60	14	1	25	0	0	35

FOOD	PORTION	CAL	PROT	FAT	CHOL	CARB	FIBER	SOD
Solid White Albacore In Spring Water	¼ cup (2 oz)	70	15	1	25	0	0	250
Tuna Fillet In Spring Water	¼ cup (2 oz)	60	13	1	30	0	0	250
FRESH								
bluefin cooked	3 oz	157	25	5	42	0	–	43
bluefin raw	3 oz	122	20	4	32	0	–	33
skipjack baked	3 oz	112	24	1	51	0	–	40
yellowfin baked	3 oz	118	25	1	49	0	–	40

TUNA DISHES
MIX
Tuna Helper

FOOD	PORTION	CAL	PROT	FAT	CHOL	CARB	FIBER	SOD
AuGratin 50% Less Fat Recipe as prep	1 cup	240	13	6	15	37	1	840
AuGratin as prep	1 cup	300	13	11	20	37	1	890
Cheesy Broccoli 50% Less Fat Recipe as prep	1 cup	240	15	5	15	38	1	820
Cheesy Broccoli as prep	1 cup	290	15	9	20	38	1	860
Cheesy Pasta 50% Less Fat Recipe as prep	1 cup	230	14	5	15	32	tr	850
Cheesy Pasta as prep	1 cup	280	14	11	20	32	tr	890
Creamy Broccoli 50% Less Fat Recipe as prep	1 cup	240	14	5	15	35	1	820
Creamy Broccoli as prep	1 cup	310	14	12	20	35	1	880
Creamy Pasta 50% Less Fat Recipe as prep	1 cup	230	14	6	15	31	1	840
Creamy Pasta as prep	1 cup	300	14	13	20	31	1	910
Fettuccine Alfredo as prep	1 cup	310	14	14	15	32	1	950
Garden Cheddar 50% Less Fat Recipe as prep	1 cup	240	13	5	15	36	1	980

FOOD	PORTION	CAL	PROT	FAT	CHOL	CARB	FIBER	SOD
Garden Cheddar as prep	1 cup	290	13	11	20	36	1	1030
Pasta Salad Low Fat Recipe as prep	⅔ cup	230	10	2	10	26	1	790
Pasta Salad as prep	⅔ cup	380	10	27	10	26	1	730
Tetrazzini 50% Less Fat Recipe as prep	1 cup	230	14	5	20	34	1	980
Tetrazzini as prep	1 cup	300	14	12	20	34	1	1040
Tuna Melt Reduced Fat Recipe as prep	1 cup	240	12	6	15	34	1	850
Tuna Melt as prep	1 cup	300	12	12	20	34	1	900
Tuna Pot Pie as prep	1 cup	440	18	24	110	40	1	1080
Tuna Romanoff 50% Less Fat Recipe as prep	1 cup	240	15	3	20	38	1	740
Tuna Romanoff as prep	1 cup	280	15	8	20	38	1	800
READY-TO-EAT								
Bumble Bee								
Tuna Salad Fat Free	1 pkg (3.5 oz)	190	9	2	15	25	0	510
Tuna Salad Kit	1 pkg (3.8 oz)	250	17	13	45	15	0	550
StarKist								
Lunch To-Go	1 pkg	310	22	13	40	26	tr	690
Ready-Mixed Tuna Salad Kit	1 pkg (3.5 oz)	190	9	6	5	25	2	420
Tuna Salad Lunch Kit	1 pkg (4.3 oz)	230	20	9	35	17	1	730
The Spreadables								
Tuna Salad	¼ can	90	–	6	13	–	–	–
Wampler								
Salad	⅓ cup	180	6	12	20	9	–	450
Salad Chunky	⅓ cup	180	8	13	20	8	–	380
TAKE-OUT								
tuna salad	1 cup	383	33	19	27	19	–	824
tuna salad	3 oz	159	14	8	11	8	–	342
TURBOT								
european baked	3 oz	104	17	3	–	0	–	163

FOOD	PORTION	CAL	PROT	FAT	CHOL	CARB	FIBER	SOD

TURKEY *(see also* DINNER, HOT DOG, TURKEY DISHES, TURKEY SUBSTITUTES*)*

CANNED

FOOD	PORTION	CAL	PROT	FAT	CHOL	CARB	FIBER	SOD
w/ broth	1 can (5 oz)	231	34	10	–	0	–	663
w/ broth	½ can (2.5 oz)	116	17	5	–	0	–	332
Mary Kitchen								
Roast Turkey Hash	1 can (14.9 oz)	420	39	11	110	42	3	1800
FRESH								
back w/ skin roasted	½ back (9 oz)	637	70	38	238	0	–	191
breast w/ skin roasted	4 oz	212	32	8	83	0	–	70
dark meat w/ skin roasted	3.6 oz	230	29	12	93	0	–	79
dark meat w/o skin roasted	3 oz	170	26	7	78	0	–	72
dark meat w/o skin roasted	1 cup (5 oz)	262	40	10	119	0	–	110
ground cooked	3 oz	188	20	11	57	0	–	68
leg w/ skin roasted	1 (1.2 lbs)	1133	152	54	466	0	–	420
leg w/ skin roasted	2.5 oz	147	20	7	61	0	–	55
light meat w/ skin roasted	4.7 oz	268	39	11	103	0	–	85
light meat w/ skin roasted	from ½ turkey (2.3 lbs)	2069	87	87	794	0	–	658
light meat w/o skin roasted	4 oz	183	35	4	81	0	–	75
neck simmered	1 (5.3 oz)	274	41	11	186	0	–	84
skin roasted	1 oz	141	13	13	36	0	–	17
skin roasted	from ½ turkey	1096	49	98	281	0	–	132
w/ skin roasted	½ turkey (4 lbs)	3857	522	181	1514	0	–	1269
w/ skin roasted	8.4 oz	498	67	23	196	0	–	164
w/ skin neck & giblets roasted	½ turkey (8.8 lbs)	4123	190	190	1920	1	–	1358
w/o skin roasted	1 cup (5 oz)	238	41	7	107	0	–	99
w/o skin roasted	7.3 oz	354	61	10	159	0	–	147
wing w/ skin roasted	1 (6.5 oz)	426	51	23	150	0	–	114
Louis Rich								
Ground	4 oz	190	20	12	90	0	0	140
Patties White	1 (4 oz)	170	19	10	65	0	0	440

FOOD	PORTION	CAL	PROT	FAT	CHOL	CARB	FIBER	SOD
Perdue								
Breast Tenderloins Butter Garlic	3 oz	100	20	1	45	2	—	830
Burger Cooked	1 (4 oz)	160	20	9	85	0	—	85
Dark Cooked	3 oz	180	20	11	85	0	—	65
Drumsticks Cooked	1 (2.2 oz)	110	14	6	80	0	—	65
Ground Cooked	3 oz	160	20	9	85	0	—	85
Tenderloins Black Pepper Cooked	3 oz	90	20	1	45	1	—	690
Thighs Cooked	1 (3.2 oz)	240	17	19	115	0	—	65
White Cooked	3 oz	150	22	7	65	0	—	45
Shady Brook								
Cutlets	4 oz	130	28	1	70	—	—	55
Drumstick	4 oz	170	22	9	70	—	—	80
Ground Breast	4 oz	120	28	1	70	0	—	55
Ground Lean	4 oz	170	20	9	90	—	—	105
Ground Turkey 85%	4 oz	220	21	15	75	—	—	75
Mesquite Seasoned Tenderloin	4 oz	110	23	1	50	—	—	360
OnlyOne Boneless Breast Roast	4 oz	130	28	1	70	—	—	55
Split Breast	4 oz	190	24	9	70	—	—	60
Tenderloin	4 oz	130	28	1	70	—	—	55
Teriyaki Seasoned Tenderloin	4 oz	120	24	1	50	—	—	460
Thigh	4 oz	220	21	15	75	—	—	75
Turkey Burgers	4 oz	170	20	9	90	—	—	105
Turkey Meatloaf Lean	4 oz	150	18	7	95	—	—	400
Whole Breast	4 oz	190	24	9	70	—	—	60
Whole Turkey	4 oz	180	23	9	75	—	—	75
Wing	4 oz	220	23	14	80	—	—	60
Zesty Lemon Seasoned Tenderlion	4 oz	120	24	1	50	—	—	200
The Turkey Store								
Breakfast Sausage Patties Mild	2 patties (2.3 oz)	160	10	13	50	1	—	420
Seasoned Cuts Turkey Breast Roast	4 oz	110	22	1	45	4	—	530

FOOD	PORTION	CAL	PROT	FAT	CHOL	CARB	FIBER	SOD
Wampler								
Boneless Breast Roast	4 oz	160	25	6	35	0	—	25
Breast Half	4 oz	160	25	6	35	0	—	25
Breast Steaks	4 oz	120	28	1	70	0	—	55
Drumsticks	4 oz	180	22	10	75	0	—	45
Ground	4 oz	210	18	15	100	0	—	70
Ground Breast	4 oz	130	28	1	70	0	—	55
Ground Lean	4 oz	160	20	8	90	0	—	70
Thighs	4 oz	170	22	10	80	0	—	40
Wings	4 oz	220	23	14	80	0	—	60
Woodfire Grill Burger	1 (3 oz)	180	21	9	65	2	—	360
FROZEN								
roast boneless seasoned light & dark meat roasted	1 pkg (1.7 lbs)	1213	167	45	413	24	—	5320
Wampler								
Burger BBQ	1 (4 oz)	240	19	17	140	3	—	240
Burgers Cracked Peppercorn & Garlic	1 (3 oz)	170	21	9	65	0	—	380
Seasoned Burgers Cracker Peppercorn & Garlic	1 (3 oz)	170	21	9	65	0	—	380
READY-TO-EAT								
bologna	1 oz	57	4	4	28	tr	—	249
breast	1 slice (0.75 oz)	23	5	tr	9	0	—	301
diced light & dark seasoned	½ lb	313	42	14	—	2	—	1928
diced light & dark seasoned	1 oz	39	5	2	—	tr	—	241
ham thigh meat	2 oz	73	11	3	—	tr	—	565
ham thigh meat	1 pkg (8 oz)	291	43	12	—	1	—	2260
pastrami	2 oz	80	10	4	—	1	—	698
pastrami	1 pkg (8 oz)	320	42	14	—	4	—	2372
patties battered & fried	1 (3.3 oz)	266	13	17	—	15	—	752

FOOD	PORTION	CAL	PROT	FAT	CHOL	CARB	FIBER	SOD
patties battered & fried	1 (2.3 oz)	181	9	12	–	10	–	512
patties breaded & fried	1 (3.3 oz)	266	13	17	–	15	–	752
patties breaded & fried	1 (2.3 oz)	181	9	12	–	10	–	512
poultry salad sandwich spread	1 tbsp	109	2	2	4	1	–	49
poultry salad sandwich spread	1 oz	238	4	4	9	2	–	107
prebasted breast w/ skin roasted	1 breast (3.8 lbs)	2175	383	60	718	0	–	6868
prebasted breast w/ skin roasted	½ breast (1.9 lbs)	1087	191	30	359	0	–	3434
prebasted thigh w/ skin roasted	1 thigh (11 oz)	494	59	27	194	0	–	1371
roll light & dark meat	1 oz	42	5	2	16	1	–	166
roll light meat	1 oz	42	5	2	12	2	–	139
salami cooked	2 oz	111	9	8	46	tr	–	569
salami cooked	1 pkg (8 oz)	446	37	31	186	1	–	2278
turkey loaf breast meat	1 pkg (6 oz)	187	38	3	69	0	–	2433
turkey loaf breast meat	2 slices (1.5 oz)	47	10	1	17	0	–	608
turkey sticks battered & fried	1 stick (2.3 oz)	178	9	11	–	11	–	536
turkey sticks breaded & fried	1 stick (2.3 oz)	178	9	11	–	11	–	536
Alpine Lace								
Breast Fat Free	2 oz	45	10	0	25	0	0	350
Boar's Head								
Breast Cracked Pepper Smoked	2 oz	60	13	1	30	1	0	460
Breast Golden Skin On	2 oz	60	11	2	25	0	0	340
Breast Golden Skinless	2 oz	60	12	1	25	tr	0	350
Breast Hickory Smoked	2 oz	70	12	2	25	tr	0	340

FOOD	PORTION	CAL	PROT	FAT	CHOL	CARB	FIBER	SOD
Breast Low Sodium Skinless	2 oz	60	12	1	25	tr	0	340
Breast Lower Sodium Skin On	2 oz	60	11	2	25	tr	0	310
Breast Maple Glazed Honey Coat	2 oz	70	14	1	30	2	0	440
Breast Ovengold Skin On	2 oz	60	12	2	35	1	0	360
Breast Ovengold Skinless	2 oz	60	13	1	20	0	0	350
Breast Roasted Mesquite Smoked Skinless	2 oz	60	13	1	25	0	0	440
Breast Roasted Salsalito	2 oz	60	13	1	25	1	0	460
Pastrami Seasoned	2 oz	60	13	1	25	1	0	440
Carl Buddig								
Honey Roasted Turkey Breast	1 pkg (2.5 oz)	120	12	7	40	3	—	780
Lean Slices Honey Roasted Breast	1 pkg (2.5 oz)	70	13	1	30	4	—	980
Lean Slices Oven Roasted Breast	1 pkg (2.5 oz)	70	15	1	30	1	—	980
Lean Slices Smoked Breast	1 pkg (2.5 oz)	70	15	1	30	1	—	880
Oven Roasted Breast	1 pkg (2.5 oz)	110	12	7	40	1	—	780
Smoked Breast	1 pkg (2.5 oz)	110	12	7	40	1	—	780
Turkey Ham	1 pkg (2.5 oz)	100	13	5	40	1	—	1020
Healthy Choice								
Deli-Thin Roasted Breast	6 slices (2 oz)	60	11	2	25	1	0	550
Deli-Thin Smoked Breast	6 slices (2 oz)	60	11	2	25	1	0	420
Deli-Thin Turkey Ham	6 slices (2 oz)	60	11	2	40	1	0	550
Fresh-Trak Honey Roast & Smoked Breast	1 slice (1 oz)	35	5	1	10	1	0	200
Fresh-Trak Oven Roasted Breast	1 slice (1 oz)	35	6	1	15	1	0	270

FOOD	PORTION	CAL	PROT	FAT	CHOL	CARB	FIBER	SOD
Honey Roasted & Smoked	1 slice (1 oz)	35	5	1	15	1	0	220
Oven Roasted Breast	1 slice (1 oz)	35	6	1	15	1	0	270
Smoked Breast	1 slice (1 oz)	30	6	1	10	0	0	230
Variety Pack Regular	3 slices (2.2 oz)	70	13	2	30	2	0	530
Hormel								
Light & Lean 97 Breast Sliced	1 slice (1 oz)	30	5	1	15	0	0	380
Light & Lean 97 Mesquite Smoked Breast	1 slice (1 oz)	30	5	1	15	0	0	370
turkey pepperoni	17 slices (1 oz)	80	9	4	40	0	0	550
Jordan's								
Healthy Trim Fat Free Oven Roasted Breast	1 slice (1 oz)	20	4	0	15	0	0	180
Louis Rich								
Bologna	1 slice (28 g)	50	3	4	20	1	0	270
Breaded Nuggets	4 (3.2 oz)	260	13	16	35	15	0	640
Breaded Patties	1 (3 oz)	220	12	13	35	13	0	530
Breaded Sticks	3 (3 oz)	230	12	15	35	12	0	580
Breast Skinless Hickory Smoked	2 oz	50	11	0	25	1	0	720
Breast Skinless Honey Roasted	2 oz	60	11	0	20	3	0	660
Breast Skinless Oven Roasted	2 oz	50	11	0	20	1	0	660
Breast Skinless Rotisserie	2 oz	50	11	0	20	1	0	670
Breast Slices Hickory Smoked	1 slice (2 oz)	50	11	0	25	1	0	720
Breast Slices Honey Roasted	1 slice (2 oz)	60	11	0	20	3	0	660
Breast Slices Oven Roasted	1 slice (2 oz)	50	11	0	20	1	0	660
Breast Slices Rotisserie	1 slice (2 oz)	50	11	0	20	1	0	670
Carving Board Hickory Smoked	2 slices (1.6 oz)	40	9	1	20	0	0	540

FOOD	PORTION	CAL	PROT	FAT	CHOL	CARB	FIBER	SOD
Carving Board Oven Roasted Thin	6 slices (2.1 oz)	60	12	1	25	1	0	710
Carving Board Oven Roasted Traditional	2 slices (1.6 oz)	40	9	1	20	0	0	540
Carving Board Rotisserie	2 slices (1.6 oz)	40	9	1	20	0	0	460
Cotto Salami	1 slice (28 g)	40	4	3	25	0	0	280
Deli-Thin Oven Roasted	4 slices (1.8 oz)	50	9	1	20	2	0	580
Deli-Thin Smoked	4 slices (1.8 oz)	50	9	2	20	1	0	480
Fat Free Hickory Smoked Breast	1 slice (1 oz)	25	4	0	10	1	0	300
Fat Free Oven Roasted Breast	1 slice (1 oz)	25	4	0	10	1	0	330
Fat Free Oven Roasted Deli-Thin Breast	4 slices (1.8 oz)	45	8	0	15	2	0	620
Fat Free Turkey Ham Honey	2 slices (1.7 oz)	35	7	0	15	2	0	600
Fat Free Turkey Ham Smoked	2 slices (1.7 oz)	35	7	0	15	1	0	580
Hickory Smoked	1 slice (1 oz)	30	5	1	10	1	0	260
Oven Roasted	1 slice (1 oz)	30	5	1	10	1	0	310
Pastrami	1 slice (1 oz)	30	5	1	20	1	0	380
Smoked	1 slice (1 oz)	30	5	1	15	0	0	280
Turkey Ham	1 slice (1 oz)	30	5	1	20	1	0	380
Turkey Ham Chopped	1 slice (1 oz)	45	5	3	20	1	0	350
Turkey Ham Honey Cured	1 slice (1 oz)	30	5	1	20	1	0	350
Oscar Mayer								
Free Oven Roasted Breast	4 slices (1.8 oz)	40	8	0	15	2	0	670
Free Smoked Breast	4 slices (1.8 oz)	40	8	0	15	2	0	570
Oven Roasted White	1 slice (1 oz)	30	4	1	10	1	0	300
Smoked White	1 slice (1 oz)	30	4	1	10	1	0	310
Perdue								
Breast Sliced Cajun Style	2 oz	50	9	1	20	1	—	800

FOOD	PORTION	CAL	PROT	FAT	CHOL	CARB	FIBER	SOD
Breast Sliced Honey Smoked	2 oz	50	10	0	20	2	–	510
Breast Sliced Pan Roasted	2 oz	70	14	2	30	0	–	390
Ham Hickory Smoked	2 oz	60	9	3	40	1	–	770
Healthsense Breast Sliced Oven Roasted	2 oz	60	10	0	20	3	–	290
Pastrami Hickory Smoked	2 oz	70	9	3	40	2	–	670
Shady Brook								
Black Forest Turkey Ham	2 oz	70	10	3	30	–	–	470
Browned Homestyle Oven Roasted Breast	2 oz	60	11	1	20	–	–	400
Browned Slow Roasted Breast	2 oz	60	11	0	20	–	–	400
Carved Breast Italian Seasoned	2 oz	60	12	0	20	–	–	490
Carved Breast Natural Roast	2 oz	60	12	0	20	–	–	470
Carved Breast Peppered	2 oz	60	12	0	20	–	–	450
Hickory Smoked Breast	2 oz	50	11	0	25	–	–	470
Honey Roasted Breast	2 oz	60	11	1	30	–	–	400
Honey Roasted Breast Covered w/ Cracked Pepper	2 oz	60	11	0	25	–	–	470
Meatballs Italian Style	3 (3 oz)	130	12	7	45	5	1	350
Smoked Drumstick	3 oz	180	22	8	70	–	–	620
Smoked Neck	3 oz	150	22	6	65	–	–	700
Smoked Whole Turkey	3 oz	150	24	4	60	–	–	660
Smoked Wing	3 oz	200	22	10	65	–	–	680

FOOD	PORTION	CAL	PROT	FAT	CHOL	CARB	FIBER	SOD
Wampler								
Bologna	2 oz	130	8	11	50	1	—	550
Dark Cured	2 oz	80	8	5	30	2	—	600
Deli Roast Breast	2 oz	50	12	1	25	0	—	250
Deli Roast Classic Spiced Breast	2 oz	70	16	1	25	1	—	380
Deli Roast Pan Roasted Breast	2 oz	70	13	2	20	1	—	400
Deli Roast Pan Roasted Skinless Breast	2 oz	50	12	0	20	1	—	400
Deli Roast Peppered Breast	21 oz	40	8	0	20	1	—	520
Deli Roast Rotisserie Breast	2 oz	50	9	2	20	1	—	500
Pastrami	2 oz	90	9	5	40	1	—	220
Salami	2 oz	90	9	6	55	1	—	560
Turkey Ham	2 oz	60	10	3	40	0	—	590
TURKEY DISHES								
gravy & turkey	1 cup (8.4 oz)	160	14	6	—	11	—	1328
gravy & turkey	1 pkg (5 oz)	95	8	4	—	7	—	786
Banquet								
Sandwich Toppers Gravy & Sliced Turkey	1 pkg (5 oz)	160	8	11	30	6	0	670
Dinty Moore								
Microwave Cup Stew	1 pkg (7.5 oz)	130	9	3	10	16	2	760
Stew	1 cup (8.5 oz)	140	10	3	20	19	2	910
Mosey's								
Turkey Breast w/ Gravy	1 serv (5 oz)	140	30	1	90	4	0	540
Shady Brook								
Meatloaf	1 serv (16 oz)	470	38	17	175	—	—	900
Spreadables								
Turkey Salad	¼ can	100	—	6	20	—	—	—
Wampler								
Turkey Ham Salad	⅓ cup	150	7	10	30	9	—	500

FOOD	PORTION	CAL	PROT	FAT	CHOL	CARB	FIBER	SOD
TURKEY SUBSTITUTES								
Lightlife								
Smart Deli Turkey	3 slices (1.5 oz)	40	9	0	0	1	0	290
Soy Is Us								
Turkey Not!	½ cup (1.75 oz)	140	25	2	0	15	9	5
Tofurkey								
Deli Slices Hickory	1.5 oz	120	13	2	0	14	2	286
Deli Slices Original	1.5 oz	120	13	2	0	14	2	286
Deli Slices Peppered	1.5 oz	120	13	2	0	14	2	286
Drummettes	1 (3 oz)	105	11	2	0	11	4	380
Giblet Gravy	1 serv (3.5 oz)	42	4	2	0	5	1	340
Stuffed Tofu Roast	1 serv (4 oz)	193	26	5	0	10	2	310
Worthington								
Smoked Turkey Meatless	3 slices (2 oz)	140	10	10	0	3	2	620
Turkee Slices	3 slices (3.3 oz)	130	13	14	0	3	2	580
Yves								
Veggie Turkey Deli Slices	1 serv (2.2 oz)	85	18	0	0	4	1	480
TURNIPS								
canned greens	½ cup	17	2	tr	0	3	–	325
cooked mashed	½ cup (4.2 oz)	47	2	tr	0	10	–	25
cubed cooked	½ cup (3 oz)	33	1	tr	0	7	–	17
frzn greens cooked	½ cup	24	3	tr	0	4	2	12
greens chopped cooked	½ cup	15	1	tr	0	3	2	21
greens raw chopped	½ cup	7	tr	tr	0	2	1	11
raw cubed	½ cup (2.4 oz)	25	1	tr	0	6	–	14
Birds Eye								
Greens w/ Diced Turnip	1 cup (3 oz)	25	2	0	0	2	2	20
TURTLE								
raw	3.5 oz	85	18	1	–	0	–	–
TUSK FISH								
raw	3.5 oz	79	17	tr	–	0	–	113
VANILLA								
Virginia Dare								
Vanilla Extract	1 tsp	10	–	0	0	–	–	–

FOOD	PORTION	CAL	PROT	FAT	CHOL	CARB	FIBER	SOD
VEAL (see also DINNER, VEAL DISHES)								
cutlet lean only braised	3 oz	172	31	4	115	0	—	57
cutlet lean only fried	3 oz	156	28	4	91	0	—	65
ground broiled	3 oz	146	21	6	87	0	—	70
loin chop w/ bone lean & fat braised	1 chop (2.8 oz)	227	24	14	94	0	—	64
loin chop w/ bone lean only braised	1 chop (2.4 oz)	155	23	6	86	0	—	58
shoulder w/ bone lean only braised	3 oz	169	29	5	110	0	—	83
sirloin w/ bone lean & fat roasted	3 oz	171	21	9	87	0	—	71
sirloin w/ bone lean only roasted	3 oz	143	22	5	89	0	—	72
VEAL DISHES								
TAKE-OUT								
parmigiana	4.2 oz	279	22	18	136	6	2	545
VEGETABLE JUICE								
Dole								
Vegetable Blend	1 bottle (12 oz)	90	4	0	0	19	2	820
Hunt's								
Cocktail	1 can (6 oz)	20	2	0	0	7	2	630
Muir Glen								
Organic	5.5 oz	50	1	0	0	10	2	420
V8								
Lightly Tangy	8 oz	58	2	1	—	11	2	345
Low Sodium	8 oz	53	2	tr	—	11	2	95
Original	8 oz	51	2	1	—	10	2	615
Picante Vegetable	8 oz	51	2	tr	—	10	2	673
Spicy Hot	8 oz	49	2	tr	—	10	2	780
Splash Tropical Blend	8 fl oz	120	0	0	0	30	—	20
VEGETABLES MIXED								
CANNED								
Chi-Chi's								
Diced Tomatoes & Green Chilies	¼ cup (2.5 oz)	20	0	0	0	4	0	340

FOOD	PORTION	CAL	PROT	FAT	CHOL	CARB	FIBER	SOD
Chun King								
Chow Mein Vegetables	⅔ cup (3 oz)	14	1	tr	0	3	1	323
Del Monte								
Mixed	½ cup (4.4 oz)	40	2	0	0	8	2	360
Mixed No Salt Added	½ cup (4.4 oz)	40	2	0	0	8	2	25
Peas And Carrots	½ cup (4.5 oz)	60	2	0	0	11	2	360
Green Giant								
Garden Medley	½ cup (4.2 oz)	40	1	0	0	9	2	360
Mixed	½ cup (4.3 oz)	60	2	0	0	12	2	460
Sweet Peas & Carrots	½ cup (4.3 oz)	50	2	0	0	11	3	410
Sweet Peas & Tiny Pearl Onion	½ cup (4.4 oz)	60	4	0	0	11	4	520
House Of Tsang								
Vegetables & Sauce Cantonese Classic	½ cup (4.2 oz)	70	1	1	0	14	1	960
Vegetables & Sauce Hong Kong Sweet & Sour	½ cup (4.5 oz)	160	0	0	0	40	0	580
Vegetables & Sauce Szechuan Hot & Spicy	½ cup (4.2 oz)	70	1	1	0	14	1	1130
Vegetables & Sauce Tokyo Teriyaki	½ cup (4.4 oz)	100	1	0	0	23	1	1240
La Choy								
Chop Suey Vegetables	½ cup (2.2 oz)	10	1	tr	0	2	1	241
LeSueur								
Early Peas w/ Mushrooms & Pearl Onions	½ cup (4.3 oz)	60	3	0	0	11	2	380
S&W								
Mixed	½ cup (4.4 oz)	35	1	0	0	7	2	370
Peas & Carrots	½ cup (4.5 oz)	60	2	0	0	11	2	360
Peas & Onions	½ cup (4.3 oz)	40	3	0	0	11	3	530
FROZEN								
mixed vegetables cooked	½ cup	54	3	tr	0	12	2	32
peas & carrots cooked	½ cup	38	3	tr	0	8	–	55

FOOD	PORTION	CAL	PROT	FAT	CHOL	CARB	FIBER	SOD
peas & onions cooked	½ cup	40	2	tr	0	8	—	—
succotash cooked	½ cup	79	4	1	0	17	—	38
Amy's Organic								
Pocket Sandwich Mediterranean Vegetables	1 (4.5 oz)	220	9	7	15	33	3	540
Pocket Sandwich Roasted Vegetables	1 (4.5 oz)	220	6	8	0	35	4	480
Pocket Sandwich Vegetable Pie	1 (5 oz)	230	7	6	0	37	2	420
Birds Eye								
Baby Sweet Peas & Pearl Onions	⅔ cup (3.2 oz)	60	4	1	0	12	4	85
Bavarian Vegetables	1 cup (5.5 oz)	150	5	8	30	15	3	460
Broccoli Cauliflower Carrots w/ Cheese	½ cup (3.9 oz)	70	3	4	5	7	2	460
Broccoli Cauliflower & Red Peppers	½ cup	20	2	0	0	5	2	20
Broccoli & Cauliflower	½ cup	20	2	0	0	4	2	20
Broccoli Carrots & Water Chestnuts	½ cup (3.3 oz)	30	2	0	0	7	3	30
Broccoli Corn & Red Peppers	½ cup	50	3	0	0	12	3	15
Broccoli Red Peppers Onions & Mushrooms	½ cup	25	2	0	0	5	2	20
Broccoli & Cauliflower & Carrots	½ cup	25	2	0	0	5	2	30
Brussels Sprouts Cauliflower & Carrots	½ cup	30	2	0	0	7	3	20
California Style Vegetables	½ cup (3 oz)	100	3	5	10	9	3	240
Cauliflower Nuggets Corn Carrots & Snow Peas Pods	½ cup (3.2 oz)	30	2	0	0	6	2	25

FOOD	PORTION	CAL	PROT	FAT	CHOL	CARB	FIBER	SOD
Chicken Viola! Italian Pesto Chicken	2 cups (6.6 oz)	240	15	9	25	24	1	690
Chicken Viola! Three Cheese Chicken	1¾ cups (5.6 oz)	220	14	8	20	24	1	570
French Style	⅔ cup (4.4 oz)	110	2	6	10	10	2	290
Gumbo Blend	¾ cup (3 oz)	40	2	0	0	10	2	30
Italian Style Vegetables & Bow Tie Pasta	1 cup (5.8 oz)	150	3	9	10	13	2	380
Mixed Vegetables	⅓ cup	50	–	0	0	–	3	35
New England Style Vegetables & Pasta Shells	1 pkg (7.9 oz)	260	6	14	15	29	3	480
Peas & Pearl Onions	⅔ cup (4.2 oz)	90	5	1	0	18	5	520
Peas & Potatoes In Cream Sauce	½ cup (4.4 oz)	90	4	3	10	13	2	350
Radiatore Pasta & Vegetables	1 cup (4.6 oz)	200	6	8	5	27	1	430
Roasted Potatoes & Broccoli	⅔ cup (3.9 oz)	100	3	4	5	15	1	470
Roletti Pasta & Vegetables	1 cup (4.4 oz)	190	5	8	5	11	1	350
Stir Fry Asparagus	2 cups (5.8 oz)	90	5	1	0	16	3	35
Stir Fry Broccoli	1 cup (3.4 oz)	30	2	0	0	5	2	30
Stir Fry Pepper	1 cup (3 oz)	25	1	0	0	5	2	15
Stir Fry Sugar Snap	¾ cup	35	1	0	0	5	1	20
Stir Fry Whole Green Bean	1¾ cup (5.3 oz)	100	4	1	0	19	2	25
Stir Fry Style Vegetables	½ cup (3.6 oz)	60	2	4	10	5	1	270
Vegetables For Stew	⅔ cup (2.9 oz)	40	1	0	0	9	1	40
Green Giant								
Alfredo Vegetables	¾ cup	70	4	3	5	9	3	440
American Mixtures Broccoli Carrots Cauliflower	¾ cup (2.6 oz)	25	1	0	0	5	2	30

FOOD	PORTION	CAL	PROT	FAT	CHOL	CARB	FIBER	SOD
American Mixtures Broccoli Carrots Waterchestnuts	¾ cup (3 oz)	30	1	0	0	6	3	30
American Mixtures Carrots Green Bean Cauliflower	¾ cup (2.7 oz)	25	1	0	0	5	2	20
American Mixtures Corn Broccoli Red Pepper	¾ cup (3.1 oz)	60	2	0	0	13	2	10
American Mixtures Sweet Peas Potatoes Carrots	⅔ cup (3 oz)	70	2	2	0	12	3	70
Butter Sauce Broccoli Pasta Sweet Peas Corn Red Peppers	¾ cup (3.5 oz)	70	3	2	<5	11	2	280
Butter Sauce Mixed	¾ cup (3.6 oz)	70	2	2	<5	11	3	240
Cheese Sauce Broccoli Cauliflower Carrots	⅔ cup (4.3 oz)	80	3	3	<5	11	2	560
Harvest Fresh Broccoli Cauliflower Carrots	1 cup (3.4 oz)	30	2	0	0	5	3	125
Harvest Fresh Mixed Vegetables	⅔ cup (3.1 oz)	50	2	0	0	10	3	125
Harvest Fresh Sweet Peas & Pearl Onions	½ cup (2.7 oz)	55	3	0	0	10	3	170
Mixed	¾ cup (2.9 oz)	50	2	0	0	11	3	35
Select Sweet Peas & Pearl Onions	⅔ cup (3.1 oz)	60	4	0	0	12	4	125
Health Is Wealth								
Veggie Munchees	2 (1 oz)	50	2	1	0	9	1	170
La Choy								
Fancy Chinese Mixed Vegetables	½ cup (2.9 oz)	9	1	tr	0	1	1	31
Tree Of Life								
Mixed	½ cup (3 oz)	65	3	0	0	13	3	60

FOOD	PORTION	CAL	PROT	FAT	CHOL	CARB	FIBER	SOD
TAKE-OUT								
buddha's delight	1 serv (16 oz)	174	17	5	35	17	3	1368
caponata	¼ cup	28	–	1	0	–	–	–
curry	1 serv (7.7 oz)	398	4	33	–	22	–	–
gyoza potstickers vegetable	8 (4.9 oz)	210	8	4	0	34	5	500
pakoras	1 (2 oz)	108	5	5	–	12	3	–
ratatouille	1 serv (3.5 oz)	96	2	7	0	7	4	812
samosa	2 (4 oz)	519	3	46	–	25	3	–
succotash	½ cup	111	5	1	0	23	–	16
VENISON								
roasted	3 oz	134	26	3	95	0	–	46
VINEGAR								
balsamic	1 tbsp (0.5 oz)	5	0	0	0	2	–	0
cider	1 tbsp	tr	tr	0	0	1	–	tr
Eden								
Organic Brown Rice	1 tbsp	2	0	0	0	0	0	0
Ume Plum	1 tsp	2	0	0	0	0	0	1050
Progresso								
Balsamic	2 tbsp (0.5 oz)	10	0	0	0	2	0	0
Victoria								
Balsamic	1 tbsp (0.5 oz)	5	0	0	0	2	–	0
White House								
Apple Cider	1 tbsp (0.5 oz)	0	0	0	0	0	0	0
White	1 tbsp (0.5 oz)	0	0	0	0	0	–	0
WAFFLES								
FROZEN								
buttermilk	1 4 in sq (1.2 oz)	88	2	3	–	14	1	262
plain	1 4 in sq (1.2 oz)	88	2	3	–	14	1	262
Eggo								
Apple Cinnamon	2 (2.7 oz)	220	5	8	20	33	1	450
Banana Bread	2 (2.7 oz)	200	5	7	0	32	2	280
Blueberry	2 (2.7 oz)	220	5	9	20	32	1	460
Buttermilk	2 (2.7 oz)	220	5	8	25	31	1	460
Golden Oat	2 (2.7 oz)	150	6	3	0	29	3	340
Homestyle	2 (2.7 oz)	220	5	8	25	32	1	480
Minis Cinnamon Toast	12 (3.2 oz)	290	5	10	25	45	2	470

FOOD	PORTION	CAL	PROT	FAT	CHOL	CARB	FIBER	SOD
Minis Homestyle	12 (3.3 oz)	260	7	9	25	38	2	600
Nut & Honey	2 (2.7 oz)	240	6	10	25	31	2	450
Nutri-Grain	2 (2.7 oz)	190	5	6	0	30	4	450
Nutri-Grain Multi-Bran	2 (2.7 oz)	180	5	6	0	32	6	410
Nutri-Grain Raisin & Bran	2 (2.9 oz)	210	5	6	0	36	5	430
Special K	2 (2 oz)	120	6	0	0	26	1	280
Strawberry	2 (2.7 oz)	220	6	8	20	32	1	460
Kellogg's								
Homestyle Low Fat	2 (2.7 oz)	180	6	3	20	34	1	340
Nutri-Grain Low Fat	2 (2.7 oz)	160	5	3	0	31	3	480
Nutri-Grain Low Fat Blueberry	2 (2.7 oz)	160	5	2	0	33	3	460
Kid Cuisine								
Wave Rider Waffle Sticks	1 meal (6.6 oz)	380	3	8	30	75	3	580
Van's								
7 Grain Belgain	2	152	7	4	0	9	8	160
Belgian Original	2	145	5	4	0	30	2	108
Belgian Original Toaster	2	145	5	4	0	24	2	92
Blueberry Toaster	2	157	5	4	0	24	2	92
Blueberry Wheat Free Toaster	2	225	4	5	0	32	5	390
Fat Free	2	155	5	2	0	30	7	230
Mini	4	107	3	4	0	18	6	275
Multigrain Toaster	2	160	6	4	0	25	6	135
Organic Whole Wheat	2	190	6	5	0	30	6	230
Organic Whole Wheat Blueberry	2	190	6	5	0	30	6	230
Wheat Free Cinnamon Apple Toaster	2	220	4	5	0	32	5	390
Wheat Free Toaster	2	220	4	5	0	32	5	390
MIX								
plain as prep	1 7 in diam (2.6 oz)	218	5	10	39	26	1	458

FOOD	PORTION	CAL	PROT	FAT	CHOL	CARB	FIBER	SOD
READY-TO-EAT								
Thomas'								
Buttermilk	1 (1.6 oz)	130	3	5	0	18	tr	490
WALNUTS								
black dried chopped	1 cup	759	30	71	0	15	–	2
english dried	1 oz	182	4	18	0	5	1	3
english dried chopped	1 cup	770	17	74	0	22	6	12
halves	14 (1 oz)	190	4	19	0	4	2	tr
Planters								
Black	1 pkg (2 oz)	340	14	31	0	8	3	0
Gold Measure Halves	1 pkg (2 oz)	380	8	38	0	8	2	0
Halves	⅓ cup (1.2 oz)	220	5	22	0	5	1	0
Pieces	¼ cup (1 oz)	190	4	20	0	4	1	0
WASABI (see HORSERADISH)								
WATER								
Absopure								
Natural Spring	8 fl oz	0	0	0	0	0	–	0
Aquafina								
Drinking Water	8 fl oz	0	0	0	0	0	–	0
Aquess								
Purified Water w/ Soluble Fiber	1 bottle (18 oz)	30	0	0	0	8	5	0
Castellina								
Sparking Spring	8 fl oz	0	0	0	0	0	0	<5
Crystal Geyser								
Spring Water	8 fl oz	0	0	0	0	0	0	0
Dasani								
Purified Water	8 oz	0	0	0	0	0	–	0
Diamond Spring								
Water	1 qt	0	0	0	0	0	–	–
Ferrarelle								
Sparkling	8 fl oz	0	0	0	0	0	1	10
Gerolsteiner								
Sparkling Mineral	8 fl oz	0	0	0	0	0	0	30
Glaceau								
Smartwater	8 oz	0	0	0	0	0	0	0

FOOD	PORTION	CAL	PROT	FAT	CHOL	CARB	FIBER	SOD
Vitamin Water Tropical Citrus	1 cup (8 oz)	40	0	0	0	9	–	0
Glacier Springs								
Drinking Water	8 fl oz	0	0	0	0	0	0	0
Glennpatrick								
Irish Spring Pure	8 oz	0	0	0	0	0	0	–
LaCroix								
Spring	1 bottle (12 oz)	0	0	0	0	0	0	<8
Meridian								
Clear All Flavors	8 oz	100	0	0	0	25	–	0
Mountain Valley								
Mineral Water	1 qt	0	0	0	0	0	–	–
Mt Shasta								
Natural Spring	1 bottle (20 oz)	0	0	0	0	0	0	<13
Propel								
Fitness Water Berry	8 fl oz	10	0	0	0	3	–	35
Fitness Water Black Cherry	8 fl oz	10	0	0	0	3	–	35
Reebok								
Fitness Water Berry	1 bottle (24 oz)	30	0	0	0	0	0	0
Fitness Water Natural	1 bottle (24 oz)	0	0	0	0	0	0	0
San Pellegrino								
Acqua Panna	8 fl oz	0	0	0	0	0	0	0
Saratoga								
Spring	8 oz	0	0	0	0	0	–	0
Snapple								
Natural Spring	8 fl oz	0	0	0	0	0	0	0
Veryfine								
Fruit 2 O Lemon	8 oz	0	0	0	0	0	–	5
Fruit 2 O Lemon Lime	8 fl oz	0	0	0	0	0	–	5
Fruit 2 O Orange	8 fl oz	0	0	0	0	0	–	5
Fruit 2 O Raspberry	8 fl oz	0	0	0	0	0	–	5
Volvic								
Spring Water	8 oz	0	0	0	0	0	0	<5
Water Joe								
Caffeine Enhanced	8 fl oz	0	0	0	0	0	–	0
WATER CHESTNUTS								
chinese sliced canned	½ cup	35	1	tr	0	9	–	6
fresh sliced	½ cup	66	1	tr	0	15	–	9

FOOD	PORTION	CAL	PROT	FAT	CHOL	CARB	FIBER	SOD
Chun King								
Sliced	2 tbsp (0.8 oz)	11	tr	tr	0	3	1	3
Whole	2 (0.7 oz)	10	tr	tr	0	2	1	2
La Choy								
Chopped	2 tbsp (0.6 oz)	9	tr	tr	0	2	1	2
Sliced	2 tbsp (0.8 oz)	11	tr	tr	0	3	1	3
Whole	2 (0.7 oz)	10	tr	tr	0	2	1	2
WATERCRESS								
raw chopped	½ cup	2	tr	tr	0	tr	tr	7
WATERMELON								
cut up	1 cup	50	1	1	0	11	1	3
seeds dried	1 oz	158	8	13	0	4	–	28
seeds dried	1 cup	602	8	51	0	17	–	28
wedge	1/16	152	3	2	0	35	2	10
WATERMELON JUICE								
Kool-Aid								
Splash Drink	1 serv (8 oz)	110	0	0	0	30	0	35
WAX BEANS								
CANNED								
Del Monte								
Cut Golden	½ cup (4.2 oz)	20	1	0	0	4	2	360
Owatonna								
Cut	½ cup	20	–	0	0	–	–	–
S&W								
Cut	½ cup (4.2 oz)	20	1	0	0	4	2	360
WHALE								
raw	3.5 oz	134	23	3	–	0	–	100
WHEAT *(see also* BULGUR, BRAN, CEREAL, COUSCOUS, FLOUR, WHEAT GERM*)*								
sprouted	1 cup (3.8 oz)	214	8	1	0	46	1	17
starch	3.5 oz	348	tr	tr	–	86	–	2
Lightlife								
Savory Seitan Barbecue	4 oz	160	24	2	0	12	0	360
Savory Seitan Teriyaki	4 oz	160	26	2	0	10	0	320

FOOD	PORTION	CAL	PROT	FAT	CHOL	CARB	FIBER	SOD
Sonoma								
Wheat Nuts Salted	2 tbsp (0.5 oz)	60	0	3	0	8	1	140
WHEAT GERM								
plain toasted	¼ cup (1 oz)	108	8	3	0	14	4	1
plain toasted	1 cup	431	33	12	0	56	–	4
w/ brown sugar & honey toasted	1 oz	107	6	2	–	17	–	1
w/ brown sugar & honey toasted	1 cup	426	25	9	–	69	–	3
Kretschmer								
Original Toasted	2 tbsp (0.5 oz)	50	4	1	0	6	2	0
WHEY								
acid dry	1 tbsp (3 g)	10	tr	tr	–	2	–	28
acid fluid	1 cup (8 fl oz)	59	25	tr	–	13	–	118
sweet dry	1 tbsp (8 g)	26	1	tr	–	6	–	80
sweet fluid	1 cup (8 fl oz)	66	2	1	–	13	–	132
whey cheese	1 oz	126	4	8	–	9	0	146
WHIPPED TOPPINGS								
cream pressurized	1 tbsp (3 g)	8	tr	tr	2	tr	–	4
cream pressurized	1 cup (2.1 oz)	154	2	13	46	7	–	78
nondairy frzn	1 tbsp	13	tr	1	0	1	–	1
nondairy powdered as prep w/ whole milk	1 cup	151	3	10	8	13	–	53
nondairy powdered as prep w/ whole milk	1 tbsp (4 g)	8	tr	tr	tr	1	–	3
nondairy pressurized	1 tbsp (4 g)	11	tr	1	0	1	–	2
nondairy pressurized	1 cup	184	1	16	0	11	–	43
Cool Whip								
Extra Creamy	2 tbsp (0.3 oz)	25	0	2	0	2	0	5
Free	2 tbsp (0.3 oz)	15	0	0	0	3	0	5
Lite	2 tbsp (0.3 oz)	20	0	1	0	2	0	0
Original	2 tbsp (0.3 oz)	25	0	2	0	2	0	0
Dream Whip								
Mix as prep	2 tbsp (0.3 oz)	20	0	1	0	2	0	5
Estee								
Whipped Topping	1 serv	10	0	1	0	1	0	5

FOOD	PORTION	CAL	PROT	FAT	CHOL	CARB	FIBER	SOD
Kraft								
Dairy Whip Light Cream	2 tbsp (0.2 oz)	10	0	1	<5	tr	0	0
Fat Free	1 tbsp (0.3 oz)	15	0	0	0	2	0	5
WHITE BEANS								
canned	1 cup	306	19	1	0	58	–	13
dried cooked	1 cup	249	17	1	0	45	–	11
dried small cooked	1 cup	253	16	1	0	46	–	4
Progresso								
Cannellini	½ cup (4.6 oz)	100	5	1	0	18	5	270
WHITEFISH								
baked	3 oz	146	21	6	65	0	–	56
smoked	1 oz	39	7	tr	9	0	–	285
smoked	3 oz	92	20	1	28	0	–	866
WHITING								
cooked	3 oz	98	20	1	71	0	–	113
raw	3 oz	77	16	1	57	0	–	61
WILD RICE								
cooked	1 cup (5.7 oz)	166	7	1	0	35	3	5
Haddon House								
Extra Fancy	¼ cup (1.6 oz)	170	6	1	0	35	2	0
WINE *(see also* CHAMPAGNE*)*								
japanese plum	3 oz	139	tr	tr	0	16	0	–
japanese sake	1 oz	33	tr	0	0	2	0	1
madeira	3.5 oz	169	0	0	–	10	0	–
port	3.5 oz	156	tr	0	–	11	0	4
red	3½ oz	74	tr	0	0	2	–	6
rose	3½ oz	73	tr	0	0	2	–	5
sherry	2 oz	84	tr	0	0	5	–	–
sweet dessert	2 oz	90	tr	0	0	7	–	5
vermouth dry	3½ oz	105	–	0	0	1	–	–
vermouth sweet	3½ oz	167	–	0	0	12	–	–
white	3½ oz	70	tr	0	0	1	–	5
Eden								
Mirin Rice Cooking Wine	1 tbsp	25	0	0	0	7	0	130

FOOD	PORTION	CAL	PROT	FAT	CHOL	CARB	FIBER	SOD
WINGED BEANS								
dried cooked	1 cup	252	18	10	0	26	—	22
WOLFFISH								
atlantic baked	3 oz	105	19	3	50	0	—	93
WRAPS *(see* BREAD*)*								
YAM *(see also* SWEET POTATO*)*								
CANNED								
S&W								
Candied	½ cup (4.9 oz)	170	2	0	0	46	4	360
FRESH								
mountain yam hawaii cooked	½ cup	59	1	tr	0	14	—	9
yam cubed cooked	½ cup	79	1	tr	0	19	—	6
YAMBEAN								
cooked	¾ cup	38	1	tr	0	9	—	4
YARDLONG BEANS								
dried cooked	1 cup	202	14	1	0	36	—	9
YAUTIA (TANNIER)								
raw sliced	1 cup (4.7 oz)	132	2	1	0	32	2	28
root raw	1 (10.7 oz)	299	4	1	0	72	5	64
YEAST								
baker's compressed	1 cake (0.6 oz)	18	1	tr	0	3	2	5
baker's dry	1 pkg (¼ oz)	21	3	tr	0	3	—	—
baker's dry	1 tbsp	35	5	1	0	5	3	—
brewer's dry	1 tbsp	25	3	tr	0	3	—	10
Fleischmann's								
Active Dry	1 pkg (7 g)	23	—	3	—	—	—	10
Bread Machine	1 pkg (7 g)	26	—	2	—	—	—	10
RapidRise	1 pkg (7 g)	26	—	2	—	—	—	10
Hodgson Mill								
Fast Rise	1 tsp (9 g)	25	3	0	0	4	1	0
YELLOW BEANS								
canned	½ cup	13	1	tr	0	3	1	170
canned low sodium	½ cup	13	1	tr	0	3	1	1
dried cooked	1 cup	254	16	2	0	45	—	8
fresh cooked	½ cup	22	1	tr	0	5	—	2

FOOD	PORTION	CAL	PROT	FAT	CHOL	CARB	FIBER	SOD
fresh raw	½ cup	17	1	tr	0	4	–	3
frozen cooked	½ cup	18	1	tr	0	4	–	9

YELLOWEYE BEANS
CANNED
B&M
| Baked | ½ cup (4.6 oz) | 170 | 8 | 2 | <5 | 28 | 7 | 460 |

YELLOWTAIL
| baked | 3 oz | 159 | 25 | 6 | – | 0 | – | 42 |

YOGURT (see also YOGURT FROZEN)
coffee lowfat	8 oz	194	11	3	11	31	–	149
fruit lowfat	8 oz	225	9	3	10	42	–	121
fruit lowfat	4 oz	113	5	1	5	21	–	60
plain	8 oz	139	8	7	29	11	–	105
plain lowfat	8 oz	144	12	4	14	16	–	159
plain no fat	8 oz	127	13	tr	4	17	–	174
vanilla lowfat	8 oz	194	11	3	11	31	–	149

Breyers
Blended Blueberry	4.4 oz	130	4	1	10	25	0	60
Blended Peach	4.4 oz	130	4	1	10	26	0	65
Blended Strawberry	4.4 oz	130	4	1	10	26	0	60
Light Nonfat Apple Pie A La Mode	8 oz	120	7	0	10	22	0	105
Light Nonfat Berry Banana Split	8 oz	120	8	0	10	21	0	105
Light Nonfat Black Cherry Jubilee	8 oz	120	8	0	10	23	0	100
Light Nonfat Blueberries N' Cream	8 oz	120	8	0	10	23	0	100
Light Nonfat Cherry Bon-Bon	8 oz	120	8	0	10	22	0	105
Light Nonfat Cherry Vanilla Cream	8 oz	120	8	0	10	22	0	105
Light Nonfat Classic Strawberry	8 oz	120	8	0	10	22	0	100
Light Nonfat Key Lime Pie	8 oz	120	8	0	10	22	0	100

FOOD	PORTION	CAL	PROT	FAT	CHOL	CARB	FIBER	SOD
Light Nonfat Lemon Chiffon	8 oz	120	7	0	10	22	0	100
Light Nonfat Peaches N' Cream	8 oz	120	8	0	10	22	0	115
Light Nonfat Raspberries N' Cream	8 oz	120	8	0	10	22	0	105
Light Nonfat Strawberry Cheesecake	8 oz	120	8	0	10	22	tr	100
Lowfat Black Cherry	8 oz	240	9	3	15	44	0	125
Lowfat Blueberry	8 oz	230	9	3	15	43	0	125
Lowfat Mixed Berry	8 oz	320	9	3	15	43	0	125
Lowfat Peach	8 oz	240	9	3	15	43	0	125
Lowfat Pineapple	8 oz	240	9	3	15	45	0	125
Lowfat Red Raspberry	8 oz	230	9	3	15	43	2	125
Lowfat Strawberry	8 oz	230	9	3	15	43	0	125
Lowfat Strawberry Banana	8 oz	240	9	3	15	44	tr	125
Lowfat Vanilla	8 oz	220	10	3	20	38	0	135
Smooth & Creamy Apple Cobbler	8 oz	230	8	2	20	46	0	140
Smooth & Creamy Black Cherry Parfait	8 oz	240	9	2	20	46	0	130
Smooth & Creamy Black Cherry Parfait	4.4 oz	130	5	1	10	26	0	70
Smooth & Creamy Blueberries 'N Cream	8 oz	240	9	2	20	46	0	125
Smooth & Creamy Blueberries 'N Cream	4.4 oz	130	5	1	10	26	0	70
Smooth & Creamy Classic Strawberry	8 oz	230	9	2	20	45	0	125
Smooth & Creamy Classic Strawberry	4.4 oz	130	5	1	10	25	0	70

FOOD	PORTION	CAL	PROT	FAT	CHOL	CARB	FIBER	SOD
Smooth & Creamy Orange Vanilla Cream	8 oz	230	9	2	20	45	0	125
Smooth & Creamy Peaches 'N Cream	4.4 oz	130	5	1	10	25	0	70
Smooth & Creamy Peaches 'N Cream	8 oz	230	9	2	20	46	0	125
Smooth & Creamy Raspberries 'N Cream	8 oz	230	9	2	20	45	0	135
Smooth & Creamy Strawberry Banana Split	8 oz	240	8	2	10	48	tr	125
Smooth & Creamy Strawberry Cheesecake	8 oz	240	9	2	20	46	0	125
Colombo								
99% Fat Free Peach	4 oz	110	3	1	5	22	0	60
99% Fat Free Strawberry	4 oz	110	3	1	5	22	0	60
Dannon								
Chunky Fruit Nonfat Apple Cinnamon	6 oz	160	7	0	5	33	0	100
Chunky Fruit Nonfat Blueberry	6 oz	160	7	0	5	32	0	110
Chunky Fruit Nonfat Cherry Vanilla	6 oz	160	7	0	5	31	0	100
Chunky Fruit Nonfat Peach	6 oz	160	7	0	5	33	0	100
Chunky Fruit Nonfat Strawberry	6 oz	160	7	0	5	32	0	105
Chunky Fruit Nonfat Strawberry Banana	6 oz	160	7	0	5	32	0	105
Danimals Lowfat Tropical Punch	4.4 oz	130	6	1	5	25	0	95
Danimals Lowfat Blueberry	4.4 oz	130	6	1	5	24	0	100

FOOD	PORTION	CAL	PROT	FAT	CHOL	CARB	FIBER	SOD
Danimals Lowfat Grape Lemonade	4.4 oz	120	6	1	5	22	0	90
Danimals Lowfat Lemon Ice	4.4 oz	120	6	1	5	22	0	100
Danimals Lowfat Orange Banana	4.4 oz	130	6	1	5	24	0	90
Danimals Lowfat Strawberry	4.4 oz	130	6	1	5	24	0	90
Danimals Lowfat Vanilla	4.4 oz	120	6	1	5	23	0	90
Danimals Lowfat Wild Raspberry	4.4 oz	120	6	1	5	22	0	90
Double Delights Banana Creme Strawberry	6 oz	160	7	1	10	32	0	100
Double Delights Bavarian Creme Raspberry	6 oz	170	7	1	10	34	0	125
Double Delights Cheesecake Cherry	6 oz	170	7	1	10	34	0	100
Double Delights Cheesecake Strawberry	6 oz	170	7	1	10	33	0	100
Double Delights Chocolate Cheesecake	6 oz	220	8	1	10	45	0	150
Double Delights Chocolate Dipped Strawberry	6 oz	210	8	1	10	45	0	150
Double Delights Chocolate Eclair	6 oz	220	8	1	10	45	0	150
Double Delights Vanilla Strawberry	6 oz	170	7	1	10	33	0	100
Double Delights Vanilla Peach & Apricot	6 oz	170	7	1	10	33	0	100

FOOD	PORTION	CAL	PROT	FAT	CHOL	CARB	FIBER	SOD
Fruit On The Bottom Lowfat Apple Cinnamon	8 oz	240	9	3	15	46	1	140
Fruit On The Bottom Lowfat Blueberry	8 oz	240	9	3	15	46	1	140
Fruit On The Bottom Lowfat Boysenberry	8 oz	240	9	3	15	45	1	150
Fruit On The Bottom Lowfat Cherry	8 oz	240	9	3	15	46	1	135
Fruit On The Bottom Lowfat Minipack Mixed Berry	4.4 oz	130	5	2	10	25	tr	80
Fruit On The Bottom Lowfat Minipack Strawberry	4.4 oz	130	5	2	10	25	tr	75
Fruit On The Bottom Lowfat Mixed Berries	8 oz	240	9	3	15	45	1	150
Fruit On The Bottom Lowfat Orange	8 oz	240	9	3	15	45	0	135
Fruit On The Bottom Lowfat Peach	8 oz	240	9	3	15	45	1	140
Fruit On The Bottom Lowfat Raspberry	8 oz	240	9	3	15	45	1	150
Fruit On The Bottom Lowfat Strawberry	8 oz	240	9	3	15	46	1	135
Fruit On The Bottom Lowfat Strawberry Banana	8 oz	240	9	3	15	43	1	140
LaCreme Vanilla	1 pkg (4.4 oz)	140	5	5	20	20	–	75
Light 'N Crunchy Mint Chocolate Chip	8 oz	140	8	0	5	27	0	150
Light 'N Crunchy Nonfat Caramel Apple Crunch	8 oz	140	8	0	<5	26	0	340
Light 'N Crunchy Nonfat Lemon Blueberry Cobbler	8 oz	140	8	0	<5	25	0	135

FOOD	PORTION	CAL	PROT	FAT	CHOL	CARB	FIBER	SOD
Light 'N Crunchy Nonfat Mocha Cappuccino	8 oz	140	8	0	<5	26	0	150
Light 'N Crunchy Nonfat Raspberry w/ Granola	8 oz	140	9	0	<5	26	2	120
Light 'N Crunchy Nonfat Vanilla Chocolate Crunch	8 oz	130	8	0	<5	23	0	140
Light Duets Cherry Cheesecake	6 oz	90	5	0	0	18	0	70
Light Duets Peaches N' Cream	6 oz	90	5	0	0	18	0	70
Light Duets Raspberry Royale	6 oz	90	5	0	0	17	0	75
Light Duets Strawberry Cheesecake	6 oz	90	5	0	0	18	0	70
Light Nonfat Banana Cream Pie	8 oz	100	8	0	<5	15	0	120
Light Nonfat Blueberry	8 oz	100	8	0	<5	18	0	115
Light Nonfat Cappuccino	8 oz	100	8	0	5	16	0	120
Light Nonfat Cherry Vanilla	8 oz	100	8	0	<5	18	0	120
Light Nonfat Coconut Cream Pie	8 oz	100	8	0	5	16	0	120
Light Nonfat Creme Caramel	8 oz	100	8	0	<5	15	0	120
Light Nonfat Lemon Chiffon	8 oz	100	8	0	5	15	0	120
Light Nonfat Mint Chocolate Cream Pie	8 oz	100	8	0	<5	17	0	120
Light Nonfat Peach	8 oz	100	8	0	<5	16	0	115
Light Nonfat Raspberry	8 oz	100	8	0	<5	17	0	120

FOOD	PORTION	CAL	PROT	FAT	CHOL	CARB	FIBER	SOD
Light Nonfat Strawberry	8 oz	100	8	0	<5	16	0	115
Light Nonfat Strawberry Banana	8 oz	100	8	0	<5	17	0	120
Light Nonfat Strawberry Kiwi	8 oz	100	8	0	5	16	0	120
Light Nonfat Tangerine Chiffon	8 oz	100	8	0	5	15	0	120
Light Nonfat Vanilla	8 oz	100	8	0	<5	15	0	120
Lowfat Coffee	8 oz	210	10	3	15	36	0	160
Lowfat Cranberry Raspberry	8 oz	210	10	3	15	36	0	160
Lowfat Lemon	8 oz	210	10	3	15	36	0	160
Lowfat Vanilla	8 oz	210	10	3	15	36	0	160
Minipack Blended Nonfat Blueberry	4.4 oz	120	5	0	5	25	0	80
Minipack Blended Nonfat Cherry	4.4 oz	110	5	0	5	24	0	80
Minipack Blended Nonfat Peach	4.4 oz	120	5	0	5	23	0	80
Minipack Blended Nonfat Raspberry	4.4 oz	120	5	0	5	24	0	80
Minipack Blended Nonfat Strawberry	4.4 oz	120	5	0	5	23	0	85
Minipack Blended Nonfat Strawberry Banana	4.4 oz	120	5	0	5	23	0	85
Sprinkl'ins Cherry Vanilla	1 (4.1 oz)	130	5	2	5	24	0	85
Sprinkl'ins Strawberry	1 (4.1 oz)	130	5	2	5	24	0	85
Sprinkl'ins Strawberry Banana	1 (4.1 oz)	130	5	2	5	24	0	80
Sprinkl'ins Vanilla w/ Cherry Crystals	1 (4.1 oz)	110	5	1	5	21	0	85
Sprinkl'ins Vanilla w/ Orange Crystals	1 (4.1 oz)	110	5	1	5	21	0	85

FOOD	PORTION	CAL	PROT	FAT	CHOL	CARB	FIBER	SOD
Horizon Organic								
Fat Free Apricot Mango	¾ cup (6 oz)	120	7	0	<5	23	0	100
Fat Free Honey	1 cup (8 oz)	160	9	0	<5	32	0	135
Jell-O								
Lowfat Cherry	4.4 oz	130	4	1	10	25	0	65
Lowfat Grape	4.4 oz	130	4	1	10	25	0	65
Lowfat Raspberry	4.4 oz	130	4	1	10	25	0	65
Lowfat Tropical Berry Twist	4.4 oz	130	4	1	10	25	0	65
Lowfat Tropical Punch	4.4 oz	130	4	1	10	25	0	65
Lowfat Watermelon	4.4 oz	130	4	1	10	25	0	65
Lowfat Wild Berry	4.4 oz	130	4	1	10	25	0	65
Lowfat Wild Strawberry	4.4 oz	130	4	1	10	25	0	65
Light N'Lively								
Free Blueberry	4.4 oz	70	4	0	5	13	0	55
Free Peach	4.4 oz	70	4	0	5	12	0	65
Free Strawberry	4.4 oz	70	4	0	5	12	0	55
Free Strawberry Banana Cream	4.4 oz	70	4	0	5	13	0	55
Free Strawberry Fruit Cup	4.4 oz	70	4	0	5	13	0	55
Lowfat Blueberry	4.4 oz	130	4	1	10	25	0	60
Lowfat Peach	4.4 oz	130	4	1	10	26	0	65
Lowfat Pineapple	4.4 oz	130	4	1	10	26	0	60
Lowfat Red Raspberry	4.4 oz	120	5	1	10	23	0	65
Lowfat Strawberry	4.4 oz	130	4	1	10	26	0	60
Lowfat Strawberry Banana Cream	4.4 oz	130	4	1	10	25	0	60
Lowfat Strawberry Fruit Cup	4.4 oz	130	4	1	10	25	0	60
Oberweis								
Peach	1 pkg (8 oz)	210	10	3	15	39	0	140
Pascual								
Nonfat Cherries & Berries	1 pkg (4.4 oz)	100	4	0	0	19	5	70
Nonfat Peach	1 pkg (4.4 oz)	100	4	0	0	19	5	70

FOOD	PORTION	CAL	PROT	FAT	CHOL	CARB	FIBER	SOD
Stonyfield Farm								
Creamy Maple	1 pkg	160	6	6	25	19	0	90
Mocho-Ccino	1 pkg	170	6	6	20	23	0	95
Nonfat Apricot Mango	1 pkg (8 oz)	160	8	0	0	31	tr	125
Nonfat Black Cherry	1 pkg (8 oz)	160	8	0	0	31	tr	130
Nonfat Cappuccino	1 pkg (8 oz)	160	9	0	0	31	0	135
Nonfat Cherry Vanilla	1 pkg (8 oz)	190	7	0	0	43	tr	120
Nonfat Chocolate Underground	1 pkg (8 oz)	200	8	0	0	46	tr	135
Nonfat French Vanilla	1 pkg (8 oz)	180	9	0	0	30	0	135
Nonfat Lotsa Lemon	1 pkg (8 oz)	160	9	0	0	30	0	140
Nonfat Peach	1 pkg (8 oz)	150	8	0	0	30	tr	130
Nonfat Plain	1 pkg (8 oz)	100	10	08	<5	15	0	150
Nonfat Raspberry	1 pkg (8 oz)	160	8	0	0	31	tr	130
Nonfat Strawberry	1 pkg (8 oz)	180	8	0	0	32	tr	130
Organic French Vanilla	1 pkg	170	6	6	20	23	0	85
Organic Wild Blueberry	1 pkg	160	5	6	20	22	tr	85
Organic Lowfat Blueberry	1 pkg (6 oz)	130	5	2	5	23	1	90
Organic Lowfat Luscious Lemon	1 pkg (6 oz)	130	5	2	5	23	1	115
Organic Lowfat Maple Vanilla	1 pkg (6 oz)	120	6	2	6	19	0	90
Organic Lowfat Mocha Latte	1 pkg (6 oz)	120	6	2	5	20	0	85
Organic Lowfat Plain	1 cup (8 oz)	110	9	2	10	14	0	135
Organic Lowfat Raspberry	1 pkg (6 oz)	130	6	2	5	23	1	100
Organic Lowfat Strawberry	1 pkg (6 oz)	130	5	2	5	23	1	115
Organic Lowfat Vanilla	1 pkg (6 oz)	120	6	2	5	20	0	100
Strawberries & Cream	1 pkg	160	5	5	20	23	tr	110
Vanilla Truffle	1 pkg	220	7	5	20	37	tr	100

FOOD	PORTION	CAL	PROT	FAT	CHOL	CARB	FIBER	SOD
YoSelf Organic Chocolate	1 (4 oz)	110	4	1	0	21	2	65
YoSelf Organic Creme Carmel	1 (4 oz)	110	4	1	5	21	2	65
Yosqueeze Strawberry	1 tube (2 oz)	60	2	1	5	11	1	30
Total								
Greek Yogurt	1 pkg (5 oz)	180	10	12	25	10	0	180
Greek Yogurt 0% Fat	1 pkg (5 oz)	80	15	0	0	6	0	110
Greek Yogurt 1% Fat	1 pkg (5 oz)	120	8	8	25	8	0	120
Yoplait								
99% Fat Free Blueberry	6 oz	180	6	2	10	34	0	80
99% Fat Free Boysenberry	6 oz	180	6	2	10	34	0	80
99% Fat Free Cherry	6 oz	180	6	2	10	34	0	80
99% Fat Free Harvest Peach	6 oz	120	4	1	5	23	0	55
99% Fat Free Harvest Peach	6 oz	180	6	2	10	34	0	80
99% Fat Free Key Lime Pie	6 oz	180	6	2	10	34	0	80
99% Fat Free Lemon	6 oz	180	6	2	10	34	0	80
99% Fat Free Mixed Berry	6 oz	120	4	1	5	23	0	55
99% Fat Free Mixed Berry	6 oz	180	6	2	10	34	0	80
99% Fat Free Orange	6 oz	180	6	2	10	34	0	80
99% Fat Free Pina Colada	6 oz	180	6	2	10	34	0	80
99% Fat Free Pineapple	6 oz	180	6	2	10	34	0	80
99% Fat Free Raspberry	6 oz	180	6	2	10	34	0	80
99% Fat Free Strawberry	6 oz	180	6	2	10	43	0	80
99% Fat Free Strawberry	6 oz	120	4	1	5	23	0	55

FOOD	PORTION	CAL	PROT	FAT	CHOL	CARB	FIBER	SOD
99% Fat Free Strawberry Banana	6 oz	180	6	2	10	34	0	80
99% Fat Free Strawberry Banana	6 oz	120	4	1	5	23	0	55
99% Fat Free Strawberry Cheesecake	6 oz	180	6	2	10	34	0	80
Custard Style Banana	6 oz	190	7	4	15	32	0	100
Custard Style Blueberry	6 oz	190	7	4	15	32	0	100
Custard Style Cherry Vanilla	6 oz	190	7	4	15	32	0	100
Custard Style Key Lime Pie	6 oz	190	7	4	15	32	0	100
Custard Style Lemon	6 oz	190	7	4	15	32	0	100
Custard Style Peaches'n Cream	6 oz	190	7	4	15	32	0	100
Custard Style Raspberry	6 oz	190	7	4	15	32	0	100
Custard Style Raspberry Cheesecake	6 oz	190	7	4	15	32	0	100
Custard Style Strawberry	6 oz	190	7	4	15	32	0	100
Custard Style Strawberry Banana	6 oz	190	7	4	15	32	0	100
Custard Style Strawberry Vanilla	4 oz	120	5	2	10	21	0	70
Custard Style Vanilla	6 oz	190	8	4	15	32	0	95
Go-Gurt Strawberry Banana Burst	1 pkg (2.25 oz)	80	2	2	5	12	0	40
Go-Gurt Watermelon Meltdown	1 pkg (2.25 oz)	80	2	2	5	12	0	40

FOOD	PORTION	CAL	PROT	FAT	CHOL	CARB	FIBER	SOD
Light Amaretto Cheesecake	6 oz	90	6	0	5	16	0	95
Light Apricot Mango	6 oz	90	5	0	5	16	0	75
Light Banana Cream	6 oz	90	6	0	5	16	0	95
Light Blueberry	6 oz	90	5	0	5	16	0	75
Light Boston Cream Pie	6 oz	90	6	0	5	16	0	95
Light Caramel Apple	6 oz	90	6	0	5	16	0	95
Light Cherry	6 oz	90	5	0	5	16	0	75
Light Key Lime Pie	6 oz	90	6	0	5	16	0	95
Light Lemon Cream Pie	6 oz	90	6	0	5	16	0	95
Light Peach	6 oz	90	5	0	5	16	0	75
Light Peach Melba	6 oz	90	5	0	5	16	0	75
Light Raspberry	6 oz	90	5	0	5	16	0	75
Light Strawberry	6 oz	90	5	0	5	16	0	75
Light Strawberry Banana	6 oz	90	5	0	5	16	0	75
Light White Chocolate Strawberry	6 oz	90	5	0	5	16	0	75
Original Cafe Au Lait	6 oz	170	6	2	10	31	0	80
Original Coconut Cream Pie	6 oz	200	6	4	10	35	0	80
Original French Vanilla	6 oz	180	6	2	10	34	0	90
Trix Rainbow Punch	6 oz	190	6	2	10	36	0	85
Trix Raspberry Rainbow	6 oz	190	6	2	10	36	0	85
Trix Strawberry Banana Bash	6 oz	190	6	2	10	36	0	85
Trix Strawberry Punch	4 oz	130	4	2	5	24	0	55
Trix Triple Cherry	6 oz	190	6	2	10	36	0	85
Trix Watermelon Burst	4 oz	130	4	2	5	24	0	55
Trix Wild Berry Blue	4 oz	130	4	2	5	24	0	55
Whips! Orange Creme	1 pkg (4 oz)	140	5	3	10	23	–	75

FOOD	PORTION	CAL	PROT	FAT	CHOL	CARB	FIBER	SOD
Whips! Raspberry Mousse	1 pkg (4 oz)	140	5	3	10	23	—	75

YOGURT FROZEN

FOOD	PORTION	CAL	PROT	FAT	CHOL	CARB	FIBER	SOD
chocolate soft serve	½ cup (4 fl oz)	115	3	4	3	18	—	71
vanilla soft serve	½ cup (4 fl oz)	114	3	4	2	17	—	63
Ben & Jerry's								
Cherry Garcia	½ cup	170	4	3	20	32	0	80
Chocolate Cherry Garcia	½ cup	190	5	4	15	35	1	65
Chocolate Chip Cookie Dough	½ cup	200	4	5	10	35	0	120
Chocolate Fudge Brownie	½ cup	190	5	3	5	36	1	105
Chocolate Heath Bar Crunch	½ cup	210	5	6	10	35	1	115
Chunky Monkey	½ cup	200	4	6	5	34	tr	65
Pop Cherry Garcia	1	260	5	14	15	31	2	70
Breyers								
Chocolate	½ cup (2.6 oz)	130	3	3	10	23	tr	45
Fat Free Chocolate	½ cup (2.6 oz)	100	3	0	<5	23	0	40
Fat Free Cookies N Cream	½ cup (2.6 oz)	110	3	0	0	25	tr	75
Fat Free Peach	½ cup (2.6 oz)	90	3	0	0	20	0	40
Fat Free Strawberry	½ cup (2.6 oz)	100	2	0	0	22	0	40
Fat Free Take Two Vanilla Chocolate	½ cup (2.6 oz)	100	2	0	0	23	tr	45
Fat Free Vanilla	½ cup (2.6 oz)	100	3	0	0	23	tr	50
Fat Free Vanilla Fudge Twirl	½ cup (2.6 oz)	110	3	0	0	25	0	45
Vanilla	½ cup (2.6 oz)	120	3	3	10	22	0	40
Vanilla Chocolate Strawberry	½ cup (2.6 oz)	120	3	3	10	22	0	40
Dannon								
Light Cappuccino	½ cup (2.8 oz)	80	4	0	0	20	0	60
Light Cherry Vanilla Swirl	½ cup (2.8 oz)	90	4	0	0	21	0	55
Light Chocolate	½ cup (2.7 oz)	80	4	0	0	21	tr	55

FOOD	PORTION	CAL	PROT	FAT	CHOL	CARB	FIBER	SOD
Light Mint Chocolate Fudge	½ cup (2.8 oz)	90	4	0	0	23	0	60
Light Peach Raspberry Melba	½ cup (2.8 oz)	90	4	0	0	20	0	60
Light Strawberry Cheesecake	½ cup (2.8 oz)	90	3	0	0	21	0	70
Light Vanilla	½ cup (2.8 oz)	80	4	0	0	20	0	60
Light Duets Strawberry Sundae	6 oz	90	5	0	0	18	0	70
Light'N Crunchy Banana Cream Pie	½ cup (2.8 oz)	110	3	1	0	23	0	65
Light'N Crunchy Carmel Toffee Crunch	½ cup (2.8 oz)	110	3	1	0	26	0	75
Light'N Crunchy Mocha Chocolate Chunk	½ cup (2.8 oz)	110	4	1	0	23	0	60
Light'N Crunchy Peanut Chocolate Crunch	½ cup (2.8 oz)	110	4	1	0	24	0	65
Light'N Crunchy Rocky Road	½ cup (2.8 oz)	110	3	1	0	27	tr	60
Light'N Crunchy Triple Chocolate	½ cup (2.8 oz)	110	4	1	0	25	tr	60
Light'N Crunchy Vanilla Streusel	½ cup (2.8 oz)	110	3	1	0	25	0	80
Haagen-Dazs								
Lowfat Dulce De Leche	½ cup	190	6	3	5	35	0	75
Nonfat Chocolate	½ cup	140	7	0	<5	28	tr	45
Nonfat Coffee	½ cup	140	7	0	<5	29	0	45
Nonfat Strawberry	½ cup	140	5	0	<5	31	0	40
Nonfat Vanilla	½ cup	140	6	0	<5	29	0	45
Nonfat Vanilla Raspberry Swirl	½ cup	130	4	0	<5	29	tr	30
Nonfat Vanilla Fudge	½ cup	160	6	0	<5	34	0	105

FOOD	PORTION	CAL	PROT	FAT	CHOL	CARB	FIBER	SOD
Turkey Hill								
Black Raspberry	½ cup	110	–	3	10	20	–	60
Caramel Cashew Crunch	½ cup	160	–	9	25	18	–	60
Chocolate Chip Cookie Dough	½ cup	140	3	5	10	23	0	120
Clark Bar	½ cup	140	–	5	10	22	–	95
Fat Free Chocolate Cherry Cordial	½ cup	100	4	0	0	24	0	70
Fat Free Chocolate Marshmallow	½ cup	130	3	0	0	30	0	40
Fat Free Mint Cookie 'N Cream	½ cup	110	4	0	0	24	0	80
Fat Free Neapolitan	½ cup	100	3	0	0	22	0	50
Fat Free Orange Swirl	½ cup	100	–	0	0	22	–	40
Fat Free Vanilla Fudge	½ cup	110	3	0	0	24	0	80
Peach Raspberry	½ cup	110	3	2	10	20	0	60
Tin Roof Sundae	½ cup	140	4	5	10	21	0	100
Vanilla & Chocolate	½ cup	110	3	3	10	19	0	70
Vanilla Bean	½ cup	110	4	3	10	17	0	70
ZUCCHINI								
baby raw	1 (0.5 oz)	3	tr	tr	0	1	tr	0
canned italian style	½ cup	33	1	tr	0	8	–	427
frzn cooked	½ cup	19	1	tr	0	4	–	2
raw sliced	½ cup	9	1	tr	0	2	1	2
sliced cooked	½ cup	14	1	tr	0	4	1	2
Progresso								
Italian Style	½ cup (4.2 oz)	50	2	2	0	7	2	400
TAKE-OUT								
indian paalkora	1 serv	46	2	2	1	7	2	141

PART TWO

Restaurant Chains

FOOD	PORTION	CAL	PROT	FAT	CHOL	CARB	FIBER	SOD
APPLEBEE'S								
DESSERTS								
Apple Betty Cobbler Ala Mode	1 serv	598	7	22	31	94	2	197
Fudge Brownie Sundae	1 serv	739	9	40	66	87	6	332
Low Fat Bikini Banana Strawberry Shortcake	1 serv	248	6	2	8	48	2	223
Low Fat Brownie Sundae	1 serv	415	11	2	3	82	3	417
Low Fat Marble Cheesecake	1 serv	261	10	2	10	50	4	378
MAIN MENU SELECTIONS								
Applebee's Burger w/ Fries	1 serv	1274	55	79	263	90	7	2713
Basic Hamburger w/ Fries	1 serv	980	31	58	118	86	6	1814
Beef Fajita Quesadilla	1 serv	1205	51	86	159	58	6	2969
Bourbon Street Steak w/ Fried New Potatoes	1 serv	1115	60	94	168	50	–	3542
Low Fat Asian Chicken Salad	1 med serv (2.5 oz)	370	19	6	40	64	7	1431
Low Fat Asian Chicken Salad	1 serv (5 oz)	623	35	9	76	107	14	2487
Low Fat Blackened Chicken Salad	1 med serv (2.5 oz)	287	40	3	43	27	6	1763
Low Fat Blackened Chicken Salad	1 serv (5 oz)	411	56	5	82	39	11	2188
Low Fat Garlic Chicken Pasta	1 serv	587	41	8	39	89	9	1551
Low Fat Lemon Chicken Pasta	1 serv	528	33	11	50	78	8	2438
Low Fat Quesadilla Chicken Fajita	1 serv	518	42	11	35	63	2	2244
Low Fat Quesadilla Veggie	1 serv	344	27	8	8	46	3	1138

FOOD	PORTION	CAL	PROT	FAT	CHOL	CARB	FIBER	SOD
Mozzarella Stix	8 pieces	963	41	57	64	74	1	1990
Quesadillas	1 serv	684	31	46	99	40	4	2175
Riblet Basket w/ Fries	1 serv	1317	78	92	219	45	7	2697
Salad Dinner w/o Dressing	1 serv	303	22	18	277	13	3	661
Salad Santa Fe Chicken	1 med	724	33	42	96	56	7	2409
Sandwich Bacon Cheese Chicken Grill w/o Fries	1	746	46	46	133	36	1	1722
Sandwich Gyro	1	880	24	69	15	44	3	2015
Stir Fry Chicken	1 serv	566	38	7	76	89	5	2470

ARBY'S

BEVERAGES

FOOD	PORTION	CAL	PROT	FAT	CHOL	CARB	FIBER	SOD
Chocolate Shake	1 (14 oz)	480	10	16	45	84	0	370
Hot Chocolate	1 serv (8.6 oz)	110	2	1	0	23	0	120
Jamocha Shake	1 (14 oz)	470	10	15	45	82	0	390
Milk	1 serv (8 oz)	120	8	5	20	12	0	120
Orange Juice	1 serv (10 oz)	140	1	0	0	34	0	0
Strawberry Shake	1 (14 oz)	500	11	13	15	87	0	340
Vanilla Shake	1 (14 oz)	470	10	15	45	83	0	360

BREAKFAST SELECTIONS

FOOD	PORTION	CAL	PROT	FAT	CHOL	CARB	FIBER	SOD
Add Egg To Breakfast	1 serv (2 oz)	110	5	9	175	2	0	170
Add Swiss Cheese Slice	1 slice (0.5 oz)	45	3	3	10	—	0	220
Biscuit w/ Bacon	1 (3.4 oz)	360	9	24	10	27	1	220
Biscuit w/ Butter	1 (2.9 oz)	280	5	17	0	27	1	780
Biscuit w/ Ham	1 (4.3 oz)	330	12	20	30	28	1	830
Biscuit w/ Sausage	1 (4.2)	460	12	33	25	28	1	300
Croissant w/ Bacon	1 (2.7 oz)	340	10	23	30	28	1	520
Croissant w/ Ham	1 (3.7 oz)	310	13	19	11	29	0	1130
Croissant w/ Sausage	1 (3.6 oz)	440	13	32	45	29	0	600
Maple Syrup	1 serv (0.5 oz)	130	0	0	0	32	0	45
Sourdough w/ Bacon	1 (5.1 oz)	420	16	10	10	66	3	960
Sourdough w/ Ham	1 (6.1 oz)	390	19	6	30	67	2	1570
Sourdough w/ Sausage	1 (5.9 oz)	520	19	19	25	67	2	1040
Toastix w/o Syrup	6 pieces (4.4 oz)	370	7	17	0	48	4	440

FOOD	PORTION	CAL	PROT	FAT	CHOL	CARB	FIBER	SOD
DESSERTS								
Apple Turnover Iced	1 (4.5 oz)	420	4	16	0	65	2	230
Cherry Turnover Iced	1 (4.5 oz)	410	4	16	0	63	1	250
MAIN MENU SELECTIONS								
Arby's Sauce	1 serv (0.5 oz)	15	0	0	0	4	0	180
Au Jus Sauce	1 serv (3 oz)	5	tr	tr	0	1	tr	386
BBQ Dipping Sauce	1 serv (1 oz)	40	0	0	0	10	0	350
Baked Potato Broccoli'N Cheddar	1 (14 oz)	540	12	24	50	71	7	680
Baked Potato Deluxe	1 (13 oz)	650	20	34	90	67	6	750
Baked Potato w/ Butter & Sour Cream	1 (11.2 oz)	500	8	24	55	65	6	170
Bronco Berry Sauce	1 serv (1.5 oz)	90	0	0	0	23	0	35
Caesar Salad w/o Dressing	1 serv (8 oz)	90	7	4	10	8	3	170
Cheddar Curly Fries	1 serv (6 oz)	460	6	24	5	54	4	1290
Chicken Finger 4-Pak	1 serv (6.77 oz)	640	31	38	70	42	0	1590
Chicken Finger Salad w/o Dressing	1 serv (13 oz)	570	30	34	65	39	3	1300
Chicken Finger Snack	1 serv (6.4 oz)	580	19	32	35	55	3	1450
Curly Fries	1 med (4.5 oz)	400	5	20	0	50	4	990
Curly Fries	1 lg (7 oz)	620	8	30	0	78	7	1540
Curly Fries	1 sm (3.8 oz)	310	4	15	0	39	3	770
German Mustard	1 pkg (0.25 oz)	5	0	0	0	0	0	60
Grilled Chicken Caesar Salad w/o Dressing	1 serv (12 oz)	230	33	8	80	8	3	920
Homestyle Fries	1 med (5 oz)	370	4	16	0	53	4	710
Homestyle Fries	1 lg (7.5 oz)	560	6	24	0	79	6	1070
Homestyle Fries	1 sm (4 oz)	300	3	13	0	42	3	570
Homestyle Fries Child-Size	1 serv (3 oz)	220	3	10	0	32	3	430
Honey Mustard	1 serv (1 oz)	130	0	12	10	5	0	160
Horsey Sauce	1 pkg (0.5 oz)	60	0	5	0	3	0	150
Jalapeno Bites	1 serv (4 oz)	330	7	21	40	29	2	670
Ketchup	1 pkg (0.3 oz)	10	0	0	0	2	0	100

FOOD	PORTION	CAL	PROT	FAT	CHOL	CARB	FIBER	SOD
Light Grilled Chicken Salad	1 (16.3 oz)	210	30	5	65	14	6	800
Marinara Sauce	1 serv (1.5 oz)	35	1	1	0	4	0	260
Mayonnaise	1 pkg (0.4 oz)	90	0	10	10	0	0	65
Mayonnaise Light Cholesterol Free	1 pkg (0.4 oz)	20	0	2	0	1	0	110
Mozzarella Sticks	1 serv (4.8 oz)	470	18	29	60	34	2	1330
Onion Petals	1 serv (4 oz)	410	4	24	0	43	2	300
Potato Cakes	2 (3.5 oz)	250	2	16	0	26	3	490
Roast Beef Sandwich Arby's Melt w/ Cheddar	1 (5.2 oz)	320	16	14	45	36	2	850
Roast Beef Sandwich Arby-Q	1 (6.4 oz)	360	16	14	70	40	2	1530
Roast Beef Sandwich Beef'N Cheddar	1 (6.9 oz)	460	23	23	50	43	2	1170
Roast Beef Sandwich Big Montana	1 (11 oz)	560	47	27	50	42	3	1900
Roast Beef Sandwich Giant	1 (7.9 oz)	440	32	20	45	42	3	1330
Roast Beef Sandwich Junior	1 (4.4 oz)	290	16	12	40	34	2	700
Roast Beef Sandwich Regular	1 (5.4 oz)	330	21	14	45	35	2	890
Roast Beef Sandwich Super	1 (8.5 oz)	450	22	21	45	48	3	1060
Sandwich Chicken Bacon'N Swiss	1 (7.4 oz)	610	31	33	110	49	2	1550
Sandwich Chicken Breast Fillet	1 (7.2 oz)	550	24	30	90	47	2	1160
Sandwich Chicken Cordon Bleu	1 (8.4 oz)	630	34	35	120	47	2	1820
Sandwich Grilled Chicken Deluxe	1 (8.7 oz)	450	29	22	110	37	2	1050
Sandwich Hot Ham 'N Swiss	1 (5.9 oz)	340	23	13	90	35	1	1450
Sandwich Light Roast Chicken Deluxe	1 (7.2 oz)	260	23	5	40	33	3	1010
Sandwich Light Roast Turkey Deluxe	1 (7.2 oz)	260	23	5	40	33	3	1030

FOOD	PORTION	CAL	PROT	FAT	CHOL	CARB	FIBER	SOD
Sandwich Market Fresh Roast Beef & Swiss	1 (12.5 oz)	780	37	40	80	74	6	1690
Sandwich Market Fresh Roast Chicken Caesar	1 (12.7 oz)	820	43	38	140	75	5	2160
Sandwich Market Fresh Roast Ham & Swiss	1 (12.5 oz)	730	36	34	125	74	5	2180
Sandwich Market Fresh Roast Turkey & Swiss	1 (12.5 oz)	760	43	33	135	75	5	1920
Sandwich Roast Chicken Club	1 (8.4 oz)	520	29	28	115	38	2	1440
Sub Sandwich French Dip	1 (10 oz)	410	26	16	45	43	2	1200
Sub Sandwich Hot Ham'N Swiss	1 (9.7 oz)	530	29	27	110	45	3	1860
Sub Sandwich Italian	1 (11 oz)	780	29	53	120	49	3	2440
Sub Sandwich Pilly Beef'N Swiss	1 (10.8 oz)	670	36	40	75	46	4	1850
Sub Sandwich Roast Beef	1 (11.6 oz)	730	35	46	76	48	3	2140
Sub Sandwich Turkey	1 (10.6 oz)	630	29	37	100	51	2	2170
Tangy Southwest Sauce	1 serv (1.5 oz)	250	0	26	30	3	0	290
SALAD DRESSINGS								
Bleu Cheese	1 serv (2 oz)	300	2	31	45	3	0	580
Buttermilk Ranch	1 serv (2 oz)	360	1	39	5	2	0	490
Buttermilk Ranch Reduced Calorie	1 serv (2 oz)	60	1	0	0	13	1	750
Caesar	1 serv (2 oz)	310	1	34	60	1	0	470
Honey French	1 serv (2 oz)	290	0	24	0	18	tr	410
Italian Reduced Calorie	1 serv (2 oz)	25	0	1	0	3	tr	1030
Thousand Island	1 serv (2 oz)	290	1	28	35	9	0	480
SALADS AND SALAD BARS								
Croutons Seasoned	1 serv (0.25 oz)	30	1	1	0	5	1	70

FOOD	PORTION	CAL	PROT	FAT	CHOL	CARB	FIBER	SOD
Croutons Cheese & Garlic	1 serv (0.63 oz)	100	3	6	–	10	0	138
Garden Salad	1 (12.3 oz)	70	4	1	0	14	6	45
Light Grilled Chicken Sandwich	1 (7.5 oz)	280	29	5	55	30	3	1170
Light Roast Chicken Salad	1 (14.8 oz)	160	20	3	40	15	6	700
Side Salad	1 (6.1 oz)	30	2	0	0	6	3	20
Turkey Club Salad w/o Dressing	1 serv (12 oz)	350	33	21	90	9	3	860

AU BON PAIN
BAKED SELECTIONS

FOOD	PORTION	CAL	PROT	FAT	CHOL	CARB	FIBER	SOD
Apple Coffee Cake	1 piece (4.6 oz)	480	6	24	96	60	2	285
Bagel Chocolate Chip	1 (5 oz)	380	12	7	5	69	3	480
Bagel Dutch Apple w/ Walnut Streussel	1 (5 oz)	360	11	5	0	77	4	480
Baguette Loaf	1 slice (1.8 oz)	140	5	5	0	29	1	350
Biscotti	1 (1.5 oz)	200	4	10	35	24	1	45
Biscotti Chocolate	1 (1.7 oz)	240	5	13	35	28	2	50
Braided Roll	1 (1.8 oz)	170	5	5	0	26	1	320
Cinnamon Roll	1 (7 oz)	710	12	26	100	110	3	740
Cookie Chocolate Chip	1 (2.1 oz)	280	3	13	40	40	2	85
Cookie Oatmeal Raisin	1 (2.1 oz)	250	3	10	30	40	2	240
Cookie Peanut Butter	1 (2.1 oz)	280	7	15	30	32	1	260
Cookie Shortbread	1 (2.4 oz)	390	3	25	65	39	1	190
Croissant Almond	1 (4.3 oz)	560	12	37	105	50	4	260
Croissant Apple	1 (3.4 oz)	280	4	10	25	46	1	180
Croissant Chocolate	1 (3.4 oz)	440	7	23	30	53	4	230
Croissant Cinnamon Raisin	1 (3.7 oz)	380	7	13	35	61	2	290
Croissant Plain	1 (2.1 oz)	270	6	15	40	30	1	240
Croissant Raspberry Cheese	1 (3.5 oz)	380	6	19	60	47	1	300
Croissant Sweet Cheese	1 (3.6 oz)	390	7	22	75	42	1	330
Danish Cheese Swirl	1 (3.8 oz)	450	7	28	95	46	1	410
Danish Lemon Swirl	1 (4 oz)	450	7	24	80	53	1	410

FOOD	PORTION	CAL	PROT	FAT	CHOL	CARB	FIBER	SOD
Danish Raspberry	1 (3.6 oz)	370	7	21	65	42	2	350
Danish Sweet Cheese	1 (3.6 oz)	420	7	26	90	42	1	380
Four Grain Loaf	1 slice (1.8 oz)	130	5	1	0	25	1	280
French Sandwich Roll	1 (1.8 oz)	120	4	5	0	25	1	320
Hazelnut Fudge Brownie	1 (4 oz)	380	5	18	100	56	4	150
Holiday Cookie Cranberry Almond Macaroon	1 (1.5 oz)	160	2	8	0	22	2	115
Holiday Cookie Cranberry Almond Macaroon w/ Chocolate	1 (1.9 oz)	210	3	11	0	27	2	120
Holiday Cookie English Toffee	1 (1.8 oz)	220	2	12	45	28	0	110
Holiday Cookie Ginger Pecan	1 (2 oz)	260	5	15	40	30	1	115
Mochaccino Bar	1 (4 oz)	404	5	24	37	44	1	294
Muffin Blueberry	1 (4.5 oz)	410	8	15	85	64	1	380
Muffin Carrot	1 (5 oz)	480	8	23	55	61	3	650
Muffin Chocolate Chip	1 (4.5 oz)	490	8	20	35	70	2	560
Muffin Corn	1 (4.6 oz)	470	8	18	65	70	2	570
Muffin Pumpkin w/ Streusel Topping	1 (5.5 oz)	470	8	18	60	74	2	550
Muffin Low Fat Chocolate Cake	1 (4 oz)	290	4	3	20	68	3	630
Muffin Low Fat Triple Berry	1 (4.2 oz)	270	5	3	25	60	2	560
Multigrain Loaf	1 slice (1.8 oz)	130	5	1	0	26	1	340
Parisienne Loaf	1 slice (1.8 oz)	120	4	5	0	25	1	300
Pear Ginger Tea Cake	1 piece (4 oz)	380	3	20	0	47	1	202
Pecan Roll	1 (6.8 oz)	900	11	48	50	111	4	480
Roll 3 Seed Pecan Raisin	1 (2.7 oz)	250	9	6	0	43	3	240
Roll Hearth Sandwich	1 (2.8 oz)	220	9	2	0	43	2	410

FOOD	PORTION	CAL	PROT	FAT	CHOL	CARB	FIBER	SOD
Roll Petit Pan	1 (2.5 oz)	200	7	1	0	41	1	570
Rye Loaf	1 slice (1.8 oz)	110	5	2	0	21	2	310
Scone Cinnamon	1 (4.1 oz)	520	10	28	145	60	1	230
Scone Current	1 (3.7 oz)	430	10	23	155	47	2	230
Scone Orange	1 (4.1 oz)	440	10	23	155	53	2	240
Sourdough Bagel Asiago Cheese	1 (4.2 oz)	380	17	6	15	66	3	690
Sourdough Bagel Cinnamon Raisin	1 (4.5 oz)	390	14	1	0	83	4	550
Sourdough Bagel Cranberry Walnut	1 (5 oz)	460	15	4	0	93	7	590
Sourdough Bagel Everything	1 (4.2 oz)	360	14	3	0	72	3	710
Sourdough Bagel Honey 8 Grain	1 (4.2 oz)	360	14	2	0	72	6	580
Sourdough Bagel Mocha Chip Swirl	1 (5 oz)	370	12	4	0	72	3	480
Sourdough Bagel Plain	1 (4 oz)	350	13	1	0	71	3	540
Sourdough Bagel Sesame	1 (4.2 oz)	380	15	4	0	71	3	540
Sourdough Bagel Wild Blueberry	1 (4.5 oz)	380	14	2	0	80	4	570
Valentine Cookie Chocolate Dipped Shortbread	1 (2.8 oz)	410	4	27	55	41	2	160
Valentine Cookie Red Sugar Shortbread Heart	1 (2.4 oz)	350	3	22	60	37	1	170
Valentine Cookie Shortbread	1 (2.4 oz)	340	3	22	60	35	1	170
BEVERAGES								
Frozen Java Blast	1 serv (16 oz)	220	7	2	10	42	0	120
Frozen Mocha Blast	1 serv (16 oz)	320	9	3	10	64	2	150
Hot Apple Cider	1 med (16 oz)	310	0	0	0	77	0	150
Hot Apple Cider	1 sm (10 oz)	190	0	0	0	47	0	95
Hot Apple Cider	1 lg (20 oz)	350	0	0	0	87	0	170
Hot Hazelnut Blast	1 serv (16 oz)	310	11	6	25	57	0	180
Hot Mocha Blast	1 lg (17 oz)	310	14	8	30	45	0	230

FOOD	PORTION	CAL	PROT	FAT	CHOL	CARB	FIBER	SOD
Hot Mocha Blast	1 med (13 oz)	260	11	6	25	41	0	180
Hot Mocha Blast	1 sm (9 oz)	160	8	4	15	23	0	120
Hot Raspberry Mocha Blast	1 serv (16 oz)	300	11	6	25	52	0	170
Hot Raspberry Mocha Blast	1 serv (10 oz)	180	14	4	15	29	0	115
Hot Raspberry Mocha Blast	1 serv (20 oz)	350	14	8	30	57	0	220
Hot Strawberry Chocolate Blast	1 serv (16 oz)	330	11	6	25	57	0	180
Hot Vanilla Chocolate Blast	1 serv (16 oz)	310	11	6	25	57	0	180
Iced Caffee Latte	1 lg (20.5 oz)	270	18	10	40	26	0	270
Iced Caffee Latte	1 sm (9 oz)	130	9	5	20	12	0	130
Iced Caffee Latte	1 med (12 oz)	150	10	6	25	15	0	150
Iced Cappuccino	1 sm (9 oz)	110	7	4	15	10	0	110
Iced Cappuccino	1 lg (20.5 oz)	270	18	10	40	26	0	270
Iced Cappuccino	1 med (12 oz)	150	10	6	25	15	0	150
Iced Cocoa	1 lg (20.5 oz)	440	20	11	40	66	0	320
Iced Cocoa	1 sm (9 oz)	200	10	6	20	27	0	160
Iced Cocoa	1 med (12 oz)	280	12	6	25	42	0	190
Iced Hazelnut Blast	1 serv (16 oz)	310	11	6	25	54	0	180
Iced Mocha Blast	1 med (12 oz)	260	11	6	25	41	0	180
Iced Mocha Blast	1 lg (20.5 oz)	360	18	10	40	50	0	280
Iced Mocha Blast	1 sm (9 oz)	180	9	5	20	25	0	135
Iced Raspberry Mocha Blast	1 serv (24 oz)	330	13	7	25	54	0	200
Iced Raspberry Mocha Blast	1 serv (16 oz)	310	11	6	25	54	0	180
Iced Raspberry Mocha Blast	1 serv (12 oz)	160	6	4	15	27	0	100
Iced Strawberry Chocolate Blast	1 serv (16 oz)	310	11	6	25	54	0	180
Iced Vanilla Chocolate Blast	1 serv (16 oz)	310	11	6	25	54	0	180
Iced Tea Peach	1 med (12 oz)	130	0	0	0	33	0	20
Iced Tea Peach	1 sm (12 oz)	90	0	0	0	22	0	15
Iced Tea Peach	1 lg (16 oz)	170	0	0	0	44	0	30
Iced Tea Raspberry	1 lg (16 oz)	150	0	0	0	38	0	30
Iced Tea Raspberry	1 med (12 oz)	110	0	0	0	29	0	20

FOOD	PORTION	CAL	PROT	FAT	CHOL	CARB	FIBER	SOD
Iced Tea Raspberry	1 sm (8 oz)	80	0	0	0	19	0	15
Whipped Cream	1 serv (1.2 oz)	160	0	11	55	11	0	0
SALAD DRESSINGS								
Bleu Cheese	1 serv (3 oz)	370	4	41	40	8	0	910
Buttermilk Ranch	1 serv (3 oz)	310	3	32	35	4	0	270
Caesar	1 serv (3 oz)	380	5	39	25	3	0	410
Fat Free Tomato Basil	1 serv (3 oz)	70	1	0	0	17	1	650
Greek	1 serv (3 oz)	440	0	50	0	2	0	820
Lemon Basil Vinaigrette	1 serv (3 oz)	330	0	32	0	15	0	460
Lite Honey Mustard	1 serv (3 oz)	280	2	17	40	30	1	560
Lite Italian	1 serv (3 oz)	230	0	20	0	15	0	570
Sesame French	1 serv (3 oz)	370	1	30	0	26	1	1010
SALADS AND SALAD BARS								
Caesar	1 serv (8.9 oz)	270	19	10	20	27	5	800
Chicken Caesar	1 serv (11.4 oz)	360	36	11	65	28	5	910
Garden	1 lg (10.6 oz)	160	7	2	0	34	6	290
Garden	1 sm (7.5 oz)	100	5	1	0	20	4	150
Mozzarella & Roasted Pepper Salad	1 serv (13.7 oz)	340	22	18	60	25	10	135
Pesto Chicken Salad	1 serv (10.7 oz)	230	20	11	45	11	4	250
Tuna	1 serv (15 oz)	490	26	27	45	40	7	750
SANDWICHES AND FILLINGS								
Bagel Spreads Lite Strawberry	1 serv (2 oz)	150	5	11	35	6	1	210
Bagel Spreads Lite Vanilla Hazelnut	1 serv (2 oz)	150	5	11	35	6	1	210
Cheddar	½ serv (1.5 oz)	170	11	14	45	1	0	260
Chicken Tarragon	1 serv (4 oz)	240	20	17	65	1	0	170
Club Sandwich Hot Roasted Turkey	1 (14.9 oz)	950	50	50	135	80	4	2240
Country Ham	1 serv (3.7 oz)	150	21	7	55	1	0	1370
Cracked Pepper Chicken	1 serv (3.9 oz)	140	27	2	72	2	0	184
Cream Cheese Lite	1 serv (2 oz)	130	5	12	35	2	1	230
Cream Cheese Lite Honey Walnut	1 serv (2 oz)	260	4	12	20	8	—	260

FOOD	PORTION	CAL	PROT	FAT	CHOL	CARB	FIBER	SOD
Cream Cheese Lite Raspberry	1 serv (2 oz)	200	6	8	20	10	—	280
Cream Cheese Lite Sun-Dried Tomato	1 serv (2 oz)	130	5	11	35	2	1	230
Cream Cheese Plain	1 serv (2 oz)	190	3	18	55	2	—	210
Cream Cheese Veggie Lite	1 serv (2 oz)	100	6	10	20	6	—	300
Grilled Chicken	1 serv (3.9 oz)	140	27	2	72	2	0	184
Hot Croissant Ham & Cheese	1 (4.2 oz)	380	16	20	70	36	1	690
Hot Croissant Spinach & Cheese	1 (3.6 oz)	270	9	16	40	27	2	330
Provolone	½ serv (1.5 oz)	150	11	11	30	1	0	370
Roast Beef	1 serv (3.7 oz)	140	22	5	50	1	0	550
Sandwich Arizona Chicken	1 (12.7 oz)	720	49	33	125	57	4	1190
Sandwich Buffalo Chicken	1 (13.7 oz)	640	41	19	85	76	3	1650
Sandwich California Chicken	1 (13.2 oz)	820	51	44	135	55	4	1200
Sandwich Fresh Mozzarella Tomato & Pesto	1 (10.5 oz)	650	30	30	55	69	4	1090
Sandwich Honey Dijon Chicken	1 (15.3 oz)	730	57	18	135	85	4	1990
Sandwich Parmesan Chicken	1 (11.1 oz)	740	42	24	70	91	5	1620
Sandwich Steak & Cheese Melt	1 (11.7 oz)	750	40	32	90	79	2	1600
Sandwich Thai Chicken	1 (8.3 oz)	420	20	6	20	72	3	1320
Swiss	½ serv (1.5 oz)	160	12	12	40	1	0	110
Tuna Salad	1 serv (4.5 oz)	360	21	29	50	3	1	520
Turkey Breast	1 serv (3.7 oz)	120	24	1	20	1	0	1110
Wraps Chicken Caesar	1 (9.9 oz)	630	36	31	80	46	2	1140
Wraps Southwestern Tuna	1 (14.4 oz)	950	41	64	110	53	4	1230
Wraps Summer Turkey	1 (11.7 oz)	340	29	9	35	36	9	1380

FOOD	PORTION	CAL	PROT	FAT	CHOL	CARB	FIBER	SOD
SOUPS								
Beef Barley	1 serv (12 oz)	112	9	3	18	16	3	980
Beef Barley	1 serv (16 oz)	150	12	4	25	22	5	1310
Beef Barley	1 serv (8 oz)	75	6	2	15	11	2	660
Beef Stew	1 serv (8 oz)	140	9	7	25	14	2	840
Bohemian Cabbage	1 serv (8 oz)	70	3	3	0	11	2	650
Bohemian Cabbage	1 serv (12 oz)	110	4	5	0	17	4	960
Bohemian Cabbage	1 serv (16 oz)	140	5	6	0	22	5	1280
Bread Bowl	1 (9 oz)	640	27	4	0	131	5	1950
Broccoli & Cheddar	1 serv (8 oz)	260	9	22	50	13	1	690
Broccoli & Cheddar	1 serv (16 oz)	520	17	44	100	25	2	1380
Broccoli & Cheddar	1 serv (12 oz)	390	13	33	75	19	2	1030
Caribbean Black Bean	1 serv (16 oz)	250	13	2	10	43	16	1540
Caribbean Black Bean	1 serv (12 oz)	180	10	2	10	32	12	1150
Caribbean Black Bean	1 serv (8 oz)	120	7	1	5	22	8	770
Chicken Chili	1 serv (12 oz)	350	21	18	65	31	5	2030
Chicken Chili	1 serv (8 oz)	240	14	12	45	21	4	1350
Chicken Chili	1 serv (16 oz)	470	28	24	90	41	8	2700
Chicken Noodle	1 serv (16 oz)	170	16	3	35	19	2	1340
Chicken Noodle	1 serv (8 oz)	80	8	2	15	10	1	670
Chicken Noodle	1 serv (12 oz)	120	12	2	25	14	2	1000
Chili	1 serv (12 oz)	340	22	14	50	32	7	910
Chili	1 serv (16 oz)	460	30	19	70	43	9	1220
Chili	1 serv (8 oz)	230	15	10	35	22	5	610
Clam Chowder	1 serv (12 oz)	400	16	29	95	24	1	1090
Clam Chowder	1 serv (16 oz)	540	22	39	125	32	1	1460
Clam Chowder	1 serv (8 oz)	270	11	19	65	16	0	730
Corn Chowder	1 serv (16 oz)	530	11	33	95	58	3	1530
Corn Chowder	1 serv (12 oz)	390	8	24	70	43	2	1150
Corn Chowder	1 serv (8 oz)	260	5	16	50	29	1	760
Cream Of Broccoli	1 serv (16 oz)	440	10	37	80	28	3	1550
Cream Of Broccoli	1 serv (12 oz)	330	8	28	60	21	2	1160
Cream Of Broccoli	1 serv (8 oz)	220	5	18	40	14	1	770
Cream Of Chicken With Wild Rice	1 serv (16 oz)	330	19	19	90	33	1	1310
French Onion	1 serv (12 oz)	120	4	5	0	17	3	1910
French Onion	1 serv (16 oz)	170	5	7	0	23	4	2550

FOOD	PORTION	CAL	PROT	FAT	CHOL	CARB	FIBER	SOD
French Onion	1 serv (8 oz)	80	2	4	0	12	2	1280
In A Bread Bowl Beef Barley	1 serv (21 oz)	760	36	7	20	147	8	2940
In A Bread Bowl Carribean Black Bean	1 serv (21 oz)	830	36	5	10	163	17	3100
In A Bread Bowl Chicken Chili	1 serv (21 oz)	990	48	22	65	162	12	3970
In A Bread Bowl Chicken Noodle	1 serv (21 oz)	760	39	6	20	146	7	2950
In A Bread Bowl Clam Chowder	1 serv (21 oz)	1050	43	32	100	155	5	3040
In A Bread Bowl Cream of Broccoli	1 serv (21 oz)	970	34	31	60	152	7	3100
In A Bread Bowl French Onion	1 serv (21 oz)	760	30	8	0	148	8	3860
In A Bread Bowl New England Potato & Cheese w/ Ham	1 serv (21 oz)	860	34	15	40	152	9	3170
In A Bread Bowl Tomato Florentine	1 serv (21 oz)	760	33	5	10	150	8	3490
In A Bread Bowl Vegetarian Chili	1 serv (21 oz)	870	36	7	0	171	8	3550
Louisiana Beans & Rice	1 serv (16 oz)	360	18	9	20	50	3	1320
Louisiana Beans & Rice	1 serv (8 oz)	180	9	5	10	25	1	660
Louisiana Beans & Rice	1 serv (12 oz)	280	13	7	15	37	2	960
New England Potato & Cheese w/ Ham	1 serv (8 oz)	150	5	8	25	14	3	820
New England Potato & Cheese w/ Ham	1 serv (12 oz)	220	7	12	40	21	4	1220
New England Potato & Cheese w/ Ham	1 serv (16 oz)	290	10	15	55	28	5	1630

FOOD	PORTION	CAL	PROT	FAT	CHOL	CARB	FIBER	SOD
Potato Leek	1 serv (12 oz)	320	6	20	70	28	2	1700
Potato Leek	1 serv (8 oz)	200	4	13	45	18	2	1060
Potato Leek	1 serv (16 oz)	400	7	25	85	36	3	2120
Sante Fe Chicken Tortilla	1 serv (16 oz)	300	12	13	30	42	4	1900
Sante Fe Chicken Tortilla	1 serv (8 oz)	150	6	7	15	21	2	950
Sante Fe Chicken Tortilla	1 serv (12 oz)	230	9	10	25	32	3	1430
Seafood Gumbo	1 serv (8 oz)	130	7	6	20	14	1	580
Seafood Gumbo	1 serv (12 oz)	190	10	9	25	21	2	870
Seafood Gumbo	1 serv (16 oz)	260	14	12	35	28	3	1160
Tomato Florentine	1 serv (8 oz)	61	4	1	5	13	2	1030
Tomato Florentine	1 serv (12 oz)	90	6	2	5	20	2	1550
Tomato Florentine	1 serv (16 oz)	122	8	2	5	27	3	2070
Tomato Tortellini	1 serv (12 oz)	90	4	2	5	15	2	1320
Tomato Tortellini	1 serv (8 oz)	60	3	1	5	11	2	950
Tomato Tortellini	1 serv (16 oz)	110	6	2	10	20	3	1770
Vegetable Stew	1 serv (8 oz)	60	3	1	5	11	2	980
Vegetable Stew	1 serv (12 oz)	100	5	2	5	16	4	1460
Vegetable Stew	1 serv (16 oz)	130	6	2	5	22	5	1950
Vegetarian Lentil	1 serv (16 oz)	270	21	1	0	47	5	1580
Vegetarian Lentil	1 serv (8 oz)	130	10	0	0	24	2	790
Vegetarian Lentil	1 serv (12 oz)	200	16	1	0	35	4	1180
Vegetarian Chili	1 serv (12 oz)	210	9	4	0	40	3	1610
Vegetarian Chili	1 serv (8 oz)	139	6	3	0	27	2	1070
Vegetarian Chili	1 serv (16 oz)	278	13	5	0	53	4	2150
Vegetarian Corn & Green Chili Bisque	1 serv (8 oz)	190	4	10	30	21	3	1140
Vegetarian Corn & Green Chili Bisque	1 serv (16 oz)	380	8	20	60	41	5	2290
Vegetarian Corn & Green Chili Bisque	1 serv (12 oz)	300	7	16	45	30	4	1830

AUNTIE ANNE'S

FOOD	PORTION	CAL	PROT	FAT	CHOL	CARB	FIBER	SOD
Caramel Dip	1 serv (1.5 oz)	135	1	3	5	27	0	110
Cheese Sauce	1 serv (1 oz)	70	3	5	15	2	0	400

FOOD	PORTION	CAL	PROT	FAT	CHOL	CARB	FIBER	SOD
Chocolate Dip	1 serv (1.25 oz)	130	1	4	2	24	1	65
Cream Cheese Light	1 serv (.75 oz)	45	2	4	15	1	0	105
Cream Cheese Pineapple	1 serv (.75 oz)	70	tr	6	20	3	0	70
Cream Cheese Strawberry	1 serv (.75 oz)	70	tr	6	20	3	0	70
Dutch Ice Kiwi Banana	1 (18 oz)	250	0	0	0	57	0	40
Dutch Ice Kiwi Banana	1 (12 oz)	160	0	0	0	38	0	25
Dutch Ice Lemonade	1 (12 oz)	270	0	0	0	66	0	0
Dutch Ice Lemonade	1 (18 oz)	405	0	0	0	99	1	0
Dutch Ice Mocha	1 (18 oz)	500	0	14	0	95	0	135
Dutch Ice Mocha	1 (12 oz)	340	0	9	0	63	0	90
Dutch Ice Orange Creme	1 (12 oz)	240	0	0	0	55	0	30
Dutch Ice Orange Creme	1 (18 oz)	360	0	0	0	83	0	45
Dutch Ice Raspberry	1 (18 oz)	220	0	0	0	51	1	40
Dutch Ice Raspberry	1 (12 oz)	150	0	0	0	34	1	25
Dutch Ice Strawberry	1 (12 oz)	190	0	0	0	43	0	35
Dutch Ice Strawberry	1 (18 oz)	280	0	0	0	65	1	50
Marinara Sauce	1 serv (1 oz)	10	0	0	0	3	0	130
Pretzel Almond w/ Butter	1	400	9	8	20	72	2	400
Pretzel Almond w/o Butter	1	350	9	2	0	72	2	390
Pretzel Cinnamon Raisin w/o Butter	1	350	9	2	0	74	2	410
Pretzel Cinnamon Sugar w/ Butter	1	450	8	9	25	83	3	430
Pretzel Garlic w/ Butter	1	350	9	5	10	68	2	850
Pretzel Garlic w/o Butter	1	320	9	1	0	66	2	830
Pretzel Glazin' Raisin w/ Butter	1	510	11	4	10	107	4	480
Pretzel Glazin' Raisin w/o Butter	1	470	11	1	0	104	3	460

FOOD	PORTION	CAL	PROT	FAT	CHOL	CARB	FIBER	SOD
Pretzel Jalapeno w/ Butter	1	310	8	5	10	59	2	940
Pretzel Jalapeno w/o Butter	1	270	8	1	0	58	2	780
Pretzel Original w/ Butter	1	370	10	4	10	72	2	930
Pretzel Original w/o Butter	1	340	10	1	0	72	3	900
Pretzel Sesame w/ Butter	1	410	12	12	15	64	7	860
Pretzel Sesame w/o Butter	1	350	11	6	0	63	3	840
Pretzel Sour Cream & Onion w/ Butter	1	340	9	5	10	66	2	930
Pretzel Sour Cream & Onion w/o Butter	1	310	9	1	0	66	2	920
Pretzel Whole Wheat w/ Butter	1	370	11	5	10	72	7	1120
Pretzel Whole Wheat w/o Butter	1	350	11	2	0	72	7	1100
Sweet Mustard	1 serv (1 oz)	60	tr	2	40	8	0	120

BASKIN-ROBBINS

FROZEN YOGURT

FOOD	PORTION	CAL	PROT	FAT	CHOL	CARB	FIBER	SOD
Maui Brownie Madness	½ cup	140	4	3	5	26	1	80
Perils Of Pauline	½ cup	140	4	3	5	25	0	105

ICE CREAM

FOOD	PORTION	CAL	PROT	FAT	CHOL	CARB	FIBER	SOD
Banana Strawberry	½ cup	130	2	7	25	17	0	40
Baseball Nut	½ cup	160	2	9	30	18	0	55
Black Walnut	½ cup	160	3	11	30	13	1	45
Cherries Jubilee	½ cup	140	2	7	30	16	0	40
Chocolate	½ cup	150	2	9	30	18	0	60
Chocolate Almond	½ cup	180	3	11	30	17	1	55
Chocolate Chip	½ cup	150	2	10	35	15	0	45
Chocolate Chip Cookie Dough	½ cup	170	2	9	35	20	0	70
Chocolate Fudge	½ cup	160	2	9	30	21	0	80
Chocolate Mousse Royale	½ cup	170	2	10	25	20	1	60

FOOD	PORTION	CAL	PROT	FAT	CHOL	CARB	FIBER	SOD
Chocolate Raspberry Truffle	½ cup	180	3	9	30	23	0	60
Chunky Heath Bar	½ cup	170	2	10	30	19	0	70
Cookies N Cream	½ cup	170	2	11	30	16	0	80
Dirt'N Worms	½ cup	160	2	8	25	22	0	80
Egg Nog	½ cup	150	2	8	40	16	0	45
Everybody's Favorite Candy Bar	½ cup	170	2	9	30	20	2	30
French Vanilla	½ cup	160	2	10	70	14	0	45
Fudge Brownie	½ cup	170	3	11	25	19	1	75
German Chocolate Cake	½ cup	180	3	10	25	20	0	75
Gold Medal Ribbon	½ cup	150	2	8	30	20	0	95
Jamoca	½ cup	140	2	9	35	14	0	45
Jamoca Almond Fudge	½ cup	140	3	9	25	17	0	40
Lemon Custard	½ cup	150	2	8	45	16	0	55
Lowfat Carmel Apple Ala Mode	½ cup	100	3	2	5	20	0	75
Lowfat Espresso'N Cream	½ cup	100	3	3	5	18	1	60
Mint Chocolate Chip	½ cup	150	3	10	35	15	0	35
No Sugar Added Call Me Nuts	½ cup	110	3	2	5	21	1	55
No Sugar Added Cherry Cordial	½ cup	100	3	2	5	18	0	55
No Sugar Added Mad About Chocolate	½ cup	100	3	2	5	19	0	40
No Sugar Added Pineapple Coconut	½ cup	90	3	2	5	16	0	60
No Sugar Added Thin Mint	½ cup	100	3	3	5	16	0	65
Nonfat Berry Innocent Cheese	½ cup	110	3	0	0	24	0	100
Nonfat Check-It-Out Cherry	½ cup	100	3	0	0	22	0	90
Nonfat Jamoca Swirl	½ cup	110	3	0	5	23	0	105

FOOD	PORTION	CAL	PROT	FAT	CHOL	CARB	FIBER	SOD
Ocean Commotion	½ cup	150	1	7	25	20	0	40
Old Fashion Butter Pecan	½ cup	160	2	11	35	13	0	35
Oregon Blueberry	½ cup	140	2	8	30	16	0	50
Peanut Butter N Chocolate	½ cup	180	3	12	30	16	1	95
Pink Bubblegum	½ cup	150	2	8	30	19	0	40
Pistachio Almond	½ cup	170	3	12	30	13	1	45
Pralines N Cream	½ cup	160	2	9	30	19	0	85
Pumpkin Pie	½ cup	130	2	7	30	16	0	50
Quarterback Crunch	½ cup	160	2	10	30	18	0	75
Reeses Peanut Butter	½ cup	180	3	11	30	17	0	70
Rocky Road	½ cup	170	3	10	30	19	0	60
Rum Raisin	½ cup	140	2	7	30	18	0	40
Strawberry Cheesecake	½ cup	150	2	9	35	17	0	65
Triple Chocolate Passion	½ cup	180	3	11	35	21	0	70
Vanilla	½ cup	140	3	8	40	14	0	40
Very Berry Strawberry	½ cup	130	1	7	25	16	0	40
Winter White Chocolate	½ cup	150	2	9	25	18	0	50
World Class Chocolate	½ cup	160	2	9	30	18	0	55
ICES AND ICE POPS								
Daiquiri Ice	½ cup	110	0	0	0	28	0	10
Sherbet Blue Raspberry	½ cup	120	1	2	5	25	0	30
Sherbet Orange	½ cup	120	1	2	5	26	0	25
Sherbet Rainbow	½ cup	120	1	2	5	26	0	25
Sorbet Pink Raspberry Lemon	½ cup	120	0	0	0	29	0	10
The Mask Ice	½ cup	120	0	0	0	29	0	10
Watermelon Ice	½ cup	110	0	0	0	28	0	10

FOOD	PORTION	CAL	PROT	FAT	CHOL	CARB	FIBER	SOD
BEN & JERRY'S								
Sugar Cone	1	48	1	tr	0	10	tr	42
FROZEN YOGURT								
Cherry Garcia	½ cup (3.3 oz)	150	4	3	15	29	tr	60
Chocolate Cherry Garcia	½ cup (3.3 oz)	170	4	4	5	37	1	55
Chocolate Fudge Brownie	½ cup (3.3 oz)	180	5	3	15	32	1	100
No Fat Black Raspberry	½ cup (3.4 oz)	140	4	0	5	30	0	60
No Fat Coffee Fudge	½ cup (3.4 oz)	140	4	0	0	30	0	65
No Fat Vanilla	½ cup (3.4 oz)	140	5	0	5	28	0	75
No Fat Vanilla Fudge Swirl	½ cup (3.4 oz)	130	3	0	0	29	0	70
ICE CREAM								
Bovinity Divinity	½ cup (3.1 oz)	240	3	14	30	24	1	50
Butter Pecan	½ cup (3.1 oz)	270	4	21	60	17	tr	105
Cherry Garcia	½ cup (3.1 oz)	210	3	12	55	20	tr	45
Chocolate Chip Cookie Dough	½ cup (3.1 oz)	180	3	11	55	17	0	45
Chocolate Fudge Brownie	½ cup (3.1 oz)	230	4	11	35	28	2	80
Chubby Hubby	½ cup (3.1 oz)	280	5	17	50	26	1	135
Chunky Monkey	½ cup (3.1 oz)	220	3	13	50	25	0	45
Coconut Almond Fudge Chip	½ cup (3.1 oz)	250	4	18	30	19	2	60
Coffee Coffee Buzz Buzz	½ cup (3.1 oz)	240	3	16	55	23	tr	60
Coffee Ole	½ cup (3.1 oz)	200	3	13	65	18	0	50
Coffee w/ Heath Bar Crunch	½ cup (3.1 oz)	250	3	16	30	25	0	105
Deep Dark Chocolate	½ cup (3.1 oz)	210	4	12	40	22	2	40
Dilbert's World Totally Nuts	½ cup (3.1 oz)	260	4	18	30	21	tr	85
Low Fat Blackberry Cobbler	½ cup (3.2 oz)	160	3	2	10	32	0	60
Low Fat Chocolate Comfort	½ cup (3.2 oz)	150	4	2	10	27	–	80

FOOD	PORTION	CAL	PROT	FAT	CHOL	CARB	FIBER	SOD
Low Fat Coconut Creme Pie	½ cup (3.2 oz)	160	4	3	15	29	0	75
Low Fat Mocha Latte	½ cup (3.2 oz)	150	4	2	10	27	—	65
Low Fat Rockin Road	½ cup (3.2 oz)	180	5	3	5	34	2	65
Low Fat Smore's	½ cup (3.2 oz)	180	4	2	5	34	1	80
Low Fat Vanilla & Chocolate Mint Patty	½ cup (3.2 oz)	170	4	3	20	32	tr	65
Maple Walnut	½ cup (3.1 oz)	240	3	13	55	19	0	40
Mint Chocolate Chunk	½ cup (3.1 oz)	240	3	16	60	24	0	55
Mint Chocolate Cookie	½ cup (3.1 oz)	230	4	14	60	24	tr	110
New York Super Fudge Chunk	½ cup (3.1 oz)	250	4	16	35	25	0	45
Peanut Butter Cup	½ cup (3.1 oz)	270	5	18	55	21	1	95
Phish Food	½ cup (3.1 oz)	230	3	12	30	30	1	70
Pistachio Pistachio	½ cup (3.1 oz)	190	3	13	35	17	0	45
Praline Pecan	½ cup (3.1 oz)	230	3	14	30	24	0	105
Southern Pecan Pie	½ cup (3.1 oz)	240	3	16	35	21	0	80
Strawberry	½ cup (3.1 oz)	180	3	10	50	20	tr	40
Sweet Cream Cookie	½ cup (3.1 oz)	230	4	14	60	23	tr	110
Triple Caramel Chunk	½ cup (3.1 oz)	240	4	13	30	28	0	95
Vanilla Caramel Fudge	½ cup (3.1 oz)	230	3	13	60	25	0	85
Vanilla Chocolate Chunk	½ cup (3.1 oz)	240	3	16	60	23	0	55
Vanilla World's Best	½ cup (3.1 oz)	200	3	13	65	17	0	50
Vanilla w/ Heath Toffee Crunch	½ cup (3.1 oz)	250	3	16	35	25	0	105
Wavy Gravy	½ cup (3.1 oz)	260	5	17	50	24	1	75
White Russian	½ cup (3.1 oz)	200	3	13	65	18	0	45
SORBETS								
Doonesberry	½ cup (3.2 oz)	100	0	0	0	27	0	10
Lemon Swirl	½ cup (3.2 oz)	100	0	0	0	25	0	10
Purple Passion Fruit	½ cup (3.2 oz)	100	0	0	0	27	0	10
Strawberry Kiwi	½ cup (3.2 oz)	110	0	0	0	27	tr	10

FOOD	PORTION	CAL	PROT	FAT	CHOL	CARB	FIBER	SOD
BIG BOY								
DESSERTS								
Frozen Yogurt Fat Free	1 serv	118	3	0	0	27	—	60
Frozen Yogurt Shake	1	156	7	1	2	33	—	120
MAIN MENU SELECTIONS								
Baked Cod w/ Salad Baked Potato Roll & Margarine	1 meal	744	57	21	76	82	—	655
Baked Potato	1	163	6	2	0	37	—	7
Breast of Chicken Pita w/ Mozzarella & Ranch Dressing	1	361	41	11	84	23	—	369
Cabbage Soup	1 bowl	40	1	5	0	7	—	347
Cabbage Soup	1 cup	34	1	4	0	6	—	295
Cajun Cod w/ Salad Baked Potato Roll & Margarine	1 meal	736	56	21	76	80	—	745
Chicken & Pasta Primavera w/ Salad Roll & Margarine	1 meal	676	53	14	65	83	—	875
Dinner Roll	1	210	0	5	0	36	—	340
Promise Margarine	1 pat	25	0	3	0	0	—	35
Rice Pilaf	1 serv	153	3	4	10	25	—	688
Scrambled Egg Beaters w/ Whole Wheat Bread & Margarine	1 meal	305	19	10	0	36	—	603
Southwest Chicken w/ Salad Baked Potato Roll & Margarine	1 meal	702	50	18	76	85	—	948
Spaghetti Marinara w/ Salad Roll & Margarine	1 meal	754	17	11	8	105	—	754
Turkey Pita w/ Ranch Dressing	1	245	25	6	83	23	—	938
Vegetable Stir Fry w/ Salad Baked Potato Roll & Margarine	1 meal	616	17	14	0	109	—	774

FOOD	PORTION	CAL	PROT	FAT	CHOL	CARB	FIBER	SOD
SALAD DRESSINGS								
Italian Fat Free	1 oz	11	0	0	0	3	—	191
Lo Cal Oriental	1 oz	20	1	2	0	4	—	189
Lo Cal Ranch	1 oz	41	1	3	8	3	—	151
SALADS AND SALAD BARS								
Chicken Breast Salad w/ Roll & Margarine	1 serv	523	44	16	73	50	—	654
Oriental Chicken Breast Salad w/ Dinner Roll & Margarine	1 serv	660	48	20	65	73	—	855
Tossed Salad	1	35	2	2	0	7	—	71
BLIMPIE								
6 INCH SUB								
5 Meatball	1 (7.8 oz)	500	23	22	25	52	2	970
Blimpie Best	1 (8.5 oz)	410	26	13	50	47	4	1480
Cheese Trio	1 (8.2 oz)	510	26	23	60	51	2	1060
Club	1 (9.8 oz)	450	30	13	40	53	3	1350
Grilled Chicken	1 (9.1 oz)	400	28	9	30	52	2	950
Ham & Swiss	1 (8.2 oz)	400	25	13	35	47	5	970
Ham Salami Provolone	1 (9.8 oz)	590	32	28	70	52	3	1880
Roast Beef	1 (8.5 oz)	340	27	5	20	47	2	870
Steak & Cheese	1 (7.1 oz)	550	27	26	70	51	2	1080
Tuna	1 (10.2 oz)	570	21	32	50	50	2	790
Turkey	1 (8.2 oz)	320	19	5	10	51	3	890
SALADS AND SALAD BARS								
Grilled Chicken Salad	1 serv (16.2 oz)	350	47	12	140	13	0	1190
BOJANGLES								
BAKED SELECTIONS								
Biscuit	1	243	4	12	2	29	2	663
Multi-Grain Roll	1	150	6	3	0	26	3	210
Sweet Biscuit Apple Cinnamon	1	330	4	13	tr	48	1	540
Sweet Biscuit Bo*Berry	1	220	3	10	tr	29	1	410
Sweet Biscuit Cinnamon	1	320	4	18	tr	37	1	560

FOOD	PORTION	CAL	PROT	FAT	CHOL	CARB	FIBER	SOD
MAIN MENU SELECTIONS								
Biscuit Sandwich Bacon	1	290	8	17	10	26	1	810
Biscuit Sandwich Bacon Egg & Cheese	1	550	17	42	160	27	1	1250
Biscuit Sandwich Cajun Filet	1	454	20	21	41	46	1	949
Biscuit Sandwich Country Ham	1	270	9	15	20	26	1	1010
Biscuit Sandwich Egg	1	400	8	30	120	26	1	630
Biscuit Sandwich Sausage	1	350	9	23	20	26	1	810
Biscuit Sandwich Smoked Sausage	1	380	10	26	20	27	1	940
Biscuit Sandwich Steak	1	649	14	49	34	13	1	1126
Bo Rounds	1 serv	235	3	11	13	31	3	328
Buffalo Bites	1 serv	180	27	5	105	5	0	720
Cajun Pintos	1 serv	110	6	0	0	18	6	480
Cajun Roast Skinfree Breast	1 serv	143	24	5	84	tr	tr	562
Cajun Roast Skinfree Leg	1 serv	161	23	8	125	tr	tr	566
Cajun Roast Skinfree Thigh	1 serv	215	20	15	95	tr	tr	428
Cajun Roast Wing	1 serv	231	22	15	117	3	tr	617
Cajun Spiced Breast	1 serv	278	18	17	75	12	tr	565
Cajun Spiced Leg	1 serv	310	15	23	67	11	tr	465
Cajun Spiced Thigh	1 serv	264	19	16	96	11	tr	530
Cajun Spiced Wing	1 serv	355	21	25	94	11	tr	630
Chicken Supremes	1 serv	337	21	16	58	26	1	629
Corn On The Cob	1 serv	140	5	2	0	34	2	20
Dirty Rice	1 serv	166	5	6	10	24	1	762
Green Beans	1 serv	25	5	0	0	25	2	710
Macaroni & Cheese	1 serv	198	7	14	26	12	tr	418
Marinated Cole Slaw	1 serv	136	1	3	0	26	3	454
Potatoes w/o Gravy	1 serv	80	2	1	0	16	1	380

FOOD	PORTION	CAL	PROT	FAT	CHOL	CARB	FIBER	SOD
Sandwich Cajun Filet w/ Mayonnaise	1	437	22	22	55	41	3	506
Sandwich Cajun Filet w/o Mayonnaise	1	337	22	11	45	41	3	401
Sandwich Cajun Steak w/ Horseradish Sauce & Pickles	1	434	18	26	55	39	2	985
Sandwich Grilled Filet w/ Mayonnaise	1	335	23	16	61	25	2	645
Sandwich Grilled Filet w/o Mayonnaise	1 serv (5.2 oz)	329	27	7	59	37	—	418
Seasoned Fries	1 serv	344	5	19	13	39	4	480
Southern Style Breast	1 serv	261	16	16	76	12	tr	702
Southern Style Leg	1 serv	254	19	15	94	11	tr	446
Southern Style Thigh	1 serv	308	16	21	78	14	tr	630
Southern Style Wing	1 serv	337	17	21	86	19	tr	684

BOSTON MARKET
BAKED SELECTIONS

FOOD	PORTION	CAL	PROT	FAT	CHOL	CARB	FIBER	SOD
Brownie	1 (3.3 oz)	450	6	27	80	47	3	190
Cinnamon Apple Pie	⅕ pie (4.8 oz)	390	2	23	0	46	2	250
Cookie Chocolate Chip	1 (2.8 oz)	340	4	17	25	48	1	240

MAIN MENU SELECTIONS

FOOD	PORTION	CAL	PROT	FAT	CHOL	CARB	FIBER	SOD
½ Chicken w/ Skin	1 serv (9.7 oz)	590	70	33	280	4	0	1010
¼ Dark Meat Chicken No Skin	1 serv (3.3 oz)	190	22	10	115	1	0	440
¼ Dark Meat Chicken w/ Skin	1 serv (4.4 oz)	320	30	21	155	2	0	500
¼ White Meat Chicken No Skin Or Wing	1 serv (4.9 oz)	170	23	4	85	2	0	480
¼ White Meat Chicken w/ Skin And Wing	1 serv (5.3 oz)	280	40	12	135	2	0	510
BBQ Baked Beans	¾ cup (7.1 oz)	270	8	5	0	48	12	540
BBQ Chicken Sandwich	1 (9.9 oz)	540	30	9	75	84	3	1690
Baked Sweet Potato Low Fat	1 (12.5 oz)	460	6	7	0	94	10	510

FOOD	PORTION	CAL	PROT	FAT	CHOL	CARB	FIBER	SOD
Black Beans And Rice	1 cup (8 oz)	300	8	10	0	45	5	1050
Boston Hearth Ham Lean	1 serv (5 oz)	210	25	9	75	9	0	1490
Broccoli Cauliflower Au Gratin	¾ cup (6.1 oz)	200	9	11	20	14	3	600
Broccoli Rice Casserole	¾ cup (6 oz)	240	5	12	40	26	2	800
Broccoli With Red Peppers	¾ cup (3.4 oz)	60	3	4	0	5	3	130
Butternut Squash Low Fat	¾ cup (6.8 oz)	160	2	6	15	25	3	580
Chicken Gravy	1 serv (1 oz)	15	0	1	0	2	0	170
Chicken Salad Sandwich	1 (11.5 oz)	680	39	30	120	63	4	1360
Chicken Sandwich w/ Cheese & Sauce	1 (12.4 oz)	750	41	33	135	72	5	1860
Chicken Sandwich w/o Cheese & Sauce Low Fat	1 (10 oz)	430	34	5	65	62	4	910
Chunky Chicken Salad	¾ cup (5.5 oz)	370	28	27	120	3	1	800
Chunky Cinnamon Apple Sauce No Fat	¾ cup (6.4 oz)	250	1	0	0	62	2	30
Cole Slaw	¾ cup (6.5 oz)	300	2	19	20	30	3	540
Corn Bread	1 (2.4 oz)	200	3	6	25	33	1	390
Coyote Bean Salad	¾ cup (5.3 oz)	190	4	9	0	24	9	210
Cranberry Relish Low Fat	¾ cup (7.9 oz)	370	2	5	0	84	5	5
Creamed Spinach	¾ cup (6.4 oz)	260	9	20	55	11	2	740
Fruit Salad Low Fat	¾ cup (5.5 oz)	70	1	1	0	15	1	10
Green Bean Casserole	¾ cup (6 oz)	130	2	9	20	10	2	440
Green Beans	¾ cup (3 oz)	80	1	6	0	5	3	200
Ham Sandwich w/ Cheese & Sauce	1 (11.8 oz)	760	38	34	100	72	5	1730

FOOD	PORTION	CAL	PROT	FAT	CHOL	CARB	FIBER	SOD
Ham Sandwich w/o Cheese & Sauce	1 (9.3 oz)	440	25	8	45	66	4	1450
Homestyle Mashed Potatoes & Gravy	¾ cup (6.6 oz)	210	4	10	25	26	1	740
Honey Glazed Carrots	¾ cup (5.4 oz)	280	1	15	0	35	4	80
Hot Cinnamon Apples	¾ cup (6.4 oz)	250	0	5	0	56	3	45
Macaroni & Cheese	¾ cup (6.7 oz)	280	13	11	30	32	1	830
Mashed Potatoes	⅔ cup (5.6 oz)	190	3	9	25	24	1	570
Meat Loaf & Brown Gravy	1 serv (7 oz)	390	30	22	120	19	1	1040
Meat Loaf & Chunky Tomato Sauce	1 serv (8 oz)	370	30	18	120	22	2	1170
Meat Loaf Sandwich w/ Cheese	1 (13.8 oz)	860	46	33	165	95	6	2270
Meat Loaf Sandwich w/o Cheese	1 (12.3 oz)	690	40	21	120	86	6	1610
New Potatoes Low Fat	¾ cup (4.6 oz)	130	3	3	0	25	2	150
Old Fashioned Potato Salad	¾ cup (6.2 oz)	340	2	24	30	30	2	870
Open Face Turkey Sandwich	1 (13.4 oz)	500	37	12	80	61	3	2170
Original Chicken Pot Pie	1 pie (14.9 oz)	780	32	46	135	61	4	1480
Oven Roasted Potato Planks Low Fat	5 pieces (5.8 oz)	180	3	5	0	32	3	370
Pastry Sandwich BBQ Chicken	1 (7.2 oz)	640	17	39	60	56	1	1260
Pastry Sandwich Broccoli Chicken Cheddar	1 (7.2 oz)	690	21	47	85	45	2	1050
Pastry Sandwich Ham & Cheddar	1 (6.6 oz)	640	19	41	60	47	1	1560
Pastry Sandwich Italian Chicken	1 (7.2 oz)	630	21	41	60	43	2	910

FOOD	PORTION	CAL	PROT	FAT	CHOL	CARB	FIBER	SOD
Red Beans And Rice Low Fat	1 cup (8 oz)	260	8	5	5	45	4	1050
Rice Pilaf	⅔ cup (5.1 oz)	180	5	5	0	32	2	600
Rotisserie Turkey Breast Skinless Low Fat	1 serv (5 oz)	170	36	1	100	1	0	850
Savory Stuffing	¾ cup (6.1 oz)	310	6	12	0	44	3	1140
Southwest Savory Chicken	1 serv (9.6 oz)	400	40	15	100	26	4	1670
Squash Casserole	¾ cup (6.6 oz)	330	7	24	70	20	3	1110
Steamed Vegetables Low Fat	⅔ cup (3.7 oz)	35	2	1	0	7	3	35
Sweet Potato Casserole	¾ cup (6.4 oz)	280	3	18	10	39	2	190
Tabasco BBQ Drumstick	1 (2.4 oz)	130	14	6	50	4	0	190
Tabasco BBQ Wing	1 (1.8 oz)	110	9	7	30	4	0	170
Teriyaki Chicken ¼ White w/ Skin	1 serv (6.8 oz)	340	40	12	135	17	0	890
Teriyaki Chicken ¼ w/ Skin	1 serv (5.9 oz)	380	30	21	155	17	0	870
Triple Topped Chicken	1 serv (9.2 oz)	470	50	22	155	20	1	1350
Turkey Club Sandwich	1 (11.1 oz)	650	39	26	105	64	4	1590
Turkey Sandwich w/ Cheese & Sauce	1 (11.8 oz)	710	45	28	110	68	4	1390
Turkey Sandwich w/o Cheese & Sauce	1 (9.3 oz)	400	45	4	60	61	4	1070
Whole Kernel Corn	¾ cup (5.8 oz)	180	5	4	0	30	2	170
Zucchini Marinara Low Fat	¾ cup (6.6 oz)	60	1	3	0	7	2	330
SALADS AND SALAD BARS								
Caesar Salad Entree	1 serv (10 oz)	510	17	42	35	17	3	1130
Caesar Salad w/o Dressing	1 serv (8 oz)	230	16	12	20	14	3	500
Caesar Side Salad	1 (4 oz)	200	7	17	15	7	1	450

FOOD	PORTION	CAL	PROT	FAT	CHOL	CARB	FIBER	SOD
Chicken Caesar Salad	1 serv (13 oz)	650	43	45	105	17	3	1580
Tossed Salad w/ Caesar Dressing	1 serv (8 oz)	380	5	31	15	18	3	810
Tossed Salad w/ Fat Free Ranch	1 serv (8 oz)	160	5	3	0	29	4	940
Tossed Salad w/ Old Venice Dressing	1 serv (8 oz)	340	4	27	0	20	3	1110
SOUPS								
Chicken Chili	1 cup (8.7 oz)	220	18	7	40	21	6	1000
Chicken Noodle	1 cup (8.4 oz)	130	11	5	40	12	2	1310
Chicken Tortilla	1 cup (8.4 oz)	220	10	11	35	19	2	1410
Potato	1 cup (8 oz)	270	8	16	40	24	2	1020
Tomato Bisque	1 cup (8 oz)	280	4	23	50	16	2	1280

BOSTON PIZZA
CHILDREN'S MENU SELECTIONS

FOOD	PORTION	CAL	PROT	FAT	CHOL	CARB	FIBER	SOD
Corkscrews n' Cheese	1 serv	870	30	33	—	112	—	760
Dino Fingers & Fries w/ Ketchup	1 serv	680	22	35	—	87	—	1270
Grill Cheese Sandwich w/ Fries & Ketchup	1 serv	770	25	32	—	103	—	1450
Mini Lasagna	1 serv	400	19	14	—	48	—	630
Pint Sized Ham Pizza	1 serv	430	22	8	—	66	—	850
Potato Smiles	1 serv	580	8	30	—	84	—	1470
Stuffed Pizza w/ Fries & Ketchup	1 serv	850	30	31	—	124	—	1520
Super Spaghetti	1 serv	340	10	6	—	61	—	660
MAIN MENU SELECTIONS								
BBQ Ribs w/ Fries	1 serv	2220	71	148	—	140	—	2420
BBQ Ribs w/ Garlic Mashed Potatoes	1 serv	1760	65	122	—	94	—	3090
BBQ Ribs w/ Spaghetti	1 serv	1870	74	121	—	113	—	2570
Baked Onion Soup	1 serv	210	11	7	—	28	—	1130
Bayou Chicken Strips w/ Dipping Sauce	1 serv	370	43	16	—	6	—	3740

FOOD	PORTION	CAL	PROT	FAT	CHOL	CARB	FIBER	SOD
Boston's Extreme Double Order	1 serv	1660	159	107	–	15	–	7990
Boston's Extreme Starter Order	1 serv	940	90	61	–	10	–	5400
Bruschetta	1 serv	640	17	39	–	55	–	1590
Buffalo Chicken Fingers w/ Caesar Salad	1 serv	650	37	38	–	42	–	2790
Buffalo Chicken Fingers w/ Fries	1 serv	1430	45	82	–	122	–	3440
Buffalo Chicken Fingers w/ Light Ranch	1 serv	600	35	34	–	40	–	3260
Cactus Cuts & Dip	1 serv	1380	21	83	–	136	–	1110
Cheese Toast	1 basket	800	36	41	–	64	–	1310
Cheese Toast	1 serv	400	18	21	–	32	–	670
Chicken & Rib Combo	1 serv	1470	68	90	–	94	–	2910
Chicken & Rib Combo w/ Fries	1 serv	1920	74	116	–	140	–	2250
Chicken & Rib Combo w/ Spaghetti	1 serv	1590	78	90	–	113	–	2440
Chicken Fingers w/ Caesar Salad	1 serv	640	37	38	–	38	–	980
Chicken Fingers w/ Fries	1 serv	1420	45	82	–	118	–	1630
Chicken Fingers w/ Light Ranch	1 serv	590	34	34	–	36	–	1440
Chips & Salsa	1 serv	830	11	41	–	109	–	1620
Deluxe Cheese Bread	1 basket	890	37	42	–	84	–	6450
Deluxe Cheese Toast	1 serv	420	19	21	–	35	–	1140
Fries	1 serv	700	10	33	–	87	–	450
Garlic Toast w/ Garlic Margarine	1 slice	170	4	6	–	22	–	240
Garlic Twist Bread	1 basket	1080	33	30	–	168	–	1180
Garlic Twist Bread	1 serv	540	17	15	–	84	–	590
Italian Pizza Bread w/ Dip	1 serv	1000	32	53	–	98	–	830
Ketchup	1 serv (2 oz)	20	1	1	–	16	–	490

FOOD	PORTION	CAL	PROT	FAT	CHOL	CARB	FIBER	SOD
Mashed Potatoes	1 serv	240	4	8	–	41	–	1110
Mexican Beef w/ Sour Cream	1 serv	970	49	57	–	66	–	1820
Mini Tortellini	1 serv	490	17	15	–	73	–	850
NY Steak Sandwich w/ Fries	1 serv	1580	54	96	–	118	–	970
Nachos	1 full order	1540	52	95	–	127	–	2370
Nachos Beef	1 full order	1760	73	106	–	129	–	2720
Nachos Chicken	1 full order	1630	68	96	–	129	–	3720
Pizza Bread w/o Meat Sauce	1 serv	520	15	14	–	84	–	520
Potato Skins	1 full order	860	28	53	–	70	–	610
Quesadilla Chicken w/ Sour Cream	1 serv	770	36	40	–	67	–	1890
Quesadilla Garden Veggie w/ Sour Cream	1 serv	750	29	40	–	70	–	1560
Quesadilla Sundried Tomato w/ Sour Cream	1 serv	890	67	50	–	39	–	1870
Shrimp Dinner w/ Fries	1 serv	1510	51	82	–	135	–	1330
Shrimp Dinner w/ Garlic Mashed Potatoes	1 serv	1050	45	57	–	89	–	1990
Shrimp Dinner w/ Spaghetti	1 serv	1180	55	56	–	108	–	1520
Side Tossed Salad w/ House Dressing	1 serv	170	2	14	–	10	–	340
Sirloin Steak Dinner w/ Fries	1 serv	1910	95	113	–	117	–	790
Sirloin Steak Dinner w/ Garlic Mashed Potatoes	1 serv	1450	89	88	–	71	–	1450
Sirloin Steak Dinner w/ Spaghetti	1 serv	1580	100	87	–	90	–	980
Spaghetti w/ Meatsauce	1 serv	370	14	8	–	60	–	650
Spinach & Artichoke Dip w/ Tortilla Chips	1 serv	890	21	57	–	81	–	1290

FOOD	PORTION	CAL	PROT	FAT	CHOL	CARB	FIBER	SOD
Steak & Shrimp Dinner w/ Fries	1 serv	1760	65	108	–	129	–	1550
Steak & Shrimp Dinner w/ Garlic Mashed Potatoes	1 serv	1310	59	83	–	83	–	2210
Steak & Shrimp Dinner w/ Spaghetti	1 serv	1430	69	82	–	102	–	1740
The Ribber w/ Fries	1 serv	1470	46	85	–	121	–	1650
The Ribber w/ Garlic Mashed Potatoes	1 serv	1010	40	60	–	74	–	2310
The Ribber w/ Spaghetti	1 serv	1140	50	60	–	94	–	1850
Veal Pamigan w/ Fries	1 serv	1550	46	88	–	138	–	1430
Veal Parmigan w/ Garlic Mashed Potatoes	1 serv	1090	40	63	–	92	–	2100
Veal Parmigan w/ Spaghetti	1 serv	1220	50	62	–	112	–	1450
Wings BBQ Double Order	1 serv	1700	159	107	–	26	–	3200
Wings BBQ Starter Size	1 serv	960	90	61	–	13	–	1810
Wings Cajun Double Order	1 serv	1610	158	107	–	5	–	4940
Wings Cajun Starter Size	1 serv	910	89	60	–	3	–	2680
Wings Honey Garlic Double Order	1 serv	1720	158	107	–	32	–	3370
Wings Honey Garlic Starter Size	1 serv	970	89	60	–	17	–	1890
Wings Screamin' Hot Double Order	1 serv	1630	158	107	–	10	–	5620
Wings Screamin' Hot Starter Size	1 serv	920	89	60	–	5	–	3020
Wings Teriyaki Double Order	1 serv	1690	159	107	–	21	–	4660
Wings Teriyaki Starter Size	1 serv	950	90	60	–	11	–	2540
Wings Thai Double Order	1 serv	1870	164	123	–	27	–	3200

FOOD	PORTION	CAL	PROT	FAT	CHOL	CARB	FIBER	SOD
Wings Thai Starter Size	1 serv	1040	92	69	–	14	–	1810
PIZZA								
Bacon Double Cheeseburger Individual	1 pie	1210	77	56	–	94	–	2170
Bacon Double Cheeseburger Large	1 slice	350	23	15	–	30	–	650
Bacon Double Cheeseburger Medium	1 slice	300	19	13	–	25	–	550
Boston Royal Individual	1 pie	770	45	23	–	96	–	1980
Boston Royal Large	1 slice	230	13	6	–	31	–	590
Boston Royal Medium	1 slice	200	11	6	–	26	–	540
Cajun Chicken Individual	1 pie	780	41	25	–	99	–	2140
Cajun Chicken Large	1 slice	250	13	8	–	31	–	610
Cajun Chicken Medium	1 slice	200	10	7	–	26	–	530
Californian Individual	1 pie	580	23	8	–	109	–	960
Californian Large	1 slice	190	8	3	–	35	–	320
Californian Medium	1 slice	160	6	2	–	30	–	290
Four Cheese Individual	1 pie	800	45	29	–	89	–	1580
Four Cheese Large	1 slice	260	14	10	–	29	–	540
Four Cheese Medium	1 slice	240	14	10	–	24	–	510
Great White Individual	1 pie	880	53	34	–	89	–	1820
Great White Large	1 slice	260	16	9	–	29	–	560
Great White Medium	1 slice	220	13	8	–	24	–	490
Hawaiian Individual	1 pie	690	39	16	–	97	–	1460
Hawaiian Large	1 slice	220	13	5	–	31	–	490
Hawaiian Medium	1 slice	180	10	4	–	26	–	420
Meat Lovers Individual	1 pie	1120	64	55	–	89	–	2450
Meat Lovers Large	1 slice	330	19	15	–	28	–	680
Meat Lovers Medium	1 slice	280	15	14	–	24	–	600
Pepperoni Individual	1 pie	760	39	27	–	89	–	1500

FOOD	PORTION	CAL	PROT	FAT	CHOL	CARB	FIBER	SOD
Pepperoni Large	1 slice	240	13	9	–	28	–	490
Pepperoni Medium	1 slice	200	10	7	–	24	–	430
Pepperoni & Mushroom Individual	1 pie	760	90	27	–	40	–	1500
Pepperoni & Mushroom Large	1 slice	250	13	9	–	29	–	490
Pepperoni & Mushroom Medium	1 slice	200	10	7	–	24	–	430
Perogy Individual	1 pie	1010	50	45	–	102	–	1020
Perogy Large	1 slice	330	16	15	–	33	–	340
Perogy Medium	1 slice	280	13	13	–	28	–	280
Popeye Individual	1 pie	730	41	21	–	94	–	1390
Popeye Large	1 slice	240	14	7	–	30	–	490
Popeye Medium	1 slice	200	11	6	–	26	–	420
Rustic Italian Individual	1 pie	940	50	37	–	102	–	4250
Rustic Italian Large	1 slice	310	16	12	–	33	–	1420
Rustic Italian Medium	1 slice	250	13	10	–	28	–	1250
Sante Fe Chicken Individual	1 pie	800	47	27	–	94	–	1650
Sante Fe Chicken Large	1 slice	260	15	9	–	30	–	550
Sante Fe Chicken Medium	1 slice	220	12	7	–	25	–	470
Super Veggie Individual	1 pie	850	42	29	–	108	–	2020
Super Veggie Large	1 slice	280	14	10	–	35	–	670
Super Veggie Medium	1 slice	230	11	7	–	30	–	580
Thai Chicken Individual	1 pie	870	45	29	–	106	–	850
Thai Chicken Large	1 slice	280	15	10	–	34	–	280
Thai Chicken Medium	1 slice	240	12	8	–	29	–	230
The Basic Individual	1 pie	620	34	15	–	89	–	1050
The Basic Large	1 slice	200	11	5	–	28	–	350

FOOD	PORTION	CAL	PROT	FAT	CHOL	CARB	FIBER	SOD
The Basic Medium	1 slice	160	9	4	–	24	–	290
The Deluxe Individual	1 pie	780	43	26	–	92	–	1830
The Deluxe Large	1 slice	240	14	7	–	30	–	540
The Deluxe Medium	1 slice	190	11	6	–	25	–	460
Tropical Chicken Individual	1 pie	1060	57	50	–	94	–	1930
Tropical Chicken Large	1 slice	340	18	16	–	30	–	610
Tropical Chicken Medium	1 slice	280	15	13	–	25	–	520
Tuscan Individual	1 pie	900	49	32	–	108	–	2060
Tuscan Large	1 slice	290	16	11	–	35	–	690
Tuscan Medium	1 slice	240	13	8	–	30	–	590
Vegetarian Individual	1 pie	670	36	15	–	100	–	1060
Vegetarian Large	1 slice	220	12	5	–	31	–	350
Vegetarian Medium	1 slice	170	9	4	–	26	–	300
Zorba The Greek Individual	1 pie	810	43	27	–	99	–	1780
Zorba The Greek Large	1 slice	270	14	9	–	32	–	610
Zorba The Greek Medium	1 slice	220	11	7	–	27	–	510
SALADS AND SALAD BARS								
Boston's Cobb Salad	1 serv	1100	25	80	–	66	–	2280
Caesar Salad	1 reg	260	5	21	–	15	–	410
Caesar Salad Meal Sized	1 serv	690	13	48	–	52	–	1060
Greek Salad	1 serv	500	10	44	–	19	–	2380
Greek Salad Meal Sized	1 serv	1110	22	90	–	53	–	3680
House Dressing	1 serv (2 oz)	136	tr	13	–	4	–	340
Spinach Salad	1 serv	190	10	14	–	6	–	470
Spinach Salad Meal Sized	1 serv	500	20	31	–	32	–	1050
Taco Salad Beef w/ Sour Cream & Salsa	1 serv	640	33	41	–	40	–	1130

FOOD	PORTION	CAL	PROT	FAT	CHOL	CARB	FIBER	SOD
Taco Salad Chicken w/ Sour Cream & Salsa	1 serv	520	28	28	—	39	—	2130
Thai Chicken Salad	1 serv	730	44	21	—	90	—	1150
Tossed Garden Greens w/ House Dressing	1 serv	170	2	14	—	10	—	350
Veggie Plate w/ Low Fat Ranch Dressing	1 serv	180	6	7	—	26	—	115
SANDWICHES								
BBQ Beef w/ Fries	1 serv	1580	66	62	—	179	—	2220
Beef Dip w/ Fries & Au Jus	1 serv	1560	64	72	—	151	—	1360
Boston Cheesesteak w/ Fries & Au Jus	1 serv	1790	80	87	—	172	—	2200
Boston Brute w/ Fries	1 serv	1420	48	60	—	163	—	3260
Buffalo Chicken w/ Fries	1 serv	1720	85	80	—	187	—	4470
Chicken Foccacia w/ Fries	1 serv	1350	45	65	—	140	—	1320
Spicy Italian Sausage w/ Caesar Salad	1 serv	1070	47	51	—	104	—	1580
Stromboli Chicken w/ Caesar Salad	1 serv	1020	53	44	—	101	—	1490
Stromboli Perogy w/ Caesar Salad	1 serv	1120	41	58	—	109	—	1550
Stromboli Sante Fe w/ Caesar Salad	1 serv	1000	44	45	—	104	—	2000
Super Ham & Cheese w/ Fries	1 serv	1370	39	71	—	137	—	2130
Tango Chicken Wrap w/ Caesar Salad	1 serv	740	37	42	—	55	—	1460
BROWN'S CHICKEN								
Breadsticks w/ Garlic Butter	1	199	6	4	tr	36	—	2213
Breast	3.5 oz	284	26	15	67	12	—	529
Coleslaw	3.5 oz	131	2	10	6	9	—	211
Corn Fritters	3.5 oz	415	5	25	4	42	—	552

FOOD	PORTION	CAL	PROT	FAT	CHOL	CARB	FIBER	SOD
Corn On Cob	1 ear (3 inch)	126	3	3	1	22	—	23
Fettucini Alfredo	1 serv (12 oz)	1507	56	64	51	173	—	3018
French Fries	3.5 oz	503	5	22	1	44	—	235
Gizzard	3.5 oz	387	24	20	88	26	—	795
Leg	3.5 oz	287	26	16	52	9	—	542
Liver	3.5 oz	341	23	19	147	19	—	704
Mostaccioli w/ Meat	1 serv (12 oz)	835	27	14	17	44	—	898
Mostaccioli w/o Meat	1 serv (12 oz)	792	24	10	0	146	—	842
Mushrooms	3.5 oz	289	6	16	1	30	—	671
Potato Salad	3.5 oz	94	2	4	11	13	—	639
Ravioli w/ Meat	1 serv (12 oz)	865	30	20	17	138	—	934
Ravioli w/o Meat	1 serv (12 oz)	822	27	16	0	140	—	878
Shrimp	3.5 oz	277	13	10	31	34	—	778
Thigh	3.5 oz	355	21	24	63	13	—	574
Wing	3.5 oz	385	23	25	81	17	—	654

BRUEGGER'S BAGELS

FOOD	PORTION	CAL	PROT	FAT	CHOL	CARB	FIBER	SOD
Blueberry	1	300	10	2	0	60	2	480
Cinnamon Raisin	1	290	10	2	0	60	3	400
Egg	1	280	10	1	25	67	3	510
Everything	1	290	11	2	0	55	2	700
Garlic	1	280	10	2	0	57	2	440
Honey Grain	1	300	11	3	0	58	3	390
Onion	1	280	10	2	0	57	2	430
Orange Cranberry	1	290	10	1	0	61	2	470
Pesto	1	280	10	2	0	55	2	480
Plain	1	280	10	2	0	56	2	430
Poppy Seed	1	280	11	2	0	57	2	440
Pumpernickel	1	280	11	2	0	56	4	390
Salt	1	270	10	2	0	55	2	1670
Sesame	1	290	11	3	0	57	2	440
Spinach	1	280	11	1	0	56	3	490
Sun Dried Tomato	1	280	10	2	0	58	3	490
Wheat Bran	1	280	10	2	0	55	5	410

BURGER KING
BEVERAGES

FOOD	PORTION	CAL	PROT	FAT	CHOL	CARB	FIBER	SOD
Cocoa Cola Classic	1 med (22 fl oz)	280	0	0	0	70	0	—
Coffee	1 serv (12 oz)	5	0	0	0	1	0	5
Diet Coke	1 med (22 fl oz)	1	0	0	0	tr	0	—
Milk 2%	1 (8 oz)	130	8	5	20	12	0	120

FOOD	PORTION	CAL	PROT	FAT	CHOL	CARB	FIBER	SOD
Shake Chocolate	1 med (13.9 oz)	440	12	10	30	75	4	330
Shake Chocolate	1 sm (10.7 oz)	330	9	7	25	58	3	250
Shake Chocolate Syrup Added	1 med (15.9 oz)	570	14	10	30	105	3	520
Shake Chocolate Syrup Added	1 sm (11.7 oz)	390	10	7	20	72	2	350
Shake Strawberry Syrup Added	1 med (15.9 oz)	550	13	9	30	104	2	350
Shake Strawberry Syrup Added	1 sm (11.7 oz)	390	10	7	20	72	1	260
Shake Vanilla	1 med (13.9 oz)	430	13	9	50	73	2	330
Shake Vanilla	1 sm (10.7 oz)	330	10	7	20	56	1	250
Sprite	1 med (22 fl oz)	260	0	0	0	66	0	–
Tropicana Orange Juice	1 serv (10 oz)	140	2	0	0	33	0	0
BREAKFAST SELECTIONS								
AM Express Dip	1 serv (1 oz)	80	0	0	0	21	–	20
AM Express Grape Jam	1 serv (0.4 oz)	30	0	0	0	7	–	0
AM Express Strawberry Jam	1 serv (0.4 oz)	30	0	0	0	8	–	0
Bacon	3 strips (0.3 oz)	40	3	3	10	0	–	170
Biscuit	1 (3.3 oz)	300	6	15	0	35	1	830
Biscuit w/ Bacon Egg & Cheese	1 (6.6 oz)	620	20	43	185	37	1	1650
Biscuit w/ Egg	1 (4.6 oz)	380	11	21	140	37	tr	1010
Biscuit w/ Sausage	1 (4.6 oz)	490	13	33	35	36	1	1240
Cini-minis w/o Icing	4 (3.8 oz)	440	6	23	25	51	1	710
Croissan'wich Sausage Egg & Cheese	1 (5.3 oz)	530	18	41	185	23	1	1120
Croissan'wich w/ Sausage & Cheese	1 (3.7 oz)	450	13	35	45	21	1	940
French Toast Sticks	5 sticks (4 oz)	440	7	23	2	51	3	490
Ham	1 serv (1.2 oz)	35	6	1	15	0	–	770
Hash Browns	1 sm (2.6 oz)	240	2	15	0	25	2	440
Land O'Lakes Whipped Classic Blend	1 serv (0.4 oz)	65	0	7	0	0	–	75
Vanilla Icing Cini-Minis	1 serv (1 oz)	110	0	3	0	20	–	40

FOOD	PORTION	CAL	PROT	FAT	CHOL	CARB	FIBER	SOD
MAIN MENU SELECTIONS								
American Cheese	2 slices (0.9 oz)	90	6	8	25	0	—	420
BK Big Fish Sandwich	1 (8.8 oz)	720	23	43	80	59	3	1180
BK Broiler Chicken Breast Patty	1 (3.5 oz)	140	21	4	90	4	—	570
BK Broiler Chicken Sandwich	1 (8.7 oz)	530	29	16	105	45	2	1060
BK Broiler Chicken Sandwich w/o Mayo	1 (8.7 oz)	370	29	9	105	45	2	1060
Bacon Cheeseburger	1 (4.9 oz)	400	24	22	70	27	1	940
Bacon Double Cheeseburger	1 (7.2 oz)	630	41	38	125	28	1	1230
Big King Sandwich	1 (7.6 oz)	640	38	42	125	28	1	980
Bull's Eye Barbecue Sauce	1 serv (0.5 oz)	20	0	0	0	5	—	140
Cheeseburger	1 (4.7 oz)	360	21	19	60	27	1	760
Chick'N Crisp Sandwich	1 (4.9 oz)	460	16	27	35	37	3	890
Chick'N Crisp Sandwich w/o Mayo	1 (4.9 oz)	360	16	16	35	37	3	890
Chicken Sandwich	1 (8 oz)	710	26	43	60	54	2	1400
Chicken Sandwich w/o Mayo	1 (8 oz)	500	26	20	60	54	2	1400
Chicken Tenders	4 (2.2 oz)	180	11	11	30	9	0	470
Chicken Tenders	8 (4.3 oz)	350	22	22	65	17	1	940
Chicken Tenders	5 (2.7 oz)	230	14	14	40	11	tr	590
Dipping Sauce Barbecue	1 serv (1 oz)	35	0	0	0	9	—	400
Dipping Sauce Honey	1 serv (1 oz)	90	0	0	0	23	—	10
Dipping Sauce Honey Mustard	1 serv (1 oz)	90	0	6	10	10	—	150
Dipping Sauce Ranch	1 serv (1 oz)	170	0	17	0	2	—	200
Dipping Sauce Sweet & Sour	1 serv (1 oz)	45	0	0	0	11	—	50
Double Cheeseburger	1 (6.9 oz)	580	38	36	120	27	1	1060
Double Whopper	1 (12.2 oz)	920	49	59	155	47	3	980
Double Whopper w/ Cheese	1 (13.1 oz)	1010	55	67	180	47	3	1460

FOOD	PORTION	CAL	PROT	FAT	CHOL	CARB	FIBER	SOD
Double Whopper w/o Mayo	1 (12.2 oz)	760	49	42	155	47	3	980
Dutch Apple Pie	1 serv (4 oz)	300	3	15	0	39	2	230
French Fries No Salt	1 king size (6 oz)	590	5	30	0	74	5	1110
French Fries No Salt	1 sm (2.6 oz)	250	2	13	0	32	2	480
French Fries No Salt	1 med (4.1 g)	400	3	21	0	50	4	760
French Fries Salted	1 med (4.1 oz)	400	3	21	0	50	4	820
French Fries Salted	1 sm (2.6 oz)	250	2	13	0	32	2	550
French Fries Salted	1 king size (6 oz)	590	5	30	0	74	5	1180
Hamburger	1 (4.2 oz)	320	19	15	50	27	1	520
Hamburger Bun	1 (4.6 oz)	130	5	2	0	24	–	250
Hamburger Patty	1 (1.9 oz)	170	14	13	50	0	–	55
Hash Browns	1 lg (4.5 oz)	410	3	26	0	42	4	750
Ketchup	1 serv (0.5 oz)	15	0	0	0	4	–	180
King Sauce	1 serv (0.5 oz)	70	0	7	4	2	–	70
Lettuce	1 leaf (0.7 oz)	0	0	0	0	0	–	0
Mustard	1 serv (3 g)	0	0	0	0	0	–	40
Onion	1 serv (0.5 oz)	5	0	0	0	1	–	0
Onion Rings	1 med serv (3.3 oz)	380	5	19	2	46	4	550
Onion Rings	1 king serv (5.3 oz)	600	8	30	4	74	6	880
Pickles	4 slices (0.5 oz)	0	0	0	0	0	–	140
Tartar Sauce	1 serv (1.5 oz)	260	0	29	20	0	–	330
Tomato	2 slices (1 oz)	5	0	0	0	1	–	0
Whopper	1 (9.5 oz)	660	29	40	85	47	3	900
Whopper Bun	1 (2.7 oz)	220	8	4	0	39	–	370
Whopper Jr.	1 (5.5 oz)	400	19	24	55	28	2	530
Whopper Jr. w/ Cheese	1 (6 oz)	450	22	28	65	28	2	770
Whopper Jr. w/ Cheese w/o Mayo	1 (6 oz)	370	22	19	65	28	2	770
Whopper Jr. w/o Mayo	1 (5.5 oz)	320	19	15	55	28	2	530
Whopper Patty	1 (2.8 oz)	250	20	19	70	0	–	85
Whopper w/ Cheese	1 (10.4 oz)	760	35	48	110	47	3	1380
Whopper w/ Cheese w/o Mayo	1 (10.4 oz)	600	35	31	110	47	3	1380
Whopper w/o Mayo	1 (9.5 oz)	510	29	23	85	47	3	900

FOOD	PORTION	CAL	PROT	FAT	CHOL	CARB	FIBER	SOD

CARL'S JR.
BAKED SELECTIONS

FOOD	PORTION	CAL	PROT	FAT	CHOL	CARB	FIBER	SOD
Cheese Danish	1 (4.1 oz)	400	5	22	15	49	1	390
Cheesecake Strawberry Swirl	1 serv (3.5 oz)	300	6	17	55	31	0	220
Chocolate Cake	1 serv (3 oz)	300	3	10	13	49	4	260
Chocolate Chip Cookie	1 (2.5 oz)	370	3	19	25	49	1	350
Cinnamon Roll	1 (4.2 oz)	420	9	13	15	68	4	570
Muffin Blueberry	1 (4.2 oz)	340	5	14	40	49	1	340
Muffin Bran	1 (4.7 oz)	370	7	13	45	61	6	410
BEVERAGES								
Coca-Cola Classic	1 reg (16 fl oz)	190	0	0	0	51	0	50
Coffee	1 reg (12 oz)	10	0	0	0	1	0	25
Diet 7UP	1 reg (16 oz)	0	0	0	0	0	0	90
Diet Coke	1 reg (16 oz)	0	0	0	0	0	0	40
Dr. Pepper	1 reg (16 oz)	200	0	0	0	52	0	30
Hot Chocolate	1 reg (12 oz)	110	1	1	<5	24	tr	125
Iced Tea	1 reg (14 fl oz)	5	0	0	0	0	—	55
Milk 1%	1 (10 fl oz)	150	14	3	15	18	0	180
Minute Maid Orange Soda	1 reg (16 oz)	230	0	0	0	59	0	30
Orange Juice	1 (6 fl oz)	90	1	0	0	20	0	0
Ramblin' Root Beer	1 reg (16 oz)	230	0	0	0	61	0	75
Shake Chocolate	1 sm (13.5 oz)	390	9	7	30	74	0	280
Shake Strawberry	1 sm (13.5 oz)	400	9	7	30	77	0	240
Shake Vanilla	1 sm (13.5 fl oz)	330	11	8	35	54	0	250
Sprite	1 reg (16 fl oz)	190	0	0	0	48	0	90
BREAKFAST SELECTIONS								
Bacon	2 strips (0.3 oz)	40	3	4	10	0	0	125
Breakfast Burrito	1 (5.3 oz)	430	22	26	460	29	tr	810
Breakfast Quesadilla Cheese	1 (5.2 oz)	300	14	14	225	27	1	750
English Muffin w/ Margarine	1 (2.6 oz)	230	5	10	0	30	2	330
French Toast Dips w/o Syrup	1 serv (3.7 oz)	410	6	25	0	40	3	380
Grape Jelly	1 serv (0.5 oz)	35	0	0	0	9	0	0
Hash Brown Nuggets	1 serv (3.3 oz)	270	3	17	0	27	2	410
Sausage	1 patty (1.8 oz)	200	7	18	35	0	0	530

FOOD	PORTION	CAL	PROT	FAT	CHOL	CARB	FIBER	SOD
Scrambed Eggs	1 serv (3.5 oz)	160	13	11	425	1	0	125
Strawberry Jam	1 serv (0.5 oz)	35	0	0	0	9	0	0
Sunrise Sandwich	1 (4.6 oz)	370	14	21	225	31	2	710
Table Syrup	1 serv (1 oz)	90	0	0	0	22	0	22
MAIN MENU SELECTIONS								
American Cheese	1 slice (0.5 oz)	60	3	5	15	0	0	270
BBQ Chicken Sandwich	1 (6.7 oz)	310	31	6	55	34	3	830
BBQ Sauce	1 serv (1.1 oz)	50	tr	0	0	11	0	270
Big Burger	1 (6.8 oz)	470	25	20	55	46	2	810
Breadstick	1 (0.3 oz)	35	1	1	0	7	1	60
Carl's Catch Fish Sandwich	1 (7.5 oz)	560	17	30	60	54	5	1220
Chicken Club Sandwich	1 (8.8 oz)	550	35	29	85	37	3	1160
Chicken Stars	6 pieces (3 oz)	230	13	14	85	11	0	450
CrissCut Fries	1 lg (5.7 oz)	550	7	34	0	55	3	1280
Croutons	1 serv (7 g)	35	tr	1	0	5	0	65
Double Western Bacon Cheeseburger	1 (11.5 oz)	970	56	57	145	58	2	1810
Famous Big Star Hamburger	1 (8.6 oz)	610	26	38	70	42	2	890
French Fries	1 reg (4.4 oz)	370	4	20	0	44	3	240
Great Stuff Potato Bacon & Cheese	1 (14.2 oz)	630	20	29	40	76	6	1720
Great Stuff Potato Broccoli & Cheese	1 (14.2 oz)	530	11	22	15	76	8	930
Great Stuff Potato Plain	1 (9.4 oz)	290	6	0	0	68	6	40
Great Stuff Potato Sour Cream & Chive	1 (10.9 oz)	430	8	14	10	70	6	160
Hamburger	1 (3.1 oz)	200	11	8	25	23	1	500
Honey Sauce	1 serv (1 oz)	90	0	0	0	23	0	5
Hot & Crispy Sandwich	1 (5 oz)	400	14	22	45	35	2	980
Mustard Sauce	1 serv (1 oz)	45	0	1	0	10	0	150
Onion Rings	1 serv (5.3 oz)	520	8	26	0	63	3	840
Salsa	1 serv (0.9 oz)	10	0	0	0	2	0	160

FOOD	PORTION	CAL	PROT	FAT	CHOL	CARB	FIBER	SOD
Sante Fe Chicken Sandwich	1 (7.9 oz)	530	30	30	85	36	3	1230
Super Star Hamburger	1 (11.2 oz)	820	43	53	120	41	2	1030
Sweet N'Sour Sauce	1 serv (1 oz)	50	0	0	0	11	0	60
Swiss Cheese	1 slice (0.5 oz)	45	3	4	10	0	0	220
Western Bacon Cheeseburger	1 (8.1 oz)	870	34	35	90	59	2	1490
Zucchini	1 serv (5.9 oz)	380	7	23	0	38	3	1040
SALAD DRESSINGS								
1000 Island	2 fl oz	250	tr	24	20	7	0	540
Blue Cheese	2 fl oz	310	2	34	25	1	0	360
French Fat Free	2 fl oz	70	0	0	0	18	1	760
House	2 fl oz	220	1	22	20	3	0	440
Italian Fat Free	2 fl oz	15	0	0	0	4	0	800
SALADS AND SALAD BARS								
Salad-To-Go Charbroiled Chicken	1 serv (12 oz)	260	28	9	70	11	4	530
Salad-To-Go Garden	1 (4.8 oz)	50	3	3	5	4	2	75

CARVEL

FROZEN YOGURT

FOOD	PORTION	CAL	PROT	FAT	CHOL	CARB	FIBER	SOD
Vanilla Low Fat No Sugar Added	4 fl oz	110	4	2	—	22	—	90
ICE CREAM								
Brown Bonnet Cone	1 (4.7 oz)	380	6	21	40	43	1	150
Brown Bonnet Cone No Fat Vanilla	1 (4.7 oz)	300	5	11	—	47	—	95
Cake	1 pkg (7 oz)	450	8	23	45	54	1	230
Cake	1 pkg (4 oz)	270	5	14	30	33	tr	160
Cake Cheesecake	1 serv (4 oz)	280	5	14	30	34	—	190
Cake Cookies & Cream	1 serv (4 oz)	270	5	14	35	32	1	160
Cake Fudge Drizzle	1/8 cake (4 oz)	310	6	17	30	35	1	170
Cake Fudgie The Whale	1/14 cake (3.6 oz)	290	5	16	30	33	1	180
Cake Holiday	1/15 cake (3.4 oz)	240	4	12	30	30	1	100
Cake S'mores	1 serv (4 oz)	270	5	14	25	33	1	150
Cake Sinfully Chocolate	1 serv (4 oz)	280	5	14	25	34	1	150

FOOD	PORTION	CAL	PROT	FAT	CHOL	CARB	FIBER	SOD
Cake Strawberries & Cream	⅛ cake (3.8 oz)	240	4	12	35	31	1	100
Chocolate	4 fl oz	190	4	10	25	22	0	100
Chocolate No Fat	4 fl oz	120	2	0	0	28	0	40
Flying Saucer Chocolate	1 (4 oz)	230	5	9	30	33	2	140
Flying Saucer Chocolate w/ Sprinkles	1 (4 oz)	330	5	14	30	49	2	150
Flying Saucer Low Fat Chocolate	1 (4 oz)	190	3	3	0	38	1	130
Flying Saucer Low Fat Vanilla	1 (4 oz)	180	4	3	0	36	1	140
Flying Saucer Vanilla	1 (4 oz)	240	5	10	40	33	1	150
Flying Saucer Vanilla w/ Sprinkles	1 (4 oz)	340	5	14	40	49	1	160
Lil'Love Cake All Vanilla	1 piece (4.4 oz)	330	6	16	35	41	tr	200
Lil'Love Cake Chocolate & Vanilla	1 piece (4 oz)	260	5	13	30	31	tr	140
Nature's Crunch	1 (4.2 g)	450	5	25	20	55	2	240
Olde Fashion Sundae Butterscotch	1 (8 oz)	500	7	17	60	80	1	340
Olde Fashion Sundae Chocolate	1 (8 oz)	470	8	19	55	71	1	280
Olde Fashion Sundae Strawberry	1 (8 oz)	420	7	15	55	64	2	230
Sinful Love Bar	1 (4.2 oz)	460	8	29	20	48	3	240
Thick Shake Chocolate	1 (16 oz)	719	18	31	116	96	tr	418
Thick Shake Low Fat Chocolate	1 (16 oz)	490	16	1	15	108	1	330
Thick Shake Low Fat Strawberry	1 (16 oz)	460	15	1	15	96	1	290
Thick Shake Low Fat Vanilla	1 (16 oz)	460	15	1	15	98	1	280
Thick Shake No Fat Chocolate	1 (16 oz)	524	17	8	36	100	1	346

FOOD	PORTION	CAL	PROT	FAT	CHOL	CARB	FIBER	SOD
Thick Shake No Fat Strawberry	1 (16 oz)	453	16	7	36	82	1	285
Thick Shake No Fat Vanilla	1 (16 oz)	462	16	7	36	84	1	278
Thick Shake Strawberry	1 (16 oz)	648	17	30	116	77	tr	358
Thick Shake Vanilla	1 (16 oz)	657	17	30	116	79	tr	350
Vanilla	4 fl oz	200	5	10	40	21	0	110
Vanilla No Fat	4 fl oz	120	4	0	0	25	0	55
SHERBET								
Black Raspberry	½ cup (3.4 oz)	150	1	1	5	33	0	35
Blueberry	½ cup (3.4 oz)	150	1	1	5	33	0	30
Lemon	½ cup (3.5 oz)	150	1	1	5	31	0	30
Lime	½ cup (3.5 oz)	150	1	1	5	31	0	30
Mango	½ cup (3.5 oz)	140	1	1	5	30	0	25
Orange	½ cup (3.5 oz)	150	1	1	5	31	0	30
Peach	½ cup (3.4 oz)	150	1	1	5	32	0	35
Pineapple	½ cup (3.5 oz)	150	1	1	5	33	0	40
Strawberry	½ cup (3.5 oz)	150	1	1	5	32	0	35

CHICK-FIL-A

FOOD	PORTION	CAL	PROT	FAT	CHOL	CARB	FIBER	SOD
BEVERAGES								
Coca-Cola Classic	1 serv (9 oz)	110	0	0	0	28	0	10
Diet Coke	1 serv (9 oz)	0	0	0	0	0	0	10
Diet Lemonade	1 serv (9 oz)	5	0	0	0	2	0	4
Ice Tea Sweetened	1 serv (9 oz)	150	0	0	0	38	0	50
Iced Tea Unsweetened	1 serv (9 oz)	0	0	0	0	0	0	50
Lemonade	1 sm (9 oz)	90	0	0	0	23	0	4
DESSERTS								
Cheesecake + One Side	1 slice (3.1 oz)	300	6	21	115	23	0	200
Fudge Nut Brownie	1 (2.6 oz)	350	10	16	30	41	0	650
Ice Cream Cone	1 sm (4.5 oz)	140	11	4	40	16	0	240
Lemon Pie	1 slice (3.5 oz)	280	1	22	5	19	0	550
MAIN MENU SELECTIONS								
Barbecue Sauce	1 serv (1 oz)	45	0	0	0	11	0	190
Carrot & Raisin Salad	1 sm (2.7 oz)	150	5	2	6	28	2	650
Chargrilled Chicken Club Sandwich	1 (8.2 oz)	390	33	12	70	38	2	980

FOOD	PORTION	CAL	PROT	FAT	CHOL	CARB	FIBER	SOD
Chargrilled Chicken Garden Salad	1 serv (9.8 oz)	190	26	5	83	12	4	800
Chargrilled Chicken Sandwich	1 (5.3 oz)	280	27	3	40	36	1	640
Chick-n-Strips	4 (4.2 oz)	230	29	8	20	10	0	380
Chick-n-Strips Salad	1 serv (11.7 oz)	370	32	17	113	21	4	725
Chicken Sandwich	1 (5.9 oz)	290	24	9	50	29	1	870
Chicken Caesar Salad	1 serv (8.1 oz)	230	31	10	85	5	2	940
Chicken Salad Sandwich	1 (5.9 oz)	320	25	5	10	42	1	810
Cole Slaw	1 sm (2.8 oz)	130	6	6	15	11	1	430
Dijon Honey Sauce	1 serv (0.4 oz)	60	0	1	5	2	0	70
Hearty Breast of Chicken Soup	1 cup (7.6 oz)	110	16	1	45	10	1	760
Honey Mustard Sauce	1 serv (1 oz)	45	0	0	0	11	0	150
Nuggets	8 (3.9 oz)	290	28	14	60	12	0	770
Polynesian Sauce	1 serv (1 oz)	110	0	6	0	13	0	210
Side Salad	1 serv (4.6 oz)	70	5	0	0	13	1	0
Waffle Potato Fries	1 sm (3 oz)	290	1	10	5	49	0	960
SALAD DRESSINGS								
Basil Vinaigrette	1 serv (1.5 oz)	250	0	26	0	5	0	190
Blue Cheese	1 serv (1.5 oz)	230	0	24	30	2	0	450
Buttermilk Ranch	1 serv (1.5 oz)	220	1	24	10	2	0	420
Fat Free Dijon Honey Mustard	1 serv (1.5 oz)	70	1	1	0	17	1	230
House	1 serv (1.6 oz)	190	0	17	5	9	1	380
Light Italian	1 serv (1.5 oz)	20	0	1	0	2	0	770
Spicy	1 serv (1.2 oz)	210	0	22	10	2	0	170
Thousand Island	1 serv (1.5 oz)	210	0	20	20	6	0	360

CHILI'S

DESSERTS

FOOD	PORTION	CAL	PROT	FAT	CHOL	CARB	FIBER	SOD
Diet By Chocolate Cake	1 serv	370	10	2	0	79	8	670
Diet By Chocolate Cake w/ Yogurt	1 serv	465	13	2	3	99	8	622
Diet By Chocolate Cake w/ Yogurt & Fudge Topping	1 serv	534	14	3	3	116	8	703

FOOD	PORTION	CAL	PROT	FAT	CHOL	CARB	FIBER	SOD
MAIN MENU SELECTIONS								
Guiltless Grill Chicken Fijitas	1 serv	726	45	13	44	108	24	4759
Guiltless Grill Chicken Platter	1 serv	563	38	7	58	83	12	3284
Guiltless Grill Chicken Salad w/ Dressing	1 serv	254	29	3	47	27	6	1475
Guiltless Grill Chicken Sandwich	1	527	44	7	43	70	18	2923
Guiltless Grill Veggie Pasta	1 serv	590	25	11	55	98	16	964
Guiltless Grill Veggie Pasta w/ Chicken	1 serv	696	44	13	97	102	17	1399
CHURCH'S CHICKEN								
Apple Pie	1 serv (3.1 oz)	280	2	12	<5	41	1	340
Biscuit	1 (2.1 oz)	250	2	16	<5	26	1	640
Breast	1 serv (2.8 oz)	200	19	12	65	4	0	510
Cajun Rice	1 serv (3.1 oz)	130	1	7	5	16	tr	260
Cole Slaw	1 serv (3 oz)	92	4	6	0	8	2	230
Corn On The Cob	1 serv (5.7 oz)	139	4	3	0	24	9	15
French Fries	1 serv (2.7 oz)	210	3	11	0	29	2	60
Leg	1 serv (2 oz)	140	13	9	45	2	0	160
Okra	1 serv (2.8 oz)	210	3	16	0	19	4	520
Potatoes & Gravy	1 serv (3.7 oz)	90	1	3	0	14	1	520
Tender Strip	1 (1.1 oz)	80	6	4	15	5	1	140
Thigh	1 serv (2.8 oz)	230	16	16	80	5	0	520
Wing	1 serv (3.1 oz)	250	19	16	60	8	0	540
CINNABON								
Caramel Pecanbon	1	890	—	41	—	—	—	—
Cinnabon	1 reg	670	—	34	—	—	—	—
DAIRY QUEEN								
FOOD SELECTIONS								
Chicken Breast Fillet Sandwich	1 (6.7 oz)	430	24	20	55	37	2	760
Chicken Strip Basket	1 serv (14.5 oz)	1000	35	50	55	102	5	2510
Chili 'n' Cheese Dog	1 (5 oz)	330	14	21	45	22	2	1090

FOOD	PORTION	CAL	PROT	FAT	CHOL	CARB	FIBER	SOD
DQ Homestyle Bacon Double Cheeseburger	1 (8.9 oz)	610	41	36	130	31	2	1380
DQ Homestyle Cheeseburger	1 (5.3 oz)	340	20	17	55	29	2	850
DQ Homestyle Double Cheeseburger	1 (7.7 oz)	540	35	31	115	30	2	1130
DQ Homestyle Hamburger	1 (4.8 oz)	290	17	12	45	29	2	630
DQ Ultimate Burger	1 (9.4 oz)	670	40	43	135	29	2	1210
French Fries	1 sm (4 oz)	350	4	18	0	42	3	880
French Fries	1 med (3.9 oz)	440	5	23	0	53	4	1110
Grilled Chicken Sandwich	1 (6.5 oz)	310	24	10	50	30	3	1040
Hot Dog	1 (3.5 oz)	240	9	14	25	19	1	730
Onion Rings	1 serv (4 oz)	320	5	16	0	39	3	180
The Great Steakmelt Basket	1 serv (13.2 oz)	770	32	38	75	72	5	2290
ICE CREAM								
Banana Split	1 (12.9 oz)	510	8	12	30	96	3	180
Blizzard Chocolate Sandwich Cookie	1 med (11.4 oz)	640	12	23	45	97	1	500
Blizzard Chocolate Sandwich Cookie	1 sm (12 oz)	520	10	18	40	79	1	380
Blizzard Chocolate Chip Cookie Dough	1 med (15.4 oz)	950	17	36	75	143	2	660
Blizzard Chocolate Chip Cookie Dough	1 sm (12 oz)	660	12	24	55	99	1	440
Breeze Heath	1 med (14.2 oz)	710	15	18	20	123	1	580
Breeze Heath	1 sm (10.2 oz)	470	11	10	10	85	1	380
Breeze Strawberry	1 sm (12 oz)	320	10	1	5	68	1	190
Breeze Strawberry	1 med (13.4 oz)	460	13	1	10	99	1	270
Buster Bar	1 (5.2 oz)	450	10	28	15	41	2	280
Chocolate Malt	1 sm (14.7 oz)	650	15	16	55	111	0	370
Chocolate Malt	1 med (19.9 oz)	880	19	22	70	153	0	500
Cone Chocolate	1 med (6.9 oz)	340	8	11	30	53	0	160
Cone Chocolate	1 sm (5 oz)	240	6	8	20	37	0	115
Cone Vanilla	1 med (6.9 oz)	330	8	9	30	53	0	160
Cone Vanilla	1 lg (8.9 oz)	410	10	12	40	65	0	200

FOOD	PORTION	CAL	PROT	FAT	CHOL	CARB	FIBER	SOD
Cone Vanilla	1 sm (5 oz)	230	6	7	20	38	0	115
Cone Yogurt	1 med (6.9 oz)	260	9	1	5	56	0	160
Cone Dipped	1 med (7.7 oz)	490	9	24	30	59	1	190
Cone Dipped	1 sm (5.5 oz)	340	6	17	20	42	1	130
Cup Of Yogurt	1 med (6.7 oz)	230	8	1	5	48	0	150
DQ 8 Inch Round Cake Undecorated	1/8 of cake (6.2 oz)	340	7	13	25	56	1	280
DQ Fudge Bar No Sugar Added	1 (2.3 oz)	50	4	0	0	13	0	70
DQ Lemon Freez'r	1/2 cup (3.2 oz)	80	0	0	0	20	0	10
DQ Nonfat Frozen Yogurt	1/2 cup (3 oz)	100	3	0		21	0	70
DQ Sandwich	1 (2.1 oz)	200	4	6	10	31	1	140
DQ Soft Serve Chocolate	1/2 cup (3.3 oz)	150	4	5	15	22	0	75
DQ Soft Serve Vanilla	1/2 cup (3.3 oz)	140	3	5	15	22	0	70
DQ Treatzza Pizza Heath	1/8 of pie (2.3 oz)	180	3	7	5	28	1	160
DQ Treatzza Pizza M&M	1/8 of pie (2.4 oz)	190	3	7	5	29	1	160
DQ Vanilla Orange Bar No Sugar Added	1 (2.3 oz)	60	2	0	0	17	0	40
Dilly Bar Chocolate	1 (3 oz)	210	3	13	10	21	0	75
Frozen Hot Chocolate	1 (20.9 oz)	860	14	35	50	127	3	350
Misty Slush	1 sm (15.9 oz)	220	0	0	0	56	0	20
Misty Slush	1 med (20.9 oz)	290	0	0	0	74	0	30
Peanut Buster Parfait	1 (10.7 oz)	730	16	31	35	99	2	400
Pecan Mudslide Treat	1 (4.6 oz)	650	11	30	35	85	2	420
S'more Galore Parfait	1 (10.7 oz)	730	11	30	30	111	3	340
Shake Chocolate	1 sm (13.9 oz)	560	13	15	50	94	0	310
Shake Chocolate	1 med (18.9 oz)	770	17	20	70	130	0	420
Starkiss	1 (3 oz)	80	0	0	0	21	0	10
Strawberry Shortcake	1 (8.5 oz)	430	7	14	60	70	1	360
Sundae Chocolate	1 med (8.2 oz)	400	8	10	30	71	0	210
Sundae Chocolate	1 sm (5.7 oz)	280	5	7	20	49	0	140
Yogurt Sundae Strawberry	1 med (8.2 oz)	280	8	1	5	61	1	160

FOOD	PORTION	CAL	PROT	FAT	CHOL	CARB	FIBER	SOD

D'ANGELO'S SANDWICH SHOP
SALADS AND SALAD BARS

FOOD	PORTION	CAL	PROT	FAT	CHOL	CARB	FIBER	SOD
Antipasto Salad w/o Dressing	1	420	—	14	40	56	—	1400
Caesar Salad w/ Dressing	1	740	—	45	70	61	—	2270
Caesar Salad w/o Dressing	1	490	—	20	15	60	—	1310
Chicken Caesar Salad w/ Dressing	1	860	—	48	130	62	—	2820
Chicken Caesar Salad w/o Dressing	1	600	—	23	70	60	—	1870
Chicken Salad D'Lite	1	325	—	4	49	34	—	980
Chicken Salad w/o Dressing	1	390	—	5	60	56	—	1200
D'Lite Turkey	1 serv	355	—	2	79	—	—	714
Greek Salad w/ Dressing	1	940	—	71	50	63	—	1320
Greek Salad w/ Tuna & Dressing	1	1010	—	72	65	63	—	1510
Greek Salad w/ Tuna w/o Dressing	1	490	—	15	65	58	—	1510
Greek Salad w/o Dressing	1	420	—	15	50	58	—	1310
Roast Beef Salad D'Lite	1	350	—	5	63	33	—	890
Roast Beef Salad w/o Dressing	1	400	—	6	50	55	—	920
Tossed Garden Salad w/o Dressing	1	270	—	2	0	55	—	650
Tuna Salad D'Lite	1	305	—	2	32	33	—	805
Tuna Salad w/o Dressing	1	330	—	3	15	55	—	840
Turkey Salad w/o Dressing	1	400	—	3	80	55	—	700

SANDWICHES

FOOD	PORTION	CAL	PROT	FAT	CHOL	CARB	FIBER	SOD
BLT w/ Cheese	1	1170	—	62	165	88	—	3310
BLT w/ Cheese Medium Sub	1	870	—	47	125	64	—	2490
BLT w/ Cheese Pokket	1	570	—	31	90	41	—	1690

FOOD	PORTION	CAL	PROT	FAT	CHOL	CARB	FIBER	SOD
BLT w/ Cheese Small Sub	1	600	–	33	90	–	–	1730
Barbecue Curls	1	480	–	19	70	45	–	650
Buffalo Chicken Wrap w/ Blue Cheese Dressing	1	621	–	28	93	51	–	1831
Buffalo Chicken Wrap w/o Dressing	1	417	–	13	78	48	–	1551
Caesar Salad w/ Dressing Pokket	1	590	–	26	40	68	–	1690
Caesar Salad w/o Dressing Pokket	1	460	–	13	10	68	–	1210
Caesar Salad w/ Chicken w/ Dressing Pokket	1	700	–	28	100	69	–	2240
Caesar Salad w/ Chicken w/ Dressing Pokket	1	570	–	16	70	68	–	1760
Caesar Wrap w/ Dressing	1	484	–	15	10	66	–	2135
Caesar Wrap w/ Fat Free Dressing	1	484	–	15	10	66	–	2135
Capicola Ham & Cheese Large Sub	1	740	–	23	85	89	–	2540
Capicola Ham & Cheese Medium Sub	1	550	–	17	65	64	–	1900
Capicola Ham & Cheese Pokket	1	350	–	11	45	41	–	1260
Capicola Ham & Cheese Small Sub	1	390	–	13	45	45	–	1310
Cheeseburger Large Sub	1	1060	–	49	165	87	–	2090
Cheeseburger Medium Sub	1	780	–	37	125	63	–	1560
Cheeseburger Pokket	1	490	–	23	80	40	–	1000

FOOD	PORTION	CAL	PROT	FAT	CHOL	CARB	FIBER	SOD
Cheeseburger Small Sub	1	530	—	25	80	44	—	1040
Chicken Salad Large Sub	1	1370	—	78	155	89	—	1570
Chicken Salad Medium Sub	1	970	—	55	110	64	—	1120
Chicken Salad Pokket	1	650	—	38	80	41	—	740
Chicken Salad Small Sub	1	690	—	39	80	44	—	790
Chicken Stir Fry D'Lite Pokket	1	360	—	5	70	46	—	1240
Chicken Stir Fry D'Lite Sub	1	280	—	6	70	47	—	1280
Chicken Stir Fry Large Sub	1	800	—	12	160	93	—	2730
Chicken Stir Fry Medium Sub	1	560	—	9	110	68	—	1890
Chicken Stir Fry Pokket	1	360	—	5	70	46	—	1240
Chicken Stir Fry Small Sub	1	380	—	6	70	47	—	1280
Classic Vegetable D'Lite Pokket	1	340	—	10	23	48	—	960
Classic Vegetable Large Sub	1	860	—	33	80	104	—	2450
Classic Vegetable Medium Sub	1	610	—	23	55	74	—	1700
Classic Vegetable Pokket	1	400	—	15	40	48	—	1180
Classic Vegetable Small Sub	1	430	—	15	40	52	—	1220
Crunchy Vegetable D'Lite Pokket	1	350	—	10	23	52	—	1000
Crunchy Vegetable D'Lite Small Sub	1	385	—	11	23	56	—	1045
Crunchy Vegetable Large Sub	1	880	—	33	80	106	—	2520
Crunchy Vegetable Pokket	1	410	—	15	40	50	—	1220

FOOD	PORTION	CAL	PROT	FAT	CHOL	CARB	FIBER	SOD
Crunchy Vegetables Medium Sub	1	620	—	23	55	76	—	1750
Crunchy Vegetables Small Sub	1	440	—	16	40	53	—	1260
Ginger Chicken Stir Fry D'Lite Pokket	1	400	—	5	72	55	—	1240
Greek Pokket	1	910	—	71	50	57	—	1120
Grilled Spicy Steak D'Lite Pokket	1	425	—	11	41	59	—	735
Grilled Steak Cheese Large Sub	1	1160	—	54	195	87	—	1970
Grilled Steak Cheese Medium Sub	1	820	—	38	135	63	—	1460
Grilled Steak Cheese Pokket	1	550	—	26	100	40	—	1010
Grilled Steak Cheese Small Sub	1	580	—	28	100	44	—	1050
Grilled Steak Combo Large Sub	1	1170	—	54	195	92	—	2200
Grilled Steak Combo Medium Sub	1	830	—	38	135	67	—	1630
Grilled Steak Combo Pokket	1	550	—	26	100	43	—	1120
Grilled Steak Combo Small Sub	1	590	—	28	100	46	—	1170
Grilled Steak D'Lite Pokket	1	390	—	11	41	51	—	735
Grilled Steak Large Sub	1	990	—	40	155	87	—	1320
Grilled Steak Medium Sub	1	680	—	27	105	63	—	940
Grilled Steak Mushrooms Large Sub	1	1000	—	40	155	—	—	1570
Grilled Steak Mushrooms Medium Sub	1	690	—	27	105	65	—	1120
Grilled Steak Mushrooms Pokket	1	450	—	18	70	41	—	720

FOOD	PORTION	CAL	PROT	FAT	CHOL	CARB	FIBER	SOD
Grilled Steak Mushrooms Small Sub	1	480	–	19	70	45	–	770
Grilled Steak Onion Large Sub	1	1000	–	40	155	91	–	1330
Grilled Steak Onion Medium Sub	1	700	–	27	105	66	–	940
Grilled Steak Onion Small Sub	1	480	–	19	70	45	–	650
Grilled Steak Onions Pokket	1	450	–	17	70	42	–	600
Grilled Steak Peppers	1	690	–	27	105	65	–	940
Grilled Steak Peppers Large Sub	1	1000	–	40	155	90	–	1330
Grilled Steak Peppers Pokket	1	540	–	17	70	42	–	600
Grilled Steak Pokket	1	440	–	17	70	40	–	600
Grilled Steak Small Sub	1	470	–	19	70	43	–	650
Ham & Cheese Large Sub	1	760	–	25	105	88	–	3030
Ham & Cheese Medium Sub	1	550	–	19	75	63	–	2170
Ham & Cheese Pokket	1	370	–	13	55	40	–	1550
Ham & Cheese Small Sub	1	400	–	14	55	44	–	1600
Ham Salami & Cheese Large Sub	1	870	–	36	110	88	–	3000
Ham Salami & Cheese Medium Sub	1	630	–	27	80	64	–	2190
Ham Salami & Cheese Pokket	1	420	–	18	60	41	–	1500
Ham Salami & Cheese Small Sub	1	450	–	20	60	44	–	1550
Hamburger Large Sub	1	920	–	38	130	87	–	1570
Hamburger Medium Sub	1	680	–	28	95	63	–	1150
Hamburger Pokket	1	430	–	18	65	40	–	740

FOOD	PORTION	CAL	PROT	FAT	CHOL	CARB	FIBER	SOD
Hamburger Small Sub	1	460	—	19	65	43	—	780
Italian Cold Cut Large Sub	1	1130	—	61	155	92	—	3580
Italian Cold Cut Medium Sub	1	820	—	44	110	68	—	2600
Italian Cold Cut Pokket	1	550	—	30	80	42	—	1790
Italian Cold Cut Small Sub	1	580	—	32	80	46	—	1830
Meatball Large Sub	1	1010	—	42	135	102	—	2600
Meatball Medium Sub	1	750	—	32	100	76	—	1980
Meatball Pokket	1	480	—	20	65	50	—	1360
Meatball Small Sub	1	520	—	21	65	54	—	1400
Meatball w/ Cheese Large Sub	1	1170	—	54	165	103	—	3000
Meatball w/ Cheese Medium Sub	1	880	—	41	125	77	—	2300
Meatball w/ Cheese Pokket	1	580	—	28	85	51	—	1600
Meatball w/ Cheese Small Sub	1	620	—	29	85	54	—	1650
Pastrami Large Sub	1	1250	—	69	175	87	—	2920
Pastrami Medium Sub	1	860	—	46	115	63	—	2010
Pastrami Pokket	1	550	—	30	75	40	—	1310
Pastrami Small Sub	1	580	—	31	75	44	—	1350
Pastrami w/ Cheese Large Sub	1	1640	—	102	270	89	—	4420
Pastrami w/ Cheese Medium Sub	1	1170	—	73	195	64	—	3210
Pastrami w/ Cheese Pokket	1	780	—	49	135	41	—	2210
Pastrami w/ Cheese Small Sub	1	820	—	51	135	45	—	2250
Roast Beef D'Lite Pokket	1	330	—	6	48	42	—	710
Roast Beef D'Lite Small Sub	1	365	—	7	48	45	—	755

FOOD	PORTION	CAL	PROT	FAT	CHOL	CARB	FIBER	SOD
Roast Beef Large Sub	1	710	–	14	95	87	–	1510
Roast Beef Medium Sub	1	520	–	10	70	63	–	1100
Seafood Salad Large Sub	1	1210	–	68	50	118	–	2890
Seafood Salad Medium Sub	1	860	–	48	35	85	–	2050
Seafood Salad Pokket	1	570	–	33	25	56	–	1400
Seafood Salad Small Sub	1	610	–	34	25	59	–	1440
Stuffed Turkey D'Lite Pokket	1	510	–	8	82	71	–	880
Stuffed Turkey D'Lite Small Sub	1	545	–	9	82	75	–	920
Stuffed Turkey Large Sub	1	1070	–	19	165	146	–	1850
Stuffed Turkey Medium Sub	1	790	–	14	120	107	–	1360
Tuna Salad Large Sub	1	1510	–	102	120	90	–	2200
Tuna Salad Medium Sub	1	1070	–	72	85	65	–	1570
Tuna Salad Pokket	1	720	–	50	60	41	–	1060
Turkey D'Lite Pokket	1	330	–	2	79	40	–	490
Turkey D'Lite Small Sub	1	365	–	4	79	43	–	535
Turkey Large Sub	1	710	–	7	160	87	–	1070
Turkey Medium Sub	1	520	–	5	115	63	–	780
Turkey Club Large Sub	1	860	–	20	180	87	–	1470
Turkey Club Medium Sub	1	630	–	15	130	63	–	1080
Turkey Club Pokket	1	400	–	9	90	40	–	690
Turkey Club Small Sub	1	430	–	10	90	43	–	740

DELTACO
BEVERAGES

FOOD	PORTION	CAL	PROT	FAT	CHOL	CARB	FIBER	SOD
Coffee	1 serv (8 oz)	0	0	0	0	1	0	5

FOOD	PORTION	CAL	PROT	FAT	CHOL	CARB	FIBER	SOD
Coke Classic	1 sm (10 oz)	120	0	0	0	29	0	10
Coke Classic	1 med (12 oz)	150	0	0	0	37	0	15
Coke Classic	1 lg (20 oz)	230	0	0	0	59	0	25
Coke Classic Best Value	1 serv (27 oz)	320	0	0	0	81	0	30
Diet Coke	1 lg (20 oz)	5	1	0	0	1	0	35
Diet Coke	1 med (12 oz)	0	0	0	0	0	0	15
Diet Coke	1 sm (10 oz)	0	0	0	0	0	0	15
Diet Coke Best Value	1 serv (27 oz)	10	1	0	0	1	0	45
Iced Tea	1 sm (10 oz)	0	0	0	0	0	0	10
Iced Tea	1 lg (20 oz)	5	0	0	0	2	0	15
Iced Tea	1 med (12 oz)	0	0	0	0	1	0	10
Iced Tea Best Value	1 serv (27 oz)	10	0	0	0	2	0	25
Milk 1% Lowfat	1 serv (11 oz)	130	10	3	10	15	0	150
Mr Pibb	1 lg (20 oz)	230	0	0	0	59	0	55
Mr Pibb	1 sm (10 oz)	120	0	0	0	29	0	30
Mr Pibb	1 med (12 oz)	150	0	0	0	37	0	10
Mr Pibb Best Value	1 serv (27 oz)	320	0	0	0	81	0	80
Orange Juice	1 serv (11 oz)	140	2	0	0	34	1	0
Shake Chocolate	1 lg (15 oz)	680	16	16	45	117	1	350
Shake Chocolate	1 sm (11.4 oz)	520	12	12	35	89	1	270
Shake Strawberry	1 lg (15 oz)	540	14	8	40	100	1	280
Shake Strawberry	1 sm (11.4 oz)	410	11	6	30	76	1	220
Shake Vanilla	1 lg (15 oz)	550	16	10	50	97	1	320
Shake Vanilla	1 sm (11.4 oz)	420	12	7	35	75	1	250
Sprite	1 med (12 oz)	140	0	0	0	37	0	40
Sprite	1 lg (20 oz)	230	0	0	0	59	0	60
Sprite	1 sm (10 oz)	110	0	0	0	29	0	30
Sprite Best Value	1 serv (27 oz)	310	0	0	0	81	0	85
BREAKFAST SELECTIONS								
Burrito Breakfast	1 (3.8 oz)	250	10	11	160	24	1	520
Burrito Egg & Cheese	1 (7.5 oz)	450	23	24	530	39	3	740
Burrito Macho Bacon & Egg	1 (15.9 oz)	1030	40	60	790	82	6	1760
Burrito Steak & Egg	1 (9 oz)	580	33	34	560	41	3	1270
Quesadilla Bacon & Egg	1 (6.1 oz)	450	21	23	260	40	2	920
Side of Bacon	2 strips (0.3 oz)	50	3	4	10	0	0	170

FOOD	PORTION	CAL	PROT	FAT	CHOL	CARB	FIBER	SOD
MAIN MENU SELECTIONS								
Beans 'n Cheese Cup	1 serv (7.7 oz)	260	16	3	5	44	16	1810
Burrito Combo	1 (8.2 oz)	490	26	21	55	53	8	1380
Burrito Del Beef	1 (8 oz)	550	31	30	90	42	3	1090
Burrito Del Classic Chicken	1 (8.5 oz)	580	24	38	70	42	3	1100
Burrito Deluxe Combo	1 (10.7 oz)	530	27	25	60	56	9	1390
Burrito Deluxe Del Beef	1 (10.5 oz)	590	32	33	95	45	4	1110
Burrito Green	1 (5 oz)	280	11	8	15	38	6	1030
Burrito Macho Beef	1 (18.9 oz)	1170	60	62	190	89	7	2190
Burrito Macho Combo	1 (19.4 oz)	1050	49	44	115	113	17	2760
Burrito Red	1 (5 oz)	270	11	8	15	38	6	1020
Burrito Red Regular	1 (7.5 oz)	390	18	12	20	59	11	1439
Burrito Regular Green	1 (7.5 oz)	400	18	12	10	59	10	1450
Burrito Spicy Chicken	1 (8.7 oz)	480	23	16	40	65	8	1620
Burrito The Works	1 (10.2 oz)	480	18	18	25	69	9	1500
Cheeseburger	1 (4.6 oz)	330	16	13	35	37	3	870
Del Cheeseburger	1 (5.6 oz)	430	16	25	45	35	4	710
Double Del Cheeseburger	1 (7.1 oz)	560	26	35	85	35	4	960
Fries	1 sm (3 oz)	210	2	14	0	20	2	160
Fries	1 reg (5 oz)	350	3	23	0	34	3	270
Fries Best Value	1 serv (7 oz)	490	5	32	0	47	5	380
Fries Chili Cheese	1 serv (10.5 oz)	670	17	46	45	51	5	880
Fries Deluxe Chili Cheese	1 serv (11.9 oz)	710	17	49	50	53	6	880
Get A Lot Meals #1 Combo Burrito Fries Drink	1 meal	980	29	44	55	124	11	1670
Get A Lot Meals #2 Del Classic Chicken Burrito Fries Drink	1 meal	1080	28	61	70	113	7	1390
Get A Lot Meals #3 Regular Red Burrito Fries Drink	1 meal	890	21	35	20	130	14	1710

FOOD	PORTION	CAL	PROT	FAT	CHOL	CARB	FIBER	SOD
Get A Lot Meals #4 Two Chicken Soft Tacos Fries Drink	1 meal	910	25	46	60	102	5	1330
Get A Lot Meals #5 Taco Combo Burrito Drink	1 meal	790	32	31	75	101	9	1540
Get A Lot Meals #6 Two Tacos Quesadilla Drink	1 meal	960	37	47	115	98	3	1170
Get A Lot Meals #7 Macho Combo Burrito Fries Drink	1 meal	1530	52	67	115	183	20	3050
Get A Lot Meals #8 Two Big Fat Tacos Fries Drink	1 meal	802	35	45	70	148	10	1640
Get A Lot Meals #9 Double Del Cheeseburger Fries Drink	1 meal	1050	29	58	85	106	7	1250
Nachos	1 serv (4 oz)	380	5	24	5	40	2	630
Nachos Macho	1 serv (17 oz)	1200	33	66	55	130	16	2720
Quesadilla Chicken	1 (6.8 oz)	580	33	31	104	41	2	1240
Quesadilla Regular	1 (5.3 oz)	500	23	27	75	39	2	860
Quesadilla Spicy Jack Chicken	1 (6.8 oz)	570	32	30	105	40	2	1300
Quesadilla Spicy Jack Regular	1 (5.3 oz)	490	23	26	75	38	2	920
Rice Cup	1 serv (4 oz)	150	3	2	2	28	1	600
Soft Taco	1 (2.8 oz)	160	8	8	20	16	1	330
Soft Taco Chicken	1 (3.3 oz)	210	11	12	30	16	1	520
Taco	1 (2.2 oz)	160	7	10	20	11	1	150
Taco Big Fat	1 (5.4 oz)	320	16	11	35	39	3	680
Taco Big Fat Chicken	1 (5.4 oz)	340	18	13	45	38	3	840
Taco Big Fat Steak	1 (5.4 oz)	390	18	19	45	38	3	960

FOOD	PORTION	CAL	PROT	FAT	CHOL	CARB	FIBER	SOD
Taco Salad Deluxe	1 (18.8 oz)	760	31	37	70	76	14	2010
Tostada Salad	1 (4.5 oz)	210	9	9	15	24	6	640

DENNY'S
BEVERAGES

FOOD	PORTION	CAL	PROT	FAT	CHOL	CARB	FIBER	SOD
2% Milk	1 serv (10 oz)	151	10	6	22	15	0	152
Chocolate Milk	1 serv (10 oz)	235	9	9	37	30	0	189
Coffee French Vanilla	1 serv (8 oz)	76	0	1	2	16	0	4
Coffee Hazelnut	1 serv (8 oz)	66	0	1	2	14	0	4
Coffee Irish Cream	1 serv (8 oz)	73	0	1	2	16	0	4
Grapefruit Juice	1 serv (10 oz)	115	0	0	0	29	0	0
Hot Chocolate	1 serv (8 oz)	90	4	2	0	18	0	153
Lemonade	1 serv (16 oz)	150	0	0	0	35	0	38
Orange Juice	1 serv (10 oz)	126	2	0	0	31	0	31
Raspberry Ice Tea	1 serv (16 oz)	78	0	0	0	21	0	0
Tomato Juice	1 serv (10 oz)	56	2	0	0	11	2	921

BREAKFAST SELECTIONS

FOOD	PORTION	CAL	PROT	FAT	CHOL	CARB	FIBER	SOD
All American Slam	1 serv (15 oz)	1028	48	87	724	24	2	1942
Applesauce	1 serv (3 oz)	60	0	0	0	15	1	13
Bacon	4 strips (1 oz)	162	12	18	36	1	0	640
Bagel Dry	1 (3 oz)	235	9	1	0	46	0	495
Banana	1 (4 oz)	110	1	0	0	29	4	0
Banana Strawberry Medley	1 serv (4 oz)	108	1	1	0	27	2	6
Biscuit Plain	1 (3 oz)	375	5	22	0	40	0	750
Biscuit w/ Sausage Gravy	1 serv (7 oz)	570	11	38	24	45	0	1475
Blueberry Topping	1 serv (3 oz)	106	0	0	0	26	0	15
Canadian Bacon	1 serv (3 oz)	110	17	5	43	1	0	1039
Cantaloupe	1 serv (3 oz)	32	1	0	0	8	1	16
Cheddar Cheese Omelette	1 serv (13 oz)	770	34	62	675	24	2	1133
Cherry Topping	1 serv (3 oz)	86	0	0	0	21	0	5
Chicken Fried Steak & Eggs	1 serv (14 oz)	723	28	56	452	31	8	1505
Country Scramble	1 serv (16 oz)	795	20	50	409	67	2	1819
Cream Cheese	1 oz	100	2	10	31	1	0	6
Egg	1 (2 oz)	134	6	12	205	1	0	61

FOOD	PORTION	CAL	PROT	FAT	CHOL	CARB	FIBER	SOD
Egg Beaters	1 serv (2.3 oz)	71	5	5	1	1	0	138
Eggs Benedict	1 serv (19 oz)	860	35	56	525	55	3	1943
English Muffin Dry	1 (4 oz)	125	5	1	0	24	1	198
Farmer's Omelette	1 serv (18 oz)	912	34	69	633	38	3	1816
French Slam	1 serv (14 oz)	1029	44	71	777	58	2	1428
French Toast	2 pieces (8 oz)	510	19	25	317	51	2	413
Fresh Fruit Mix	1 serv (3 oz)	36	1	0	0	9	1	16
Grapefruit	½ (5 oz)	60	1	0	0	16	6	0
Grapes	1 serv (3 oz)	55	1	1	0	15	1	0
Grits	1 serv (4 oz)	80	2	0	0	18	0	520
Ham	1 serv (3 oz)	94	15	3	23	2	0	761
Ham'n'Cheddar Omelette	1 serv (14 oz)	743	36	55	657	24	2	1518
Hashed Browns	1 serv (4 oz)	218	2	14	0	20	2	424
Hashed Browns Covered	1 serv (6 oz)	318	9	23	30	21	2	604
Hashed Browns Covered & Smothered	1 serv (8 oz)	359	9	26	30	26	2	790
Honeydew	1 serv (3 oz)	31	1	0	0	8	1	22
Junior Meals Basic Breakfast	1 serv (9 oz)	558	18	39	230	38	3	1103
Junior Meals Junior French Slam	1 serv (7 oz)	461	21	35	386	18	1	663
Junior Meals Junior Grand Slam	1 serv (5 oz)	397	17	25	230	33	1	1118
Junior Meals Junior Waffle Supreme	1 serv (4 oz)	190	3	11	73	20	0	102
Meat Lover's Sampler	1 serv (14 oz)	806	42	62	481	24	2	2211
Moon Over My Hammy	1 serv (12 oz)	807	44	48	430	46	2	2247
Muffin Blueberry	1 (3 oz)	309	4	14	0	42	0	190
Oatmeal	1 serv (4 oz)	100	5	2	0	18	3	175
Original Grand Slam	1 serv (10 oz)	795	34	50	460	65	2	2237
Pancakes	3 (5 oz)	491	12	7	0	95	3	1818

FOOD	PORTION	CAL	PROT	FAT	CHOL	CARB	FIBER	SOD
Pork Chop & Eggs	1 serv (12 oz)	555	33	36	469	21	2	968
Porterhouse Steak & Eggs	1 serv (18 oz)	1223	70	95	570	21	2	1369
Ready To Eat Cereal	1 serv (1 oz)	100	2	0	0	23	1	276
Sausage	4 links (3 oz)	354	16	32	64	0	0	944
Sausage Cheddar Omelette	1 serv (16 oz)	1036	46	86	721	24	2	1841
Scram Slam	1 serv (18 oz)	974	42	80	694	30	4	1750
Senior Belgian Waffle Slam	1 serv (6 oz)	399	16	33	302	12	0	612
Senior Omelette	1 serv (12 oz)	623	23	47	439	27	3	1194
Senior Starter	1 serv (7 oz)	336	11	24	205	36	2	541
Senior Triple Play	1 serv (8 oz)	537	20	25	409	64	2	1445
Sirloin Steak & Eggs	1 serv (13 oz)	808	37	64	474	21	2	952
Slim Slam	1 serv (14 oz)	638	34	12	34	98	1	1772
Southern Slam	1 serv (13 oz)	1065	37	84	484	47	0	2449
Strawberries w/ Sugar	1 serv (3 oz)	115	1	1	0	26	1	12
Strawberry Topping	1 serv (3 oz)	115	1	1	0	26	1	12
Sunshine Slam	1 serv (8 oz)	537	20	25	409	64	2	1445
Super Play It Again Slam	1 serv (15 oz)	1192	51	75	690	98	3	3555
Syrup	3 tbsp (1.5 oz)	143	0	0	0	36	0	26
Syrup Reduced Calorie	1 serv (1.5 oz)	25	0	0	0	6	0	96
T-Bone Steak & Eggs	1 serv (16 oz)	1045	56	82	530	21	2	1191
Toast Dry	1 slice (1 oz)	92	3	1	0	17	1	166
Ultimate Omelette	1 serv (17 oz)	780	31	62	639	29	4	1360
Veggie Cheese Omelette	1 serv (16 oz)	714	28	53	644	29	4	955
Waffle	1 (6 oz)	304	7	21	146	23	0	200
Whipped Margarine	1 serv (0.5 oz)	87	0	10	0	0	0	117
Whipped Cream	1 serv (2 oz)	23	0	2	7	2	0	3
DESSERTS								
Apple Pie	1 serv (7 oz)	430	3	20	<5	59	1	390
Apple Pie w/ Equal	1 serv (7 oz)	370	3	20	<5	43	2	360
Banana Split	1 serv (19 oz)	894	15	43	78	121	6	177
Blueberry Topping	1 serv (3 oz)	106	0	0	0	26	0	15
Cheesecake Pie	1 serv (4 oz)	470	8	27	90	48	0	280
Cherry Topping	1 serv (3 oz)	86	0	0	0	21	0	5

FOOD	PORTION	CAL	PROT	FAT	CHOL	CARB	FIBER	SOD
Cherry Pie	1 serv (7 oz)	540	5	21	<5	83	2	430
Chocolate Topping	1 serv (2 oz)	317	2	25	0	27	0	83
Chocolate Cake	1 serv (4 oz)	370	4	17	29	53	2	374
Chocolate Pecan Pie	1 serv (6 oz)	790	6	37	70	107	3	460
Chocolate Shake	1 serv (10 oz)	579	12	27	108	77	0	278
Coconut Cream Pie	1 serv (7 oz)	480	5	26	15	58	1	440
Double Scoop Sundae	1 serv (6 oz)	375	6	27	74	29	0	86
Dutch Apple Pie	1 serv (7 oz)	440	3	19	0	65	1	290
French Silk Pie	1 serv (6 oz)	650	6	43	165	60	2	220
Fudge Topping	1 serv (2 oz)	201	1	10	3	30	1	96
German Chocolate Pie	1 serv (7 oz)	580	7	33	15	66	2	460
Hot Fudge Cake Sundae	1 serv (8 oz)	687	9	38	62	83	3	486
Ice Cream Float	1 serv (12 oz)	280	3	10	39	47	0	109
Key Lime Pie	1 serv (6 oz)	600	10	27	35	79	0	300
Lemon Meringue Pie	1 serv (7 oz)	460	5	17	95	71	1	310
Pecan Pie	1 serv (6 oz)	600	5	28	50	81	2	430
Single Scoop Sundae	1 serv (3 oz)	188	3	14	37	14	0	43
Strawberry Topping	1 serv (3 oz)	115	1	1	0	26	1	12
Vanilla Shake	1 serv (11 oz)	581	11	27	108	77	0	236
MAIN MENU SELECTIONS								
BBQ Sauce	1 serv (1.5 oz)	47	0	1	0	11	0	595
Bacon Cheddar Burger	1 (14 oz)	935	53	63	164	43	3	1732
Bacon Lettuce & Tomato Sandwich	1 (6 oz)	634	18	46	54	37	3	1116
Baked Potato Plain	1 (6 oz)	186	4	0	0	43	4	14
Battered Cod Dinner w/ Tartar Sauce	1 serv (9 oz)	732	30	47	105	48	3	1335
Broccoli In Butter Sauce	2 serv (4 oz)	50	3	2	5	7	3	280
Brown Gravy	1 serv (1 oz)	13	0	0	0	2	0	184
Buffalo Chicken Strips	1 serv (10 oz)	734	48	42	96	43	0	1673
Buffalo Wings	12 pieces (15 oz)	856	92	54	500	1	1	5552
Carrots In Honey Glaze	2 serv (4 oz)	80	1	3	0	12	3	220

FOOD	PORTION	CAL	PROT	FAT	CHOL	CARB	FIBER	SOD
Charleston Chicken Sandwich	1 (11 oz)	632	35	32	81	53	4	1967
Chicken Fried Chicken	1 serv (6 oz)	327	25	18	65	16	1	993
Chicken Fried Steak w/ Gravy	1 serv (4 oz)	265	15	17	27	14	1	668
Chicken Gravy	1 serv (1 oz)	14	0	1	2	2	0	139
Chicken Melt Sandwich	1 (7 oz)	520	26	29	39	43	2	1096
Chicken Quesadilla	1 serv (16 oz)	827	50	55	181	43	2	1982
Chicken Strip w/ Dressing	1 serv (10 oz)	635	47	25	95	55	0	1510
Chicken Strips	5 pieces (10 oz)	720	47	33	95	56	0	1666
Classic Burger	1 (11 oz)	673	37	40	106	42	3	1142
Classic Burger w/ Cheese	1 (13 oz)	836	47	53	137	43	3	1595
Club Sandwich	1	485	29	35	90	40	–	1385
Corn In Butter Sauce	2 serv (4 oz)	120	3	4	5	19	5	260
Cornbread Stuffing Plain	1 serv (2 oz)	182	4	9	0	20	0	405
Cottage Cheese	1 serv (3 oz)	72	9	3	10	2	0	281
Country Gravy	1 serv (1 oz)	17	0	1	0	2	0	93
Delidinger Sandwich	1 (14 oz)	852	56	45	80	62	3	3142
Deluxe Grilled Cheese Sandwich	1 (7 oz)	482	18	26	1	44	2	1135
Dinner Roll	1 (1.5 oz)	132	4	2	0	26	1	265
French Fries Unsalted	1 serv (4 oz)	323	5	14	0	44	0	130
Fried Fish Sandwich	1 (11 oz)	905	29	56	69	74	4	1704
Gardenburger Patty	1 patty (3.4 oz)	160	11	3	10	22	3	390
Gardenburger Patty w/ Bun & Fat Free Honey Mustard Dressing	1 serv (11.1 oz)	653	21	32	26	72	6	1017
Green Beans w/ Bacon	2 serv (4 oz)	60	1	4	5	6	3	390
Green Peas In Butter Sauce	2 serv (4 oz)	100	5	2	5	14	4	360

FOOD	PORTION	CAL	PROT	FAT	CHOL	CARB	FIBER	SOD
Grilled Alaskan Salmon	1 serv (7 oz)	296	43	14	102	1	0	257
Grilled Chicken Breast	1 serv (4 oz)	130	24	4	67	0	0	566
Grilled Chicken Dinner	1 serv (4 oz)	130	24	4	67	0	0	560
Grilled Chicken Sandwich	1 (11 oz)	509	34	19	83	52	3	1809
Grilled Chopped Steak w/ Gravy	1 serv (10 oz)	400	30	26	91	12	2	447
Grilled Mushrooms	1 serv (2 oz)	14	2	0	0	2	1	0
Ham & Swiss On Rye	1 (9 oz)	533	23	31	36	40	5	1638
Hashed Browns	1 serv (4 oz)	218	2	14	0	20	2	424
Herb Toast	1 serv (2 oz)	200	4	11	0	21	1	372
Horseradish Sauce	1 serv (1.5 oz)	170	1	20	43	3	0	227
Junior Meals Junior Burger	1 serv (3 oz)	261	14	15	41	16	0	115
Junior Meals Junior Chicken Strips	1 serv (5 oz)	318	25	12	48	28	0	755
Junior Meals Junior Fried Fish	1 serv (5 oz)	465	15	34	68	25	1	743
Junior Meals Junior Grilled Cheese	1 serv (4 oz)	375	12	22	1	35	1	811
Junior Meals Junior Shrimp Basket	1 serv (4 oz)	291	10	16	60	27	2	774
Lunch Basket Charleston Chicken Ranch Melt	1 serv (14 oz)	975	47	59	96	68	4	2479
Lunch Basket Chicken Strips	1 serv (8 oz)	568	34	26	70	45	0	1239
Lunch Basket Classic Burger	1 serv (12 oz)	674	38	39	121	42	3	1161
Lunch Basket Delidinger	1 serv (14 oz)	852	56	45	80	62	3	3142
Lunch Basket Five Star Philly	1 serv (10 oz)	657	41	29	97	55	4	652
Lunch Basket Patty Melt	1 serv (8 oz)	696	39	42	129	39	2	1026
Mashed Potatoes Plain	1 serv (6 oz)	105	3	1	0	21	2	378

FOOD	PORTION	CAL	PROT	FAT	CHOL	CARB	FIBER	SOD
Mayonnaise	2 tbsp (1 oz)	200	0	22	16	1	0	159
Mozzarella Sticks w/ Sauce	8 pieces (10 oz)	756	37	43	48	56	7	5423
Onion Ring Basket	1 serv (5 oz)	439	6	27	7	44	1	1158
Onion Rings	1 serv (3 oz)	264	3	16	4	27	0	695
Patty Melt Sandwich	1 (8 oz)	695	38	44	114	39	2	1007
Pork Chop Dinner w/ Gravy	1 serv (8 oz)	386	39	24	121	0	0	844
Porterhouse Steak	1 (14 oz)	708	56	54	161	0	0	713
Pot Roast Dinner w/ Gravy	1 serv (7 oz)	260	39	11	140	5	0	1085
Rice Pilaf	1 serv (3 oz)	112	2	2	0	21	0	328
Roast Turkey & Stuffing	1 serv (12 oz)	701	47	27	100	63	0	2346
Sampler	1 serv (15 oz)	1120	44	59	69	104	5	3430
Seasoned Fries	1 serv (4 oz)	261	5	12	0	35	0	556
Senior Battered Cod	1 serv (5 oz)	465	15	34	68	25	1	743
Senior Chicken Fried Steak	1 serv (8 oz)	341	16	18	27	29	2	943
Senior Grilled Cheese Sandwich	1 serv	360	16	25	50	21	—	1190
Senior Grilled Chicken Breast	1 serv (6 oz)	219	26	6	67	16	0	880
Senior Liver w/ Bacon & Onions	1 serv (8 oz)	322	22	19	270	20	2	643
Senior Pork Chop	1 serv (4 oz)	193	19	12	60	0	0	422
Senior Pot Roast	1 serv (5 oz)	149	20	6	71	6	0	818
Senior Roast Turkey & Stuffing	1 serv (8 oz)	596	29	25	51	61	0	1750
Senior Turkey Sandwich	1	340	24	27	75	26	—	1000
Senior Sandwich Ham & Swiss	1 serv (9 oz)	497	22	30	36	34	4	1537
Shrimp Dinner	1 serv (8 oz)	558	19	32	135	49	3	1114
Sirloin Steak Dinner	1 serv (5.5 oz)	271	22	21	62	0	0	273
Sliced Tomatoes	3 slices (2 oz)	13	1	0	0	3	1	6
Sour Cream	1 serv (1.5 oz)	91	1	9	19	2	0	23
Steak & Shrimp Dinner w/ Gravy	1 serv (9 oz)	645	36	42	150	31	2	1143

FOOD	PORTION	CAL	PROT	FAT	CHOL	CARB	FIBER	SOD
Super Bird Sandwich	1 (9 oz)	620	35	32	60	48	2	1880
T-Bone Steak Dinner	1 serv (10 oz)	530	42	40	121	0	0	534
Turkey Breast On Multigrain	1 (9 oz)	476	23	26	57	39	5	1107
SALAD DRESSINGS								
Bleu Cheese	1 oz	124	4	12	18	4	0	405
Caesar	1 oz	142	1	15	2	1	0	340
Creamy Italian	1 oz	106	0	10	0	4	0	306
Fat Free Honey Mustard	1 oz	38	0	0	0	9	0	121
French	1 oz	106	0	10	7	3	0	274
Oriental Peanut Dressing	1 serv (1 oz)	106	1	8	0	6	0	399
Ranch	1 oz	101	1	11	8	1	0	215
Reduced Calorie French	1 oz	76	0	5	0	8	0	265
Reduced Calorie Italian	1 oz	32	0	1	0	3	0	515
Thousand Island	1 oz	104	0	10	21	2	0	208
SALADS AND SALAD BARS								
Buffalo Chicken Salad	1 serv (17 oz)	615	39	37	88	36	3	1258
Fried Chicken Salad	1 serv (13 oz)	506	38	31	94	30	3	1174
Garden Chicken Delight Salad	1 serv (16 oz)	277	30	5	67	30	6	785
Grilled Chicken Caesar Salad w/ Dressing	1 serv (13 oz)	655	37	47	86	23	4	1728
Oriental Chicken Salad w/ Dressing	1 serv (20 oz)	568	33	26	67	49	7	1656
Side Caesar w/ Dressing	1 serv (6 oz)	338	8	25	7	20	3	725
Side Garden Salad w/ Dressing	1 serv (7 oz)	113	3	4	0	16	3	147
SOUPS								
Cheese	1 serv (8 oz)	293	6	23	19	13	4	895
Chicken Noodle	1 serv (8 oz)	60	2	2	10	8	0	640
Clam Chowder	1 serv (8 oz)	214	5	11	5	22	1	903
Cream Of Broccoli	1 serv (8 oz)	193	4	12	0	15	2	818
Cream of Potato	1 serv (8 oz)	222	4	12	0	23	2	761
Split Pea	1 serv (8 oz)	146	8	6	5	18	2	819
Vegetable Beef	1 serv (8 oz)	79	6	1	5	11	2	820

FOOD	PORTION	CAL	PROT	FAT	CHOL	CARB	FIBER	SOD
DOMINO'S PIZZA								
12 INCH MEDIUM PIZZAS								
Add A Topping Anchovies	1 topping serv	23	3	1	9	0	0	395
Add A Topping Bacon	1 topping serv	81	4	7	12	tr	0	226
Add A Topping Banana Peppers	1 topping serv	3	tr	tr	—	1	—	92
Add A Topping Canned Mushrooms	1 topping serv	4	tr	tr	0	1	tr	75
Add A Topping Cheddar Cheese	1 topping serv	57	4	5	15	tr	0	88
Add A Topping Cooked Beef	1 topping serv	56	3	5	11	tr	tr	154
Add A Topping Extra Cheese	1 topping serv	48	3	4	7	1	tr	150
Add A Topping Fresh Mushrooms	1 topping serv	4	tr	tr	0	1	tr	1
Add A Topping Green Olives	1 topping serv	12	tr	1	0	tr	tr	255
Add A Topping Green Peppers	1 topping serv	3	tr	tr	0	1	tr	tr
Add A Topping Ham	1 topping serv	18	2	1	7	tr	0	162
Add A Topping Italian Sausage	1 topping serv	55	2	4	11	2	tr	171
Add A Topping Onion	1 topping serv	4	tr	tr	0	1	tr	tr
Add A Topping Pepperoni	1 topping serv	62	3	6	13	tr	tr	199
Add A Topping Pineapple Tidbits	1 topping serv	10	tr	0	0	2	tr	1
Add A Topping Ripe Olives	1 topping serv	14	tr	1	0	1	tr	71
Deep Dish Cheese	2 slices (6.3 oz)	477	18	22	19	50	3	1085
Hand Tossed Cheese	2 slices (5.2 oz)	347	14	11	15	49	3	723
Thin Crust Cheese	¼ pie (3.7 oz)	271	12	12	15	31	2	809

FOOD	PORTION	CAL	PROT	FAT	CHOL	CARB	FIBER	SOD
14 INCH LARGE PIZZAS								
Add A Topping Anchovies	1 topping serv	23	3	1	tr	0	0	395
Add A Topping Anchovies	1 topping serv	23	3	1	9	0	0	395
Add A Topping Bacon	1 topping serv	75	4	6	11	tr	0	207
Add A Topping Banana Peppers	1 topping serv	3	tr	tr	–	1	–	81
Add A Topping Canned Mushrooms	1 topping serv	3	tr	tr	0	1	tr	50
Add A Topping Cheddar Cheese	1 topping serv	48	3	4	12	tr	0	73
Add A Topping Cheddar Cheese	1 topping serv	48	3	4	12	tr	0	73
Add A Topping Cooked Beef	1 topping serv	44	2	4	8	tr	tr	123
Add A Topping Extra Cheese	1 topping serv	45	3	4	7	1	tr	140
Add A Topping Extra Cheese	1 topping serv	45	3	4	7	1	tr	140
Add A Topping Fresh Mushrooms	1 topping serv	3	tr	tr	0	1	tr	tr
Add A Topping Green Olives	1 topping serv	11	tr	1	0	tr	tr	63
Add A Topping Green Peppers	1 topping serv	2	tr	tr	0	1	tr	tr
Add A Topping Ham	1 topping serv	17	2	1	7	tr	0	156
Add A Topping Italian Sausage	1 topping serv	44	2	3	9	1	tr	137
Add A Topping Onion	1 topping serv	3	tr	tr	0	1	tr	tr
Add A Topping Pepperoni	1 topping serv	55	2	5	12	tr	tr	177
Add A Topping Pineapple Tidbits	1 topping serv	8	2	0	0	tr	tr	1

FOOD	PORTION	CAL	PROT	FAT	CHOL	CARB	FIBER	SOD
Add A Topping Ripe Olives	1 topping serv	12	tr	1	0	1	tr	63
Deep Dish Cheese	2 slices (6.1 oz)	455	18	20	18	54	3	1029
Hand-Tossed Cheese	2 slices (4.8 oz)	317	13	10	14	45	3	669
Thin Crust Cheese	⅙ pie (3.5 oz)	253	11	11	14	29	2	757
6 INCH DEEP DISH PIZZAS								
Add A Topping Anchovies	1 topping serv	45	6	2	18	0	0	790
Add A Topping Bacon	1 topping serv	82	4	7	12	tr	0	226
Add A Topping Banana Peppers	1 topping serv	3	tr	tr	–	tr	–	73
Add A Topping Canned Mushrooms	1 topping serv	2	tr	tr	0	tr	tr	36
Add A Topping Cheddar Cheese	1 topping serv	86	5	7	22	tr	0	132
Add A Topping Cooked Beef	1 topping serv	44	2	4	8	tr	tr	122
Add A Topping Extra Cheese	1 topping serv	57	4	5	9	1	tr	180
Add A Topping Fresh Mushrooms	1 topping serv	2	tr	tr	0	tr	tr	tr
Add A Topping Green Olives	1 topping serv	10	tr	1	0	tr	tr	204
Add A Topping Green Peppers	1 topping serv	2	tr	tr	0	tr	tr	tr
Add A Topping Ham	1 topping serv	17	2	1	7	tr	0	156
Add A Topping Italian Sausage	1 topping serv	44	1	3	9	1	tr	137
Add A Topping Onion	1 topping serv	3	tr	tr	0	1	tr	tr
Add A Topping Pepperoni	1 topping serv	50	2	5	10	tr	tr	159
Add A Topping Pineapple Tidbits	1 topping serv	5	tr	0	0	1	tr	tr

FOOD	PORTION	CAL	PROT	FAT	CHOL	CARB	FIBER	SOD
Add A Topping Ripe Olives	1 topping serv	11	tr	1	0	tr	tr	57
Cheese	1 pie (7.6 oz)	595	23	27	23	68	4	1300
MAIN MENU SELECTIONS								
Breadstick	1 (0.8 oz)	78	2	3	0	11	tr	158
Buffalo Wings Barbeque	1 piece (0.9 oz)	50	6	2	26	2	tr	175
Buffalo Wings Hot	1 piece (0.9 oz)	45	5	2	26	1	tr	354
Cheesy Bread	1 piece (1 oz)	103	3	5	5	11	tr	187
Garden Salad	1 lg (7.7 oz)	39	2	tr	0	8	3	26
Garden Salad	1 sm (4.3 oz)	22	1	tr	0	4	2	14
SALAD DRESSINGS								
Marzetti Blue Cheese	1 serv (1.5 oz)	220	2	24	40	2	0	440
Marzetti Creamy Caesar	1 serv (1.5 oz)	200	1	22	10	2	0	470
Marzetti Fat Free Ranch	1 serv (1.5 oz)	40	0	0	0	10	1	560
Marzetti Honey French	1 serv (1.5 oz)	210	0	18	0	14	0	300
Marzetti House Italian	1 serv (1.5 oz)	220	0	24	0	1	0	440
Marzetti Light Italian	1 serv (1.5 oz)	20	–	1	0	2	0	780
Marzetti Ranch	1 serv (1.5 oz)	260	0	29	5	1	0	380
Marzetti Thousand Island	1 serv (1.5 oz)	200	0	20	25	5	0	320

DUNKIN' DONUTS

BAGELS AND CREAM CHEESE

FOOD	PORTION	CAL	PROT	FAT	CHOL	CARB	FIBER	SOD
Bagel Blueberry	1	340	10	1	0	75	tr	670
Bagel Cinnamon Raisin	1	340	10	1	0	74	1	480
Bagel Egg	1	350	11	2	25	72	0	610
Bagel Everything	1	360	11	2	0	74	0	710
Bagel Garlic	1	360	11	1	0	76	0	720
Bagel Onion	1	330	10	1	0	70	0	660
Bagel Plain	1	340	10	1	0	73	0	710
Bagel Poppyseed	1	360	11	3	0	74	tr	710
Bagel Pumpernickel	1	350	11	2	0	75	2	560
Bagel Salt	1	340	10	1	0	73	0	3030
Bagel Sesame	1	380	12	5	0	74	0	720

FOOD	PORTION	CAL	PROT	FAT	CHOL	CARB	FIBER	SOD
Bagel Wheat	1	330	12	2	0	73	4	670
Cream Cheese Chive	1 pkg	190	3	19	55	3	tr	220
Cream Cheese Garden Vegetable	1 pkg	180	3	17	45	3	tr	310
Cream Cheese Lite	1 pkg	130	5	11	30	3	0	250
Cream Cheese Plain	1 pkg	200	4	19	60	3	0	230
Cream Cheese Salmon	1 pkg	180	5	17	50	2	0	150
BAKED SELECTIONS								
Bow Tie Donut	1	300	4	17	0	34	tr	340
Cake Donut Blueberry	1	290	3	16	10	35	tr	400
Cake Donut Butternut	1	300	3	16	0	36	tr	360
Cake Donut Chocolate Coconut	1	300	4	19	0	31	1	370
Cake Donut Chocolate Frosted	1	300	3	16	0	38	tr	370
Cake Donut Chocolate Glazed	1	290	3	16	0	33	1	370
Cake Donut Cinnamon	1	270	3	15	0	31	tr	360
Cake Donut Coconut	1	290	3	17	0	33	tr	360
Cake Donut Double Chocolate	1	310	3	17	0	37	2	370
Cake Donut Glazed	1	270	3	15	0	33	tr	360
Cake Donut Old Fashioned	1	250	3	15	0	26	tr	360
Cake Donut Powdered	1	270	3	15	0	32	tr	350
Cake Donut Toasted Coconut	1	300	3	17	0	35	tr	370
Cake Donut Whole Wheat Glazed	1	310	4	19	0	32	2	380
Chocolate Frosted Donut	1	200	3	9	0	29	tr	260
Chocolate Kreme Filled Donut	1	270	3	13	0	35	tr	260
Cinnamon Bun	1	510	8	15	10	85	0	420
Coffee Roll	1	270	4	14	0	33	1	340
Coffee Roll Chocolate Frosted	1	290	4	15	0	36	1	340

FOOD	PORTION	CAL	PROT	FAT	CHOL	CARB	FIBER	SOD
Coffee Roll Maple Frosted	1	290	4	14	0	36	1	340
Coffee Roll Vanilla Frosted	1	290	4	14	0	36	1	340
Cookie Chocolate Chocolate Chunk	1	210	3	11	35	26	2	110
Cookie Chocolate Chunk	1	220	3	11	35	28	1	105
Cookie Chocolate Chunk w/ Nut	1	230	3	12	35	27	1	110
Cookie Chocolate White Chocolate Chunk	1	230	3	12	35	28	1	160
Cookie Oatmeal Raisin Pecan	1	220	3	10	30	29	1	110
Cookie Peanut Butter Chocolate Chunk w/ Nuts	1	240	4	14	25	24	2	125
Cookie Peanut Butter w/ Nuts	1	240	5	14	30	24	1	150
Croissant Almond	1	350	6	22	5	34	2	270
Croissant Chocolate	1	400	5	25	5	37	2	240
Croissant Plain	1	290	5	18	5	26	tr	270
Cruller Glazed	1	290	3	15	0	37	tr	350
Cruller Glazed Chocolate	1	280	3	15	0	35	1	360
Cruller Plain	1	240	3	15	0	25	tr	340
Cruller Powdered	1	270	3	15	0	30	tr	340
Cruller Sugar	1	250	3	15	0	27	tr	340
Donut Apple Crumb	1	230	3	10	0	34	tr	270
Donut Apple N' Spice	1	200	3	8	0	29	tr	270
Donut Bavarian Kreme	1	210	3	9	0	30	tr	270
Donut Black Raspberry	1	210	3	8	0	32	tr	280
Donut Blueberry Crumb	1	240	3	10	0	36	tr	260
Donut Boston Kreme	1	240	3	9	0	36	tr	280

FOOD	PORTION	CAL	PROT	FAT	CHOL	CARB	FIBER	SOD
Donut Chocolate Iced Bismark	1	340	3	15	0	50	tr	290
Dunkin' Donut	1	240	3	15	0	25	tr	340
Eclair Donut	1	270	3	11	0	39	tr	290
Fritter Glazed	1	260	4	14	0	31	1	330
Glazed Donut	1	180	3	8	0	25	tr	250
Jelly Filled Donut	1	210	3	8	0	32	tr	280
Jelly Stick	1	290	3	12	0	44	tr	390
Lemon Donut	1	200	3	9	0	28	tr	270
Maple Frosted Donut	1	210	3	9	0	30	tr	260
Marble Frosted Donut	1	200	3	9	0	29	tr	260
Muffin Apple Cinnamon Pecan	1	510	8	21	70	74	1	590
Muffin Apple N'Spice	1	350	5	12	35	57	2	390
Muffin Banana Nut	1	360	7	15	35	52	3	490
Muffin Blueberry	1 (4 oz)	320	6	12	35	49	3	480
Muffin Blueberry	1 (6 oz)	490	8	17	75	78	2	610
Muffin Bran	1	390	11	12	20	60	3	620
Muffin Cherry	1	340	6	12	40	53	2	510
Muffin Chocolate Hazelnut	1	610	10	26	70	87	3	610
Muffin Chocolate Chip	1 (6 oz)	590	8	24	75	88	3	560
Muffin Chocolate Chip	1 (4 oz)	400	6	17	35	58	4	440
Muffin Corn	1 (4 oz)	390	8	15	55	57	2	590
Muffin Corn	1 (6 oz)	500	10	16	80	78	1	920
Muffin Cranberry Orange	1	470	8	15	75	76	2	600
Muffin Cranberry Orange Nut	1	350	6	15	35	52	3	500
Muffin Honey Raisin Bran	1 (3.3 oz)	330	5	10	15	57	4	360
Muffin Lemon Poppyseed	1	360	5	13	35	56	1	530
Muffin Oat Bran	1	370	11	13	20	55	3	620
Muffin Lowfat Apple & Spice	1	240	4	2	0	54	tr	460

FOOD	PORTION	CAL	PROT	FAT	CHOL	CARB	FIBER	SOD
Muffin Lowfat Banana	1	250	4	2	0	57	tr	430
Muffin Lowfat Blueberry	1	250	4	2	0	55	1	430
Muffin Lowfat Bran	1	240	4	1	0	57	4	430
Muffin Lowfat Cherry	1	250	4	2	0	56	tr	430
Muffin Lowfat Chocolate	1	250	4	3	0	53	2	470
Muffin Lowfat Corn	1	240	3	3	45	52	0	480
Muffin Lowfat Cranberry Orange	1	240	4	2	0	55	1	430
Muffin Reduced Fat Blueberry	1	450	8	12	65	77	2	590
Muffin Reduced Fat Corn	1	460	10	11	75	79	1	900
Munchkins Chocolate Cake Glazed	3	200	2	10	0	26	tr	250
Munchkins Cake Butternut	3	200	2	11	0	25	tr	240
Munchkins Cake Cinnamon	4	250	3	14	0	29	tr	350
Munchkins Cake Coconut	3	200	2	12	0	23	tr	240
Munchkins Cake Glazed	3	200	2	10	0	27	0	250
Munchkins Cake Plain	4	220	2	14	0	22	tr	310
Munchkins Cake Powdered	4	250	2	14	0	29	tr	310
Munchkins Cake Sugared	4	240	2	14	0	28	tr	310
Munchkins Cake Toasted Coconut	3	200	2	11	0	24	tr	—
Munchkins Yeast Glazed	5	200	3	9	0	27	tr	220
Munchkins Yeast Jelly Filled	5	210	3	9	0	30	tr	240
Munchkins Yeast Lemon Filled	4	170	2	8	0	23	0	190

FOOD	PORTION	CAL	PROT	FAT	CHOL	CARB	FIBER	SOD
Munchkins Yeast Sugar Raised	7	220	4	12	0	26	tr	290
Strawberry Frosted Donut	1	210	3	9	0	30	tr	260
Strawberry Donut	1	210	3	8	0	32	tr	260
Sugar Raised Donut	1	170	3	8	0	22	tr	250
Sugared Cake Donut	1	250	3	15	0	27	tr	350
Vanilla Frosted Donut	1	210	3	9	0	30	tr	260
Vanilla Kreme Filled Donut	1	270	3	13	0	36	tr	250
BEVERAGES								
Coffee Coolatta w/ 2% Milk	1 (16 oz)	240	4	2	10	52	0	80
Coffee Coolatta w/ Cream	1 (16 oz)	410	3	22	75	51	0	65
Coffee Coolatta w/ Milk	1 (16 oz)	260	4	4	15	52	0	75
Coffee Coolatta w/ Skim Milk	1 (16 oz)	230	4	0		52	0	80
Coolatta Orange Mango Fruit	1 (16 oz)	290	tr	0	0	71	tr	30
Coolatta Pink Lemonade Fruit	1 (16 oz)	350	07	0	0	88	0	30
Coolatta Raspberry Lemonade	1 (16 oz)	280	0	0	0	68	0	35
Coolatta Strawberry Fruit	1 (16 oz)	280	0	0	0	70	1	30
Coolatta Vanilla	1 (16 oz)	450	1	7	0	94	0	170
Cream	1 serv (1 oz)	60	1	5	20	1	0	10
Dark Roast Coffee	1 serv (10 oz)	5	0	0	0	1	0	5
Decaf Coffee	1 serv (10 oz)	0	0	0	0	0	0	0
Dunkaccino	1 (10 oz)	250	2	11	10	34	tr	240
Dunkaccino	1 (20 oz)	510	4	23	20	71	1	500
Dunkaccino	1 (18.75 oz)	480	4	22	20	67	1	470
Dunkaccino	1 (14 oz)	360	3	17	15	51	1	360
French Vanilla Coffee	1 serv (10 oz)	5	0	0	0	1	0	5
Hazelnut Coffee	1 serv (10 oz)	5	0	0	0	1	0	10
Hot Cocoa	1 (20 oz)	470	5	16	0	79	3	640
Hot Cocoa	1 (10 oz)	230	2	8	0	38	2	310

FOOD	PORTION	CAL	PROT	FAT	CHOL	CARB	FIBER	SOD
Hot Cocoa	1 (18.75 oz)	440	4	15	0	75	3	610
Hot Cocoa	1 (14 oz)	330	3	11	0	57	2	460
Regular Coffee	1 serv (10 oz)	5	0	0	0	1	0	5
SANDWICHES								
Breakfast Sandwich Ham Egg Cheese	1	320	22	12	195	31	2	1340
Omwich Bagel Bacon Cheddar	1	600	26	21	295	79	tr	1630
Omwich Bagel Spanish Cheese	1	570	24	18	280	79	tr	1370
Omwich Bagel Three Cheese	1	610	25	22	305	78	tr	1630
Omwich Croissant Spanish Cheese	1	530	19	36	285	33	1	930
Omwich Croissant Bacon Cheddar	1	560	21	38	295	33	1	1190
Omwich Croissant Three Cheese	1	560	20	39	305	33	1	1200
Omwich English Muffin Bacon Cheddar	1	400	21	21	295	33	2	1440
Omwich English Muffin Spanish Cheese	1	370	18	18	280	34	2	1180
Omwich English Muffin Three Cheese	1	400	19	22	305	33	2	1450
EINSTEIN BROS BAGELS								
BAGELS								
Bagel Chips Cinnamon Raisin Swirl	1 serv (1 oz)	90	3	1	0	19	1	120
Bagel Chips Plain	1 serv (1 oz)	90	3	0	0	18	1	14
Bagel Chips Sourdough Dill	1 serv (1 oz)	90	3	1	0	18	1	120
Bagel Chips Sun Dried Tomato	1 serv (1 oz)	90	3	1	0	17	1	130
Bagel Chips Sunflower	1 serv (1 oz)	100	3	2	0	8	1	190
Bagel Chips Wild Blueberry	1 serv (1 oz)	90	3	1	0	19	1	105

FOOD	PORTION	CAL	PROT	FAT	CHOL	CARB	FIBER	SOD
Chocolate Chip	1 (4 oz)	380	11	3	0	78	2	480
Chopped Garlic	1 (4.2 oz)	377	14	4	0	81	5	593
Chopped Onion	1 (4 oz)	340	11	3	0	72	2	500
Cinnamon Raisin Swirl	1 (4 oz)	360	11	1	0	78	2	480
Cinnamon Sugar	1	330	10	0	0	72	2	510
Dark Pumpernickel	1 (3.8 oz)	330	11	1	0	72	5	710
Everything	1 (4 oz)	342	13	2	0	74	2	653
Honey 8 Grain	1 (4 oz)	320	11	1	0	71	4	500
Nutty Banana	1 (4 oz)	370	11	3	0	77	2	500
Plain	1 (3.7 oz)	330	11	1	0	72	2	520
Poppy Dip'd	1 (3.9 oz)	346	12	2	0	73	2	520
Salt	1 (3.9 oz)	330	11	1	0	72	2	1626
Sesame Dip'd	1 (4.1 oz)	381	11	5	0	74	3	523
Spinach Herb	1 (3.8 oz)	320	11	1	0	71	3	510
Sun Dried Tomato	1 (3.8 oz)	320	11	1	0	70	3	520
Veggie Confetti	1 (3.8 oz)	330	10	1	0	71	3	480
Wild Blueberry	1 (4 oz)	360	11	1	0	79	3	510
SANDWICHES AND FILLINGS								
Butter & Margarine Blend	1 serv (0.4 oz)	60	0	7	0	0	0	75
Capers	1 tbsp	0	0	0	0	0	0	320
Cheddar Cheese	1 serv (0.75 oz)	110	7	9	30	1	0	180
Classic New York Lox & Bagel	1 (11.4 oz)	560	24	24	75	31	3	1120
Cream Cheese Cheddarpeno	1 serv (1 oz)	90	2	8	30	2	0	150
Cream Cheese Chive	1 serv (1 oz)	90	1	9	35	2	0	125
Cream Cheese Maple Walnut Raisin	1 serv (1 oz)	100	1	8	25	7	0	95
Cream Cheese Plain	1 serv (1 oz)	100	1	9	35	2	0	130
Cream Cheese Smoked Salmon	1 serv (1 oz)	90	2	8	35	2	0	130
Cream Cheese Strawberry	1 serv (1 oz)	90	1	8	30	4	0	105
Cream Cheese Sun Dried Tomato	1 serv (1 oz)	90	1	8	35	3	0	160
Cucumbers	1 serv (1 oz)	0	0	0	0	1	0	0

FOOD	PORTION	CAL	PROT	FAT	CHOL	CARB	FIBER	SOD
Fruit Spreads	1 tbsp	40	0	0	0	10	0	10
Ham	1 serv (2.5 oz)	75	10	2	20	1	0	560
Ham & Cheese Sandwich	1 (9.9 oz)	520	31	15	70	63	3	1280
Honey	1 tbsp	64	0	0	0	18	0	1
Hummus	2 tbsp	60	2	3	0	4	1	105
Hummus Sandwich	1 (6 oz)	440	13	7	0	62	4	590
Lettuce	1 leaf	0	0	0	0	0	0	0
Lite Cream Cheese Plain	1 serv (1 oz)	60	2	5	20	2	0	150
Lite Cream Cheese Spinach Dill	1 serv (1 oz)	60	2	5	20	2	0	150
Lite Cream Cheese Veggie	1 serv (1 oz)	60	2	5	20	3	0	170
Lite Cream Cheese Wildberry	1 serv (1 oz)	70	2	4	15	7	0	85
Lowfat Chicken Salad Sandwich	1 (11.6 oz)	440	26	9	45	63	3	940
Lowfat Tuna Salad Sandwich	1 (11.6 oz)	440	29	8	30	62	3	970
Marshall's Lox	1 serv (2 oz)	90	12	4	10	2	0	400
Mayonnaise Lite Reduced Calorie	1 serv (0.5 oz)	50	0	5	5	1	0	115
Peanut Butter	1 serv (1.1 oz)	190	7	16	0	8	2	140
Peanut Butter & Jelly Sandwich	1 (6 oz)	595	18	17	0	99	4	663
Scrambled Egg Sandwich	1 (7.7 oz)	480	25	17	385	56	2	630
Scrambled Egg Sandwich w/ Meat & Cheese	1 (8.9 oz)	520	32	31	8	57	2	1000
Smoked Turkey	1 serv (2.5 oz)	75	13	1	20	0	0	550
Smoked Turkey Sandwich	1 (9.9 oz)	480	28	14	45	59	3	1180
Spouts Alfalfa	1 serv (0.5 oz)	0	0	0	0	3	1	10
Sweet Onions	1 serv (1 oz)	0	0	0	0	2	0	0
Swiss Cheese	1 serv (0.75 oz)	100	8	8	25	0	0	60
Tasty Turkey Sandwich	1 (10 oz)	530	25	22	90	61	2	1210

FOOD	PORTION	CAL	PROT	FAT	CHOL	CARB	FIBER	SOD
Tomato	1 serv (1.5 oz)	0	0	0	0	2	1	0
Turkey Pastrami 99% Fat Free	1 serv (2.5 oz)	75	12	6	0	2	0	510
Turkey Pastrami Sandwich	1 (9.7 oz)	460	29	12	20	60	3	—
Veg Out Sandwich	1 (8.9 oz)	350	12	17	3	62	3	570
Whitefish Salad Sandwich	1 (9.2 oz)	630	22	23	45	59	3	1020

EL POLLO LOCO
MAIN MENU SELECTIONS

FOOD	PORTION	CAL	PROT	FAT	CHOL	CARB	FIBER	SOD
Broccoli Slaw	1 serv (5 oz)	203	3	17	0	14	3	365
Burrito BRC	1 (9.3 oz)	482	16	15	15	72	9	1250
Burrito Classic Chicken	1 (9.3 oz)	556	30	22	117	61	8	1499
Burrito Grilled Steak	1 (11.3 oz)	705	39	32	77	68	10	1689
Burrito Loco Grande	1 (13.1 oz)	632	33	26	129	67	8	1649
Burrito Smokey Black Bean	1 (9.3 oz)	566	16	22	22	78	9	1337
Burrito Spicy Hot Chicken	1 (9.8 oz)	559	30	22	117	61	8	1503
Burrito Whole Wheat Chicken	1 (10.8 oz)	592	31	26	146	60	8	1199
Chicken Breast	1 piece (3 oz)	160	26	6	110	0	0	390
Chicken Leg	1 piece (1.75 oz)	90	11	5	75	0	0	150
Chicken Soft Taco	1 (4 oz)	224	16	12	66	15	0	585
Chicken Thigh	1 piece (2 oz)	180	16	12	130	0	0	230
Chicken Wing	1 (1.5 oz)	110	12	6	80	0	0	220
Chicken Tamale	1 (3.5 oz)	190	6	8	10	23	2	480
Cole Slaw	1 serv (5 oz)	206	2	16	11	12	2	358
Corn-On-Cob	1 ear (5.5 oz)	146	5	2	0	33	2	18
Cornbread Stuffing	1 serv (6 oz)	281	6	12	0	40	6	832
Crispy Green Beans	1 serv (5 oz)	41	1	2	0	6	3	667
Cucumber Salad	1 serv (4.2 oz)	34	2	0	0	7	1	11
Fiesta Corn	1 serv (5 oz)	152	4	6	0	25	6	397
Flame Broiled Chicken Salad	1 serv (14.9 oz)	167	27	5	56	11	4	765
French Fries	1 serv (4.4 oz)	323	5	14	0	44	0	330
Garden Salad	1 serv (6.4 oz)	29	3	0	0	6	2	20

FOOD	PORTION	CAL	PROT	FAT	CHOL	CARB	FIBER	SOD
Gravy	1 serv (1 oz)	14	0	0	2	2	0	139
Honey Glazed Carrots	1 serv (5 oz)	104	1	6	0	14	3	403
Lime Parfait	1 serv (5 oz)	125	1	3	0	25	0	107
Macaroni & Cheese	1 serv (6 oz)	238	10	12	31	22	1	919
Mashed Potatoes	1 serv (5 oz)	97	3	1	0	21	2	369
Pinto Beans	1 serv (6 oz)	185	11	4	0	29	8	744
Polo Bowl	1 serv (19 oz)	504	37	13	56	69	9	2068
Potato Salad	1 serv (6 oz)	256	3	14	15	30	3	527
Rainbow Pasta Salad	1 serv (5 oz)	157	6	1	0	30	2	533
Salad Shell	1 (5.6 oz)	440	7	27	0	42	0	610
Smokey Black Beans	1 serv (5 oz)	255	6	13	11	29	4	609
Southwest Cole Slaw	1 serv (5 oz)	178	2	13	8	15	3	267
Spanish Rice	1 serv (4 oz)	130	2	3	0	24	1	397
Spiced Apples	1 serv (5 oz)	146	0	0	0	39	0	139
Steak Bowl	1 serv (15.2 oz)	616	37	26	68	62	8	1743
Taco Al Carbon Chicken	1 serv (4.4 oz)	265	10	12	28	30	3	223
Taco Al Carbon Steak	1 (4.4 oz)	394	20	22	46	30	3	473
Taquito	1 serv (5 oz)	370	15	17	25	43	3	690
Tortilla Corn	1 (1.1 oz)	70	1	1	0	14	1	35
Tortilla Flour	1 (1 oz)	90	3	3	0	13	0	224
Tortilla Wrap Chicken Caesar	1 (10.47 oz)	518	28	19	48	59	3	1709
Tortilla Wrap Southwest	1 (11.97 oz)	632	30	27	61	69	5	1792
Tostada Salad Chicken	1 serv (14.7 oz)	332	35	14	80	26	4	1280
Tostado Salad Steak	1 serv (13.2 oz)	525	40	31	100	26	4	1206
SALAD DRESSINGS								
Blue Cheese	1 serv (2 oz)	300	2	32	50	2	0	590
Light Italian	1 serv (2 oz)	25	0	1	0	3	0	990
Ranch	1 serv (2 oz)	350	1	39	5	2	0	500
Thousand Island	1 serv (2 oz)	270	1	27	30	9	0	460

FAZOLI'S
DESSERTS

FOOD	PORTION	CAL	PROT	FAT	CHOL	CARB	FIBER	SOD
Cheesecake Plain	1 slice	339	7	26	110	20	–	260
Cheesecake Turtle	1 slice	373	8	27	104	28	–	252
Cookie Milk Chocolate Chunk	1	300	6	15	30	54	–	345

FOOD	PORTION	CAL	PROT	FAT	CHOL	CARB	FIBER	SOD
Lemon Ice	1 serv (12 oz)	142	0	0	0	36	–	9
Strawberry Topping	1 serv (1 oz)	33	0	0	0	8	–	38
MAIN MENU SELECTIONS								
Baked Spaghetti Parmesan	1 serv	697	38	26	60	76	–	767
Baked Ziti	1 sm	486	23	17	35	56	–	575
Baked Ziti	1 reg	748	36	26	54	87	–	864
Breadstick	1	173	4	8	0	19	–	516
Breadstick Dry	1	100	4	1	0	18	–	180
Broccoli Fettuccine Alfredo	1 reg	826	28	23	21	125	–	265
Broccoli Fettuccine Alfredo	1 sm	563	20	15	14	85	–	190
Broccoli Lasagna	1 serv	423	21	18	138	45	–	761
Cheese Ravioli w/ Meat Sauce	1 serv	511	20	17	73	65	–	795
Cheese Ravioli w/ Tomato Sauce	1 serv	476	21	15	66	65	–	534
Chicken Parmesan	1 serv	468	42	9	86	47	–	682
Fettuccine Alfredo	1 reg	798	25	22	21	119	–	232
Fettuccine Alfredo	1 sm	535	17	15	14	80	–	169
Lasagna	1 serv	437	22	19	144	41	–	968
Minestrone Soup	1 serv	123	1	1	2	23	–	910
Pizza Cheese Double Slice	1 serv	465	24	15	39	58	–	971
Pizza Combination Double Slice	1 serv	572	29	25	60	63	–	1369
Pizza Pepperoni Double Slice	1 serv	526	27	22	53	61	–	1226
Sampler Platter	1 serv	708	26	21	97	97	–	733
Shrimp & Scallop Fettuccine	1 serv	649	32	20	103	80	–	355
Spaghetti w/ Meat Sauce	1 reg	553	26	12	30	90	–	223
Spaghetti w/ MeatSauce	1 sm	372	17	8	20	60	–	161
Spaghetti w/ Meatballs	1 sm	718	28	31	62	80	–	726
Spaghetti w/ Meatballs	1 reg	1022	39	42	62	119	–	968

FOOD	PORTION	CAL	PROT	FAT	CHOL	CARB	FIBER	SOD
Spaghetti w/ Tomato Sauce	1 reg	512	16	10	0	93	–	244
Spaghetti w/ Tomato Sauce	1 sm	358	12	8	0	62	–	231
SALAD DRESSINGS								
Honey French	1 serv	146	0	12	0	9	–	208
House Italian	1 serv	106	tr	9	0	5	–	509
Ranch	1 serv	155	0	17	3	1	–	215
Reduced Calorie Italian	1 serv	55	0	5	0	3	–	393
Thousand Island	1 serv	129	0	13	17	4	–	223
SALADS AND SALAD BARS								
Garden Salad	1	30	2	tr	0	6	–	19
Italian Chef Salad	1	262	15	21	47	13	–	1446
Pasta Salad	1 serv	599	19	26	24	69	–	2019

FOSTERS FREEZE

FOOD	PORTION	CAL	PROT	FAT	CHOL	CARB	FIBER	SOD
Soft Serve Vanilla	1 serv (4 oz)	152	–	4	9	–	–	100

FRIENDLY'S
FROZEN YOGURT

FOOD	PORTION	CAL	PROT	FAT	CHOL	CARB	FIBER	SOD
Lowfat Simply Vanilla	½ cup (2.6 oz)	120	4	3	10	19	0	70
Mint Chocolate Chip	½ cup (2.6 oz)	130	4	4	10	21	0	65
ICE CREAM								
Purely Pistachio	½ cup	160	3	10	35	16	0	50
Vanilla	½ cup	150	26	8	35	16	0	40

GODFATHER'S PIZZA

FOOD	PORTION	CAL	PROT	FAT	CHOL	CARB	FIBER	SOD
Golden Crust Cheese	⅒ lg (3.5 oz)	242	12	9	14	28	–	363
Golden Crust Cheese	⅛ med (3.1 oz)	212	10	8	12	26	–	311
Golden Crust Combo	⅛ med (4.4 oz)	271	13	12	22	28	–	562
Golden Crust Combo	⅒ lg (4.9 oz)	305	16	14	25	31	–	674
Original Crust Cheese	⅒ jumbo (5.8 oz)	382	22	9	27	53	–	580
Original Crust Cheese	¼ mini (1.9 oz)	131	7	3	8	19	–	183
Original Crust Cheese	⅛ med (3.5 oz)	231	13	5	14	24	–	338
Original Crust Cheese	⅒ lg (4 oz)	258	15	6	18	36	–	396
Original Crust Combo	¼ mini (2.9 oz)	176	10	7	16	21	–	382
Original Crust Combo	⅒ lg (5.6 oz)	338	19	12	31	38	–	740
Original Crust Combo	⅛ med (5.1 oz)	306	17	11	27	36	–	660
Original Crust Combo	⅒ jumbo (8.3 oz)	503	29	18	47	56	–	1096

FOOD	PORTION	CAL	PROT	FAT	CHOL	CARB	FIBER	SOD
GODIVA								
Chocolatier Dark Chocolate w/ Raspberry	1 bar (1.5 oz)	220	2	11	3	28	0	10
Chocolatier Milk Chocolate	1 bar (1.5 oz)	230	3	13	10	26	0	30
Mochaccino Mousse	2 pieces (1.25 oz)	210	2	15	4	17	0	10
Truffle Assorted	2 pieces (1.5 oz)	220	2	13	10	24	0	15
GREAT STEAK & POTATO COMPANY NY								
Baked Potato w/ Broccoli & Cheese	1 serv (12 oz)	340	—	5	—	—	—	340
Chicken Philadelphia	1 serv (10 oz)	640	—	27	—	—	—	620
Chicken Teriyaki	1 serv (11 oz)	580	—	17	—	—	—	1470
Fresh Cut Fries	1 reg	540	—	29	—	—	—	440
Fresh Cut Fries	1 sm	460	—	24	—	—	—	380
Fresh Cut Fries	1 serv	920	—	48	—	—	—	760
Great Potato w/ Steak	1 serv (14 oz)	600	—	32	—	—	—	600
Great Potato w/ Turkey	1 serv (14 oz)	610	—	28	—	—	—	620
Great Salad Experience w/ Chicken w/o Dressing	1 serv (15 oz)	260	—	9	—	—	—	490
Great Steak	1 serv (11 oz)	660	—	34	—	—	—	400
Great Steak	1 lg (18 oz)	1070	—	55	—	—	—	610
Ham Delight	1 serv (11 oz)	710	—	33	—	—	—	1590
Turkey Philadelphia	1 serv (10 oz)	690	—	28	—	—	—	290
Veggi Delight	1 serv (7 oz)	570	—	29	—	—	—	440
HAAGEN-DAZS								
FROZEN YOGURT								
Pinapple Coconut	½ cup	230	4	13	90	25	0	55
Soft Serve Nonfat Chocolate	½ cup	110	4	0	0	23	0	65
Soft Serve Nonfat Chocolate Mousse	½ cup	80	5	0	0	24	1	65
Soft Serve Nonfat Coffee	½ cup	110	5	0	<5	22	0	70
Soft Serve Nonfat Strawberry	½ cup	110	4	0	0	24	0	60

FOOD	PORTION	CAL	PROT	FAT	CHOL	CARB	FIBER	SOD
Soft Serve Nonfat Vanilla	½ cup	110	5	0	<5	22	0	75
Soft Serve Nonfat Vanilla Mousse	½ cup	70	4	0	<5	23	0	65
Soft Serve Nonfat White Chocolate	½ cup	110	5	0	<5	22	0	75
Vanilla Fudge	½ cup	160	6	0	<5	34	0	100
Vanilla Raspberry Swirl	½ cup	130	4	0	<5	29	tr	30
ICE CREAM								
Bailey's Irish Cream	½ cup	270	5	17	115	23	0	70
Bar Chocolate	1 (2.7 oz)	200	4	12	85	16	tr	55
Bar Chocolate & Dark Chocolate	1 (3.6 oz)	350	5	24	85	28	2	45
Bar Coffee	1 (2.7 oz)	190	3	13	85	15	0	65
Bar Coffee & Almond Crunch	1 (3.7 oz)	370	5	27	90	27	tr	80
Bar Vanilla	1 (2.7 oz)	190	3	13	85	15	0	50
Bar Vanilla & Almonds	1 (3.7 oz)	380	6	28	90	26	1	70
Bar Vanilla & Milk Chocolate	1 (3.5 oz)	340	5	24	90	25	tr	65
Belgian Chocolate Chocolate	½ cup	330	5	21	85	29	2	85
Brownies A La Mode	½ cup	280	5	16	90	28	tr	135
Butter Pecan	½ cup	300	5	22	105	20	tr	110
Cappuccino Commotion	½ cup	310	5	21	100	25	1	90
Chocolate	½ cup	269	5	17	110	21	1	60
Chocolate Chocolate Chip	½ cup	300	5	19	100	26	2	55
Chocolate Chocolate Mint	½ cup	300	5	20	95	25	1	50
Chocolate Swiss Almond	½ cup	300	5	20	100	24	2	55
Coffee	½ cup	250	5	17	115	20	0	65
Coffee Mocha Chip	½ cup	270	4	19	105	24	tr	75
Cookie Dough Dynamo	½ cup	310	4	20	95	29	0	125
Cookies & Cream	½ cup	270	5	17	105	23	0	95

FOOD	PORTION	CAL	PROT	FAT	CHOL	CARB	FIBER	SOD
Cookies & Fudge	½ cup	180	7	3	15	33	tr	115
Deep Chocolate Peanut Butter	½ cup	350	8	24	80	26	4	85
Dulce De Leche Caramel	½ cup	270	5	16	95	27	0	90
Lowfat Coffee Fudge	½ cup	170	5	3	25	32	0	95
Macadamia Brittle	½ cup	280	4	19	105	24	0	105
Macadamia Nut	½ cup	320	5	24	110	20	0	100
Mint Chip	½ cup	280	4	18	105	25	tr	85
Pistachio	½ cup	280	5	19	110	21	tr	80
Pralines & Cream	½ cup	280	4	17	95	28	0	160
Rum Raisin	½ cup	260	4	17	105	21	0	55
Strawberry	½ cup	250	4	16	90	22	tr	90
Vanilla	½ cup	250	4	17	115	20	0	65
Vanilla Chocolate Chip	½ cup	290	5	19	100	25	tr	70
Vanilla Swiss Almond	½ cup	290	5	20	100	23	tr	70
SORBET								
Bar Raspberry & Vanilla	1 (2.5 oz)	90	2	0	0	21	tr	15
Mango	½ cup	120	0	0	0	31	tr	0
Orange	½ cup	120	0	0	0	30	tr	0
Raspberry	½ cup	120	0	0	0	30	2	0
Soft Serve Raspberry	½ cup	110	0	0	0	28	2	0
Strawberry	½ cup	120	0	0	0	30	1	0
Zesty Lemon	½ cup	120	0	0	0	31	tr	0
HARDEE'S								
BEVERAGES								
Orange Juice	1 serv (11 oz)	140	2	tr	0	34	—	5
Shake Chocolate	1 (12.2 oz)	370	13	5	30	67	—	270
Shake Peach	1 (12.1 oz)	390	10	4	25	77	—	290
Shake Strawberry	1 (12.7 oz)	420	11	4	20	83	—	270
Shake Vanilla	1 (12.2 oz)	350	12	5	20	65	—	300
BREAKFAST SELECTIONS								
Apple Cinnamon 'N' Raisin Biscuit	1 (2.18 oz)	200	2	8	0	30	—	350
Bacon & Egg Biscuit	1 (5.5 oz)	570	22	33	275	45	—	1400
Bacon Egg & Cheese Biscuit	1 (5.9 oz)	610	24	37	280	45	—	1630

FOOD	PORTION	CAL	PROT	FAT	CHOL	CARB	FIBER	SOD
Big Country Breakfast Bacon	1 serv (9.4 oz)	820	33	49	535	62	—	1870
Big Country Breakfast Sausage	1 serv (11.4 oz)	1000	41	66	570	62	—	3210
Biscuit 'N' Gravy	1 (7.8 oz)	510	10	28	15	55	—	1500
Country Ham Biscuit	1 (3.8 oz)	430	15	22	25	45	—	1930
Frisco Breakfast Sandwich Ham	1 (7.4 oz)	500	24	25	290	46	—	1370
Ham Biscuit	1 (4 oz)	400	9	20	15	47	—	1340
Ham Egg & Cheese Biscuit	1 (6.5 oz)	540	20	30	285	48	—	1660
Hash Rounds	1 serv (2.8 oz)	230	3	14	0	24	—	560
Jelly Biscuit	1 (3.5 oz)	440	6	21	0	57	—	1000
Rise 'N' Shine Biscuit	1 (2.9 oz)	390	6	21	0	44	—	1000
Sausage Biscuit	1 (4.1 oz)	510	14	31	25	44	—	1360
Sausage & Egg Biscuit	1 (6.3 oz)	630	23	40	285	45	—	1480
Three Pancakes	1 serv (4.8 oz)	280	8	2	15	56	—	890
Ultimate Omelet Biscuit	1 (5.8 oz)	570	22	33	120	45	—	1370
DESSERTS								
Big Cookie	1 (2.0 oz)	280	4	12	15	41	—	150
Cone Chocolate	1 (4.1 oz)	180	5	2	15	34	—	110
Cone Vanilla	1 (4.1 oz)	170	4	2	10	34	—	130
Cool Twist Cone Vanilla/ Chocolate	1 (4.1 oz)	180	4	2	10	34	—	120
Peach Cobbler	1 serv (6 oz)	310	2	7	0	60	—	360
Sundae Hot Fudge	1 (5.5 oz)	290	7	6	20	51	—	310
Sundae Strawberry	1 (5.8 oz)	210	5	2	10	43	—	140
MAIN MENU SELECTIONS								
Baked Beans	1 serv (5 oz)	170	8	1	0	32	—	600
Big Roast Beef Sandwich	1 (6.5 oz)	460	26	24	70	35	—	1230
Cheeseburger	1 (4.3 oz)	310	16	14	40	30	—	890
Chicken Fillet Sandwich	1 (7.5 oz)	480	26	18	55	54	—	1280
Cole Slaw	1 serv (4 oz)	240	2	20	10	13	—	340
Cravin' Bacon Cheeseburger	1 (8.1 oz)	690	30	46	95	38	—	1150
Fisherman's Fillet	1 (8.3 oz)	560	26	27	65	54	—	1330

FOOD	PORTION	CAL	PROT	FAT	CHOL	CARB	FIBER	SOD
French Fries	1 lg (6 oz)	430	6	18	0	59	–	190
French Fries	1 sm (3.4 oz)	240	4	10	0	33	–	100
French Fries	1 med (5 oz)	350	5	15	0	49	–	150
Fried Chicken Breast	1 piece (5.2 oz)	370	29	15	75	29	–	1190
Fried Chicken Leg	1 piece (2.4 oz)	170	13	7	45	15	–	570
Fried Chicken Thigh	1 piece (4.2 oz)	330	19	15	60	30	–	1000
Fried Chicken Wing	1 piece (2.3 oz)	200	10	8	30	23	–	740
Frisco Burger	1 (8.1 oz)	720	33	46	95	43	–	1340
Gravy	1 serv (1.5 oz)	20	tr	tr	0	3	–	260
Grilled Chicken Sandwich	1 (7.1 oz)	350	25	11	65	38	–	950
Hamburger	1 (3.9 oz)	270	14	11	35	29	–	670
Hot Ham 'N' Cheese	1 (5.1 oz)	310	16	12	50	34	–	1410
Mashed Potatoes	1 serv (4 oz)	70	2	tr	0	14	–	330
Mesquite Bacon Cheeseburger	1 (4.5 oz)	370	19	18	45	32	–	970
Mushroom 'N' Swiss Burger	1 (6.8 oz)	490	28	25	80	39	–	1100
Quarter Pound Double Cheeseburger	1 (6 oz)	470	27	27	80	31	–	1290
Regular Roast Beef	1 (4.3 oz)	320	17	16	43	26	–	820
The Boss	1 (7 oz)	570	37	33	85	42	–	910
The Works Burger	1 (8.1 oz)	530	25	30	80	41	–	1030
SALAD DRESSINGS								
French Fat Free	1 serv (2 oz)	70	0	0	0	18	0	300
Ranch	1 serv (2 oz)	290	1	29	25	6	–	510
Thousand Island	1 serv (2 oz)	250	1	23	35	9	–	540
SALADS AND SALAD BARS								
Garden Salad	1 (10.2 oz)	220	12	13	40	11	–	350
Grilled Chicken Salad	1 (11.5 oz)	150	20	3	60	11	–	610
Side Salad	1 (4.6 oz)	25	1	tr	0	4	–	45
HOT SAM'S PRETZELS								
Bavarian	1 lg (5.1 oz)	390	14	0	0	83	4	780
Bavarian	1 reg (2.5 oz)	200	7	0	0	42	2	390
Bavarian Stix	10 (5 oz)	390	14	0	0	83	4	780
Sweet Dough	1 (4.5 oz)	360	11	3	0	73	4	780
Sweet Dough Blueberry	1 (4.5 oz)	400	11	4	0	81	2	610

FOOD	PORTION	CAL	PROT	FAT	CHOL	CARB	FIBER	SOD
IHOP								
Pancake Buckwheat	1 (2.5 oz)	134	4	5	61	19	1	372
Pancake Buttermilk	1 (2 oz)	108	3	3	31	17	tr	459
Pancake Country Griddle	1 (2.25 oz)	134	4	4	38	22	1	497
Pancake Egg	1 (2 oz)	102	2	5	66	12	tr	213
Pancake Harvest Grain 'N Nut	1 (2.25 oz)	160	4	8	38	18	1	391
Waffle	1 (4 oz)	305	6	15	70	37	1	468
Waffle Belgian	1 (6 oz)	408	9	20	146	49	1	882
Waffle Belgian Harvest Grain 'N Nut	1 (6 oz)	445	10	28	147	40	3	876
JACK IN THE BOX								
BEVERAGES								
2% Milk	1 serv (8 fl oz)	130	9	5	20	14	0	85
Barq's Root Beer	1 reg (20 fl oz)	180	0	0	0	50	0	50
Classic Ice Cream Shake Chocolate	1 reg (11 fl oz)	630	11	27	85	85	tr	330
Classic Ice Cream Shake Oreo Cookie	1 reg (12 oz)	740	13	36	95	91	tr	490
Classic Ice Cream Shake Strawberry	1 reg (10 fl oz)	640	10	28	85	85	0	300
Classic Ice Cream Shake Vanilla	1 reg (11 oz)	610	12	31	95	73	0	320
Classice Ice Cream Shake Cappuccino	1 reg (11 oz)	630	11	29	90	80	0	320
Coca-Cola Classic	1 reg (20 fl oz)	170	0	0	0	46	0	40
Coffee	1 reg (12 fl oz)	5	0	0	0	1	0	5
Diet Coke	1 reg (20 fl oz)	0	0	0	0	0	0	15
Dr Pepper	1 reg (20 fl oz)	190	0	0	0	49	0	25
Iced Tea	1 reg (20 fl oz)	0	0	0	0	0	0	0
Minute Maid Lemonade	1 reg (20 fl oz)	190	0	0	0	48	0	90
Orange Juice	1 serv (10 oz)	150	2	0	0	34	1	20
Sprite	1 reg (20 fl oz)	160	0	0	0	41	0	40
BREAKFAST SELECTIONS								
Breakfast Jack	1 (4.2 oz)	300	18	12	185	30	0	890
Country Crock Spread	1 pat (5 g)	25	0	3	0	0	0	40
Grape Jelly	1 serv (0.5 oz)	40	0	0	0	9	0	5

FOOD	PORTION	CAL	PROT	FAT	CHOL	CARB	FIBER	SOD
Hash Browns	1 serv (2 oz)	160	1	11	—	14	1	310
Pancake Syrup	1 serv (1.5 oz)	120	0	0	0	30	0	5
Pancakes w/ Bacon	1 serv (5.6 oz)	400	13	12	30	59	3	980
Sausage Croissant	1 (6.4 oz)	670	21	48	250	39	2	940
Sourdough Breakfast Sandwich	1 (5.2 oz)	380	21	21	355	31	0	1120
Supreme Croissant	1 (6 oz)	570	21	20	235	39	2	1240
Ultimate Breakfast Sandwich	1 (8.5 oz)	620	36	36	245	39	tr	1800
DESSERTS								
Carrot Cake	1 serv (3.5 oz)	370	3	16	35	54	2	340
Cheesecake	1 serv (3.5 oz)	310	8	18	65	29	2	210
Double Fudge Cake	1 serv (3 oz)	300	3	10	50	50	1	320
Hot Apple Turnover	1 (3.8 oz)	340	4	18	0	41	2	510
MAIN MENU SELECTIONS								
¼ lb Burger	1 (6 oz)	510	26	27	65	39	0	1080
American Cheese	1 slice (0.4 oz)	45	2	4	10	0	0	200
Bacon & Cheddar Potato Wedges	1 serv (9.3 oz)	800	20	58	55	49	4	1470
Bacon Ultimate Cheeseburger	1 (10.4 oz)	1150	57	89	230	31	0	1770
Barbeque Dipping Sauce	1 serv (1 fl oz)	45	1	0	0	11	0	300
Cheeseburger	1 (4 oz)	330	15	15	60	32	2	760
Chicken & Fries	1 serv (9.3 oz)	730	26	34	65	79	5	1690
Chicken Caesar Sandwich	1 (8.3 oz)	520	27	26	55	44	4	1050
Chicken Fajita Pita	1 (6.6 oz)	280	24	9	75	25	3	840
Chicken Sandwich	1 (5.9 oz)	450	16	26	45	38	2	1030
Chicken Strips Breaded	5 pieces (5.3 oz)	360	27	17	80	24	1	970
Chicken Supreme Sandwich	1 (8.2 oz)	680	23	45	85	46	4	1500
Chili Cheese Curly Fries	1 serv (8.1 oz)	650	12	41	25	60	13	1640
Double Cheeseburger	1 (5.3 oz)	450	24	24	75	35	0	970
Egg Rolls	3 pieces (6 oz)	440	15	24	35	40	4	1020
Egg Rolls	5 pieces (10 oz)	730	25	41	60	67	7	1700
Fish & Chips	1 serv (9 oz)	720	19	35	35	81	6	1580

FOOD	PORTION	CAL	PROT	FAT	CHOL	CARB	FIBER	SOD
French Fries	1 reg (4.1 oz)	360	4	17	0	48	3	740
Grilled Chicken Fillet Sandwich	1 (8.1 oz)	520	27	26	140	42	4	1240
Hamburger	1 (3.6 oz)	280	13	12	45	32	2	560
Jumbo Fries	1 serv (5 oz)	430	4	20	0	58	4	890
Jumbo Jack	1 (7.8 oz)	560	28	36	80	31	4	680
Jumbo Jack w/ Cheese	1 (8.6 oz)	650	32	43	105	32	4	1090
Ketchup	1 pkg (0.3 oz)	10	0	0	0	3	0	100
Monster Taco	1 (4 oz)	290	11	18	40	21	3	550
Onion Rings	1 serv (4.2 oz)	460	7	25	0	50	3	780
Pilly Cheesesteak Sandwich	1 (7.6 oz)	520	33	25	155	41	4	1980
Salsa	1 serv (1 oz)	10	0	0	0	2	0	200
Seasoned Curly Fries	1 serv (4.5 oz)	420	6	24	0	46	4	1030
Sour Cream	1 serv (1 oz)	60	1	6	20	1	0	30
Sourdough Jack	1 (7.8 oz)	670	32	43	110	39	0	1180
Soy Sauce	1 serv (0.3 oz)	5	tr	0	0	tr	0	480
Spicy Crispy Chicken Sandwich	1 (7.9 oz)	560	24	27	50	55	0	1020
Stuffed Jalapenos	10 pieces (7.6 oz)	680	20	40	75	59	5	2220
Stuffed Jalapenos	7 pieces (5.3 oz)	470	14	28	50	41	3	1560
Super Scoop French Fries	1 serv (7 oz)	610	6	28	0	82	5	1250
Sweet & Sour Dipping Sauce	1 serv (1 oz)	40	tr	0	0	11	0	160
Swiss-Style Cheese	1 slice (0.4 oz)	40	3	3	10	0	0	190
Taco	1 (2.7 oz)	190	7	11	20	15	2	410
Tartar Dipping Sauce	1 pkg (1.5 oz)	220	1	23	20	2	0	240
Teriyaki Bowl Chicken	1 serv (17.6 oz)	670	29	4	15	128	5	1620
Ultimate Cheeseburger	1 (9.8 oz)	1030	50	79	205	30	0	1200
SALAD DRESSINGS								
Blue Cheese	1 serv (2 fl oz)	210	1	18	15	11	0	750
Buttermilk House	1 serv (2 fl oz)	290	1	30	20	6	0	560
Buttermilk House Dipping Sauce	1 serv (0.9 oz)	130	tr	13	10	3	tr	240
Low Calorie Italian	1 serv (2 fl oz)	25	0	2	0	2	0	670
Thousand Island	1 serv (2 fl oz)	250	1	24	20	10	0	570

FOOD	PORTION	CAL	PROT	FAT	CHOL	CARB	FIBER	SOD
SALADS AND SALAD BARS								
Croutons	1 serv (0.4 oz)	50	1	2	0	8	0	105
Garden Chicken Salad	1 serv (8.9 oz)	200	23	9	65	8	3	420
Side Salad	1 (3 oz)	50	2	3	10	3	1	75
JAMBA JUICE								
Jambolas Honey Nut Energy	1 serv	192	5	1	—	—	2	—
Jambolas Mighty Multi Grain	1 serv	208	8	3	—	—	5	—
Jambolas Mind Over Blueberry	1 serv	170	5	1	—	—	2	—
Jambolas Pizza Protein	1 serv	199	9	3	—	—	3	—
Mango-A-Go-Go	1 reg (24 oz)	460	2	2	—	—	3	—
Orchard Oasis	1 reg (24 oz)	440	2	2	—	—	4	—
Protein Berry Pizazz	1 reg (24 oz)	470	25	1	—	—	6	—
Razzmatazz	1 reg (24 oz)	440	3	2	—	—	4	—
KENNY ROGERS ROASTERS								
MAIN MENU SELECTIONS								
½ Chicken w/ Skin	1 serv (9.06 oz)	515	65	28	301	2	—	1129
½ Chicken w/o Skin & Wing	1 serv (7.03 oz)	313	56	10	221	1	—	876
¼ Chicken Dark Meat w/ Skin	1 serv (4.35 oz)	271	29	17	165	1	—	524
¼ Chicken Dark Meat w/o Skin & Wing	1 serv (3.29 oz)	169	25	7	130	1	—	454
¼ Chicken White Meat w/ Skin	1 serv (4.71 oz)	244	35	11	136	1	—	604
¼ Chicken White Meat w/o Skin & Wing	1 serv (3.74 oz)	144	31	2	92	tr	—	422
Baked Sweet Potato	1 (9 oz)	263	4	tr	0	62	1	26
Chicken Caesar Salad	1 serv (9.4 oz)	285	34	9	122	18	1	704
Cinnamon Apples	1 serv (5.27 oz)	199	0	5	13	41	3	3
Cole Slaw	1 serv (5.05 oz)	225	1	16	13	18	2	288
Corn Muffin	1 (2 oz)	175	2	8	0	24	1	210
Corn On The Cob	1 (2.25 oz)	68	2	1	0	14	2	11

FOOD	PORTION	CAL	PROT	FAT	CHOL	CARB	FIBER	SOD
Corn Stuffing	1 serv (7.1 oz)	326	7	19	5	34	tr	765
Creamy Parmesan Spinach	1 serv (5.3 oz)	119	10	69	12	10	tr	547
Garlic Parsley Potatoes	1 serv (6.5 oz)	259	3	12	16	37	3	867
Honey Baked Beans	1 serv (5 oz)	148	6	1	0	32	tr	787
Italian Green Beans	1 serv (6.1 oz)	116	2	8	0	10	tr	374
Macaroni & Cheese	1 serv (5.51 oz)	197	6	6	26	24	1	661
Pasta Salad	1 serv (5 oz)	236	6	12	40	28	1	296
Pita BBQ Chicken	1 (7.33 oz)	401	33	7	112	51	—	1307
Pita Chicken Caesar	1 (9.2 oz)	606	36	35	122	34	1	829
Pita Roasted Chicken	1 (10.8 oz)	685	47	35	159	42	tr	1620
Pot Pie Chicken	1 (12 oz)	708	26	33	69	78	tr	1500
Potato Salad	1 serv (7.01 oz)	390	3	27	0	34	2	628
Real Mashed Potatoes	1 serv (8 oz)	295	4	14	2	39	1	478
Rice Pilaf	1 serv (5 oz)	173	3	5	0	43	0	146
Roasted Chicken Salad	1 serv (16.9 oz)	292	35	10	218	19	6	573
Sandwich Turkey	1 (9.2 oz)	385	39	12	88	30	1	923
Side Salad	1 serv (4.73 oz)	23	1	1	0	5	2	16
Sour Cream & Dill Pasta Salad	1 serv (5 oz)	233	4	16	16	20	1	432
Steamed Vegetables	1 serv (4.25 oz)	48	3	tr	0	8	4	59
Sweet Corn Niblets	1 serv (5 oz)	112	3	1	0	28	1	385
Tomato Cucumber Salad	1 serv (6 oz)	123	1	2	0	10	1	794
Turkey Sliced Breast	1 serv (4.5 oz)	158	34	2	78	—	—	586
Zucchini & Squash Santa Fe	1 serv (5 oz)	70	1	5	0	8	1	209
SALAD DRESSINGS								
Blue Cheese	1 serv (2.47 oz)	370	3	39	65	3	0	720
Buttermilk Ranch	1 serv (2.47 oz)	430	1	48	10	2	0	620
Caesar	1 serv (2.47 oz)	340	1	36	15	3	0	780
Honey French	1 serv (2.47 oz)	350	0	29	0	22	0	490
Honey Mustard	1 serv (2.47 oz)	320	1	28	40	18	1	410
Italian Fat Free	1 serv (2.47 oz)	35	0	0	0	8	0	1040
Thousand Island	1 serv (2.47 oz)	330	1	33	40	8	0	550
SOUPS								
Chicken Noodle	1 cup (6 oz)	55	4	1	13	7	1	559
Chicken Noodle	1 bowl (10 oz)	91	7	2	22	12	tr	931

FOOD	PORTION	CAL	PROT	FAT	CHOL	CARB	FIBER	SOD
KFC								
BBQ Baked Beans	1 serv (5.5 oz)	190	6	3	5	33	6	760
Biscuit	1 (2 oz)	180	4	10	0	20	tr	560
Chicken Pot Pie	1 (13 oz)	770	29	42	70	69	5	2160
Chicken Twister	1 (8.7 oz)	550	26	32	85	40	1	980
Cole Slaw	1 serv (5 oz)	180	2	9	5	21	3	280
Corn On The Cob	1 ear (5.7 oz)	150	5	2	0	35	2	20
Cornbread	1 (2 oz)	228	3	13	42	25	1	194
Crispy Strips Colonel's	3 (3.25 oz)	261	20	16	40	10	3	658
Crispy Strips Spicy Buffalo	3 (4.2 oz)	350	22	19	35	22	2	1110
Extra Tasty Crispy Breast	1 (5.9 oz)	470	31	28	80	25	1	930
Extra Tasty Crispy Drumstick	1 (2.4 oz)	190	13	11	60	8	tr	260
Extra Tasty Crispy Thigh	1 (4.2 oz)	370	19	25	70	18	2	540
Extra Tasty Crispy Whole Wing	1 (1.9 oz)	200	10	13	45	10	tr	290
Green Beans	1 serv (4.7 oz)	45	1	2	5	7	3	730
Hot & Spicy Breast	1 (6.5 oz)	530	32	35	110	23	2	1110
Hot & Spicy Drumstick	1 (2.3 oz)	190	13	11	50	10	tr	300
Hot & Spicy Thigh	1 (3.8 oz)	370	18	27	90	13	1	570
Hot & Spicy Whole Wing	1 (1.9 oz)	210	10	15	50	9	tr	340
Hot Wings	6 (4.8 oz)	471	27	33	150	18	2	1230
Macaroni & Cheese	1 serv (5.4 oz)	180	7	8	10	21	2	860
Mashed Potatoes With Gravy	1 serv (4.8 oz)	120	1	6	tr	17	2	440
Mean Greens	1 serv (5.4 oz)	70	4	3	10	11	5	650
Original Recipe Breast	1 (5.4 oz)	400	29	24	135	16	1	1116
Original Recipe Chicken Sandwich	1 (7.3 oz)	497	29	22	52	46	3	1213
Original Recipe Drumstick	1 (2.2 oz)	140	13	9	75	4	0	422
Original Recipe Thigh	1 (3.2 oz)	250	16	18	95	6	1	747
Original Recipe Whole Wing	1 (1.6 oz)	140	9	10	55	5	0	414

FOOD	PORTION	CAL	PROT	FAT	CHOL	CARB	FIBER	SOD
Potato Salad	1 serv (5.6 oz)	230	4	14	15	23	3	540
Potato Wedges	1 serv (4.8 oz)	280	5	13	5	28	5	750
Tender Roast Breast w/ Skin	1 (4.9 oz)	251	37	11	151	1	0	830
Tender Roast Breast w/o Skin	1 (4.2 oz)	169	31	4	112	1	0	797
Tender Roast Drumstick w/ Skin	1 (1.9 oz)	97	15	4	85	tr	0	271
Tender Roast Drumstick w/o Skin	1 (1.2 oz)	67	11	2	63	tr	0	259
Tender Roast Thigh w/ Skin	1 (3.2 oz)	207	19	12	120	<2	0	504
Tender Roast Thigh w/o Skin	1 (2.1 oz)	106	13	6	84	tr	0	312
Tender Roast Wing w/ Skin	1 (1.8 oz)	121	12	8	74	1	0	331
Value BBQ Chicken Sandwich	1 (5.3 oz)	256	17	8	57	28	2	782
KRISPY KREME								
Chocolate Iced	1 (2 oz)	260	3	14	<5	30	1	105
Chocolate Iced Cake	1 (2 oz)	230	3	12	15	28	tr	280
Chocolate Iced Creme Filled	1 (2.3 oz)	270	4	14	<5	32	2	150
Chocolate Iced Cruller	1 (1.7 oz)	240	2	14	10	26	tr	160
Chocolate Iced Custard Filled	1 (2.7 oz)	250	4	9	5	38	3	150
Chocolated Iced w/ Sprinkles	1 (2 oz)	220	2	10	<5	31	tr	95
Cinnamon Apple Filled	1 (2.3 oz)	210	4	9	<5	29	3	150
Cinnamon Bun	1 (2.1 oz)	220	5	11	0	26	4	160
Glazed Blueberry	1 (2.4 oz)	300	2	15	5	37	1	200
Glazed Creme Filled	1 (2.3 oz)	270	4	14	<5	32	2	150
Glazed Cruller	1 (1.5 oz)	220	2	14	10	22	0	150
Glazed Devil's Food	1 (1.9 oz)	240	2	13	10	29	3	180

FOOD	PORTION	CAL	PROT	FAT	CHOL	CARB	FIBER	SOD
Lemon Filled	1 (2.2 oz)	210	4	10	5	28	tr	150
Maple Iced	1 (1.8 oz)	200	3	9	0	28	2	100
Original Glazed	1 (1.3 oz)	180	2	10	<5	17	tr	95
Powdered Blueberry Filled	1 (2.1 oz)	200	4	9	5	26	2	160
Powdered Cake	1 (1.8 oz)	220	3	11	15	26	0	250
Raspberry Filled	1 (2 oz)	210	4	10	<5	27	3	160
Traditional Cake	1 (1.7 oz)	200	3	11	15	22	tr	280

KRYSTAL

BEVERAGES

Chocolate Shake	1 (16 fl oz)	275	8	10	32	44	—	178

BREAKFAST SELECTIONS

Biscuit	1 (2.5 oz)	244	3	12	2	31	—	437
Biscuit Bacon	1 (2.9 oz)	306	8	17	14	32	—	726
Biscuit Bacon, Egg & Cheese	1 (4.7 oz)	421	14	26	153	33	—	899
Biscuit Country Ham	1 (3.7 oz)	334	14	17	23	31	—	1147
Biscuit Egg	1 (4 oz)	327	8	19	134	32	—	481
Biscuit Gravy	1 (7.5 oz)	419	7	26	23	40	—	980
Biscuit Sausage	1 (4.1 oz)	437	10	30	49	31	—	668
Sunriser	1 (3.8 oz)	259	14	17	162	17	—	544

DESSERTS

Apple Pie	1 serv (4.5 oz)	300	3	10	0	49	—	420
Donut Plain	1 (1.3 oz)	150	2	9	5	17	—	135
Donut w/ Chocolate Icing	1 (1.8 oz)	212	2	11	5	27	—	165
Donut w/ Vanilla Icing	1 (1.8 oz)	198	2	9	5	29	—	135
Lemon Meringue Pie	1 serv (4 oz)	340	7	9	50	57	—	190
Pecan Pie	1 serv (4 oz)	450	5	23	55	56	—	290

MAIN MENU SELECTIONS

Bacon Cheeseburger	1 (7.4 oz)	521	26	34	89	29	—	1083
Big K	1 (8 oz)	540	29	35	93	29	—	1283
Burger Plus	1 (6.5 oz)	415	20	26	63	28	—	614
Burger Plus w/ Cheese	1 (7.1 oz)	473	23	31	77	28	—	867
Cheese Krystal	1 (2.5 oz)	187	11	10	29	16	—	453
Chili	1 lg (12 oz)	327	16	12	28	41	—	1283
Chili	1 reg (8 oz)	218	11	8	19	27	—	855

FOOD	PORTION	CAL	PROT	FAT	CHOL	CARB	FIBER	SOD
Chili Cheese Pup	1 (2.7 oz)	211	9	13	31	14	–	642
Chili Pup	1 (2.5 oz)	182	7	10	24	13	–	597
Corn Pup	1 (2.3 oz)	214	6	14	24	17	–	710
Crispy Crunchy Chicken Sandwich	1 (5.75 oz)	467	16	24	56	48	–	949
Double Cheese Krystal	1 (4.5 oz)	337	21	19	57	25	–	815
Double Krystal	1 (4 oz)	277	18	14	43	24	–	547
Fries	1 reg (4.1 oz)	358	4	18	12	45	–	157
Fries	1 sm (3 oz)	262	3	13	9	33	–	115
Fries	1 lg (5.3 oz)	463	5	23	16	59	–	203
Krys Kross Fries	1 serv (4.3 oz)	486	5	29	31	52	–	604
Krys Kross Fries Chili Cheese	1 serv (6.8 oz)	625	12	39	61	57	–	1111
Krys Kross Fries w/ Cheese	1 serv (5.3 oz)	515	5	31	31	54	–	803
Krystal	1 (2.2 oz)	158	10	7	22	16	–	324
Plain Pup	1 (1.9 oz)	160	6	9	20	12	–	470

LITTLE CAESARS
MAIN MENU SELECTIONS

FOOD	PORTION	CAL	PROT	FAT	CHOL	CARB	FIBER	SOD
Crazy Bread	1 piece (1.4 oz)	106	3	3	0	16	1	114
Crazy Sauce	1 serv (6 oz)	170	5	tr	0	14	5	381
Deli-Style Sandwich Ham & Cheese	1 (11.6 oz)	728	30	35	54	71	3	1602
Deli-Style Sandwich Italian	1 (11.9 oz)	740	29	37	62	71	3	1831
Deli-Style Sandwich Veggie	1 (11.9 oz)	647	22	29	29	74	4	1195
Hot Oven-Baked Sandwich Cheeser	1 (12.1 oz)	822	40	39	580	75	5	2244
Hot Oven-Baked Sandwich Meatsa	1 (15 oz)	1036	55	56	130	75	5	3302
Hot Oven-Baked Sandwich Pepperoni	1 (11.2 oz)	899	43	47	58	74	4	2428
Hot Oven-Baked Sandwich Supreme	1 (13.1 oz)	894	41	46	700	77	5	2367

FOOD	PORTION	CAL	PROT	FAT	CHOL	CARB	FIBER	SOD
Hot Oven-Baked Sandwich Veggie	1 (13.7 oz)	669	33	23	58	79	6	1534

PIZZA

FOOD	PORTION	CAL	PROT	FAT	CHOL	CARB	FIBER	SOD
Baby Pan!Pan!	1 serv (8.4 oz)	616	33	24	47	67	4	1466
Pan!Pan! Cheese	1 med slice (2.9 oz)	181	9	6	15	22	1	379
Pan!Pan! Pepperoni	1 med slice (3 oz)	199	11	8	15	22	1	452
Pizza!Pizza! Cheese	1 med slice (3.2 oz)	201	11	7	17	24	1	281
Pizza!Pizza! Pepperoni	1 med slice (3.3 oz)	220	12	9	17	24	1	358

SALAD DRESSINGS

FOOD	PORTION	CAL	PROT	FAT	CHOL	CARB	FIBER	SOD
1000 Island	1 serv (1.5 oz)	183	—	17	30	6	—	542
Blue Cheese	1 serv (1.5 oz)	160	—	14	17	8	—	600
Caesar	1 serv (1.5 oz)	255	—	27	13	3	—	404
French	1 serv (1.5 oz)	166	—	16	0	5	—	553
Greek	1 serv (1.5 oz)	268	—	30	9	tr	—	202
Italian	1 serv (1.5 oz)	200	—	21	12	3	—	468
Italian Fat Free	1 serv (1.5 oz)	15	—	0	0	3	—	420
Ranch	1 serv (1.5 oz)	221	—	22	18	5	—	340

SALADS AND SALAD BARS

FOOD	PORTION	CAL	PROT	FAT	CHOL	CARB	FIBER	SOD
Antipasto Salad	1 serv (8.4 oz)	176	12	12	19	7	2	542
Caesar Salad	1 serv (5 oz)	140	9	5	11	14	2	372
Greek Salad	1 serv (10.3 oz)	168	9	10	37	12	3	653
Tossed Salad	1 serv (8.5 oz)	116	5	3	0	19	3	170

LONG JOHN SILVER'S
MAIN MENU SELECTIONS

FOOD	PORTION	CAL	PROT	FAT	CHOL	CARB	FIBER	SOD
Breaded Chicken Strips	1 piece (1.15 oz)	100	6	5	10	6	0	360
Breaded Clams	1 serv (3 oz)	300	11	17	40	31	5	670
Breaded Fish	1 piece (1.6 oz)	110	5	5	20	11	0	340
Cheese Sticks	1 serv (1.6 oz)	160	6	9	10	12	tr	360
Chicken Salsa	1 reg (11 oz)	690	18	32	20	81	5	1690
Corn Cobbette w/ Butter	1 piece (3.3 oz)	140	3	8	0	19	0	0
Corn Cobbette w/o Butter	1 (3.1 oz)	80	3	1	0	19	0	0
Fish Cajun	1 lg (23 oz)	1450	18	70	60	85	10	3630
Flavorbaked Chicken	1 piece (2.6 oz)	110	19	3	55	tr	tr	600
Flavorbaked Fish	1 piece (2.3 oz)	90	14	3	35	1	0	320
Fries	1 reg (3 oz)	250	3	15	0	28	3	500

FOOD	PORTION	CAL	PROT	FAT	CHOL	CARB	FIBER	SOD
Fries	1 lg (5 oz)	420	5	24	0	46	4	830
Honey Mustard Sauce	1 serv (0.4 oz)	20	0	0	0	5	0	60
Hushpuppy	1 (0.8 oz)	60	1	3	0	9	0	25
Ketchup	1 serv (.32 oz)	10	0	0	0	2	0	110
Popcorn Chicken Munchers	1 serv (4 oz)	380	23	23	35	20	2	1030
Popcorn Fish Munchers	1 serv (4 oz)	300	14	14	50	29	tr	1220
Popcorn Shrimp Munchers	1 serv (4 oz)	320	15	15	85	33	1	1440
Rice	1 serv (3 oz)	140	3	3	0	26	tr	210
Sandwich Batter Dipped Fish No Sauce	1 (5.4 oz)	320	17	13	30	40	6	800
Sandwich Flavorbaked Chicken	1 (5.8 oz)	290	24	10	60	27	2	970
Sandwich Flavorbaked Fish	1 (6 oz)	320	23	14	55	28	2	930
Sandwich Ultimate Fish	1 (6.4 oz)	430	18	21	35	44	3	1340
Shrimp Sauce	1 serv (0.4 oz)	15	0	0	0	3	0	180
Side Salad	1 (4.3 oz)	25	1	0	0	4	tr	15
Slaw	1 serv (3.4 oz)	140	1	6	0	20	3	260
Sweet'N'Sour Sauce	1 serv (0.4 oz)	20	0	0	0	5	0	45
Tartar Sauce	1 serv (0.4 oz)	35	0	2	0	5	0	35
Wraps Chicken Cajun	1 reg (11 oz)	720	18	35	25	83	5	1860
Wraps Chicken Cajun	1 lg (22 oz)	1440	37	71	50	165	11	3730
Wraps Chicken Ranch	1 reg (11 oz)	730	18	36	25	82	5	1810
Wraps Chicken Ranch	1 lg (22 oz)	1450	36	72	50	165	10	3620
Wraps Chicken Salsa	1 lg (22 oz)	1370	36	64	35	162	10	3370
Wraps Chicken Tartar	1 lg (22 oz)	1450	36	72	45	165	11	3560
Wraps Chicken Tartar	1 reg (11 oz)	730	18	36	25	83	6	1780
Wraps Fish Cajun	1 reg (11.5 oz)	730	18	35	30	85	5	1820
Wraps Fish Ranch	1 lg (23 oz)	1460	35	72	60	170	10	3520
Wraps Fish Ranch	1 reg (11.5 oz)	730	18	36	30	85	5	1760
Wraps Fish Salsa	1 reg (11.5 oz)	690	18	32	25	84	5	1640
Wraps Fish Salsa	1 lg (23 oz)	1380	35	64	45	167	10	3280
Wraps Fish Tartar	1 lg (23 oz)	1470	35	72	55	170	10	3460

FOOD	PORTION	CAL	PROT	FAT	CHOL	CARB	FIBER	SOD
Wraps Fish Tartar	1 reg (11.5 oz)	730	18	36	25	85	5	1730
Wraps Popcorn Shrimp Cajun	1 reg (11 oz)	720	16	35	50	86	5	1830
Wraps Popcorn Shrimp Cajun	1 lg (22 oz)	1450	32	71	95	172	10	3660
Wraps Popcorn Shrimp Ranch	1 lg (22 oz)	1460	32	72	100	171	10	3560
Wraps Popcorn Shrimp Ranch	1 reg (11 oz)	720	16	35	50	86	5	1830
Wraps Popcorn Shrimp Salsa	1 reg (11 oz)	690	16	32	40	84	5	1660
Wraps Popcorn Shrimp Salsa	1 lg (22 oz)	1380	32	64	85	169	9	3310
Wraps Popcorn Shrimp Tartar	1 reg (11 oz)	730	16	36	45	86	5	1750
Wraps Popcorn Shrimp Tartar	1 lg (22 oz)	1460	32	72	95	172	10	3500
SALAD DRESSINGS								
Fat-Free French	1 serv (1.5 oz)	50	0	0	0	14	–	360
Fat-Free Ranch	1 serv (1.5 oz)	50	2	0	0	13	–	380
Italian	1 serv (1 oz)	130	0	14	0	2	–	280
Malt Vinegar	1 serv (0.3 oz)	0	0	0	0	0	0	15
Ranch Dressing	1 serv (1 oz)	170	0	18	5	1	–	260
Thousand Island	1 serv (1 oz)	110	0	10	15	5	–	280
MANHATTAN BAGEL								
Blueberry	1	260	9	tr	0	54	2	560
Cheddar Cheese	1	270	11	4	10	48	2	560
Chocolate Chip	1	290	9	3	0	56	2	530
Cinnamon Raisin	1	280	10	tr	0	57	3	560
Egg	1	270	10	2	0	53	2	710
Everything	1	290	11	3	0	54	3	2000
Jalapeno Cheddar	1	260	16	2	0	53	2	310
Marble	1	260	10	tr	0	52	3	540
Oat Bran	1	260	10	1	0	53	3	470
Oat Bran Raisin Walnut	1	270	10	3	0	54	3	450
Onion	1	270	10	tr	0	55	2	560
Plain	1	260	10	tr	0	52	2	560
Poppy	1	300	11	4	0	54	5	560

FOOD	PORTION	CAL	PROT	FAT	CHOL	CARB	FIBER	SOD
Pumpernickel	1	250	10	1	0	52	3	530
Rye	1	260	10	1	0	52	3	560
Salt	1	260	10	tr	0	53	2	7100
Sesame	1	310	11	5	0	55	3	560
Spinach	1	270	10	tr	0	54	3	580
Sun-Dried Tomato	1	260	10	1	0	53	3	340
Whole Wheat	1	260	10	tr	0	52	3	470

MAX & ERMA'S

FOOD	PORTION	CAL	PROT	FAT	CHOL	CARB	FIBER	SOD
Black Bean Roll Up	1 serv	401	–	8	13	–	–	534
Fat Free French	2 tbsp	126	–	tr	0	–	–	1034
Fat Free Honey Mustard	2 tbsp	60	–	0	0	–	–	280
Fruit Smoothie	1 serv	114	–	tr	0	–	–	3
Garden Grill	1 serv	467	–	7	12	–	–	911
Garlic Breadstick	1	156	–	6	0	–	–	293
Gourmet Garden Grill	1 serv	484	–	8	12	–	–	912
Grilled Zucchini & Mushroom Pasta	1 serv	448	–	10	13	–	–	–
Grilled Zucchini & Mushroom Pasta w/ Chicken	1 serv	621	–	18	78	–	–	–
Hula Bowl w/ Fat Free Honey Mustard Dressing	1 serv	526	–	8	91	–	–	1309
Lo-Cal Ranch	2 tbsp	54	–	6	7	–	–	141
Tijuana Tortilla Wrap	1	692	–	15	54	–	–	1958

MCDONALD'S
BAKED SELECTIONS

FOOD	PORTION	CAL	PROT	FAT	CHOL	CARB	FIBER	SOD
Apple Pie Baked	1 (2.7 oz)	260	3	13	0	34	tr	200
Chocolate Chip Cookie	1 (1.2 oz)	170	2	10	20	22	1	120
Cinnamon Roll	1	390	6	18	65	50	–	310
Danish Apple	1	340	5	15	20	47	–	340
Danish Cheese	1	400	7	21	40	45	–	400
Lowfat Muffin Apple Bran	1 (4 oz)	300	6	3	0	61	3	380
McDonaldland Cookies	1 pkg (1.5 oz)	180	3	5	0	32	1	190

FOOD	PORTION	CAL	PROT	FAT	CHOL	CARB	FIBER	SOD
BEVERAGES								
Coca-Cola Classic	1 sm (16 oz)	150	0	0	0	40	—	15
Coca-Cola Classic	1 lg (32 oz)	310	0	0	0	86	—	30
Coca-Cola Classic	1 child serv (12 oz)	110	0	0	0	29	—	10
Coca-Cola Classic	1 med (21 oz)	210	0	0	0	58	—	20
Diet Coke	1 sm (16 oz)	1	0	0	0	0	—	30
Diet Coke	1 med (21 oz)	0	0	0	0	0	—	30
Diet Coke	1 child serv (12 oz)	0	0	0	0	0	—	20
Diet Coke	1 lg (32 oz)	0	0	0	0	0	—	60
Hi-C Orange	1 sm (16 oz)	160	0	0	0	44	—	30
Hi-C Orange	1 lg (32 oz)	350	0	0	0	94	—	60
Hi-C Orange	1 med (21 oz)	240	0	0	0	64	—	40
Hi-C Orange	1 child serv (12 oz)	120	0	0	0	32	—	20
Milk 1%	1 serv (8 oz)	100	8	3	10	13	0	115
Orange Juice	1 serv (6 oz)	80	0	0	0	20	0	20
Shake Chocolate	1 sm (14.5 oz)	360	11	9	40	60	1	250
Shake Strawberry	1 sm (14.5 oz)	360	11	9	40	60	0	180
Shake Vanilla	1 sm (14.5 oz)	360	11	9	40	59	0	250
Sprite	1 sm (16 fl oz)	150	0	0	0	39	—	55
Sprite	1 med (21 oz)	210	0	0	0	56	—	80
Sprite	1 lg (32 oz)	310	0	0	0	83	—	115
Sprite	1 child serv (12 oz)	110	0	0	0	28	—	40
BREAKFAST SELECTIONS								
Bacon Egg & Cheese Biscuit	1	540	21	34	250	36	—	1550
Bagel Ham & Egg Cheese	1	550	26	23	255	58	—	1490
Bagel Spanish Omelet	1	690	27	38	275	59	—	1560
Bagel Steak & Egg Cheese	1	660	27	31	285	59	—	1300
Biscuit	1 (2.9 oz)	290	5	15	0	34	1	780
Breakfast Burrito	1 (4.1 oz)	320	13	20	195	21	—	660
Egg McMuffin	1 (4.8 oz)	290	17	14	235	27	1	790
English Muffin	1 (1.9 oz)	140	4	2	0	25	1	210
Hash Browns	1 serv (1.9 oz)	130	1	8	0	14	1	330
Hotcakes Margarine & Syrup	1 serv	600	9	17	20	104	—	770
Hotcakes Plain	1 serv	340	9	8	20	58	—	630
Sausage	1 (1.5 oz)	170	6	16	35	0	0	290

FOOD	PORTION	CAL	PROT	FAT	CHOL	CARB	FIBER	SOD
Sausage Biscuit	1 (4.5 oz)	470	11	31	35	35	1	1080
Sausage Biscuit w/ Egg	1 (6.2 oz)	550	18	37	245	35	1	1160
Sausage McMuffin	1 (3.9 oz)	360	13	23	45	26	1	740
Sausage McMuffin w/ Egg	1 (5.7 oz)	440	19	28	255	27	1	890
Scrambled Eggs	2 (3.6 oz)	160	13	11	425	1	0	170
DESSERTS								
McFlurry Butterfinger	1	620	16	22	70	90	–	260
McFlurry M&M	1	630	16	23	75	90	–	210
McFlurry Nestle Crunch	1	630	16	24	75	89	–	230
McFlurry Oreo	1	570	15	20	70	82	–	280
Nuts For Sundaes	1 serv (7 g)	40	2	4	0	2	0	55
Reduced Fat Ice Cream Cone Vanilla	1 (3.2 oz)	150	4	5	20	23	0	75
Sundae Hot Caramel	1 (6.4 oz)	360	7	10	35	61	0	180
Sundae Hot Fudge	1 (6.3 oz)	340	8	12	30	52	1	170
Sundae Strawberry	1 (6.2 oz)	290	7	7	30	50	tr	95
MAIN MENU SELECTIONS								
Barbeque Sauce	1 pkg (1 oz)	45	0	0	0	10	0	250
Big Mac	1	570	26	32	85	45	3	1100
Big Xtra!	1	710	24	46	95	51	–	1400
Big Xtra! w/ Cheese	1	810	29	55	120	52	–	1870
Cheeseburger	1 (4.2 oz)	320	16	13	40	35	2	830
Chicken McNuggets	6 pieces (3.7 oz)	290	15	17	55	20	–	540
Chicken McNuggets	4 pieces (2.5 oz)	190	10	11	35	13	–	360
Chicken McNuggets	9 pieces	430	23	25	80	29	–	810
Crispy Chicken Deluxe	1 (7.8 oz)	500	26	25	55	43	3	1100
Filet-O-Fish	1	470	15	26	50	45	–	890
French Fries	1 sm (2.4 oz)	210	3	10	0	26	2	135
French Fries	1 lg	540	8	26	0	68	–	350
French Fries	1 med	450	6	22	0	57	–	290
French Fries	1 super	610	9	29	0	77	–	390
Grilled Chicken Deluxe	1 (7.8 oz)	440	27	20	60	38	3	1040
Grilled Chicken Deluxe Plain w/o Mayonnaise	1 (7.2 oz)	300	27	5	50	38	3	930

FOOD	PORTION	CAL	PROT	FAT	CHOL	CARB	FIBER	SOD
Grilled Chicken Salad Deluxe	1 serv (9 oz)	120	21	2	45	7	2	240
Hamburger	1	270	13	9	30	35	–	600
Honey	1 pkg (0.5 oz)	45	0	0	0	12	0	0
Honey Mustard	1 pkg (0.5 oz)	50	0	5	10	3	0	85
Hot Mustard	1 pkg (1 oz)	60	1	4	5	7	tr	240
Light Mayonnaise	1 pkg (0.4 oz)	40	0	4	5	tr	0	80
Quarter Pounder	1	430	23	21	70	37	2	840
Quarter Pounder w/ Cheese	1 (7 oz)	530	28	30	95	38	2	1310
Sweet 'N Sour Sauce	1 pkg (1 oz)	50	0	0	0	11	0	140
SALAD DRESSINGS								
Caesar	1 pkg (2.1 oz)	160	2	14	20	7	0	450
Fat Free Herb Vinaigrette	1 pkg (2.1 oz)	50	0	0	0	11	0	330
Ranch	1 pkg (2.1 oz)	230	1	21	20	10	0	550
Reduced Calorie Red French	1 pkg (2.1 oz)	160	0	8	0	23	0	490
SALADS AND SALAD BARS								
Croutons	1 pkg	50	1	1	0	9	–	105
Garden Salad	1 serv (6.2 oz)	35	2	0	0	7	2	20
MRS. FIELDS								
Brownie Double Fudge	1 (3.1 oz)	420	5	20	35	56	3	125
Brownie Fudge Walnut	1 (3.4 oz)	500	7	29	40	54	4	135
Brownie Pecan Fudge	1 (2.8 oz)	390	4	21	40	48	2	135
Brownie Pecan Pie	1 (3 oz)	400	5	21	55	48	4	160
Cookie Chewy Fudge	1 (1.7 oz)	230	3	12	25	32	1	100
Cookie Coconut Macadamia	1 (1.7 oz)	250	3	15	35	28	1	230
Cookie Milk Chocolate Chip	1 (1.7 oz)	240	3	12	35	32	1	210
Cookie Milk Chocolate Macadamia	1 (1.7 oz)	250	3	14	30	29	1	190
Cookie Milk Chocolate w/ Walnuts	1 (1.7 oz)	250	3	13	30	30	1	200

FOOD	PORTION	CAL	PROT	FAT	CHOL	CARB	FIBER	SOD
Cookie Oatmeal Raisin	1 (1.7 oz)	220	3	10	30	31	2	230
Cookie Peanut Butter	1 (1.7 oz)	240	4	13	40	27	1	280
Cookie Semi-Sweet Chocolate	1 (1.7 oz)	230	3	12	30	32	1	210
Cookie Semi-Sweet Chocolate w/ Walnuts	1 (1.8 oz)	240	3	13	30	30	2	190
Cookie Triple Chocolate	1 (1.7 oz)	230	3	12	30	31	1	210
Cookie White Chunk Macadamia	1 (1.7 oz)	260	3	15	30	29	tr	190
Muffin Banana Walnut	1 (3.9 oz)	460	9	24	45	53	5	390
Muffin Blueberry	1 (4 oz)	390	6	15	45	58	2	470
Muffin Chocolate Chip	1 (4 oz)	450	7	19	40	65	5	470
Muffin Mandarin Orange	1 (4 oz)	420	6	17	45	59	1	490
Peanut Butter Dream Bar	1 (5 oz)	750	11	40	40	85	8	270
Stokabunga Energy Cookie	1 (5 oz)	750	11	48	60	74	5	310

MY FAVORITE MUFFIN

FOOD	PORTION	CAL	PROT	FAT	CHOL	CARB	FIBER	SOD
Basic Muffin	⅓ muffin	220	3	10	0	30	0	190
Double Chocolate	⅓ muffin	190	2	8	0	30	2	230
Fat Free Bavarian	⅓ muffin	100	2	0	0	24	1	140
Fat Free Bavarian Chocolate	⅓ muffin	130	3	0	0	31	3	200

NEWPORT CREAMERY

BEVERAGES

FOOD	PORTION	CAL	PROT	FAT	CHOL	CARB	FIBER	SOD
Skim Milk	1 serv (16 oz)	206	–	5	20	–	–	–

ICE CREAM

FOOD	PORTION	CAL	PROT	FAT	CHOL	CARB	FIBER	SOD
Reduced Fat No Sugar Added Chocolate	½ cup (2.6 oz)	110	4	3	0	22	1	80
Reduced Fat No Sugar Added Coffee	½ cup (2.6 oz)	100	4	4	15	18	0	70

FOOD	PORTION	CAL	PROT	FAT	CHOL	CARB	FIBER	SOD
Soft Serve Nonfat Frozen Yogurt Cone or Dish	1 reg (5 oz)	125	–	0	0	–	–	–
SALAD DRESSINGS								
Corn Oil & Vinegar	1 tbsp	45	–	6	0	–	–	–
Fat Free Ranch	1½ oz	48	–	0	0	–	–	–
Low-Cal French	1½ oz	48	–	0	0	–	–	–
SALADS AND SALAD BARS								
Chef's Salad	1 serv	215	–	8	50	–	–	–
Chicken Fajita	1 serv	295	–	20	44	–	–	–
Grilled Chicken	1 serv	247	–	13	48	–	–	–
SANDWICHES								
Lite Chicken Salad	1	379	–	19	63	–	–	–
Lite Grilled Cheese	1	274	–	17	30	–	–	–
Lite Grilled Chicken Breast Pocket	1	327	–	12	74	–	–	–
Lite Sliced Turkey	1	288	–	12	32	–	–	–
Lite Tuna Salad	1	358	–	21	23	–	–	–
Lite Vegetarian Pocket Broccoli Cheese	1	214	–	5	15	–	–	–
Lite Vegetarian Pocket Peppers Onions Mushrooms Cheese	1	230	–	6	15	–	–	–
Low Fat Cheese	1 slice	73	–	4	15	–	–	–
Mayonnaise	2 tsp	71	–	8	5	–	–	–
Smart Sides Broccoli	1 serv	23	–	tr	0	–	–	–
Smart Sides Cottage Cheese	1 serv	90	–	4	13	–	–	–
Smart Sides Side Salad	1 serv	30	–	0	0	–	–	–

OLIVE GARDEN

FOOD	PORTION	CAL	PROT	FAT	CHOL	CARB	FIBER	SOD
Garden Fare Apple Carmellina	1 serv (12.2 oz)	560	6	2	5	131	–	190
Garden Fare Dinner Capellini Pomodoro	1 serv (21.1 oz)	610	19	16	5	98	–	940
Garden Fare Dinner Capellini Primavera	1 serv (20.1 oz)	400	18	7	15	68	–	950
Garden Fare Dinner Chicken Giardino	1 serv (20.6 oz)	550	42	11	85	71	–	1000

FOOD	PORTION	CAL	PROT	FAT	CHOL	CARB	FIBER	SOD
Garden Fare Dinner Linguine Alla Marinara	1 serv (16.3 oz)	500	16	9	0	89	—	160
Garden Fare Dinner Penne Fra Diavolo	1 serv (14.3 oz)	420	13	7	10	77	—	940
Garden Fare Dinner Shrimp Primavera	1 serv (28.4 oz)	740	48	15	290	104	—	1630
Garden Fare Lunch Capellini Pamodoro	1 serv (11.7 oz)	360	12	9	5	57	—	540
Garden Fare Lunch Capellini Primavera	1 serv (11.2 oz)	260	12	5	15	42	—	560
Garden Fare Lunch Chicken Giardino	1 serv (12.8 oz)	360	23	9	50	47	—	900
Garden Fare Lunch Linguine Alla Marinara	1 serv (10.2 oz)	310	10	6	0	54	—	105
Garden Fare Lunch Penne Fra Diavolo	1 serv (10.2 oz)	300	9	5	10	57	—	640
Garden Fare Lunch Shrimp Primavera	1 serv (15.2 oz)	410	25	8	145	60	—	840
Minestrone Soup	1 serv (6 oz)	80	4	1	0	15	—	450
PANDA EXPRESS								
Black Pepper Chicken	1 serv (5 oz)	210	—	9	—	—	—	570
Chicken w/ Mushrooms	1 serv (5 oz)	170	—	3	—	—	—	570
Chicken w/ String Beans	1 serv (5 oz)	180	—	9	—	—	—	620
Egg Flower Soup	1½ cups	80	—	0	—	—	—	640
Egg Rolls	2 (3 oz)	190	—	6	—	—	—	490
Hot & Sour Soup	1½ cups	110	—	4	—	—	—	890
Lo Mein	1 serv (8 oz)	300	—	10	—	—	—	1090
Mixed Vegetables	1 serv (5 oz)	80	—	3	0	—	—	450
Orange Chicken	1 serv (5 oz)	310	—	13	—	—	—	420
Spicy Chicen w/ Peanuts	1 serv (5 oz)	510	—	29	—	—	—	1250
Steamed Rice	1 serv (8 oz)	220	—	0	0	—	—	0
Sweet & Sour Pork	1 serv (4 oz)	310	—	20	—	—	—	250

FOOD	PORTION	CAL	PROT	FAT	CHOL	CARB	FIBER	SOD
Sweet & Sour Sauce	1 serv (2 oz)	60	—	0	0	—	—	150
Vegetable Chow Mein	1 serv (8 oz)	300	—	10	—	—	—	610
Vegetable Fried Rice	1 serv (8 oz)	410	—	19	—	—	—	440

PERKINS

FOOD	PORTION	CAL	PROT	FAT	CHOL	CARB	FIBER	SOD
Low Fat Brownie	1 (5.4 oz)	260	—	1	—	—	—	—
Low Fat Muffin Banana	1 (5.8 oz)	330	—	3	—	—	—	—
Low Fat Muffin Blueberry	1 (5.8 oz)	270	—	3	—	—	—	—
Low Fat Muffin Honey Bran	1 (5.8 oz)	270	—	3	—	—	—	—
Low Fat Muffin Plain	1 (5.8 oz)	300	—	3	—	—	—	—

PICCADILLY CAFETERIA

BAKED SELECTIONS

FOOD	PORTION	CAL	PROT	FAT	CHOL	CARB	FIBER	SOD
Corn Sticks	1 (2 oz)	165	3	10	26	17	tr	385
French Bread	1 slice	132	4	2	6	24	4	199
Garlic Bread	1 serv (15.8 oz)	1154	35	24	48	195	34	1718
Mexican Corn Bread	1 piece	220	4	14	31	21	1	547
Roll	1 (2 oz)	130	4	2	0	23	4	195
Roll Whole Wheat	1 (1.7 oz)	117	4	1	19	22	3	159
Texas Toast	1 serv (15.5 oz)	1088	35	17	48	195	34	1633

BEVERAGES

FOOD	PORTION	CAL	PROT	FAT	CHOL	CARB	FIBER	SOD
Iced Tea	1 serv (6.5 oz)	2	tr	0	0	tr	0	0
Punch	1 serv (9 oz)	133	0	0	0	34	0	1

DESSERTS

FOOD	PORTION	CAL	PROT	FAT	CHOL	CARB	FIBER	SOD
Apple Pie	1 slice (7.2 oz)	439	4	19	0	67	3	476
Cantaloupe	1 serv (9 oz)	89	2	1	0	21	3	23
Cantaloupe	1 serv (5.5 oz)	55	1	tr	0	13	2	14
Chocolate Cream Pie	1 slice (7.5 oz)	512	9	25	66	65	tr	655
Custard	1 cup (5.4 oz)	183	6	1	25	39	0	358
Custard Pie	1 slice (6.2 oz)	412	8	18	18	54	tr	630
Dole Whip Topping	1 serv (3 oz)	68	0	1	0	15	0	14
Fresh Fruit Plate	1 serv (21.1 oz)	389	13	5	11	81	9	306
Gelatin	1 serv (4.75 oz)	128	2	4	14	22	0	94
Honeydew Melon	1 serv (5.5 oz)	55	1	tr	0	14	1	16
Honeydew Melon	1 serv (9 oz)	89	1	tr	0	23	2	26
Lemon Chiffon Pie	1 slice (6.3 oz)	481	14	20	32	61	tr	645
Pound Cake	1 slice (3.8 oz)	371	5	17	76	51	0	744
Watermelon	1 serv (11 oz)	100	2	1	0	22	1	6

FOOD	PORTION	CAL	PROT	FAT	CHOL	CARB	FIBER	SOD
MAIN MENU SELECTIONS								
Au Jus	1 serv (3 oz)	5	tr	tr	0	1	0	537
Baby Lima Beans	1 serv (4.5 oz)	151	5	6	0	19	4	371
Baked Potato	1	218	4	tr	0	50	4	16
Baked Potato w/ Topping	1	350	5	15	33	51	4	119
Beef Chopped Steak Fried	1 serv (4 oz)	311	22	23	59	4	0	457
Beef Leg Roast	1 serv (4 oz)	311	34	18	92	1	tr	472
Beef Liver Fried	1 serv (4.5 oz)	430	25	29	418	15	2	404
Beef Tips Braised	1 serv (10 oz)	470	30	26	56	41	3	828
Black-eyed Peas w/ Pork Jowls	1 serv (4 oz)	108	4	6	7	9	0	386
Broccoli Buttered	1 serv (4 oz)	77	3	6	0	5	3	273
Broccoli & Rice Au Gratin	½ cup	184	7	9	18	20	1	577
Carrots Young Buttered	½ cup	90	1	6	0	9	1	512
Cauliflower Buttered	1 serv	80	2	6	0	6	2	260
Chicken Baked w/o Skin	¼ chicken	352	59	11	168	tr	0	401
Chicken Teriyaki	1 serv (4 oz)	445	45	22	124	14	tr	1432
Chicken Teriyaki Polynesian	1 serv (4 oz)	537	39	27	104	34	1	2051
Corn	1 serv (4.5 oz)	128	3	7	0	17	0	423
Cornbread Stuffing	1 serv (4.5 oz)	164	9	9	26	12	tr	597
Crackers	4 (0.4 oz)	51	1	1	–	8	tr	172
Cranberry Sauce	1 serv (1.5 oz)	64	tr	tr	0	17	tr	12
Eggplant Escalloped	½ cup	180	4	10	15	19	1	928
Fish Baked	1 serv (7 oz)	195	24	10	54	3	tr	532
Green Beans	1 serv (4.5 oz)	77	2	6	7	5	1	552
Ham Baked	1 serv (4 oz)	224	26	10	67	6	0	1703
Macaroni & Cheese	½ cup	317	15	11	22	38	2	1752
Mashed Potatoes	1 serv (4.8 oz)	120	3	3	0	20	0	62
Meatballs Baked & Spaghetti	1 serv (11.5 oz)	108	9	5	23	7	tr	419
New Potatoes Boiled	½ cup	148	2	12	0	12	tr	852
Okra Smothered	1 serv (4 oz)	121	2	10	0	9	1	633
Onion Sauce	1 serv (4 oz)	152	5	7	0	30	1	481
Rice	½ cup	99	2	tr	0	22	tr	9

FOOD	PORTION	CAL	PROT	FAT	CHOL	CARB	FIBER	SOD
Rice Polynesian	1 serv (4 oz)	140	2	6	0	20	tr	627
Spaghetti Baked	1 serv (9.5 oz)	256	9	10	13	33	2	448
Squash Baked Italian	1 serv (4.75 oz)	73	4	3	8	8	1	1072
Squash Mixed Yellow & Zucchini	1 serv (4 oz)	72	1	5	0	6	1	390
Squash Yellow Baked French Style	⅓ cup	86	3	5	5	9	1	405
Turkey Breast	1 serv (3 oz)	99	20	2	—	tr	tr	612
Vegetables Unseasoned	1 serv (5 oz)	29	2	tr	0	6	2	23
SALADS AND SALAD BARS								
Broccoli Salad	1 serv (4 oz)	202	2	20	13	6	2	252
Cabbage Combination Salad	1 serv (4.5 oz)	50	1	tr	0	15	1	1164
Carrot & Raisin Salad	1 serv (4.5 oz)	321	2	23	10	30	2	280
Cole Slaw w/ Cream	1 serv (4 oz)	182	2	18	9	5	1	344
Cucumber & Celery Salad	1 serv (4 oz)	82	1	6	0	6	1	686
Fruit Salad	1 serv (6 oz)	59	1	1	0	14	2	6
Neptune Salad	1 serv	361	10	34	25	3	1	659
Spinach Tossed Salad	1 serv (4 oz)	88	3	6	44	6	2	147
Spring Salad Bowl	1 serv (4 oz)	22	1	tr	0	5	1	21
SOUPS								
Gumbo Chicken	1 serv (8 oz)	92	9	2	22	9	1	1033
Gumbo Seafood	1 serv (8 oz)	98	10	2	45	10	1	1300
Vegetable	1 serv (8 oz)	49	2	tr	0	10	tr	998

PIZZA HUT
DESSERTS

FOOD	PORTION	CAL	PROT	FAT	CHOL	CARB	FIBER	SOD
Apple Pizza	1 slice (2.8 oz)	250	3	5	0	48	2	230
Cherry Pizza	1 slice (2.8 oz)	250	3	5	0	47	3	220
MAIN MENU SELECTIONS								
Bread Stick	1 (1.3 oz)	130	3	4	0	20	1	170
Bread Stick Dipping Sauce	1 serv (1.2 oz)	30	tr	1	0	5	tr	170
Buffalo Wings Hot	4 pieces (2.1 oz)	210	22	12	130	4	tr	900
Buffalo Wings Mild	5 pieces (2.9 oz)	200	23	12	150	tr	0	510
Cavatini Pasta	1 serv (12.5 oz)	480	21	14	8	66	9	1170
Cavatini Supreme Pasta	1 serv (13.9 oz)	560	24	19	10	73	10	1400

FOOD	PORTION	CAL	PROT	FAT	CHOL	CARB	FIBER	SOD
Garlic Bread	1 slice (1.3 oz)	150	3	8	0	16	1	240
Ham & Cheese Sandwich	1 (9.7 oz)	550	33	21	22	57	4	2150
Spaghetti Marinara	1 serv (16.6 oz)	490	18	6	0	91	8	730
Spaghetti Meat Sauce	1 serv (16.4 oz)	600	23	13	25	98	9	910
Spaghetti Meatballs	1 serv (18.8 oz)	850	37	24	17	120	10	1120
Supreme Sandwich	1 (10.2 oz)	640	34	28	28	62	4	2150
PIZZA								
Edge Chicken Supreme	1 sq (2.5 oz)	90	7	4	15	9	tr	290
Edge Meat Lover's	1 sq (2 oz)	160	7	11	20	8	tr	440
Edge The Works	1 sq (2.2 oz)	110	5	6	10	9	tr	270
Edge Veggie Lover's	1 sq (1.9 oz)	70	4	3	<5	9	tr	180
Hand Tossed Beef Topping	1 slice	330	16	17	25	29	3	880
Hand Tossed Cheese	1 slice	240	12	10	10	28	2	650
Hand Tossed Chicken Supreme	1 slice	230	13	7	15	29	2	650
Hand Tossed Ham	1 slice	260	14	10	20	28	2	800
Hand Tossed Italian Sausage	1 slice	340	16	18	30	28	2	910
Hand Tossed Meat Lover's	1 slice	320	14	17	30	28	2	900
Hand Tossed Pepperoni	1 slice	280	13	13	20	28	2	790
Hand Tossed Pepperoni Lover's	1 slice	250	11	11	15	27	2	730
Hand Tossed Pork Topping	1 slice	320	16	16	25	29	3	920
Hand Tossed Super Supreme	1 slice	290	13	14	25	29	2	850
Hand Tossed Supreme	1 slice	270	13	12	20	29	3	730
Hand Tossed Veggie Lover's	1 slice	220	9	8	5	29	2	580
Insider Cheese	1 med slice (4.9 oz)	370	17	16	30	41	3	890
Pan Beef Topping	1 med slice (4.3 oz)	330	14	18	20	29	3	690
Pan Cheese	1 med slice (3.9 oz)	290	12	14	10	28	2	590

FOOD	PORTION	CAL	PROT	FAT	CHOL	CARB	FIBER	SOD
Pan Chicken Supreme	1 med slice (4.5 oz)	270	13	12	15	29	2	580
Pan Ham	1 med slice (3.8 oz)	260	11	12	15	28	2	610
Pan Italian Sausage	1 med slice (4.3 oz)	340	13	20	25	29	2	720
Pan Meat Lover's	1 med slice (4.7 oz)	360	14	21	30	29	3	840
Pan Pepperoni	1 med slice (3.7 oz)	280	11	14	15	28	2	610
Pan Pepperoni Lover's	1 med slice (4.3 oz)	330	14	18	20	29	2	760
Pan Pork Topping	1 med slice (3.7 oz)	320	13	17	20	29	3	730
Pan Super Supreme	1 med slice (5 oz)	340	14	18	25	30	3	780
Pan Supreme	1 med slice (4.7 oz)	320	13	17	20	29	3	670
Pan Veggie Lover's	1 med slice (4.6 oz)	270	10	12	5	30	3	510
Personal Pan Beef Topping	1 pie (10.2 oz)	710	31	35	45	71	6	1580
Personal Pan Cheese	1 pie (9.2 oz)	630	23	28	25	71	6	1370
Personal Pan Ham	1 pie (9.1 oz)	580	27	23	35	70	5	1450
Personal Pan Italian Sausage	1 pie (10.2 oz)	740	31	39	55	71	6	1640
Personal Pan Pepperoni	1 pie (9 oz)	620	26	28	30	70	5	1430
Personal Pan Pork Topping	1 pie (10.2 oz)	700	31	34	40	71	6	1670
Sicilian Beef Topping	1 slice (4 oz)	260	11	11	15	31	2	640
Sicilian Cheese	1 slice (4 oz)	290	12	13	10	31	2	630
Sicilian Chicken Supreme	1 slice (4.6 oz)	270	12	11	15	32	2	620
Sicilian Ham	1 slice (3.8 oz)	257	11	10	14	30	3	745
Sicilian Italian Sausage	1 slice (4.4 oz)	333	13	18	24	31	3	855
Sicilian Meat Lover's	1 slice (4.7 oz)	350	14	19	25	31	2	830
Sicilian Pepperoni	1 slice (3.9 oz)	280	10	13	15	31	2	630
Sicilian Pepperoni Lover's	1 slice (4.4 oz)	320	13	16	20	31	2	780
Sicilian Pork Topping	1 slice (4.4 oz)	320	13	16	20	31	2	750
Sicilian Super Supreme	1 slice (5 oz)	340	13	18	20	32	2	780
Sicilian Supreme	1 slice (4.7 oz)	310	12	15	15	32	2	690
Sicilian Veggies Lover's	1 slice (4.6 oz)	270	12	11	15	32	2	620
Stuffed Crust Beef Topping	1 lg slice (5.8 oz)	390	19	18	30	40	3	1150
Stuffed Crust Cheese	1 lg slice (5.5 oz)	360	18	16	25	39	3	1090

FOOD	PORTION	CAL	PROT	FAT	CHOL	CARB	FIBER	SOD
Stuffed Crust Chicken Supreme	1 lg slice (6.5 oz)	350	21	13	35	41	3	1130
Stuffed Crust Ham	1 lg slice (5.5 oz)	330	18	13	30	39	3	1130
Stuffed Crust Italian Sausage	1 lg slice (5.8 oz)	400	19	20	35	40	3	1180
Stuffed Crust Meat Lover's	1 lg slice (6.7 oz)	470	22	25	50	13	3	1430
Stuffed Crust Pepperoni	1 lg slice (5.4 oz)	360	17	16	30	39	3	1120
Stuffed Crust Pepperoni Lover's	1 lg slice (6.2 oz)	420	21	21	40	40	3	1350
Stuffed Crust Pork Topping	1 lg slice (5.7 oz)	380	19	18	30	40	3	1190
Stuffed Crust Super Supreme	1 lg slice (7.2 oz)	430	21	22	40	41	3	1360
Stuffed Crust Supreme	1 lg slice (6.7 oz)	410	20	20	35	41	3	1220
Stuffed Crust Veggie Lover's	1 lg slice (6.6 oz)	340	16	14	20	42	3	1030
The Big New Yorker Beef Topping	1 slice (7.2 oz)	480	24	26	40	42	8	1380
The Big New Yorker Cheese	1 slice (6.1 oz)	380	19	17	20	41	7	1140
The Big New Yorker Ham	1 slice (5.9 oz)	340	18	13	25	41	7	1160
The Big New Yorker Pepperoni	1 slice (5.6 oz)	370	17	16	20	41	7	1150
The Big New Yorker Pork Topping	1 slice (7.2 oz)	470	23	25	35	42	8	1470
The Big New Yorker Sausage	1 slice (8 oz)	570	27	33	55	42	8	1620
The Big New Yorker Supreme	1 slice (7.8 oz)	450	22	23	35	43	8	1350
The Big New Yorker Veggie Lover's	1 slice (12 oz)	450	18	22	10	52	9	1340
Thin'N Crispy Cheese	1 med slice (3 oz)	200	10	9	10	22	2	590
Thin'N Crispy Chicken Supreme	1 med slice (4 oz)	200	12	7	20	23	2	620

FOOD	PORTION	CAL	PROT	FAT	CHOL	CARB	FIBER	SOD
Thin'N Crispy Ham	1 med slice (2.9 oz)	170	9	7	15	21	2	610
Thin'N Crispy Italian Sausage	1 med slice (3.7 oz)	290	12	17	30	22	2	800
Thin'N Crispy Meat Lovers	1 med slice (4.1 oz)	310	14	19	35	22	2	910
Thin'N Crispy Pepperoni	1 med slice (2.8 oz)	190	9	9	15	21	2	610
Thin'N Crispy Pepperoni Lover's	1 med slice (3.4 oz)	250	12	13	20	22	2	760
Thin'N Crispy Pork Topping	1 med slice (3.7 oz)	270	13	14	25	22	2	820
Thin'N Crispy Super Supreme	1 med slice (4.6 oz)	280	13	15	25	23	2	840
Thin'N Crispy Supreme	1 med slice (4.1 oz)	250	12	13	20	23	2	710
Thin'N Crispy Veggie Lover's	1 med slice (4 oz)	190	8	7	5	22	2	520
Thin'n Crispy Beef Topping	1 med slice (3.7 oz)	270	13	15	25	22	2	750
Twist Crust Cheese	1 lg slice (6.7 oz)	450	20	16	15	58	3	1210
Twist Crust Marinara Sauce	1 serv (3 oz)	60	2	1	0	12	2	491
Twist Crust Ranch Sauce	1 serv (3 oz)	440	2	48	20	4	0	840
Twist Crust Supreme	1 lg slice (7.5 oz)	470	20	18	25	59	3	1280

POPEYE'S

FOOD	PORTION	CAL	PROT	FAT	CHOL	CARB	FIBER	SOD
Apple Pie	1 serv (3.1 oz)	290	3	16	10	37	2	820
Biscuit	1 serv (2.3 oz)	250	4	15	<5	26	1	430
Breast Mild	1 (3.7 oz)	270	23	16	60	9	2	660
Breast Spicy	1 (3.7 oz)	270	23	16	60	9	2	590
Cajun Rice	1 serv (3.9 oz)	150	10	5	25	17	3	1260
Cole Slaw	1 serv (4 oz)	149	1	11	3	14	3	271
Corn On The Cob	1 serv (5.2 oz)	127	4	3	0	21	9	20
French Fries	1 serv (3 oz)	240	4	12	10	31	3	610
Leg Mild	1 (1.7 oz)	120	10	7	40	4	0	240
Leg Spicy	1 (1.7 oz)	120	10	7	40	4	0	240
Nuggets	1 serv (4.2 oz)	410	17	32	55	18	3	660
Nuggets Mild Tender	1 (1.2 oz)	110	6	7	15	6	1	160

FOOD	PORTION	CAL	PROT	FAT	CHOL	CARB	FIBER	SOD
Nuggets Spicy Tender	1 (1.2 oz)	110	6	7	15	6	1	215
Onion Rings	1 serv (3.1 oz)	310	5	19	25	31	2	210
Potatoes & Gravy	1 serv (3.8 oz)	100	5	6	<5	11	3	460
Red Beans & Rice	1 serv (5.9 oz)	270	8	17	10	30	7	680
Shrimp	1 serv (2.8 oz)	250	16	16	110	13	3	650
Thigh Mild	1 (3.1 oz)	300	15	23	70	9	tr	620
Thigh Spicy	1 (3.1 oz)	300	15	23	70	9	tr	450
Wing Mild	1 (1.6 oz)	160	9	11	40	7	0	290
Wing Spicy	1 (1.6 oz)	160	9	11	40	7	0	290

QUINCY'S
BAKED SELECTIONS

FOOD	PORTION	CAL	PROT	FAT	CHOL	CARB	FIBER	SOD
Banana Nut Bread	1 serv (2 oz)	165	2	7	5	22	—	195
Biscuit	1 (2.5 oz)	270	5	15	11	29	—	610
Cornbread	1 serv (2 oz)	140	3	5	0	19	—	340
Yeast Roll	1 (2 oz)	160	1	4	0	29	—	285

BREAKFAST SELECTIONS

FOOD	PORTION	CAL	PROT	FAT	CHOL	CARB	FIBER	SOD
Bacon	1 serv (0.25 oz)	35	2	3	5	0	—	100
Corned Beef Hash	1 serv (4.5 oz)	210	10	15	45	11	—	795
Country Ham	1 serv (1.5 oz)	90	9	6	35	1	—	1100
Escalloped Apples	1 serv (3.5 oz)	120	0	2	0	26	—	20
Oatmeal	1 serv (1 oz)	175	4	2	0	18	—	285
Pancakes	1 (1.5 oz)	95	3	3	30	12	—	250
Sausage Gravy	1 serv (4 oz)	70	2	6	10	3	—	150
Sausage Links	1 (2 oz)	225	7	22	20	0	—	390
Sausage Patties	1 (2 oz)	230	7	23	45	0	—	350
Scrambled Eggs	1 serv (2 oz)	95	7	7	215	1	—	270
Steak Fingers	1 serv (3.5 oz)	360	16	25	50	18	—	690
Syrup	1 oz	75	0	0	0	20	—	15

DESSERTS

FOOD	PORTION	CAL	PROT	FAT	CHOL	CARB	FIBER	SOD
Banana Pudding	1 serv (5 oz)	240	3	12	10	30	—	240
Brownie Pudding Cake	1 serv (4 oz)	310	4	5	0	66	—	395
Caramel Topping	1 serv (1 oz)	105	0	1	0	24	—	120
Chocolate Chip Cookies	1 (0.5 oz)	60	1	8	5	8	—	35
Cobbler Apple	1 serv (6 oz)	255	1	8	5	49	—	285
Cobbler Cherry	1 serv (6 oz)	410	1	8	5	55	—	185
Cobbler Peach	1 serv (6 oz)	305	1	8	5	50	—	190
Frozen Yogurt	1 serv (4 oz)	135	5	2	5	25	—	85

FOOD	PORTION	CAL	PROT	FAT	CHOL	CARB	FIBER	SOD
Fudge Topping	1 serv (1 oz)	105	1	4	0	15	–	75
Sugar Cookie	1 (0.5 oz)	60	tr	3	5	8	–	30
MAIN MENU SELECTIONS								
⅓ Pound Hamburger	1 serv (8 oz)	565	32	33	66	32	–	603
BBQ Beans	1 serv (4 oz)	114	4	1	0	21	–	604
Bacon Cheese Burger	1 (9 oz)	663	37	41	87	33	–	997
Baked Potato	1 (6 oz)	115	5	0	0	30	–	0
Broccoli	1 serv (4 oz)	34	3	0	0	5	–	50
Cheese Sauce	1 serv (1 oz)	58	2	5	11	1	–	212
Chopped Steak Steak	1 serv (8 oz)	499	31	42	89	0	–	348
Cinnamon Apples	1 serv (4 oz)	172	0	5	0	34	–	149
Corn	1 serv (4 oz)	96	3	1	0	24	–	271
Country Steak w/ Gravy	1 serv (8 oz)	530	32	25	54	44	–	1161
Cowboy Steak	1 serv (14 oz)	580	61	33	176	9	–	1308
Filet w/ Bacon	1 serv (8 oz)	340	48	17	124	2	–	311
Green Beans	1 serv (4 oz)	61	1	4	0	6	–	796
Grilled Chicken	1 reg serv (5 oz)	120	25	2	55	1	–	540
Grilled Chicken Sandwich	1 (9 oz)	324	33	4	55	39	–	1183
Grilled Salmon	1 serv (7 oz)	228	46	4	109	1	–	112
Homestyle Chicken Fillet	1 serv (3 oz)	217	13	9	25	21	–	682
Junior Sirloin Steak	1 serv (5.5 oz)	194	25	10	69	0	–	199
Large Sirloin Steak	1 serv (10 oz)	368	46	20	119	2	–	390
Mashed Potatoes	1 serv (4 oz)	54	1	6	0	11	–	195
NY Strip Steak	1 serv (10 oz)	450	53	26	148	1	–	156
Philly Cheese Steak	1 serv (11 oz)	588	37	30	87	38	–	1684
Porterhouse Steak	1 serv (17 oz)	683	67	46	154	0	–	346
Regular Sirloin Steak	1 serv (8 oz)	285	34	16	71	0	–	317
Ribeye Steak	1 serv (10 oz)	452	48	29	116	0	–	156
Rice Pilaf	1 serv (4 oz)	119	2	2	0	23	1	1283
Roasted BBQ Chicken	1 serv (14 oz)	941	70	65	340	21	–	1548
Roasted Herb Chicken	1 serv (14 oz)	875	70	65	340	4	–	1238
Sirloin Tips w/ Mushroom Gravy	1 serv (6 oz)	196	28	7	64	5	–	578

FOOD	PORTION	CAL	PROT	FAT	CHOL	CARB	FIBER	SOD
Sirloin Tips w/ Peppers & Onions	1 serv (5 oz)	203	27	8	63	4	—	793
Smothered Steak Sandwich	1 (9 oz)	429	34	15	69	36	—	846
Smothered Strip Steak	1 serv (10 oz)	622	55	41	148	12	—	239
Southern Breaded Shrimp	1 serv (7 oz)	546	19	31	135	47	—	821
Spicy BBQ Chicken Sandwich	1 (10 oz)	368	34	1	55	45	—	1608
Steak & Shrimp	1 serv (9 oz)	677	48	39	170	33	—	816
Steak Fries	1 serv (4 oz)	358	5	19	0	45	—	245
T-Bone Steak	1 serv (13 oz)	521	51	35	118	0	—	265
SALAD DRESSINGS								
Blue Cheese	1 serv (1 oz)	155	2	16	10	2	—	165
French	1 serv (1 oz)	125	0	12	0	4	—	500
Honey Mustard	1 serv (1 oz)	100	2	6	0	10	—	220
Italian	1 serv (1 oz)	135	0	14	0	3	—	230
Light Creamy Italian	1 serv (1 oz)	65	2	4	0	8	—	485
Light French	1 serv (1 oz)	85	2	4	0	13	—	285
Light Italian	1 serv (1 oz)	20	2	2	0	2	—	485
Light Thousand Island	1 serv (1 oz)	65	2	4	20	8	—	340
Parmesan Peppercorn	1 serv (1 oz)	150	1	14	0	4	—	280
Ranch	1 serv (1 oz)	110	1	11	10	1	—	195
SOUPS								
Chili With Beans	1 serv (6 oz)	235	13	11	15	21	—	920
Clam Chowder	1 serv (6 oz)	180	3	9	0	21	—	835
Cream Of Broccoli	1 serv (6 oz)	170	2	10	0	18	—	770
Vegetable Beef	1 serv (6 oz)	90	5	2	0	14	—	325
QUIZNO'S								
Sub Honey Burbon Chicken	1 sm	329	24	6	38	45	3	1494
Sub Turkey Lite	1 sm	334	17	6	19	52	3	1909
Sub Tuscan Chicken Salad	1 sm	326	21	6	35	45	4	1271

FOOD	PORTION	CAL	PROT	FAT	CHOL	CARB	FIBER	SOD

RALLY'S
BEVERAGES

FOOD	PORTION	CAL	PROT	FAT	CHOL	CARB	FIBER	SOD
Coke	1 serv (20 oz)	177	0	0	0	47	–	17
Coke	1 serv (16 oz)	132	0	0	0	35	–	13
Coke	1 serv (32 oz)	264	0	0	0	70	–	26
Coke	1 serv (42 oz)	372	0	0	0	99	–	36
Diet Coke	1 serv (42 oz)	2	0	0	0	0	–	38
Diet Coke	1 serv (32 oz)	1	0	0	0	1	–	27
Diet Coke	1 serv (20 oz)	1	0	0	0	0	–	18
Fanta Orange	1 serv (20 oz)	202	0	0	0	52	–	15
Fanta Orange	1 serv (32 oz)	301	0	0	0	77	–	22
Fanta Orange	1 serv (16 oz)	150	0	0	0	38	–	11
Fanta Orange	1 serv (42 oz)	424	0	0	0	109	–	32
Mr. Pibb	1 serv (32 oz)	237	0	0	0	60	–	33
Mr. Pibb	1 serv (42 oz)	334	0	0	0	84	–	46
Mr. Pibb	1 serv (20 oz)	159	0	0	0	40	–	22
Mr. Pibb	1 serv (16 oz)	113	0	0	0	29	–	16
Root Beer	1 serv (20 oz)	197	0	0	0	52	–	22
Root Beer	1 serv (16 oz)	146	0	0	0	38	–	16
Root Beer	1 serv (32 oz)	294	0	0	0	77	–	33
Root Beer	1 serv (42 oz)	414	0	0	0	109	–	46
Shake Banana	1 serv	399	9	11	38	70	–	223
Shake Chocolate	1 serv	411	10	12	38	73	–	262
Shake Strawberry	1 serv	399	9	11	38	70	–	223
Shake Vanilla	1 serv	320	9	11	38	49	–	197
Sprite	1 serv (20 oz)	161	0	0	0	40	–	36
Sprite	1 serv (32 oz)	264	0	0	0	66	–	59
Sprite	1 serv (16 oz)	132	0	0	0	33	–	29
Sprite	1 serv (42 oz)	338	0	0	0	84	–	76

MAIN MENU SELECTIONS

FOOD	PORTION	CAL	PROT	FAT	CHOL	CARB	FIBER	SOD
Big Buford	1	743	41	46	151	35	–	1860
Chicken Fillet Sandwich	1	399	21	15	42	43	–	790
Chili w/ Cheese & Onion	1 serv (13 oz)	669	43	41	137	37	–	2125
Chili w/ Cheese & Onion	1 serv (7 oz)	360	23	22	74	20	–	1144
French Fries	1 extra lg (8 oz)	423	7	21	13	52	–	585
French Fries	1 reg (4 oz)	211	3	11	7	26	–	293
French Fries	1 lg (6 oz)	317	5	16	10	39	–	439

FOOD	PORTION	CAL	PROT	FAT	CHOL	CARB	FIBER	SOD
Onion Rings	1 serv	210	6	2	0	45	—	855
Rallyburger	1	433	20	22	63	35	—	1176
Rallyburger w/ Cheese	1	488	23	35	27	35	—	1376
Spicy Chicken Sandwich	1	437	18	18	40	50	—	887
Super Barbecue Bacon	1	593	29	31	88	49	—	1709
Super Double Cheeseburger	1	762	41	48	154	37	—	1734

SBARRO

FOOD	PORTION	CAL	PROT	FAT	CHOL	CARB	FIBER	SOD
Baked Ziti	1 serv (14 oz)	830	—	42	—	—	—	950
Meat Lasagna	1 serv (17 oz)	730	—	38	—	—	—	1660
Pizza Cheese	1 serv (6 oz)	450	—	14	—	—	—	990
Pizza Pepperoni	1 serv (6 oz)	510	—	21	—	—	—	1240
Pizza Sausage	1 serv (10 oz)	640	—	29	—	—	—	1560
Pizza Spinach & Broccoli Stuffed	1 serv (11 oz)	710	—	26	—	—	—	1490
Pizza Supreme	1 serv (10 oz)	600	—	25	—	—	—	1580
Pizza Veggie Slice	1 serv (10 oz)	490	20	12	15	75	1	1350
Spaghetti w/ Sauce	1 serv (18 oz)	630	—	18	—	—	—	1260

SCHLOTZSKY'S DELI

SALADS AND SALAD BARS

FOOD	PORTION	CAL	PROT	FAT	CHOL	CARB	FIBER	SOD
Caesar	1 serv (7 oz)	150	—	8	—	—	—	510
Chicken Caesar	1 serv (9 oz)	250	—	10	—	—	—	940
Chinese Chicken	1 serv (9 oz)	150	—	3	—	—	—	450
Choice Potato Salad	1 serv (5 oz)	250	—	18	—	—	—	530
Country Style Cole Slaw	1 serv (4 oz)	230	—	16	—	—	—	290
Garden	1 serv (9 oz)	60	—	1	—	—	—	120
Greek	1 serv (12 oz)	220	—	12	—	—	—	560

SANDWICHES

FOOD	PORTION	CAL	PROT	FAT	CHOL	CARB	FIBER	SOD
Light & Flavorful Albacore Tuna	1 (13 oz)	530	—	16	—	—	—	1660
Light & Flavorful Chicken Breast	1 (15 oz)	540	—	10	—	—	—	2370
Light & Flavorful Dijon Chicken	1 (15 oz)	500	—	6	—	—	—	2090
Light & Flavorful Dijon Chicken	1 sm (10 oz)	330	—	4	—	—	—	1370

FOOD	PORTION	CAL	PROT	FAT	CHOL	CARB	FIBER	SOD
Light & Flavorful Pesto Chicken	1 (14 oz)	510	–	9	–	–	–	1930
Light & Flavorful Santa Fe Chicken	1 (17 oz)	640	–	19	–	–	–	2300
Light & Flavorful Smoked Turkey Breat	1 (13 oz)	500	–	7	–	–	–	2120
Light & Flavorful The Vegetarian	1 (12 oz)	520	–	17	–	–	–	1330
Original Cheese	1 (14 oz)	850	–	44	–	–	–	2110
Original Ham & Cheese	1 (17 oz)	790	–	32	–	–	–	3430
Original Turkey	1 (17 oz)	1020	–	51	–	–	–	3740
Specialty Deli Albacore Tuna Melt	1 (16 oz)	820	–	40	–	–	–	2290
Specialty Deli BLT	1 (10 oz)	580	–	24	–	–	–	1550
Specialty Deli Chicken Club	1 (16 oz)	690	–	23	–	–	–	2400
Specialty Deli Corned Beef	1 (12 oz)	590	–	15	–	–	–	2490
Specialty Deli Corned Beef Reuben	1 (15 oz)	830	–	35	–	–	–	3510
Specialty Deli Pastrami & Swiss	1 (15 oz)	860	–	37	–	–	–	3720
Specialty Deli Pastrami Reuben	1 (16 oz)	920	–	43	–	–	–	3920
Specialty Deli Roast Beef	1 (14 oz)	620	–	17	–	–	–	1730
Specialty Deli Roast Beef & Cheese	1 (17 oz)	850	–	34	–	–	–	2450
Specialty Deli Texas Schlotzsky	1 (16 oz)	820	–	37	–	–	–	3360
Specialty Deli The Philly	1 (16 oz)	820	–	32	–	–	–	2190
Specialty Deli Turkey & Bacon Club	1 (17 oz)	870	–	40	–	–	–	3010
Specialty Deli Turkey Guacamole	1 (16 oz)	680	–	24	–	–	–	2680
Specialty Deli Turkey Reuben	1 (16 oz)	860	–	39	–	–	–	3890

FOOD	PORTION	CAL	PROT	FAT	CHOL	CARB	FIBER	SOD
Specialty Deli Vegetable Club	1 (13 oz)	580	–	24	–	–	–	1440
Specialty Deli Western Vegetarian	1 (12 oz)	650	–	33	–	–	–	1160
The Original	1 (14 oz)	940	–	50	–	–	–	3170

SEE'S CANDIES

FOOD	PORTION	CAL	PROT	FAT	CHOL	CARB	FIBER	SOD
Bridge Mix	14 pieces (1.4 oz)	200	2	12	10	24	1	45
Dark Chocolate Bordeaux	2 (1.4 oz)	170	tr	27	25	27	1	40
Dark Chocolates	2 (1.2 oz)	160	2	10	10	19	2	35
Lollypop Butterscotch	1	90	0	3	10	17	0	75
Lollypop Cafe Latte	1	90	0	3	10	16	0	40
Lollypop Chocolate	1	90	tr	5	5	14	tr	40
Lollypop Peanut Butter	1	90	2	4	0	14	0	95
Marshmints	3 (1.4 oz)	140	tr	4	0	27	tr	10
Milk Chocolate Bordeaux	2 (1.4 oz)	170	1	8	15	27	tr	45
Milk Chocolate Butter	2 (1.4 oz)	190	1	9	15	27	tr	50
Milk Chocolate Buttercreams	2 (1.4 oz)	180	1	8	15	27	0	50
Milk Chocolate California Brittle	2 (1.3 oz)	220	3	16	25	19	0	115
Milk Chocolate Nuts & Chews	3 (1.7 oz)	250	4	16	15	26	2	60
Milk Chocolate Peanuts	3 (1.5 oz)	230	6	17	5	18	2	90
Milk Chocolate Soft Centers	2 (1.4 oz)	170	1	9	15	25	tr	40
Milk Chocolates	2 (1.2 oz)	160	2	9	10	20	tr	40
Nuts & Chews	3 (1.6 oz)	240	4	16	10	25	2	50
P-Nut Crunch	2 (1.4 oz)	220	4	15	10	21	1	80
Peanut Brittle	1.5 oz	230	4	16	25	21	0	280
Pecan Buds	3 (1.7 oz)	270	3	21	10	22	tr	30
Red Hot Swamp Goo	3 pieces (1.4 oz)	140	tr	4	0	27	tr	10
Soft Centers	2 (1.4 oz)	170	1	9	10	25	tr	40
Truffles Black or Gold	2 (1.4 oz)	180	2	11	10	22	1	25

FOOD	PORTION	CAL	PROT	FAT	CHOL	CARB	FIBER	SOD
Truffles Mint	3 (1.6 oz)	200	2	11	15	26	tr	30
Victoria Toffee	1.5 oz	250	4	19	20	19	1	115

SIZZLER
DESSERTS

FOOD	PORTION	CAL	PROT	FAT	CHOL	CARB	FIBER	SOD
Chocolate & Vanilla Soft Serve	4 oz	136	1	4	0	24	0	100
Chocolate Syrup	1 oz	90	0	0	0	21	0	15
Strawberry Topping	1 oz	70	0	0	0	18	0	5
Whipped Topping	1 tbsp	12	0	1	0	1	0	0

HOT BUFFET

FOOD	PORTION	CAL	PROT	FAT	CHOL	CARB	FIBER	SOD
Broccoli Cheese Soup	1 serv (4 oz)	139	2	9	8	10	0	355
Chicken Noodle Soup	1 serv (4 oz)	31	2	1	7	4	0	495
Chicken Wings	1 oz	73	4	4	20	4	0	135
Clam Chowder	1 serv (4 oz)	118	3	6	6	11	0	511
Fettucine	2 oz	80	3	1	5	15	0	5
Focaccia Bread	2 pieces	108	2	7	1	9	0	134
Marinara Sauce	1 oz	13	0	0	0	3	0	90
Meatballs	4	157	9	11	30	5	1	461
Minestrone Soup	1 serv (4 oz)	36	1	0	1	7	2	443
Nacho Cheese Soup	1 serv (4 oz)	120	5	10	30	3	0	600
Potato Skins	2 oz	160	2	8	0	22	3	463
Refried Beans	¼ cup	62	4	1	5	11	3	272
Saltine Crackers	2	25	1	1	2	4	0	74
Spaghetti	2 oz	80	3	0	0	16	1	1
Taco Filling	2 oz	103	2	9	16	3	1	232
Taco Shells	1	50	1	2	0	7	1	20
Vegetable Sirloin Soup	1 serv (4 oz)	60	6	2	10	6	0	364

MAIN MENU SELECTIONS

FOOD	PORTION	CAL	PROT	FAT	CHOL	CARB	FIBER	SOD
Buttery Dipping Sauce	1 serv (1.5 oz)	330	0	37	0	0	0	0
Cheese Toast	1 piece	273	6	21	5	16	1	494
Cocktail Sauce	1 serv (1.5 oz)	40	0	0	0	8	0	396
Dakota Ranch Steak	1 (6 oz)	316	30	20	101	—	—	253
Dakota Ranch Steak	1 (9.5 oz)	500	47	32	160	—	—	400
Dakota Ranch Steak	1 (8 oz)	421	37	27	135	—	—	337
French Fries	1 serv (4 oz)	358	5	12	0	45	4	245
Hamburger	1	626	45	33	142	36	1	335

FOOD	PORTION	CAL	PROT	FAT	CHOL	CARB	FIBER	SOD
Hibachi Chicken Breast w/ Pineapple	5 oz	193	28	3	65	13	1	666
Hibachi Sauce	1 serv (1.5 oz)	57	0	0	0	11	0	707
Lemon Herb Chicken Breast	5 oz	140	27	3	65	0	0	380
Malibu Chicken Patty	1	310	23	19	75	11	0	588
Malibu Sauce	1 serv (1.5 oz)	283	0	31	28	0	0	354
Margarine Whipped	1½ tbsp	105	0	12	0	0	0	146
Potato Baked Plain	1 (4 oz)	105	2	0	0	24	2	6
Rice Pilaf	1 serv (6 oz)	256	4	5	0	47	1	866
Salmon	8 oz	110	32	12	41	0	0	232
Sante Fe Chicken Breast	5 oz	150	30	3	65	0	0	350
Shrimp Broiled	5 oz	150	23	6	218	0	0	377
Shrimp Fried	4 pieces	223	18	2	118	35	2	706
Shrimp Mini	4 oz	152	13	1	80	24	1	480
Shrimp Scampi	5 oz	143	27	3	150	0	0	386
Sour Dressing	2 tbsp	60	0	6	0	0	0	30
Swordfish	8 oz	315	45	14	89	0	0	331
Tartar Sauce	1 serv (1.5 oz)	170	0	17	14	6	0	453
SALAD DRESSINGS								
Blue Cheese	1 oz	111	1	12	8	1	0	168
Honey Mustard	1 oz	160	0	16	10	4	0	110
Italian Lite	1 oz	14	0	0	0	2	0	350
Japanese Rice Vinegar Fat Free	1 oz	10	0	0	0	2	0	172
Parmesan Italian	1 oz	100	0	10	0	2	0	450
Ranch	1 oz	120	0	12	10	2	0	240
Ranch Reduced Calorie	1 oz	90	0	8	10	4	0	270
Thousand Island	1 oz	143	0	15	11	3	0	125
SALADS AND SALAD BARS								
Alfafa Sprouts	¼ cup	2	0	0	0	0	0	0
Avocado	½	153	2	15	0	6	3	11
Bean Sprouts	¼ cup	8	1	0	0	2	0	2
Beets	¼ cup	13	0	0	0	3	1	117
Bell Peppers	2 oz	8	1	0	0	2	1	1
Broccoli	½ cup	12	1	0	0	2	1	12

FOOD	PORTION	CAL	PROT	FAT	CHOL	CARB	FIBER	SOD
Cabbage Red	¼ cup	5	0	0	0	1	0	2
Cantoupe	½ cup	28	1	0	0	7	1	7
Carrot & Raisin Salad	2 oz	130	1	10	10	10	1	104
Carrots	¼ cup	12	0	0	0	3	1	10
Chinese Chicken Salad	2 oz	54	4	2	10	6	1	119
Chives	1 oz	62	1	6	0	1	1	181
Cottage Cheese	2 oz	51	8	1	5	2	0	230
Cucumber	2 oz	7	0	0	0	2	1	1
Eggs	1 oz	44	4	3	122	0	0	35
Garbanzo Beans	¼ cup	63	3	1	0	11	3	255
Grapes	½ cup	29	0	0	0	8	1	1
Guacamole	1 oz	42	0	4	0	2	0	425
Honeydew Melon	½ cup	30	0	0	0	8	1	9
Iceberg Lettuce	1 cup	7	1	0	0	1	1	5
Jicama	2 oz	13	1	0	0	3	0	1
Kidney Beans	¼ cup	52	3	0	0	10	4	222
Kiwifruit	2 oz	35	1	0	0	8	2	3
Mediterranean Minted Fruit Salad	2 oz	29	1	0	0	7	0	11
Mexican Fiesta Salad	2 oz	54	2	1	0	10	1	99
Mushrooms	¼ cup	4	0	0	0	1	0	1
Old Fashioned Potato Salad	2 oz	84	1	5	6	10	1	231
Onions Red	2 tbsp	8	0	0	0	2	0	1
Peaches	¼ cup	34	0	0	0	9	1	3
Peas	¼ cup	31	2	0	0	6	2	35
Pineapple	½ cup	38	0	0	0	10	1	1
Real Bacon Bits	1 tbsp	27	2	2	0	2	1	165
Red Herb Potato Salad	2 oz	121	1	9	9	9	1	271
Romaine Lettuce	1 cup	9	1	0	0	1	1	4
Salsa	1 oz	7	0	0	0	2	0	156
Seafood Louis Pasta Salad	2 oz	64	3	2	17	9	1	139
Seafood Salad	2 oz	56	3	3	7	4	0	255
Spicy Jicama Salad	2 oz	16	0	0	0	4	0	28
Spinach	½ cup	6	1	0	0	1	1	22
Strawberries	½ cup	22	0	0	0	5	2	1
Teriyaki Beef Salad	2 oz	49	4	2	7	5	1	136
Tomatoes Cherry	¼ cup	12	0	0	0	3	1	5

FOOD	PORTION	CAL	PROT	FAT	CHOL	CARB	FIBER	SOD
Tuna Pasta Salad	2 oz	133	6	10	10	6	0	188
Turkey Ham	1 oz	62	4	5	19	0	0	376
Watermelon	½ cup	26	0	0	0	6	0	2
Zucchini	¼ cup	5	0	0	0	1	1	1

SMOOTHIE KING

FOOD	PORTION	CAL	PROT	FAT	CHOL	CARB	FIBER	SOD
Activator Banana	1 (20 oz)	429	19	1	2	90	4	260
Activator Chocolate	1 (20 oz)	429	19	1	2	90	4	260
Activator Strawberry	1 (20 oz)	559	20	1	2	123	5	260
Activator Vanilla	1 (20 oz)	429	19	1	2	90	4	260
Angel Food	1 (20 oz)	330	6	1	2	79	4	71
Blackberry Dream	1 (20 oz)	343	2	tr	0	86	3	39
Caribbean Way	1 (20 oz)	392	2	tr	0	96	5	18
Celestial Cherry High	1 (20 oz)	285	1	tr	0	69	4	22
Coconut Surprise	1 (20 oz)	457	8	6	3	99	5	126
Cranberry Supreme	1 (20 oz)	577	3	1	24	139	3	120
Cranberry Cooler	1 (20 oz)	538	1	tr	0	132	3	95
GoGuava	1 (20 oz)	300	1	0	0	72	2	50
Grape Expectations	1 (20 oz)	399	3	tr	0	96	2	24
Grape Expectations II	1 (20 oz)	529	4	tr	0	129	4	24
Hawaiian Cafe Au Lei	1 (20 oz)	286	10	tr	5	62	tr	170
High Protein Almond Mocha	1 (20 oz)	402	31	13	17	45	4	245
High Protein Banana	1 (20 oz)	412	34	14	14	44	6	315
High Protein Chocolate	1 (20 oz)	401	31	13	17	45	4	244
High Protein Lemon	1 (20 oz)	390	29	13	12	41	3	177
High Protein Pineapple	1 (20 oz)	380	31	13	12	41	7	206
Hulk Chocolate	1 (20 oz)	846	23	29	102	129	6	626
Hulk Strawberry	1 (20 oz)	953	24	29	102	156	6	645
Hulk Vanilla	1 (20 oz)	846	23	29	102	129	5	646
Immune Builder	1 (20 oz)	333	5	1	24	80	4	47
Instant Vigor	1 (20 oz)	359	2	1	0	87	2	38
Island Treat	1 (20 oz)	334	2	1	0	81	5	29
Lemon Twist Banana	1 (20 oz)	339	3	tr	0	82	2	24
Lemon Twist Strawberry	1 (20 oz)	399	3	tr	0	97	2	23
Light & Fluffy	1 (20 oz)	389	2	tr	0	98	4	12
Malt	1 (20 oz)	887	17	41	166	119	tr	370

FOOD	PORTION	CAL	PROT	FAT	CHOL	CARB	FIBER	SOD
Mangofest	1 (20 oz)	320	1	0	0	78	2	50
Mo'cuccino	1 (20 oz)	440	9	12	75	71	1	190
Muscle Punch	1 (20 oz)	339	6	1	2	80	4	75
Muscle Punch Plus	1 (20 oz)	340	6	1	2	80	5	65
Peach Slice	1 (20 oz)	341	5	tr	2	80	3	93
Peach Slice Plus	1 (20 oz)	471	5	tr	2	113	5	93
Peanut Power	1 (20 oz)	502	15	21	2	72	4	88
Peanut Power Plus Grape	1 (20 oz)	703	16	21	2	119	4	87
Peanut Power Plus Strawberry	1 (20 oz)	632	15	21	2	104	5	87
Pep Upper	1 (20 oz)	334	3	1	0	80	5	39
Pineapple Pleasure	1 (20 oz)	313	2	tr	0	76	4	29
Power Punch	1 (20 oz)	430	6	1	2	102	4	91
Power Punch Plus	1 (20 oz)	499	10	2	2	113	4	91
Raspberry Sunrise	1 (20 oz)	335	3	1	0	85	4	39
Shake	1 (20 oz)	875	16	41	166	117	0	359
Slim & Trim Chocolate	1 (20 oz)	270	12	2	4	55	3	261
Slim & Trim Strawberry	1 (20 oz)	357	7	1	2	79	3	149
Slim & Trim Vanilla	1 (20 oz)	227	6	1	2	51	2	150
Super Punch	1 (20 oz)	425	2	tr	0	95	6	179
Super Punch Plus	1 (20 oz)	516	2	tr	0	118	6	195
Yogurt D'Lite	1 (20 oz)	341	13	4	14	65	2	183
Youth Fountain	1 (20 oz)	267	3	tr	0	65	5	40

STARBUCKS

ICE CREAM

FOOD	PORTION	CAL	PROT	FAT	CHOL	CARB	FIBER	SOD
Biscotte Bliss	½ cup	240	4	12	55	30	—	70
Caffe Almond Fudge	½ cup	260	5	13	55	30	—	80
Caffe Almond Roast	1 bar	280	4	18	25	26	—	45
Dark Roast Expresso Swirl	½ cup	220	4	10	55	29	—	60
Frappuccino Coffee	1 bar	110	4	2	10	20	—	50
Italian Roast Coffee	½ cup	230	5	12	65	26	—	65
Javachip	½ cup	250	4	13	60	29	—	55
Low Fat Latte	½ cup	170	5	3	10	31	—	65
Low Fat Mocha Mambo	½ cup	170	5	3	10	32	—	75

FOOD	PORTION	CAL	PROT	FAT	CHOL	CARB	FIBER	SOD
Vanilla Mochachip	½ cup	270	5	16	75	27	–	60
SNACKS								
Crunchy Honey Bar	1 (1.06 oz)	150	3	7	0	18	1	40
Lively Lemon Bar	1 (1.23 oz)	140	3	4	0	23	1	70
Tangy Apple Bar	1 (1.23 oz)	140	3	4	0	23	1	80

SUBWAY
BEVERAGES

FOOD	PORTION	CAL	PROT	FAT	CHOL	CARB	FIBER	SOD
Fruizle Smoothie Berry Lishus	1 sm (13 oz)	113	1	0	15	28	1	30
Fruizle Smoothie Berry Lishus w/ Banana	1 sm (17 oz)	221	1	1	15	56	4	30
Fruizle Smoothie Peach Pizazz	1 sm (12 oz)	103	1	0	0	26	0	25
Fruizle Smoothie Pineapple Delight w/ Banana	1 sm (17 oz)	241	1	1	0	61	4	25
Fruizle Smoothie Pineapple Delite	1 sm (13 oz)	133	1	0	0	33	1	25
Fruizle Smoothie Sunrise Refresher	1 sm (12 oz)	119	1	0	0	29	1	20
COOKIES								
Chocolate Chip	1	215	2	10	13	30	1	160
Chocolate Chunk	1	217	2	10	12	30	1	105
Double Chocolate	1	209	2	10	15	30	1	170
M&M	1	215	2	10	13	30	1	105
Oatmeal Raisin	1	210	3	8	14	30	2	180
Peanut Butter	1	221	4	12	12	26	1	200
Sugar	1	227	2	12	17	28	0	135
White Macadamia Nut	1	221	2	11	15	28	1	160
SALAD DRESSINGS								
Fat Free French	1 serv (2 oz)	70	0	0	0	17	0	390
Fat Free Italian	1 serv (2 oz)	20	0	0	0	4	0	610
Fat Free Ranch	1 serv (2 oz)	60	0	0	0	14	0	530
SALADS AND SALAD BARS								
BMT	1 serv	275	16	19	55	11	3	1590
Cold Cut Trio	1 serv	234	14	15	57	11	3	1370
Ham	1 serv	112	11	3	25	11	3	1070

FOOD	PORTION	CAL	PROT	FAT	CHOL	CARB	FIBER	SOD
Meatball	1 serv	320	17	20	56	17	4	1050
Roast Beef	1 serv	117	12	3	25	10	3	720
Roasted Chicken Breast	1 serv	130	18	3	50	9	3	630
Seafood & Crab	1 serv	197	9	11	24	17	4	970
Steak & Cheese	1 serv	181	17	8	37	12	4	890
Subway Club	1 serv	146	17	4	33	12	3	1110
Subway Melt	1 serv	203	17	10	44	11	3	1410
Tuna	1 serv	238	13	16	42	10	3	880
Turkey Breast	1 serv	105	11	2	20	11	3	820
Turkey Breast & Ham	1 serv	117	13	3	26	11	3	1030
Veggie Delight	1 serv	50	2	1	0	9	3	310
SANDWICHES								
6 Inch Steak & Cheese	1	362	23	13	37	41	4	1200
6 Inch Subway Melt	1	384	23	15	44	40	3	1720
6 Inch Sub BMT	1	456	21	24	55	40	3	1890
6 Inch Sub Cold Cut Trio	1	415	19	20	57	40	3	1670
6 Inch Sub Ham	1	261	17	5	25	39	3	1260
6 Inch Sub Meatball	1	501	23	25	56	46	4	1350
6 Inch Sub Roast Beef	1	267	17	5	20	39	3	900
6 Inch Sub Roasted Chicken Breast	1	291	21	5	46	40	3	990
6 Inch Sub Seafood & Crab	1	378	14	16	24	46	3	1270
6 Inch Sub Subway Club	1	296	22	5	33	40	3	1290
6 Inch Sub Tuna	1	419	18	21	42	39	3	1180
6 Inch Sub Turkey Breast	1	254	17	4	20	39	3	1000
6 Inch Sub Turkey Breast & Ham	1	267	18	5	26	40	3	1210
6 Inch Sub Veggie Delight	1	200	7	3	0	37	3	500
American Cheese Triangles	2	41	2	4	10	0	0	200
Asiago Caesar Sauce	1.5 tbsp	110	1	11	10	2	0	230

FOOD	PORTION	CAL	PROT	FAT	CHOL	CARB	FIBER	SOD
Bacon Strips	2	45	3	4	8	0	0	180
Breakfast Bacon & Egg	1	321	14	16	184	34	3	520
Breakfast Cheese & Egg	1	317	14	15	187	34	3	550
Breakfast Ham & Egg	1	338	21	14	201	34	3	1100
Breakfast Western Egg	1	300	14	12	182	36	3	540
Cheddar Triangles	2	59	4	5	15	0	0	95
Cucumber Slices	3	2	0	0	0	0	0	0
Deli Ham	1	210	11	4	12	35	3	770
Deli Roast Beef	1	223	13	5	13	35	3	660
Deli Tuna	1	325	13	16	26	36	3	830
Deli Turkey Breast	1	215	13	4	13	36	3	730
Deli Style Roll	1	165	6	3	0	32	3	280
Dijon Horseradish	1.5 tbsp	91	0	10	8	1	0	160
Dijon Horseradish Melt	6 inch	465	25	22	52	47	4	1620
Fat Free Red Wine Vinaigrette	1.5 tbsp	29	0	0	1	6	0	340
Fat Free Sweet Onion	1.5 tbsp	38	0	0	0	9	0	85
Green Pepper Strips	3 (0.2 oz)	2	0	0	0	0	0	0
Hearty Italian Bread	6 inch	207	8	3	0	41	3	340
Honey Mustard	1.5 tbsp	28	0	0	0	7	0	140
Honey Mustard Ham	6 inch	311	18	5	25	52	4	1260
Honey Oat Bread	6 inch	249	10	4	0	48	4	380
Italian Bread	6 inch	178	7	2	0	33	2	350
Lettuce	1 serv (0.7 oz)	3	0	0	0	0	0	0
Mayonnaise	1 tbsp	111	0	12	9	0	0	80
Mayonnaise Light	1 tbsp	46	0	5	6	1	0	100
Moneterey Cheddar Bread	6 inch	235	10	6	10	39	3	400
Mustard	2 tsp	7	0	0	0	1	0	115
Olive Oil Blend	1 tsp	45	0	5	0	0	0	0
Olive Rings	3 (3 g)	3	0	tr	0	0	0	25
Onions	1 serv (0.5 oz)	5	0	0	0	1	0	0
Parmesan Oregano Bread	6 inch	211	8	4	0	40	3	530
Pepperjack Cheese Triangles	2	40	2	4	11	0	0	210

FOOD	PORTION	CAL	PROT	FAT	CHOL	CARB	FIBER	SOD
Pickle Chips	3 pieces (0.3 oz)	1	0	0	0	0	0	125
Provolone Circles	2 havles	51	4	4	11	0	0	125
Red Wine Vinaigrette Club	6 inch	350	24	6	33	53	4	1520
Roasted Garlic Bread	6 inch	225	8	3	0	45	4	1210
Sourdough Bread	6 inch	208	8	3	0	41	3	210
Southwest Sauce	1.5 tbsp	86	0	9	7	2	0	190
Southwest Turkey Bacon	6 inch	407	21	17	35	48	4	1230
Sweet Onion Chicken Teriyaki	6 inch	374	26	5	50	59	4	1090
Swiss Triangles	2	53	4	4	13	0	0	30
Tomato Slices	3 (1.2 oz)	7	0	0	0	2	0	0
Vinegar	1 tsp	1	0	0	0	0	0	0
Wheat Sub	6 inch	186	7	2	0	36	3	360
SOUPS								
Black Bean	1 cup	180	9	5	5	27	15	1160
Brown & Wild Rice w/ Chicken	1 cup	190	6	11	20	17	2	990
Cheese w/ Ham & Bacon	1 cup	230	8	16	20	13	2	1270
Chicken & Dumplings	1 cup	130	7	5	30	16	1	1030
Cream Of Broccoli	1 cup	130	4	7	15	12	1	890
Cream Of Potato w/ Bacon	1 cup	210	5	12	20	20	4	970
Golden Broccoli Cheese	1 cup	180	6	12	10	12	9	910
Hearty Chili Beef	1 cup	250	15	7	20	31	9	1450
Minestrone	1 cup	70	3	1	5	11	0	1030
New England Clam Chowder	1 cup	140	5	5	15	19	1	900
Potato Cheese Chowder	1 cup	210	7	10	25	22	2	1010
Roasted Chicken Noodle	1 cup	90	7	4	20	7	1	1180
Tomato Bisque	1 cup	90	1	3	0	15	3	750
Vegetable Beef	1 cup	90	5	2	5	14	2	1340

FOOD	PORTION	CAL	PROT	FAT	CHOL	CARB	FIBER	SOD

TACO BELL
BEVERAGES

FOOD	PORTION	CAL	PROT	FAT	CHOL	CARB	FIBER	SOD
2% Lowfat Milk	1 serv (8 oz)	110	8	5	15	11	0	115
Coffee Black	1 serv (12 oz)	5	0	0	0	1	0	5
Diet Pepsi	1 serv (16 oz)	0	0	0	0	0	0	47
Dr. Pepper	1 serv (16 oz)	208	0	0	0	52	0	9
Lipton Iced Tea Sweetened	1 serv (16 oz)	140	0	0	0	40	0	60
Lipton Iced Tea Unsweetened	1 serv (16 oz)	0	0	0	0	0	0	60
Mountain Dew	1 serv (16 oz)	227	0	0	0	61	0	93
Orange Juice	1 serv (6 oz)	80	1	0	0	18	0	0
Pepsi Cola	1 serv (16 oz)	200	0	0	0	51	0	47
Slice	1 serv (16 oz)	200	0	0	0	53	0	73

BREAKFAST SELECTIONS

FOOD	PORTION	CAL	PROT	FAT	CHOL	CARB	FIBER	SOD
Breakfast Quesadilla Cheese	1 (5.5 oz)	380	15	21	280	33	1	1010
Breakfast Quesadilla w/ Bacon	1 (6 oz)	450	19	27	290	33	2	1200
Breakfast Quesadilla w/ Sausage	1 (6 oz)	430	17	25	285	33	1	1090
Country Breakfast Burrito	1 (4 oz)	270	8	14	195	26	2	690
Double Bacon & Egg Burrito	1 (6.25 oz)	480	18	27	405	39	2	1240
Fiesta Breakfast Burrito	1 (3.5 oz)	280	9	16	25	25	2	580
Grande Breakfast Burrito	1 (6.25 oz)	420	13	22	205	43	3	1050
Hash Brown Nuggets	1 serv (3.5 oz)	280	2	18	0	29	1	570

MAIN MENU SELECTIONS

FOOD	PORTION	CAL	PROT	FAT	CHOL	CARB	FIBER	SOD
7-Layer Burrito	1 (10 oz)	530	16	23	25	66	13	1280
BLT Soft Taco	1 (4.5 oz)	340	11	23	40	22	7	610
Bacon Cheeseburger Burrito	1 (8.5 oz)	570	27	31	70	46	6	1460
Bean Burrito	1 (7 oz)	380	13	12	10	55	13	1100
Big Beef Burrito Supreme	1 (10.5 oz)	520	24	23	55	54	11	1520
Big Beef MexiMelt	1 (4.75 oz)	290	16	15	45	23	4	850

FOOD	PORTION	CAL	PROT	FAT	CHOL	CARB	FIBER	SOD
Big Chicken Burrito Supreme	1 (9 oz)	510	23	24	95	52	4	1900
Border Sauce Fire	1 serv (0.3 oz)	0	0	0	0	0	0	110
Border Sauce Hot	1 serv (0.3 oz)	0	0	0	0	0	0	85
Border Sauce Mild	1 serv (0.3 oz)	0	0	0	0	0	0	75
Burger Sauce	1 serv (0.5 oz)	60	0	5	5	2	0	110
Burrito Supreme	1 (9 oz)	440	17	19	35	51	10	1230
Cheddar Cheese	1 serv (0.25 oz)	30	2	2	5	0	0	45
Cheese Quesadilla	1 (4.25 oz)	350	16	18	50	32	2	860
Chicken Fajita Wrap	1 (8 oz)	470	17	22	60	51	4	1290
Chicken Fajita Wrap Supreme	1 (9 oz)	520	18	25	70	53	4	1300
Chicken Quesadilla	1 (6 oz)	410	23	21	90	34	3	1170
Chicken Club Burrito	1 (8 oz)	540	20	32	80	43	4	1250
Chili Cheese Burrito	1 (5 oz)	330	14	13	35	37	5	870
Choco Taco Ice Cream Dessert	1 serv (4 oz)	310	3	17	20	37	1	100
Cinnamon Twists	1 serv (1 oz)	140	1	6	0	19	0	190
Club Sauce	1 serv (0.5 oz)	80	0	8	10	1	0	105
Double Decker Taco	1 (5.75 oz)	340	14	15	25	38	9	750
Double Decker Taco Supreme	1 (7 oz)	390	15	19	35	40	9	760
Fajita Sauce	1 serv (0.5 oz)	70	0	7	5	1	0	130
Green Sauce	1 serv (1 oz)	5	0	0	0	1	0	150
Grilled Chicken Burrito	1 (7 oz)	410	17	15	55	50	4	1380
Grilled Chicken Soft Taco	1 (4.5 oz)	240	12	12	45	21	3	1110
Grilled Steak Soft Taco	1 (4.5 oz)	230	15	10	25	20	2	1020
Grilled Steak Soft Taco Supreme	1 (5.75 oz)	290	16	14	35	24	3	1040
Guacamole	1 serv (0.75 oz)	35	0	3	0	1	1	80
Mexican Pizza	1 serv (7.75 oz)	570	21	35	45	42	8	1040
Mexican Rice	1 serv (4.75 oz)	190	5	9	15	23	1	760
Nacho Cheese Sauce	2 serv (2 oz)	120	2	10	5	5	0	470
Nachos	1 serv (3.5 oz)	320	5	18	5	34	3	570
Nachos Beef Beef Supreme	1 serv (7 oz)	450	14	24	30	45	9	810
Nachos Bellgrande	1 serv (11 oz)	770	21	39	35	84	17	1310

FOOD	PORTION	CAL	PROT	FAT	CHOL	CARB	FIBER	SOD
Picante Sauce	1 serv (0.3 oz)	0	0	0	0	0	0	110
Pico De Gallo	1 serv (0.75 oz)	5	0	0	0	1	0	65
Pintos 'n Cheese	1 serv (4.5 oz)	190	9	9	15	18	10	650
Red Sauce	1 serv (1 oz)	10	0	0	0	2	0	320
Soft Taco	1 (3.5 oz)	220	11	10	25	21	3	580
Soft Taco Supreme	1 (5 oz)	260	12	14	35	23	3	590
Sour Cream	1 serv (0.75 oz)	40	1	4	10	1	0	10
Steak Fajita Wrap	1 (8 oz)	470	20	21	40	50	3	1190
Steak Fajita Wrap Supreme	1 (9 oz)	510	21	25	50	52	3	1200
Taco	1 (2.75 oz)	180	9	10	25	12	3	330
Taco Supreme	1 (4 oz)	220	10	14	35	14	3	350
Taco Salad w/ Salsa	1 (19 oz)	850	30	52	60	65	16	1780
Taco Salad w/ Salsa w/o Shell	1 (16.5 oz)	420	24	22	60	32	15	1520
Three Cheese Blend	1 serv (0.25 oz)	25	2	2	5	0	0	50
Tostada	1 (6.25 oz)	300	10	15	15	31	12	650
Veggie Fajita Wrap	1 (8 oz)	420	10	19	20	53	3	980
Veggie Fajita Wrap Supreme	1 (9 oz)	470	11	22	30	55	3	990

TACO JOHN'S

CHILDREN'S MENU SELECTIONS

FOOD	PORTION	CAL	PROT	FAT	CHOL	CARB	FIBER	SOD
Kid's Meal Crispy Taco	1 serv (8 oz)	579	13	34	35	54	–	789
Kid's Meal Softshell Taco	1 serv (8.5 oz)	617	15	33	35	64	–	1037

DESSERTS

FOOD	PORTION	CAL	PROT	FAT	CHOL	CARB	FIBER	SOD
Choco Taco	1 serv (3.5 oz)	320	3	17	20	38	–	100
Churro	1 serv (1.5 oz)	147	2	8	4	17	–	160
Flauta Apple	1 serv (2 oz)	84	1	1	0	19	–	72
Flauta Cherry	1 serv (2 oz)	143	2	4	0	27	–	110
Flauta Cream Cheese	1 serv (2 oz)	181	2	8	10	27	–	135
Italian Ice	1 serv (4 oz)	80	0	0	0	19	–	5

MAIN MENU SELECTIONS

FOOD	PORTION	CAL	PROT	FAT	CHOL	CARB	FIBER	SOD
Bean Burrito	1 (6.5 oz)	387	15	11	18	57	–	866
Beans Refried	1 serv (9.5 oz)	357	18	9	17	53	–	1032
Beef Burrito	1 (6.5 oz)	449	23	20	52	44	–	863
Chicken Fajita Burrito	1 (6.25)	370	22	12	49	45	–	1536

FOOD	PORTION	CAL	PROT	FAT	CHOL	CARB	FIBER	SOD
Chicken Fajita Salad w/o Dressing	1 serv (12.25 oz)	557	22	33	56	44	—	1541
Chicken Fajita Softshell	1 (4.5 oz)	200	13	7	33	21	—	903
Chili	1 serv (9.25 oz)	350	20	21	56	19	—	865
Chimichanga Platter	1 serv (18 oz)	979	32	38	59	127	—	2341
Combination Burrito	1 (6.5 oz)	418	19	16	35	50	—	865
Crispy Tacos	1 serv (3.25 oz)	182	9	11	26	12	—	272
Double Enchilada Platter	1 serv (18.25 oz)	967	42	42	89	106	—	1921
Meat & Potato Burrito	1 (7.75 oz)	503	17	24	25	53	—	1341
Mexi Rolls w/ Nacho Cheese	1 serv (9.75 oz)	863	30	48	54	72	—	1392
Mexican Rice	1 serv (8 oz)	567	8	18	0	40	—	1293
Nacho Cheese	1 serv (2 oz)	300	5	10	—	0	—	600
Nachos	1 serv (3.5 oz)	333	7	21	0	27	—	611
Potato Oles	1 lg serv (6.12 oz)	484	4	30	—	50	—	1285
Potato Oles	1 serv (4.63 oz)	363	3	23	—	38	—	964
Potato Oles Bravo	1 serv (8.88 oz)	579	11	38	7	47	—	1550
Potato Oles w/ Nacho Cheese	1 serv (6.63 oz)	483	8	33	—	38	—	1564
Ranch Burrito	1 (7 oz)	447	18	23	74	44	—	804
Sampler Platter	1 serv (25.5 oz)	1406	61	61	126	156	—	2875
Sierra Chicken Fillet Sandwich	1 (8.5 oz)	534	30	29	68	40	—	1406
Smothered Burrito Platter	1 serv (19.5 oz)	1031	39	40	70	132	—	2351
Softshell Tacos	1 serv (4.25 oz)	230	14	10	26	23	—	520
Sour Cream	1 oz	60	1	5	—	1	—	15
Super Burrito	1 (8.5 oz)	465	20	19	41	53	—	922
Super Nachos	1 serv (13 oz)	919	26	56	48	72	—	1484
Taco Bravo	1 serv (6.25 oz)	346	15	14	28	39	—	677
Taco Burger	1 (5 oz)	280	15	12	32	28	—	576
Taco Salad w/o Dressing	1 (12.4 oz)	584	20	38	46	43	—	766

TACOTIME

FOOD	PORTION	CAL	PROT	FAT	CHOL	CARB	FIBER	SOD
Casita Burrito Meat	1 serv (12 oz)	647	40	31	89	54	16	1233
Cheddar Cheese	1 serv (0.75 oz)	86	5	7	22	0	0	132

FOOD	PORTION	CAL	PROT	FAT	CHOL	CARB	FIBER	SOD
Chicken	1 serv (2.5 oz)	109	11	6	33	2	0	402
Chips	1 serv (2 oz)	266	4	12	0	35	3	461
Crisp Burrito Bean	1 (5.25 oz)	427	15	18	12	53	9	453
Crisp Burrito Chicken	1 (4.75 oz)	422	17	25	54	32	2	795
Crisp Burrito Meat	1 (5.25 oz)	552	34	30	58	39	7	1000
Crisp Taco	1 (4 oz)	295	22	17	48	16	5	609
Crustos	1 serv (3.5 oz)	373	9	15	0	47	–	86
Double Soft Bean Burrito	1 (9.5 oz)	506	23	12	22	77	19	860
Double Soft Combination Burrito	1 (9.5 oz)	617	39	23	63	66	18	1343
Double Soft Meat Burrito	1 serv (6.5 oz)	726	57	33	99	55	17	1809
Empanada Cherry	1 (4 oz)	250	5	9	0	37	–	46
Enchilada Sauce	1 serv (1 oz)	12	0	0	0	3	1	133
Flour Tortilla 10 in	1 (2.75 oz)	213	6	4	0	31	6	393
Flour Tortilla 7 in	1 (1.75 oz)	88	4	1	0	16	1	42
Flour Tortilla 8 in	1 (1.25 oz)	107	5	3	0	16	2	33
Fried Flour Tortilla 10 in	1 (2.75 oz)	318	6	16	0	37	2	315
Fried Flour Tortilla 8 in	1 (1.35 oz)	205	4	11	0	24	1	203
Guacamole	1 serv (1 oz)	29	0	2	0	2	1	94
Hot Sauce	1 serv (1 oz)	10	0	0	0	2	0	120
Lettuce	1 serv (0.5 oz)	2	0	0	0	0	0	1
Mexi Fries	1 lg (8 oz)	532	6	34	0	54	–	1598
Mexi Fries	1 reg (4 oz)	266	3	17	0	27	–	799
Mexican Dressing No Fat	1 serv (2 oz)	20	0	0	0	5	–	130
Mexican Rice	1 serv (4 oz)	159	3	2	0	30	1	530
Nachos	1 serv (10.5 oz)	680	26	38	78	61	11	1250
Nachos Deluxe	1 serv (15.25 oz)	1048	46	57	109	91	17	2252
Natural Super Taco Meat	1 (11.25 oz)	627	41	27	82	60	14	915
Olives	1 serv (0.50 oz)	16	tr	2	0	1	0	124
Quesadilla Cheese	1 serv (3.25 oz)	205	11	11	30	17	1	255
Ranchero Salsa	1 serv (2 oz)	21	1	1	0	3	1	192
Refritos	1 serv (2.5 oz)	97	6	0	0	18	6	101
Refritos	1 serv (7 oz)	326	18	10	22	44	13	525

FOOD	PORTION	CAL	PROT	FAT	CHOL	CARB	FIBER	SOD
Rolled Soft Flour Taco	1 (7 oz)	512	33	23	63	46	12	1111
Shredded Beef	1 serv (2.5 oz)	70	1	7	–	1	–	31
Soft Taco Chicken	1 (7 oz)	387	21	16	48	41	7	933
Sour Cream	1 serv (1 oz)	55	1	5	19	1	0	11
Sour Cream Dressing	1 serv (1.5 oz)	137	1	14	8	2	0	207
Super Shredded Beef Soft Taco	1 (8 oz)	368	12	11	22	38	7	556
Taco Cheeseburger	1 (7.5 oz)	633	31	36	66	48	7	1291
Taco Meat	1 serv (2.5 oz)	208	22	11	38	7	5	576
Taco Salad Chicken w/o Dressing	1 serv (9 oz)	370	19	21	48	27	3	861
Taco Salad w/o Dressing	1 serv (7.75 oz)	479	30	28	63	30	7	895
Taco Shell 6 in	1 (1.25 oz)	110	2	6	0	14	2	48
Thousand Island Dressing	1 serv (1 oz)	160	0	16	10	4	0	270
Tomato	1 serv (0.5 oz)	3	0	0	0	1	0	1
Tostada Delight Salad Meat	1 (9.75 oz)	628	36	33	82	48	13	1004
Value Soft Bean Burrito	1 (6.75 oz)	380	16	10	15	58	13	715
Value Soft Meat Burrito	1 (6.75 oz)	491	31	21	56	48	12	1197
Value Soft Taco	1 (5.25 oz)	316	24	15	48	23	5	599
Veggie Burrito	1 (11 oz)	491	21	16	24	70	10	643
Wheat Tortilla 11 in	1 (3.5 oz)	175	8	3	0	33	2	84
TCBY								
Hand Dipped All Flavors 96% Fat Free	½ cup (3 oz)	140	3	3	5	26	0	26
Hand Dipped All Flavors Nonfat	½ cup (2.9 oz)	120	4	0	0	25	1	60
Lowfat Ice Cream All Flavors No Sugar Added	½ cup (2.6 oz)	110	3	3	10	19	0	60
Nonfat Ice Cream All Flavors	½ cup (2.9 oz)	120	3	0	0	26	1	55
Soft Serve All Flavors 96% Fat Free	½ cup (3.4 fl oz)	140	4	3	15	23	0	60

FOOD	PORTION	CAL	PROT	FAT	CHOL	CARB	FIBER	SOD
Soft Serve All Flavors No Sugar Added Nonfat	½ cup (2.8 oz)	80	4	0	<5	20	0	35
Soft Serve All Flavors Nonfat	½ cup (3.4 oz)	110	4	0	<5	23	0	60
Sorbet All Flavors Nonfat & Nondairy	½ cup (3.4 oz)	100	0	0	0	24	0	30
TROPIGRILL								
Banana Tropical	1 serv (7.55 oz)	498	4	14	0	90	9	7
Black Beans (combo meal portion)	1 serv (4.78 oz)	153	9	2	0	24	10	444
Black Beans (side)	1 serv (8.39 oz)	269	15	4	0	43	18	780
Boiled Yuca	1 serv (12 oz)	334	1	0	0	81	5	456
Boneless Breast	1 serv (3.14 oz)	140	26	4	83	1	tr	169
Cheese Potatoes	1 serv (7.42 oz)	177	6	6	10	25	2	779
Chicken ¼ Dark Meat	1 serv (4.52 oz)	298	33	18	187	1	tr	448
Chicken ¼ Dark Meat w/o Skin	1 serv (3.42 oz)	170	26	7	144	1	tr	312
Chicken ¼ White Meat	1 serv (5.09 oz)	295	42	14	170	1	tr	894
Chicken ¼ White Meat w/o Skin	1 serv (3.82 oz)	167	35	3	117	tr	tr	401
Chicken Caesar Sandwich	1 (6.4 oz)	457	34	20	97	36	tr	931
Chicken Sandwich	1 (7.92 oz)	442	33	19	89	35	tr	702
Congri	1 serv (7.08 oz)	439	11	13	0	69	7	786
Vegetable Kabob	1 (3.07 oz)	106	3	1	0	22	5	286
White Rice	1 serv (6.82 oz)	341	7	6	0	65	2	239
Yellow Rice	1 serv (7 oz)	294	6	5	0	56	3	371
Yucatan Fries	1 serv (5.3 oz)	440	1	24	0	54	3	84
VILLAGE INN								
French Toast Cinnamon Raisin	1 serv	809	–	16	9	–	–	740
Fruit & Nut Pancakes Low Cholesterol	1 serv	936	–	19	2	–	–	754
Omelette Chicken & Cheese	1 serv	721	–	19	120	–	–	705
Omelette Fresh Veggie	1 serv	704	–	18	102	–	–	883

FOOD	PORTION	CAL	PROT	FAT	CHOL	CARB	FIBER	SOD
Omelette Mushroom & Cheese	1 serv	680	—	18	102	—	—	688
Turkey & Vegetable Scrambled Sensation	1 serv	726	—	19	124	—	—	710

WENDY'S
BEVERAGES

FOOD	PORTION	CAL	PROT	FAT	CHOL	CARB	FIBER	SOD
Cola	11 oz	130	0	0	0	36	0	10
Diet Cola	11 oz	0	0	0	0	0	0	15
Frosty Junior	6 oz	170	4	4	20	26	0	100
Frosty Medium	16 oz	440	11	11	50	73	0	260
Frosty Small	12 oz	330	8	8	35	56	0	200
Lemon-Lime Soda	11 oz	130	0	0	0	34	0	30

CHILDREN'S MENU SELECTIONS

FOOD	PORTION	CAL	PROT	FAT	CHOL	CARB	FIBER	SOD
French Fries Kid's Meal	1 serv (3.2 oz)	270	4	13	0	35	3	85
Kid's Meal Cheeseburger	1 (4.2 oz)	310	17	12	45	33	2	800
Kid's Meal Hamburger	1 (3.9 oz)	270	14	9	30	33	1	620
Kid's Meal Chicken Nuggets	4 pieces (2.1 oz)	190	9	13	25	9	0	380

MAIN MENU SELECTIONS

FOOD	PORTION	CAL	PROT	FAT	CHOL	CARB	FIBER	SOD
¼ lb Hamburger Patty	1 (2.6 oz)	200	19	14	65	0	0	290
2 Oz Hamburger Patty	1 (1.3 oz)	100	9	7	30	0	0	150
American Cheese	1 slice (0.6 oz)	70	4	6	15	0	0	260
American Cheese Jr.	1 slice (0.4 oz)	45	3	4	10	0	0	170
Bacon	1 strip (4 g)	20	1	2	5	0	0	90
Baked Potato Chili & Cheese	1 (15.4 oz)	630	20	24	40	83	9	770
Big Bacon Classic	1 (9.9 oz)	580	34	30	100	46	3	1460
Breaded Chicken Fillet	1 (3.5 oz)	230	22	11	50	13	0	390
Cheddar Cheese Shredded	2 tbsp (0.6 oz)	70	4	6	15	1	0	110
Cheddar Shredded	2 tbsp (0.6 oz)	70	4	6	15	1	0	110
Chicken Breast Filet Sandwich	1 (7.3 oz)	430	27	16	56	46	2	750

FOOD	PORTION	CAL	PROT	FAT	CHOL	CARB	FIBER	SOD
Chicken Club Sandwich	1 (7.6 oz)	470	30	20	65	47	2	940
Chicken Nuggets	5 pieces (2.6 oz)	230	11	16	30	11	0	470
Chili	1 lg (12 oz)	310	23	10	45	32	7	1190
Chili	1 sm (8 oz)	210	15	7	30	21	5	800
Classic Single w/ Everything	1 (7.6 oz)	410	25	19	70	37	2	920
French Fries	1 Great Biggie	570	8	27	0	73	7	180
French Fries	1 med (5 oz)	420	6	20	0	50	5	130
French Fries	1 Biggie (5.6 oz)	470	7	23	0	61	6	150
Grilled Chicken Fillet	1 (2.9 oz)	110	19	3	55	1	0	400
Grilled Chicken Sandwich	1 (6.6 oz)	300	24	7	56	36	2	740
Honey Mustard Reduced Calorie	1 tsp (7 g)	25	0	2	0	2	0	40
Hot Stuffed Bake Potato Plain	1 (10 oz)	310	7	0	0	72	6	25
Hot Stuffed Baked Potato Bacon & Cheese	1 (12.6 oz)	530	16	18	25	78	7	820
Hot Stuffed Baked Potato Broccoli & Cheese	1 (14.4 oz)	470	9	14	5	80	9	470
Jr. Bacon Cheeseburger	1 (5.8 oz)	380	20	19	55	34	2	870
Jr. Cheeseburger	1 (4.5 oz)	310	17	12	45	34	2	800
Jr. Cheeseburger Deluxe	1 (6.3 oz)	360	18	16	50	36	2	860
Kaiser Bun	1 (2.5 oz)	200	6	3	0	38	2	340
Ketchup	1 tsp (7 g)	10	0	0	0	2	0	80
Lettuce	1 leaf (0.5 oz)	0	0	0	0	0	0	0
Mayonnaise	1½ tsp (9 g)	30	0	3	5	1	0	60
Mustard	½ tsp (5 g)	5	0	0	0	0	0	50
Nuggets Sauce Barbeque	1 pkg (1 oz)	45	1	0	0	10	0	160
Nuggets Sauce Honey Mustard	1 pkg (1 oz)	130	0	12	10	6	0	220
Nuggets Sauce Sweet & Sour	1 pkg (1 oz)	50	0	0	0	12	0	120

FOOD	PORTION	CAL	PROT	FAT	CHOL	CARB	FIBER	SOD
Onion	4 rings (0.5 oz)	5	0	0	0	1	0	0
Pickles	4 slices (0.4 oz)	0	0	0	0	0	0	140
Saltines	2 (0.2 oz)	25	1	1	0	4	0	80
Sandwich Bun	1 (2 oz)	160	5	2	0	31	1	300
Spicy Chicken Fillet	1 (3.6 oz)	210	22	9	60	10	0	920
Spicy Chicken Sandwich	1 (7.5 oz)	410	28	14	65	43	2	1280
Tomatoes	1 slice (0.9 oz)	5	0	0	0	1	1	0
Whipped Margarine	1 pkg (0.5 oz)	70	0	7	0	0	0	115
SALAD DRESSINGS								
Blue Cheese	1 pkg (2 oz)	360	2	36	30	1	0	350
French	1 pkg (2 oz)	250	0	21	0	13	0	670
Hidden Valley Ranch	1 pkg (2 oz)	200	1	20	25	3	0	410
Hidden Valley Ranch Reduced Fat Reduced Calorie	1 pkg (2 oz)	120	1	11	20	4	0	470
Italian Reduced Fat Reduced Calorie	1 pkg (2 oz)	80	0	7	0	6	0	690
Italian Caesar	1 pkg (1.5 oz)	230	1	24	25	1	0	350
Thousand Island	1 pkg (2 oz)	260	1	25	20	7	0	380
SALADS AND SALAD BARS								
Bacon Bits	2 tbsp (0.5 oz)	45	6	2	10	0	0	550
Ceasar Side Salad w/o Dressing	1 (3.2 oz)	110	9	5	15	6	1	360
Chicken Salad	2 tbsp (1.2 oz)	70	4	5	0	2	0	135
Deluxe Garden Salad w/o Dressing	1 (9.5 oz)	110	7	6	0	10	4	320
Grilled Chicken Salad w/o Dressing	1 (11.9 oz)	200	27	7	55	10	4	780
Side Salad w/o Dressing	1 (5.4 oz)	60	4	3	0	5	2	160
Soft Breadstick	1 (1.5 oz)	130	4	3	5	23	1	250
Taco Chips	15 (1.5 oz)	210	3	9	0	28	2	160
Taco Salad w/o Dressing	1 (16.4 oz)	380	26	19	65	28	8	1040

WHATABURGER

BAKED SELECTIONS

FOOD	PORTION	CAL	PROT	FAT	CHOL	CARB	FIBER	SOD
Biscuit	1	280	5	13	3	37	–	509
Blueberry Muffin	1	239	6	8	0	36	–	538

FOOD	PORTION	CAL	PROT	FAT	CHOL	CARB	FIBER	SOD
Cinnamon Roll	1	320	4	16	10	39	—	190
Cookie Chocolate Chunk	1	247	4	16	28	28	—	75
Cookie White Chocolate Macadamia Nut	1	269	3	16	34	31	—	80
Fried Apple Turnover	1	215	2	11	0	27	—	241
BEVERAGES								
Cherry Coke	1 reg	227	0	0	0	60	—	11
Coffee	1 sm	5	tr	0	0	1	—	5
Coke Classic	1 reg	211	0	0	0	56	—	19
Creamer	1 pkg	10	0	1	0	1	—	4
Diet Coke	1 reg	2	0	0	0	1	—	26
Dr. Pepper	1 reg	207	0	1	0	52	—	51
Iced Tea	1 reg	5	0	0	0	2	—	15
Lemon Juice	1 pkg	1	0	0	0	tr	—	1
Milk 2%	1 serv	113	8	4	18	11	—	113
Orange Juice	1 serv (10 oz)	140	2	0	0	33	—	0
Root Beer	1 reg	237	0	0	0	63	—	25
Shake Chocolate	1 junior	364	9	9	36	61	—	172
Shake Strawberry	1 junior	352	9	9	35	60	—	168
Shake Vanilla	1 junior	325	9	10	37	51	—	172
Sprite	1 reg	211	0	0	0	48	—	45
Sugar	1 pkg	15	0	0	0	4	—	0
Sweet And Low	1 pkg	4	0	0	0	1	—	0
BREAKFAST SELECTIONS								
Biscuit w/ Bacon	1	359	10	20	15	37	—	730
Biscuit w/ Bacon Egg & Cheese	1	511	18	33	213	38	—	1010
Biscuit w/ Egg & Cheese	1	434	14	26	202	38	—	797
Biscuit w/ Sausage	1	446	12	29	37	37	—	794
Biscuit w/ Sausage Egg & Cheese	1	601	21	42	236	38	—	1081
Biscuit w/ Sausage Gravy	1	479	9	27	20	48	—	1253
Breakfast Platter w/ Bacon	1 serv	695	22	44	389	54	—	1162
Breakfast Platter w/ Sausage	1 serv	785	25	53	412	54	—	1234

FOOD	PORTION	CAL	PROT	FAT	CHOL	CARB	FIBER	SOD
Breakfast On A Bun w/ Bacon	1	365	18	19	210	29	—	815
Breakfast On A Bun w/ Sausage	1	455	20	28	232	30	—	886
Butter	1 pkg	36	0	4	11	0	—	42
Egg Omelette Sandwich	1	288	13	13	198	29	—	602
Grape Jelly	1 pkg	45	0	0	0	10	—	15
Hashbrown	1 serv	150	1	9	0	16	—	228
Honey	1 pkg	25	0	0	0	7	—	0
Margarine	1 pkg	25	0	3	0	0	—	40
Pancake Syrup	1 pkg	180	0	0	0	42	—	50
Pancakes	3	259	11	6	0	40	—	842
Pancakes w/ Bacon	1 serv	335	15	12	12	40	—	1074
Pancakes w/ Sausage	1 serv	426	18	21	34	40	—	1127
Srambled Eggs	2	189	11	15	374	2	—	211
Strawberry Jam	1 pkg	40	0	0	0	9	—	15
Taquito Bacon & Egg	1	335	15	16	286	32	—	761
MAIN MENU SELECTIONS								
Bacon	1 slice	38	2	3	6	0	—	106
Cheese Slice	1 lg	89	5	7	22	tr	—	338
Cheese Slice	1 sm	46	3	4	12	tr	—	176
Chicken Strips	2	120	7	5	14	10	—	420
Club Crackers	1 pkg	30	1	2	0	4	—	75
Croutons	1 pkg	30	1	1	0	5	—	90
Fajita Beef	1	326	22	12	28	34	—	670
Fajita Grilled Chicken	1	272	18	7	33	35	—	691
French Fries	1 lg	442	7	24	0	49	—	227
French Fries	1 reg	332	5	18	0	37	—	208
French Fries	1 junior	221	4	12	0	25	—	139
Garden Salad	1	56	3	1	0	11	—	32
Grilled Chicken Salad	1 serv	150	23	1	49	14	—	434
Grilled Chicken Sandwich	1	442	34	14	66	48	—	1103
Grilled Chicken Sandwich w/o Bun Oil w/ Mustard	1	300	33	3	66	35	—	994

FOOD	PORTION	CAL	PROT	FAT	CHOL	CARB	FIBER	SOD
Grilled Chicken Sandwich w/o Bun Oil & Dressing	1	358	34	6	66	46	—	989
Grilled Chicken Sandwich w/o Dressing	1	385	34	9	66	46	—	989
Jalapeno Pepper	1	3	tr	tr	0	1	—	190
Justaburger	1	276	13	11	34	30	—	578
Ketchup	1 pkg	30	0	0	0	7	—	344
Onion Rings	1 lg	493	8	29	0	51	—	893
Onion Rings	1 reg	329	5	19	0	34	—	596
Peppered Gravy	1 serv (3 oz)	75	0	5	0	8	—	375
Picante Sauce	1 pkg	5	tr	0	0	1	—	130
Taquito Potato & Egg	1	446	14	22	281	48	—	883
Taquito Sausage & Egg	1	443	20	26	315	32	—	790
Texas Toast	1 slice	147	4	5	0	22	—	250
Whataburger	1	598	30	26	84	61	—	1096
Whataburger Double Meat	1	823	49	42	168	62	—	1298
Whataburger Jr.	1	300	14	12	34	35	—	583
Whataburger w/o bun oil	1	407	25	19	84	34	—	839
Whatacatch Sandwich	1	467	18	25	33	43	—	636
Whatachick'n Sandwich	1	501	27	23	40	51	—	1122
SALAD DRESSINGS								
Low Fat Ranch	1 pkg	66	1	3	15	9	—	607
Low Fat Vinaigrette	1 pkg	37	0	2	0	6	—	896
Ranch	1 pkg	320	0	33	50	4	—	750
Thousand Island	1 pkg	160	0	12	15	12	—	470
WHITE CASTLE								
Cheeseburger	2 (3.6 oz)	310	15	17	30	23	6	480
Grilled Chicken Sandwich	2 (4 oz)	250	17	9	20	24	5	490
Grilled Chicken Sandwich w/ Sauce	2 (4.8 oz)	290	17	9	20	24	5	600
Hamburger	2 (3.2 oz)	270	12	14	20	23	5	270

FOOD	PORTION	CAL	PROT	FAT	CHOL	CARB	FIBER	SOD

WINCHELL'S DONUTS

FOOD	PORTION	CAL	PROT	FAT	CHOL	CARB	FIBER	SOD
Apple Fritter	1 (4.25 oz)	580	4	37	—	59	—	201
Cinnamon Crumb	1 (2 oz)	240	2	11	—	34	—	208
Cinnamon Roll	1 (3 oz)	360	5	21	—	39	—	179
Glazed Jelly	1 (3 oz)	300	5	13	—	43	—	172
Glazed Round	1 (1.75 oz)	210	1	12	—	24	—	100
Glazed Twist	1 (1.75 oz)	210	1	11	—	26	—	100
Iced Chocolate Bar	1 (2 oz)	220	3	11	—	28	—	125
Iced Chocolate Cake	1 (2 oz)	230	2	10	—	31	—	218
Iced Chocolate Devil's Food	1 (2 oz)	240	3	12	—	31	—	221
Iced Chocolate French	1 (1.89 oz)	220	3	13	—	23	—	217
Iced Chocolate Raised	1 (1.75 oz)	210	3	10	—	26	—	96
Plain	1 (1.58 oz)	200	1	11	—	24	—	211
Plain Donut Hole	1 (0.4 oz)	50	tr	3	—	5	—	13

Visit the
Simon & Schuster Web site:
www.SimonSays.com

and sign up for our
mystery e-mail updates!

Keep up on the latest
new releases, author appearances,
news, chats, special offers, and more!
We'll deliver the information
right to your inbox — if it's new,
you'll know about it.

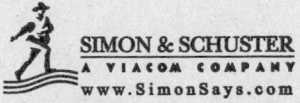

SIMON & SCHUSTER
A VIACOM COMPANY
www.SimonSays.com

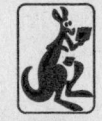

POCKET BOOKS

POCKET STAR BOOKS